CLINICAL ECHOCARDIOGRAPHY REVIEW

A Self-Assessment Tool

CLINICAL ECHOCARDIOGRAPHY REVIEW

A Self-Assessment Tool

EDITORS

Allan L. Klein, MD, FRCP(C), FACC, FAHA, FASE

Professor of Medicine
Cleveland Clinic Lerner College of Medicine of Case Western Reserve University
Director, Cardiovascular Imaging Research
Director, Center for the Diagnosis and Treatment of Pericardial Diseases
Department of Cardiovascular Medicine
Heart and Vascular Institute
Cleveland Clinic
Cleveland, Ohio

Craig R. Asher, MD, FACC

Cardiology Fellowship Director
Department of Cardiology
Cleveland Clinic Florida
Weston, Florida

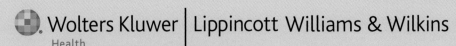

Wolters Kluwer | Lippincott Williams & Wilkins
Health

Philadelphia • Baltimore • New York • London
Buenos Aires • Hong Kong • Sydney • Tokyo

Acquisitions Editor: Frances DeStefano
Product Manager: Leanne McMillan
Production Manager: Alicia Jackson
Senior Manufacturing Manager: Benjamin Rivera
Marketing Manager: Kimberly Schonberger
Design Coordinator: Holly McLaughlin
Production Service: Aptara, Inc.

© 2011 by LIPPINCOTT WILLIAMS & WILKINS, a WOLTERS KLUWER business
Two Commerce Square
2001 Market Street
Philadelphia, PA 19103, USA
LWW.com

Printed in China

Library of Congress Cataloging-in-Publication Data

Clinical echocardiography review : a self-assessment tool / editors,
Allan L. Klein, Craig R. Asher.
    p. ; cm.
Includes bibliographical references and index.
Summary: "The book focuses on the time tested way of "the Socratic method" to teach the key concepts to busy clinical cardiologists, fellows, anesthesiologists and sonographers using a multiple choice question & answer format. The book will emphasize diagnostic interpretation rather than clinical management. This book is comprehensive with chapters ranging from fundamentals to new technologies. The format of each chapter is standardized with 3 types of questions. At the beginning, there are simple questions followed by an answer. Then, questions associated with a still frame graphic (M-Mode, 2-D or a 3-D) come next and are followed by an answer. Finally, questions are presented involving case studies associated with several questions based on movies and still frames"– Provided by publisher.
ISBN-13: 978-1-60831-054-8 (alk. paper)
ISBN-10: 1-60831-054-X (alk. paper)
1. Echocardiography–Examinations, questions, etc. I. Klein, Allan L. II. Asher, Craig R.
[DNLM: 1. Echocardiography–Examination Questions. 2. Heart Diseases–ultrasonography–Examination Questions. WG 18.2]
RC683.5.U5C567 2011
616.1'207543076–dc22

2010031605

Care has been taken to confirm the accuracy of the information presented and to describe generally accepted practices. However, the authors, editors, and publisher are not responsible for errors or omissions or for any consequences from application of the information in this book and make no warranty, expressed or implied, with respect to the currency, completeness, or accuracy of the contents of the publication. Application of the information in a particular situation remains the professional responsibility of the practitioner.

The authors, editors, and publisher have exerted every effort to ensure that drug selection and dosage set forth in this text are in accordance with current recommendations and practice at the time of publication. However, in view of ongoing research, changes in government regulations, and the constant flow of information relating to drug therapy and drug reactions, the reader is urged to check the package insert for each drug for any change in indications and dosage and for added warnings and precautions. This is particularly important when the recommended agent is a new or infrequently employed drug.

Some drugs and medical devices presented in the publication have Food and Drug Administration (FDA) clearance for limited use in restricted research settings. It is the responsibility of the health care provider to ascertain the FDA status of each drug or device planned for use in their clinical practice.

To purchase additional copies of this book, call our customer service department at (800) 638-3030 or fax orders to (301) 223-2320. International customers should call (301) 223-2300.

Visit Lippincott Williams & Wilkins on the Internet: at LWW.com. Lippincott Williams & Wilkins customer service representatives are available from 8:30 am to 6 pm, EST.

10 9 8 7 6 5 4 3 2 1

ACKNOWLEDGEMENTS

We would like to thank Marilyn, Jared, Lauren, Jordan, Jean and Sam Klein and Diann, Drew, Laura and George Asher for their encouragement during our careers and support while editing this book. We would especially like to thank Marie Campbell who put a lot of effort into putting this book together. Finally we would like to express our gratitude to Wolters Kluwer, Lippincott Williams & Wilkins publishers, and in particular Frances DeStefano and Leanne McMillan, for their guidance in making this book a great success.

CONTENTS

CONTRIBUTORS

Marianela Areces, MD
Department of Cardiology
Cleveland Clinic Florida
Weston, Florida

Craig R. Asher, MD
Cardiology Fellowship Director
Department of Cardiology
Cleveland Clinic
Weston, Florida

Gerard P. Aurigemma, MD
Professor
Departments of Medicine and Radiology
University of Massachusetts Medical School
Director, Noninvasive Cardiology
Department of Medicine/Division of
    Cardiovascular Disease
UMassMemorial Healthcare
Worcester, Massachusetts

Jeroen J. Bax, MD, PhD
Director of Noninvasive Imaging
Professor of Cardiology
Department of Cardiology
Leiden University Medical Center
Leiden, The Netherlands

Juan-Carlos Brenes, MD, FACC, FASE
Department of Cardiology
Columbia University
Co-Director, Echocardiography Laboratory
Columbia University Division of Cardiology
Mount Sinai Medical Center
Miami Beach, Florida

**Charles J. Bruce, MBChB, FCP (SA),
    FACC, FASE**
Associate Professor of Medicine
College of Medicine
Consultant
Division of Cardiovascular Diseases
Mayo Clinic
Rochester, Minnesota

Kwan-Leung Chan, MD, FRCPC, FACC
Cardiologist
University of Ottawa Heart Institute and the
    Ottawa Hospital
Professor
Department of Medicine
University of Ottawa
Ottawa, Ontario
Canada

Sonal Chandra, MD
Clinical Associate
Department of Cardiology
University of Chicago
Chicago, Illinois

**Farooq A. Chaudhry, MD, FACP, FACC,
FASE, FAHA**
Associate Professor of Medicine
Columbia University College of Physicians and
    Surgeons
Associate Chief of Cardiology
Director of Echocardiography
St. Luke's Roosevelt Hospital Center
New York, New York

Heidi M. Connolly, MD
Professor of Medicine
College of Medicine
Consultant
Division of Cardiovascular Diseases
Mayo Clinic
Rochester, Minnesota

Victoria Delgado, MD, PhD
Staff Cardiologist
Department of Cardiology
Leiden University Medical Center
Leiden, The Netherlands

Smriti Deshmukh, MD
Assistant Clinical Professor of Medicine
Department of Medicine, Division of Cardiology
Columbia University
Attending Cardiologist
Department of Medicine
The Presbyterian Hospital
New York, New York

Benjamin W. Eidem, MD, FACC, FASE
Associate Professor
Departments of Pediatrics and Pediatric
    Cardiology
Mayo Clinic
Rochester, Minnesota

Maurice Enriquez-Sarano, MD
Professor of Medicine
Division of Cardiovascular Diseases
Director
Valvular Heart Disease Clinic
Mayo Clinic and Foundation
Rochester, Minnesota

Steven B. Feinstein, MD, FACC
Professor of Medicine/Cardiology
Director of Echocardiography
Department of Medicine/Cardiology
Rush University Medical Center
Chicago, Illinois

Mario J. Garcia, MD, FACC, FACP
Professor of Medicine and Radiology
Chief, Division of Cardiology
Montefiore Medical Center-Albert Einstein College
    of Medicine Cardiology
Bronx, New York

Linda D. Gillam, MD, FACC, FAHA, FASE
Professor of Clinical Medicine
Columbia University
College of Physicians & Surgeons
Medical Director, Cardiac Valve Program
Department of Medicine
Columbia University Medical Center
New York, New York

Brian P. Griffin, MD, FACC
Director Cardiovascular Medicine Training
    Program
John and Rosemary Brown Chair in Cardiovascular
    Medicine
Department of Cardiovascular Medicine
Heart and Vascular Institute
Cleveland Clinic
Cleveland, Ohio

Shunichi Homma, MD
MM Hatch Professor of Medicine
Department of Medicine—Cardiology
Columbia University College of Physicians and
    Surgeons
Attending Physician
Department of Medicine—Cardiology
New York Presbyterian Hospital
Columbia University Medical Center
New York, New York

Susie N. Hong-Zohlman, MD
Research Fellow in Medicine
Department of Medicine
Beth Israel Deaconess Medical Center
Boston, Massachusetts

Richard A. Humes, MD
Professor
Department of Pediatrics
Wayne State University
Chief
Division of Cardiology
Children's Hospital of Michigan
Detroit, Michigan

Allan L. Klein, MD, FRCP(C), FACC, FAHA, FASE
Professor of Medicine
Cleveland Clinic Lerner College of Medicine of Case
    Western Reserve University
Director, Cardiovascular Imaging Research
Director, Center for the Diagnosis and Treatment of
    Pericardial Diseases
Department of Cardiovascular Medicine
Heart and Vascular Institute
Cleveland Clinic
Cleveland, Ohio

Itzhak Kronzon, MD, FASE
Professor of Medicine
Associate Chairman of Cardiovascular Medicine
    Director of Cardiac Imaging
Lenox Hill Heart and Vascular Institute of New York
New York, New York

Steve L. Liao, MD
The James J. Peters Veteran Affairs Medical Center
Department of Medicine, Cardiovascular Division
Bronx, New York
The Zena and Michael A. Weiner Cardiovascular
    Institute
The Mount Sinai School of Medicine
New York, New York

Warren J. Manning, MD
Professor of Medicine
Department of Medicine
Beth Israel Deaconess Medical Center
Boston, Massachusetts

Thomas H. Marwick, MD, PhD, FRACP, FRCP, FESC, FACC
Section Head Cardiovascular Imaging
Department of Cardiovascular Medicine
Heart and Vascular Institute
Cleveland Clinic
Cleveland, Ohio

Ronald Mastouri, MD
Assistant Professor of Clinical Medicine
Department of Medicine
Indiana University Medical Center
Krannert Institute of Cardiology
Indianapolis, Indiana

Victor Mor-Avi, PhD
Research Associate
Professor
Director of Cardiac Imaging Research
Department of Medicine, Section of Cardiology
University of Chicago
Chicago, Illinois

Annitta J. Morehead, BA, RDCS
Manager, Cardiovascular Imaging Core
Heart and Vascular Institute
Cleveland Clinic
Cleveland, Ohio

Sherif F. Nagueh, MD, FACC, FAHA
Professor of Medicine
Department of Cardiology
Weill Cornell Medical College
Associate Director, Echocardiography Laboratory
Methodist DeBakey Heart and Vascular Center
The Methodist Hospital
Houston, Texas

Gian M. Novaro, MD, MS
Director, Echocardiography
Department of Cardiology
Cleveland Clinic Florida
Weston, Florida

Sorin V. Pislaru, MD, PhD
Assistant Professor of Medicine
Division of Cardiovascular Diseases
Mayo Clinic and Foundation
Rochester, Minnesota

L. Leonardo Rodriguez, MD
Program Director, Advanced Fellowship Program
Department of Cardiovascular Medicine
Heart and Vascular Institute
Cleveland Clinic
Cleveland, Ohio

Muhamed Saric, MD, PhD
Associate Professor of Medicine
Department of Medicine
New York University School of Medicine;
Associate Director
Noninvasive Cardiology Laboratory
New York University Medical Center
New York, New York

Stephen G. Sawada, MD
Department of Medicine
Indiana University Medical Center
Krannert Institute of Cardiology
Indianapolis, Indiana

Partho P. Sengupta, MD, DM
Associate Professor of Medicine
Director of Noninvasive Cardiology
Department of Medicine
University of California Irvine
Irvine, California

Roxy Senior, MD, DM, FRCP, FESC, FACC
Consultant Cardiologist
Director of Cardiac Research
Northwick Park Hospital
Honorary Professor, Middlesex University, London
Honorary Senior Lecturer, Imperial College, London
Middlesex, Harrow, United Kingdom

James B. Seward, MD, FACC
Professor of Medicine and Pediatrics
Division of Cardiovascular Research
Mayo Clinic Rochester
Rochester, Minnesota

Nishant Shah, MD
Assistant Professor
Department of Pediatrics
Wayne State University
Children's Hospital of Michigan Detroit
Detroit, Michigan

Ying T. Sia, MD, MSc, FRCRC
Associate Professor
Department of Medicine
University of Montreal
Attending
Department of Medicine, Service of Cardiology
Centre Hospitalier de l'University of Montreal
Montreal, Quebec, Canada

David I. Silverman, MD
Professor of Medicine
University of Connecticut School of Medicine
Director, Echocardiography Laboratory
Hartford Hospital
Hartford, Connecticut

William J. Stewart, MD, FACC, FASE
Professor of Medicine
Director, Cardiovascular Curriculum
Cleveland Clinic Lerner College of Medicine
Staff Cardiologist
Department of Cardiovascular Medicine
Heart and Vascular Institute
Cleveland Clinic
Cleveland, Ohio

Lissa Sugeng, MD, MPH
Associate Professor of Medicine
Section of Cardiovascular Medicine
Yale School of Medicine
New Haven, CT

Imran S. Syed, MD
Instructor in Medicine
College of Medicine
Senior Associate Consultant
Division of Cardiovascular Diseases
Mayo Clinic
Rochester, Minnesota

Dennis A. Tighe, MD
Professor
Department of Medicine
UMass Medical School
Associate Director
Non-invasive Cardiology
UMass-Memorial Medical Center
Worcester, Massachusetts

David Verhaert, MD
Staff Cardiologist
Ziekenhuis Oost-Limburg
Genk, Belgium

Shepard D. Weiner, MD
Clinical Fellow
Department of Medicine—Cardiology
New York Presbyterian Hospital
Columbia University Medical Center
New York, New York

Lynn Weinert, BS, RDCS
Sonographer
Department of Cardiology
University of Chicago
Chicago, Illinois

Omar Wever-Pinzon, MD
Division of Cardiology
St. Luke's-Roosevelt Hospital Center
Columbia University, College of Physicians &
    Surgeons
New York, New York

Andrew O. Zurick III, MD
Cardiac Imaging Fellow
Department of Cardiovascular Medicine
Heart and Vascular Institute
Cleveland Clinic
Cleveland, Ohio

FOREWORD

The field of cardiovascular ultrasound had experienced a progressive increase in technical capability and clinical application. The earliest texts on echocardiography dealt only with M-mode tracings, while the most recent versions include two- and three-dimensional imaging as well as blood and tissue Doppler recordings. Not surprisingly, the size of these texts has increased proportionately, representing a challenge to anyone who seeks to master every aspect of cardiac ultrasound. Not surprisingly, new approaches to teaching/learning echocardiography have been sought.

One of the time honored techniques for transmitting information in the clinical setting employs the Socratic method. Whether on rounds or in a laboratory or operating room, attending physicians traditionally pose questions to their trainees about the cases they are overseeing. The concept is that one will best remember that information which they were unable to provide in response to a question. This method also enables the teacher to assess the student and, importantly, enables the trainee to assess their own knowledge and direct future educational efforts.

The current text by Klein, Asher and coauthors exploits the attributes of the Socratic method as an educational tool for cardiac ultrasound. Each aspect of echocardiography is covered by a series of questions which calibrates one's knowledge of the field. More importantly, the explanations of the correct answers provide new information in a format that will not likely be soon forgotten. Many of the questions are based upon actual images and recordings, simulating the setting in which this knowledge would be needed clinically. The net effect is to keep one's interest with challenging queries and immediately enforce the acquisition of new information.

There is little doubt that cardiac ultrasound will continue to progress and play an increasing role in clinical care. In addition, the availability of small handheld devices should expand the application of echocardiography to noncardiologists. Thus, there will be a continuing need for tools to transmit information and to enable self-assessment. The text by Klein, Asher and coauthors serves that purpose very well and is a welcome addition to the cardiac ultrasound literature.

Anthony DeMaria
Judith and Jack White Chair in Cardiology
University of California, San Diego
Editor-in-Chief, Journal of the American
College of Cardiology
San Diego, California

FOREWORD

In 1953, Swedish physician Dr. Inge Edler, using an industrial ultrasound device, generated the first images of the human heart and published his experience the following year in a manuscript entitled "The use of ultrasonic reflecto-scope for continuous recording of the movements of heart valves." The next five decades have seen an unrelenting series of advances in the imaging modality, soon named "echocardiography" by its proponents. Amplitude mode imaging gave way to two-dimensional (2D) echocardiography, then 3D echocardiography, Doppler imaging, transesophageal imaging, contrast ultrasound, tissue Doppler, and much more. What began as an exercise in scientific curiosity eventually transformed the profession of cardiovascular medicine, becoming, without question, the most important noninvasive diagnostic technique used in the practice of cardiology.

However, with each passing decade, the challenges of mastering echocardiography have become increasingly daunting for each new generation of students and practitioners. The physicists who develop ultrasound equipment have been astonishingly creative, devising increasingly complex mathematical approaches to ultrasound imaging that empower practitioners with increasingly powerful diagnostic tools. However, the price we pay for technological advances are the formidable obstacles to learning how to apply echocardiography in clinical practice. Dr. Allan Klein and his coauthors, top leaders and educators in this field, have sought to make learning of echocardiography easier and, frankly, more fun.

This learning tool does not attempt to educate the reader in detail about the physics of ultrasound or the nuances of esoteric research. Rather, this text uses a more user-friendly approach based upon the "question and answer" approach to education. Both educators and students, when interviewed, invariably favor such an approach. I own several textbooks of ultrasound that I keep next to my bed in case I suffer from insomnia. A few minutes of reading is usually all it takes for me to fall asleep. That cannot happen with the "Clinical Review of Echocardiography." Using a question and answer format, the reader is engaged from the very beginning. The questions cover a range of difficulty that allows the beginner and advanced student to increase their knowledge and self-confidence. The problem-oriented learning is particularly appealing because it simulates the clinical environment so well that it is easy to forget that you are reading a textbook.

The topics covered range from the mundane to the esoteric, including basic imaging methods, such as systolic function assessment, as well as sophisticated areas such as optimization of cardiac resynchronization therapy. Although not a substitute for a comprehensive reference book, this textbook is ideal for review and re-certification. It is equally useful for individuals who want to assess their skills or increase their knowledge to keep pace with the advancing technology of echocardiographic imaging. Of equal importance, you will find that this approach is simply a fun way to learn. Once you start, you may have trouble putting this book aside.

Steven Nissen, MD, MACC
Chairman, Department of Cardiovascular Medicine
Staff, Molecular Cardiology
Director, Joseph J. Jacobs Center for Thrombosis and
Vascular Biology
Department of Cardiovascular Medicine
Heart and Vascular Institute
Cleveland Clinic
Cleveland, Ohio

PREFACE

We are delighted with this new interactive and contemporary text book entitled *Clinical Echocardiography Review: A Self-Assessment Tool.* In 2011, echocardiography is seeing a major renaissance in interest and growth. We are now in the modern era of miniaturization, 3D and dyssynchrony echocardiography, speckle tracking, real-time TEE, and molecular imaging with contrast. At the same time, reimbursement for imaging is decreasing and there is competing technology. The busy clinician and fellow have to keep up with the latest in the changing clinical practice of echocardiography. This book focuses on the time tested way of "the Socratic method" to teach the key concepts to busy clinical cardiologists, fellows, anesthesiologists, and sonographers using a multiple-choice question & answer format. The book will emphasize diagnostic interpretation rather than clinical management.

This book is comprehensive with 28 state-of-the-art chapters ranging from fundamentals to new technologies. The format of each chapter is standardized with three types of questions. At the beginning, there are simple questions followed by an answer. Then, questions associated with a still frame graphic (M-mode, 2D, or a 3D) come next and are followed by an answer. Finally, questions are presented involving case studies associated with several questions based on movies and still frames. The reader will need to go to the Web site to work with these questions in either study mode or test mode.

We have chosen leading national and international experts as well as educators in the field of echocardiography. We will cover the basics from a sonographer approach to the echocardiography examination, physics and artifacts to more clinically oriented topics including atrial fibrillation, prosthetic valves, cardiomyopathies, and pericardial disease and then new technologies such as dyssynchrony assessment, strain, and strain rate. We have emphasized key take home points after each of the cases. This book uses the question & answer method which is similar to how we teach our fellows to read echocardiograms. Also, it will be useful for the clinical cardiologist who wants to hone their echocardiographic skills in day-to-day practice.

Clinical Echocardiography Review: A Self-Assessment Tool may be the largest echocardiography review book out there with over 1,000 questions and answers as well as key references for each chapter. There are ample graphs, tables and figures, and detailed explanations to answer the questions.

We hope that you enjoy the basics as well as the "latest and greatest" of echocardiography in the 21st century.

Allan L. Klein and Craig R. Asher

CLINICAL ECHOCARDIOGRAPHY REVIEW

A Self-Assessment Tool

CHAPTER 1

Physics of Ultrasound, Technique and Instrumentation

Victor Mor-Avi

1. Sound waves cannot travel through one of the following:
   A. Water.
   B. Air.
   C. Metal.
   D. Vacuum.

2. Ultrasound is a pressure wave with a frequency above the audible range of human hearing, which is:
   A. 200 Hz.
   B. 2 kHz.
   C. 20,000 Hz.
   D. 200 kHz.

3. The frequency of a sound wave is measured in Hz as the:
   A. Inverse of the wavelength.
   B. Maximal amplitude of particle vibration.
   C. Number of times particles vibrate each second in the direction perpendicular to wave propagation.
   D. Number of times particles vibrate each second in the direction of wave propagation.

4. Ultrasound imaging is usually performed using frequencies in the range of:
   A. 1–30 kHz.
   B. Below 5 MHz.
   C. Above 0.5 MHz.
   D. 1–30 MHz.

5. Assuming that sound velocity in muscle tissue is 1,600 m/sec, the wavelength of a sound wave with the frequency of 1.6 MHz is:
   A. 1 mm.
   B. 1 cm.
   C. 1 m.
   D. 0.1 mm.

6. As an ultrasound wave travels through the human body, the type of tissue that results in the fastest loss of its strength is:
   A. Fat.
   B. Bone.
   C. Lung.
   D. Blood.

7. The main goal of the gel used during ultrasound imaging is to:
   A. Disinfect the transducer.
   B. Cool the transducer.
   C. To numb the skin and thus reduce patient's discomfort caused by pressure.
   D. To improve the contact between transducer surface and the skin.

8. Materials that respond to acoustic waves by generating electric signals and vice versa are known as:
   A. Doppler crystals.
   B. Acoustic coupling gels.
   C. Piezoelectric crystals.
   D. Chronotropic agents.

9. Doppler effect refers to:
   A. Change in strength of a sound wave reflected by a moving target.
   B. Change in frequency of a sound wave reflected by a moving target.
   C. Change in shape of a sound wave reflected by a moving target.
   D. Loss of ultrasound energy as a result of wave dissipation by flow.

10. Doppler angle is the angle between:
   A. The flow and the long axis of the left ventricle.
   B. The ultrasound beam and the long axis of the left ventricle.
   C. The flow and the transmitted ultrasound beam.
   D. The flow and the central axis of the transducer.

11. A positive Doppler shift indicates that the reflector is moving:
   A. Faster than the sound wave propagates.
   B. Directly toward the transducer.
   C. Directly away from the transducer.
   D. So that the angle between the transmitted beam and the direction of motion is >90 degrees.

12. Doppler shift of zero indicates that the reflector is stationary or:
   A. Moving in a direction perpendicular to the beam.
   B. Moving in a direction parallel to the beam.
   C. Moving in a direction perpendicular to the central axis of the transducer.
   D. Moving too fast to register.

13. Time gain compensation is part of the ultrasound image formation aimed at correcting intensity for variations to the extent to which different media result in ultrasound _____:
   A. Scattering.
   B. Absorption.
   C. Reflection.
   D. Attenuation.

14. The strength of the transmitted ultrasound wave is controlled by adjusting the:
   A. Time gain compensation controls.
   B. Compression control.
   C. Power control.
   D. Overall gain control.

15. The spatial resolution of an ultrasound image is defined as the:
   A. Smallest distance between two objects that allows distinction between them.
   B. Size of the smallest object that can be clearly visualized in its entirety.
   C. Smallest cluster of pixels that can define a single object.
   D. Smallest difference in the size of an object that can be visually detected.

16. The spatial resolution of an ultrasound image is equal to the:
   A. Gap between two adjacent pixels.
   B. Twice the wavelength.
   C. Size of a pixel in the relevant direction.
   D. One-half of the wavelength.

17. The temporal resolution of a sequence of ultrasound images is defined by the:
   A. Shortest duration of an event that can be detected with confidence.
   B. Shortest time in which image information can change completely.
   C. Shortest time between two events that allows distinction between them.
   D. Shortest time in which pixel values can change.

18. The temporal resolution of a sequence of ultrasound images is equal to the:
   A. Inverse of transducer frequency.
   B. Inverse of frame rate.
   C. One cycle of the ultrasound wave.
   D. Inverse of the number of frames in the sequence.

19. The dynamic range of echoes displayed on the screen is adjusted by the:
   A. Time gain compensation control.
   B. Compression control.
   C. Transmit power control.
   D. Overall gain control.

20. As the frequency of ultrasound increases, the maximum imaging depth in the human body:
    A. Increases.
    B. Decreases.
    C. Remains unchanged.
    D. May increase or decrease depending on the mechanical index used.

21. After capturing the image shown in Figure 1-1A, another image was obtained by increasing imaging frequency (Fig. 1-1B). Figure 1-1B has:

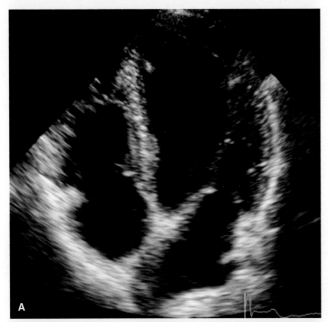

Fig. 1-1A

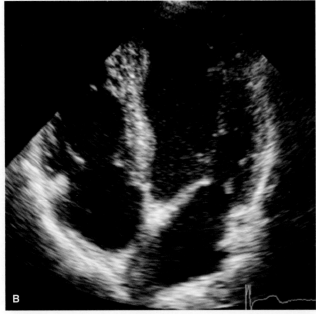

Fig. 1-1B

A. Bigger imaging depth.
B. Better temporal resolution.
C. Better spatial resolution.
D. Less acoustic shadowing.

22. After capturing the image shown in Figure 1-2A, another image was obtained by switching to the harmonic mode (Fig. 1-2B). Figure 1-2B was created from reflections of ultrasound of:

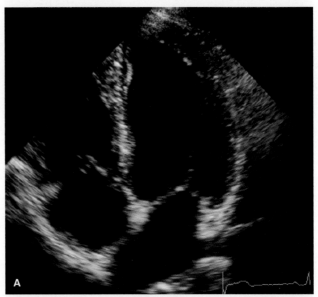

Fig. 1-2A

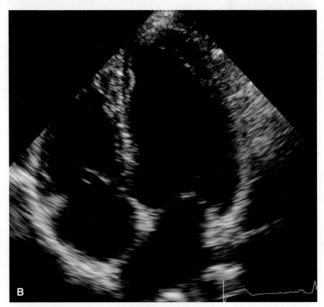

Fig. 1-2B

A. Double the frequency of the transmitted waves.
B. Half the frequency of the transmitted waves.
C. Same frequency of the transmitted waves generated by resonating particles.
D. Half the frequency of the transmitted waves generated by nonlinear reflectors.

23. After capturing the image shown in Figure 1-3A, another image was obtained by reducing imaging depth (Fig. 1-3B). Which of the two images has a lower frame rate?

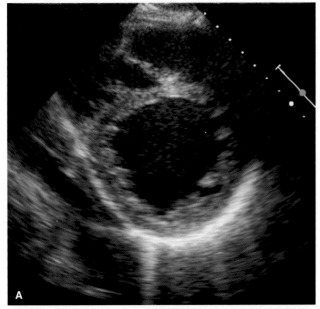

Fig. 1-3A

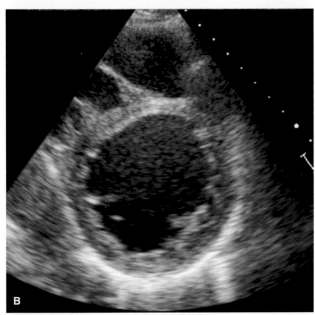

Fig. 1-3B

A. Figure 1-3A.
B. Figure 1-3B.
C. Both image sequences have identical frame rates.
D. Impossible to determine without knowing how wavelength responded to the change.

24. After capturing the image sequence shown in Figure 1-4A, another sequence was obtained by reducing the sector angle (Fig. 1-4B). The sequence in Figure 1-4B has:

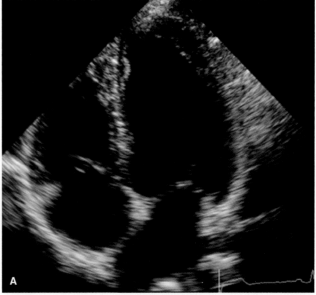

Fig. 1-4A

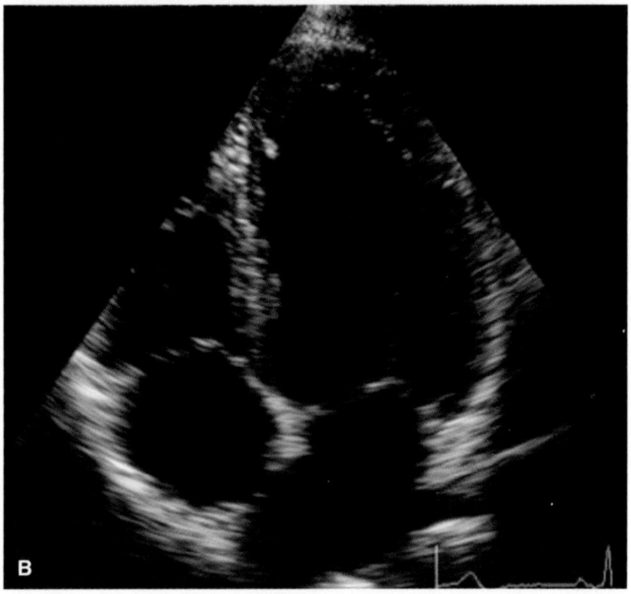

Fig. 1-4B

A. Better spatial resolution.
B. Lower temporal resolution.
C. Higher frame rate.
D. More scan lines per pixel.

25. Figure 1-5 DOES NOT:

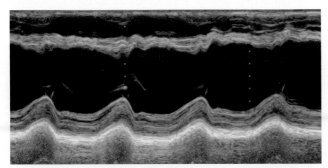

Fig. 1-5

A. Display ultrasound reflections along a single scan line over time.
B. Display power spectrum of velocities measured along a single scan line over time.
C. Have higher temporal resolution than two-dimensional imaging.
D. Allow simultaneous visualization of different anatomical structures.

26. Figure 1-6 DOES NOT:

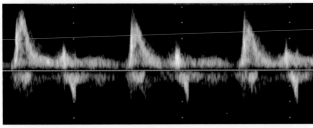

Fig. 1-6

A. Display ultrasound reflections along a single scan line over time.
B. Display power spectrum of velocities measured along a single scan line over time.
C. Have higher temporal resolution than two-dimensional imaging.
D. Have to obtain information about distribution of flow velocities.

27. Continuous spectral Doppler imaging displays the strength of each velocity component by assigning to them:
A. Different gray-scale levels.
B. Different heights of the deflections.
C. Different slopes of the deflections.
D. Different colors in the color Doppler image.

28. The color pattern characterizing turbulent flow in this color-flow Doppler image (Fig. 1-7) can be described as:

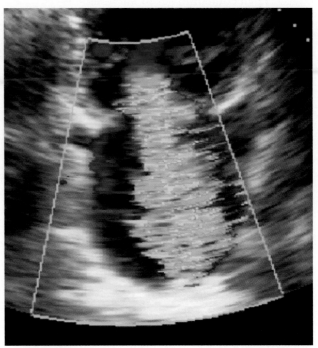

Fig. 1-7

A. Disorganized.
B. Spiral-shaped.
C. Mosaic.
D. Broken.

29. "Laminar flow" in a blood vessel means that flow velocities are:
A. Completely disorganized and do not follow the laws of hydrodynamics.
B. Highest along the central axis of the vessel and gradually decrease toward the walls.
C. Low everywhere except when swirling around the central axis of the vessel.
D. Same everywhere in the vessel.

30. Phased-array transducers use differences in phase of pulses transmitted by individual elements to:
A. Allow imaging the heart throughout the different phases of the cardiac cycle.
B. Steer the ultrasound beam in different directions and thus scan a "slice" rather than a single line.
C. Interrogate a range of flow velocities inside the heart by determining phase shifts caused by moving targets.
D. Quickly switch the transducer between transmit and receive phases.

31. Echocardiographic contrast agents are based on the idea that ultrasound reflection is augmented by the:
   A. High content of gas in microbubbles.
   B. Added gas-liquid interface in the presence of microbubbles.
   C. High speed of sound waves in gas.
   D. Rapid motion of the microbubbles in blood.

32. One well-known artifact of ultrasound imaging is frequently referred to as "acoustic shadowing," depicted in Figure 1-8. The main cause of this artifact is the inability of the imaging system to accurately compensate for:

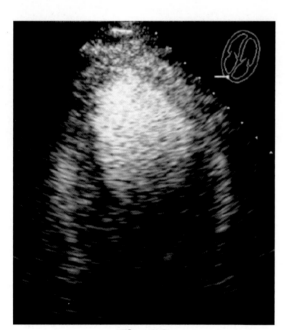

Fig. 1-8

   A. Increased attenuation by a structure such as a ventricular cavity.
   B. Reduced attenuation by structures such as a ventricular cavity.
   C. Increased attenuation by structures such as a contrast-filled ventricular cavity.
   D. Increased attenuation secondary to a temporary surge in frequency associated with the presence of contrast material.

33. Shadowing artifacts (Fig. 1-9A) can be effectively reduced as shown (Fig. 1-9B) by using:

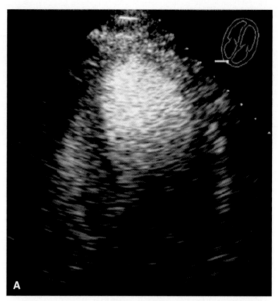

Fig. 1-9A

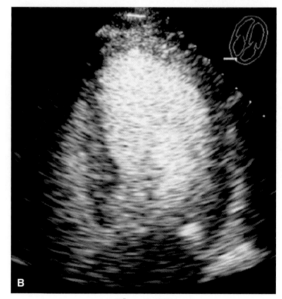

Fig. 1-9B

   A. Lower compression setting.
   B. Lower overall gain.
   C. Higher transmit power that destroys microbubbles.
   D. Less contrast material.

ANSWERS

1. ANSWER: D. Sound waves cannot travel in a vacuum, as pressure waves can only be transmitted through physical media consisting of molecules that interact with each other. Water, air, and metal are all such media, and therefore sound waves can and indeed do travel in them.

2. ANSWER: C. The upper limit of the audible range of human hearing is 20,000 Hz or 20 kHz. There are animals that can hear sounds in different ranges than humans. For example, bats' hearing includes sounds in a much higher frequency range. This is known as supersonic hearing. They produce these sound waves, which then echo back to them by bouncing off objects so that they know how far something is, just like a sonar on a submarine.

3. ANSWER: D. Frequency in general is measured in Hz (abbreviation for Hertz), which is defined as 1/sec. The frequency of a wave is defined as the number of times a particle in a conducting medium vibrates per unit time. Thus, frequency is the inverse of the period. Since sound waves are pressure disturbances traveling in the medium in the direction of the particle vibrations, they are called longitudinal waves. In other words, sound waves are vibrations in the direction of wave propagation, and therefore the correct answer.

4. ANSWER: D. Ultrasound imaging is usually performed using frequencies in the range of 1–30 MHz. The lower frequencies in this range are used to image large organs or deeper structures that require significant penetration depth, while the higher frequencies are used for smaller and more superficial structures that require less depth but better spatial resolution.

5. ANSWER: A. Wavelength, λ is defined as the distance a wave travels during a single cycle. Wavelength can be calculated as the product of velocity, c, and the period, T, or, alternatively, the ratio of velocity and frequency, f:

$$\lambda = c \cdot T = \frac{c}{f} = \frac{1600 \text{ m/sec}}{1.6 \text{ MHz}} = \frac{1.6 \cdot 10^3 \text{ m/sec}}{1.6 \cdot 10^6 \text{ 1/sec}} = 10^{-3} = 1 \text{ mm}$$

6. ANSWER: C. Because of the high content of air and the abundance of highly reflective tissue/air interfaces, the sound waves dissipate in the lung so fast that the lungs are virtually opaque to ultrasound.

7. ANSWER: D. The main goal of the coupling gel is to improve the contact between transducer surface and the skin by eliminating any tissue/air interfaces, which are highly reflective and thus prevent ultrasound transmission into the body.

8. ANSWER: C. Materials that respond to electric signals by vibrating and generating acoustic waves, and vice versa, respond to acoustic waves by generating electric signals, are knows as piezoelectric crystals. These materials are the basis for medical ultrasound imaging, which relies on transmitting waves by "exciting" the crystals in the transducer by an electrical stimulus, and then receiving the ultrasound waves reflected by structures inside the body and translating them back into electrical signals that are used to form an image of the reflecting structures.

9. ANSWER: B. Doppler effect refers to a change in the frequency of a sound wave reflected by a moving target. We are all familiar with the Doppler effect from our daily life: sounds coming from a moving object have higher pitch when the object approaches us than when the same object moves away from us. This is how we can tell if a train is approaching the station or leaving before we can actually see it.

10. ANSWER: C. Doppler angle is the angle between the direction of flow (in Figure 1-10, flow through the tricuspid valve indicated by the blue arrow) and that of the ultrasound beam (green line). The orientation of either the ventricle (long axis indicated by the pink line) or the transducer (central axis indicated by the brown line) has no role in the interaction between ultrasound and moving blood cells that reflect ultrasound at a frequency that depends on the direction of blood flow along the beam.

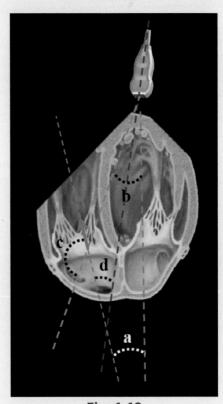

Fig. 1-10

Like the train, blood cells moving away from the transducer reflect sound with lower frequency than those moving toward the transducer. What determines whether it is the former or the latter is the angle between the flow and the direction of the transmitted beam: when the angle is <90 degrees, then the flow is away from the transducer, and vice versa, when the angle is >90 degrees, then the flow is toward the transducer.

11. *ANSWER: D.* A positive Doppler shift indicates that the reflector is moving so that the angle between the transmitted beam and the direction of flow is >90 degrees, i.e., the reflectors are getting closer, but not necessarily moving directly toward the transducer.

12. *ANSWER: A.* Doppler shift of zero indicates that the reflector is stationary or moving in a direction perpendicular to the beam. Importantly, when the Doppler angle is 90 degrees, the flow is neither toward nor away from the transducer, but perpendicular to the beam and thus will produce no Doppler shift, or, in other words, will reflect ultrasound at the same frequency that was transmitted.

13. *ANSWER: D.* The combined result of ultrasound scattering, absorption, and reflection is attenuation. Time gain compensation aims at providing a correction for the loss of intensity (or attenuation) by all these different mechanisms. This is done assuming that attenuation in different types of tissue in the heart is the same, which is a reasonably accurate assumption. However, it may become quite inaccurate when there are materials with drastically different acoustic properties such as contrast agents that cause much stronger attenuation. This is the reason why acoustic shadowing artifacts are frequently seen distal to contrast-filled blood pools, such as ventricles or atria.

14. *ANSWER: C.* The strength of the transmitted ultrasound wave is controlled by adjusting the power control. Gain control determines to what extent the received signal is amplified, and the compression determines the dynamic range of received signals that are used to create the image. Time gain compensation has nothing to do with the strength of the transmitted power: it is part of postprocessing of the reflections designed to correct for beam attenuation as it travels through the body.

15. *ANSWER: A.* The spatial resolution of an ultrasound image is defined as the smallest distance between two objects that allows distinction between them. This is the definition of spatial resolution. Understandably, the spatial resolution also determines the size of the smallest object that can be visualized. However, the change in the size of an object is certainly not the definition of resolution.

16. *ANSWER: C.* While spatial resolution along the ultrasound beam is directly related to wavelength, it is affected by other factors in other directions. However, it can be easily determined by the size of a pixel in the relevant direction, if that is known. The gap between two adjacent pixels is a nonsensical answer designed to confuse you, since there is no gap between adjacent pixels.

17. *ANSWER: C.* Similar to spatial resolution, temporal resolution of a sequence of ultrasound images is defined by the shortest time between two events that allows distinction between them. Similarly, temporal resolution determines the shortest duration of an event that can be detected, but "with confidence" is a subjective term that makes answer (A) incorrect. Answers (B) and (D) are nonsense.

18. *ANSWER: B.* The temporal resolution of a sequence of ultrasound images is equal to the inverse of the frame rate. The inverse of the transducer frequency is a period (duration of a single cycle) of the ultrasound wave, and is in the order of magnitude of microseconds. The temporal resolution of a sequence of images is nowhere near: it is hundreds of thousands of times longer. Answer (D) is nonsense, as one can create a sequence of any number of frames, which has nothing to do with temporal resolution.

19. *ANSWER: B.* The dynamic range of echoes displayed on the screen is adjusted by the compression control. This control can be used to include or suppress weak echoes.

20. *ANSWER: B.* Sound waves of higher frequencies dissipate in conducting media faster than those with lower frequencies, due to a variety of mechanisms. Thus, of two sound waves transmitted with identical intensities but at different frequencies, the intensity of the wave with the higher frequency that reaches a certain depth is smaller than that of the wave with the lower frequency. In other words, increased frequency translates into smaller imaging depth.

21. *ANSWER: C.* Figure 1-1B was obtained using higher frequency, which equates to smaller wavelength that allows differentiation between two distinct objects located closer to each other. Thus, Figure 1-1B has better spatial resolution.

22. *ANSWER: A.* Harmonic imaging (or more precisely, second harmonic imaging) uses ultrasound reflections that have twice the frequency of the transmitted waves. It is also possible to use higher harmonics, such as third, fourth, and so on for image formation, but typically only second harmonic imaging is available in commercial systems, because higher harmonic images are noisier and have not been shown to be useful.

23. ANSWER: A. To increase the frame rate, the operator should decrease imaging depth, as it takes less time for ultrasound waves to reach more superficial structures and return to the transducer. Thus, it takes less time to create and image with smaller depth and, consequently, more frames can be created every second, resulting in a higher frame rate.

24. ANSWER: C. By reducing the sector angle, one reduces the number of scan lines used to generate an image. This results in shorter total time necessary to transmit waves and then receive and process the reflections from the scanned sector, i.e., shorter time to create a single frame. This also translates into a larger number of frames per second, or higher frame rate.

25. ANSWER: B. M-mode imaging does not display power spectrum of velocities measured along a single scan line over time, which can be obtained using the spectral Doppler mode. It does indeed display ultrasound reflections along a single scan line over time. It has higher temporal resolution than two-dimensional imaging because it is essentially one-dimensional: one scan line only which allows formation of a much larger number of lines per second than the number of full frames combined of hundreds of lines each in a two-dimensional image. M-mode does allow simultaneous visualization of different anatomical structures, as long as they can be connected by a straight line going through the transducer.

26. ANSWER: A. Spectral Doppler imaging does not display ultrasound reflections along a single scan line over time, which is what the M-mode does. It does indeed display the power spectrum of velocities measured along a single scan line over time, which provides information about the distribution of flow velocities.

27. ANSWER: A. Continuous spectral Doppler imaging displays the strength of each velocity component by assigning to them different gray-scale levels. Each vertical line represents a power spectrum of the Doppler signal at one time point, while the x-axis represents time. The lowest velocities are shown closer to the baseline, while higher velocities are shown further away from the baseline. The brightness of each point indicates how predominant the specific velocity is at that moment. Thus, a higher deflection at a certain moment in time means that higher velocities were detected, and the brightest point along the deflection indicates the strongest, most predominant velocity.

28. ANSWER: C. The color pattern characterizing turbulent flow in color-flow Doppler imaging can be described as mosaic. This is a common term used frequently by echocardiographers.

29. ANSWER: B. "Laminar" in Latin means "smooth" or "regular." "Laminar flow" in a blood vessel refers to a smooth flow pattern, where flow velocities are highest along the central axis of the vessel and gradually decrease toward the walls.

30. ANSWER: B. Phased-array transducers use differences in phase of pulses transmitted by individual elements to steer the ultrasound beam in different directions and thus scan a "slice" rather than a single line.

31. ANSWER: B. Echocardiographic contrast agents are based on the idea that ultrasound reflection is increased by the added gas-liquid interface in the presence of microbubbles.

32. ANSWER: C. The main source of acoustic shadowing is the inability of the imaging system to accurately compensate for increased attenuation by a structure such as a contrast-filled ventricular cavity.

33. ANSWER: D. Shadowing artifacts can be effectively reduced by using less contrast material.

SUGGESTED READINGS

Evans D. *Doppler Ultrasound—Physics, Instrumentation and Clinical Applications*. New York, NY: John Wiley & Sons; 1989.

Gonzalez RC, Wintz P. *Digital Image Processing*. Reading, MA: Addison Wesley; 1977.

Goss S, Johnston R, Dunn F. Comprehensive compilation of empirical ultrasonic properties of mammalian tissue. *J Acoust Soc Am*. 1978;64:423.

Hagen-Ansert L. *Textbook of Diagnostic Ultrasonography*. St. Louis, MO: Mosby; 1995.

Hedrick WR, Hykes DL, Starchman DE. *Ultrasound Physics and Instrumentation*. St. Louis, MO: Mosby; 1995.

Kremkau F. *Diagnostic Ultrasound—Principles, Instrumentation and Exercises*. Orlando, FL: Grune & Stratton; 1993.

Rumack CM, Wilson SR, Charboneau JW. *Diagnostic Ultrasound*. St. Louis, MO: Mosby; 1991.

Smith H, Zagzebski JA. *Doppler Ultrasound*. Madison, WI: Medical Physics Publishing; 1991.

Wells PNT. *Biomedical Ultrasonics*. New York, NY: Academic Press; 1977.

Zagzebski JA. *Essentials of Ultrasound Physics*. St. Louis, MO: Mosby; 1996.

Cardiac Ultrasound Artifacts

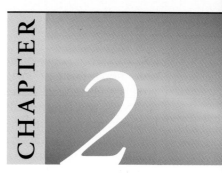

CHAPTER 2

Juan-Carlos Brenes and Craig R. Asher

1. Which of the following fundamental principles of echocardiography is assumed to be correct when interpreting an ultrasound image?
   A. All reflections are received from each pulse after the next pulse is sent.
   B. The distance to the reflecting object is inversely proportional to the round-trip travel time.
   C. The sound emitted by the transducer travels in straight lines.
   D. Sound travels in tissue at a speed of 900 m/sec.

2. Linear artifacts within the ascending aorta:
   A. Produce interruption of the pattern of blood in the ascending aorta when color Doppler imaging is applied.
   B. May extend through the aortic wall.
   C. Display rapid oscillatory movement.
   D. Usually have clearly defined borders.

3. Which of the following statements regarding the development of ascending aorta artifacts during transesophageal echocardiography is correct?
   A. Linear artifacts within the ascending aorta are most commonly caused by ultrasound refraction.
   B. Artifacts are more likely to appear when the aortic diameter is smaller than the left atrial diameter.
   C. A linear structure located at half the distance from the transducer as from the anterior aortic wall is most likely an artifact.
   D. M-mode echocardiography has proven to be useful in distinguishing artifacts from true aortic flaps.

4. Which of the following statements regarding reverberation-type artifacts is correct?
   A. Multiple path artifacts are the result of reverberations between weakly reflective surfaces.
   B. The larger the impedance mismatch between media, the higher the likelihood of reflections to occur.
   C. Interfaces oriented parallel to the direction of sound propagation have the highest probability of creating reflections.
   D. The intensity of the reverberation lines increases as the distance from the transducer increases.
   E. Reverberations cannot be eliminated from the field of view.

5. Which of the following statements regarding tissue harmonic imaging is correct?
   A. A significant proportion of harmonics is produced by side lobes.
   B. Artifacts are more common to develop with harmonic imaging than with fundamental imaging.
   C. Tissue harmonic signals pass only through the body wall one time.
   D. Reverberation artifacts are more common to develop with harmonic imaging.

6. Which of the following statements regarding the development of beam-width artifacts is correct?
   A. The lateral resolution diminishes as the depth decreases.
   B. The ultrasound beam reaches its narrowest diameter in the focal zone.

C. Focusing can increase the chance of development of beam-width artifacts.

D. A beam-width artifact can make real structures, such as struts on a prosthetic valve, look smaller than the actual size.

7. Which of the following statements regarding artifacts within the ascending aorta is correct?
   A. The utilization of M-mode echocardiography has been shown to increase the false-positive diagnosis of an ascending aorta dissection.
   B. Artifacts within the ascending aorta are less likely to appear when the aortic diameter exceeds the left atrial diameter.
   C. Linear artifacts are usually found at half the distance between the transducer and the atrial-aortic interface.
   D. Artifacts within the ascending aorta are more likely to move with less amplitude as the aortic wall.
   E. An ascending aorta diameter of >5 cm along with an atrial/aortic ratio of ≤0.6 are important determinants of artifact appearance.

8. Which of the following statements regarding side lobe artifacts is correct?
   A. Side lobe artifacts involve the presence of a weakly reflective object which is close to the central beam of ultrasound.
   B. In a side lobe artifact, an image will appear at the wrong location but in the same direction of the main beam.
   C. Side lobe artifacts are created after echoes are returned from highly reflective objects located within the pathway of the central (main) beam.
   D. All the energy emitted from an ultrasound transducer remains within the central (main) beam.

9. Which of the following statements regarding a refraction type of artifact is correct?
   A. Refraction develops when the ultrasound beam is completely reflected.
   B. Two different media with the same propagation speed create a refraction type of artifact.
   C. Refraction can cause the appearance of a double image (side by side).

D. Refraction makes structures appear closer to the transducer.

10. Which of the following statements regarding range ambiguity is true?
    A. Range ambiguity occurs when echoes from deep structures created by a first pulse arrive at the transducer before the second pulse has been emitted.
    B. Range ambiguity occurs when echoes from deep structures created by a first pulse arrive at the transducer after the second pulse has been emitted.
    C. The pulse repetition frequency (PRF) is not affected by the imaging depth.
    D. To avoid range ambiguity, PRF is increased when scanning deeper structures.

11. Which of the following statements regarding mirror-imaging artifact in spectral Doppler echocardiography is correct?
    A. It usually appears when the Doppler gains are set too low.
    B. It consists in the development of a symmetric spectral image on the opposite side of the baseline from the true signal.
    C. The mirror image is usually more intense but otherwise very similar to the true signal.
    D. It can be reduced by increasing the power output and better alignment of the Doppler beam with the flow direction.

12. Which of the following techniques can help distinguish a left ventricular thrombus from an artifact (near-field clutter)?
    A. Increasing the depth.
    B. Increasing the transducer frequency.
    C. Using a single view.
    D. Increasing the mechanical index.

13. True structures, as opposed to artifacts, are characterized by the following:
    A. Ill-defined borders.
    B. Visualization in a single view.
    C. Not crossing anatomical borders.
    D. Lack of attachments to nearby structures.

14. A mirror-image artifact in two-dimensional echocardiography develops when:
   A. A structure is located behind a weak reflector leading to partial reflection of the ultrasound beam.
   B. A structure is located in front of a highly reflective surface, which produces near total reflection of the ultrasound beam.
   C. The ultrasound beam is deflected from the expected straight-line path.
   D. Structures located outside the main beam are interrogated.

15. Which of the following statements is correct regarding a ring-down artifact?
   A. It is a type of reverberation artifact that is indistinguishable from a comet tail artifact.
   B. It is caused by a resonating pocket of air bubbles surrounding fluid.
   C. It is a type of ultrasound machine artifact caused when the transducer crystal is defective.
   D. It is a type of artifact that is not seen in cardiac imaging.

16. The arrow in Figure 2-1 is pointing to an artifact generated due to:

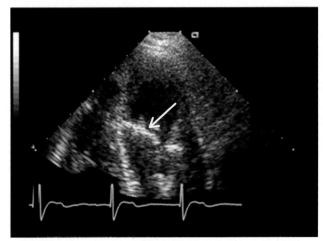

Fig. 2-1

   A. Side lobes.
   B. Acoustic shadowing.
   C. Beam width.
   D. Range ambiguity.
   E. Refraction.

17. On Figure 2-2, the arrow is pointing to which of the following types of artifacts?

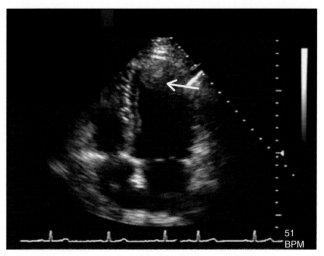

Fig. 2-2

   A. Shadowing.
   B. Refraction.
   C. Near-field clutter.
   D. Beam-width.
   E. Side lobes.

18. The artifact seen in Figure 2-3 corresponds to:

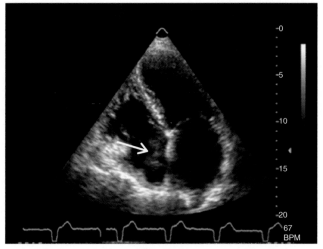

Fig. 2-3

   A. Shadowing.
   B. Refraction.
   C. Near-field clutter.
   D. Range ambiguity.
   E. Beam-width artifact.

19. The spectral tracing in Figure 2-4 was obtained from the suprasternal notch using continuous-wave Doppler with the sample volume in the proximal descending aorta. Which of the following statements is correct?

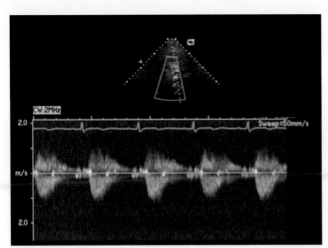

Fig. 2-4

A. The tracing corresponds to a near-field clutter type of artifact.
B. The superimposition of adjacent flows is due to a beam-width artifact.
C. The spectral tracing results from a ghosting artifact.
D. This is an example of the shadowing type of artifact.

20. The image within the left atrium in Figure 2-5 corresponds to a:

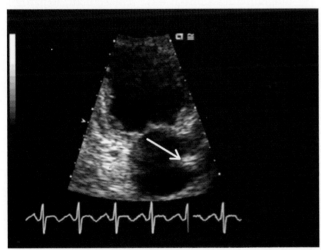

Fig. 2-5

A. Refraction type of artifact.
B. Near-field clutter.
C. Shadowing artifact.
D. Side lobe artifact.

21. Which of the following is the best explanation for the M-mode image in Figure 2-6?

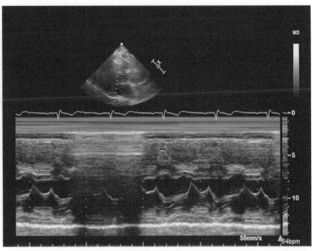

Fig. 2-6

A. There is shadowing of the mitral valve due to near-field clutter.
B. There is shielding of the mitral valve due aortic valve calcification.
C. There is attenuation of the mitral valve due to inspiration.
D. There is no artifact in this image.

22. Describe the type of artifact seen in the left atrium of this patient with a mechanical aortic valve (Fig. 2-7).

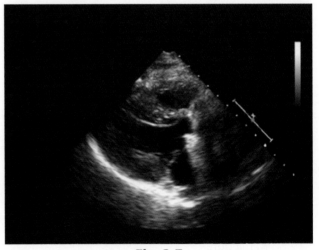

Fig. 2-7

A. Shadowing.
B. Ghosting.
C. Attenuation.
D. Shielding.
E. Refraction.

23. The arrow in Figure 2-8 is pointing to an artifact called:

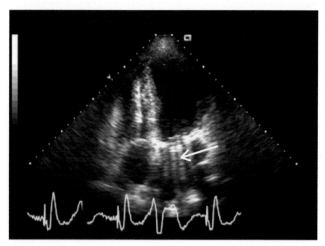

Fig. 2-8

A. Near-field clutter.
B. Reverberation.
C. Shadowing.
D. Refraction.

24. Describe the type of artifact present in this parasternal long-axis image of a patient with a mechanical mitral valve prosthesis (Fig. 2-9):

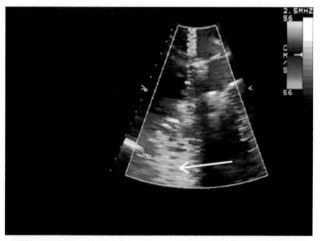

Fig. 2-9

A. Shielding.
B. Refraction.
C. Ghosting.
D. Beam-width.
E. Side lobe.

25. The arrow in Figure 2-10 is pointing to which of the following types of artifacts?

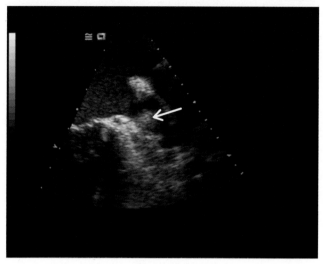

Fig. 2-10

A. Refraction.
B. Near-field clutter.
C. Reverberation.
D. Ghosting.

CASE 1:

26. A 75-year-old man underwent a follow-up echocardiogram after a mitral valve replacement. Regarding the artifact images present in the left atrium in Video 2.1, which of the following statements is correct?
A. Shadowing is a reverberation-type artifact.
B. Shadowing refers to the increase in echo amplitude from reflectors that lie behind a strongly reflecting structure.
C. In the presence of shadowing, an alternate acoustic window can help assess the region of interest.
D. Shadowing and reverberations limit the evaluation of structures in the near field.

CASE 2:

27. After scanning the short-axis at the level of the aortic valve, the sonographer calls you to help with the interpretation of this image (Video 2.2). This corresponds to:
A. A dilated sinus of Valsalva.
B. A patient with a heterotopic heart transplant.
C. A refraction-type artifact.
D. A mirror-type artifact.
E. A large mobile vegetation.

CASE 3:

28. A 60-year-old woman presented for a routine echocardiogram due to a heart murmur. She recently underwent cosmetic surgery. Video 2.3 shows:
    A. A refraction type of artifact.
    B. An artifact secondary to breast implants.
    C. A near-field clutter type of artifact.
    D. A beam-width type of artifact.

CASE 4:

29. Video 2.4 displays an example of an artifact known as:
    A. Mirror image.
    B. Background noise.
    C. Intercept angle.
    D. Ghosting.
    E. Shadowing.

CASE 5:

30. Regarding the imaging artifact present posterior to the inferolateral wall of the left ventricle (Video 2.5), which of the following statements is correct?
    A. This is an example of a refraction type of artifact.
    B. It results from the presence of a weak reflector (specular reflector).
    C. The angle at which the sound gets reflected equals the angle of its incidence.
    D. This video corresponds to a patient with a heterotopic heart transplant.

ANSWERS

1. ANSWER: C. Echocardiography is a diagnostic ultrasound test used to evaluate cardiac anatomy and physiology. As such, it is based on the physical principles of sound which travels through a medium in the form of a propagating wave. There are several assumptions behind the concept of ultrasound imaging that apply to echocardiography, and the violation of any of these can result in an artifact. Artifacts are images that are not real; located in the wrong place; have an inappropriate brightness, shape, or size; or represent structures that are missing.

Basic assumptions of ultrasound include the following: The ultrasonic wave emitted by the ultrasound probe travels along a straight line path to and from the transducer and makes only one path forward and back. All the echoes that are detected along that straight line originate from the axis of the main beam only. All reflections are received from each pulse before the next pulse is sent. Sound travels in tissue at a speed of 1540 m/sec. The distance to the reflecting object is determined by the elapsed time between the transmitted pulse and the detected echo. This distance is proportional to the round-trip travel time. The amplitude of returning echoes is related directly to the reflecting or scattering properties of distant objects.

2. ANSWER: B. Clinically, it is essential to be able to distinguish artifacts from an intimal flap associated with an aortic dissection. The utilization of criteria to define artifacts in this scenario has been shown to improve the specificity of transesophageal echocardiography in the diagnosis of aortic dissection. Linear artifacts within the ascending aorta usually lack rapid oscillatory movements, which are usually associated with intimal flaps. They also may extend "through" the aortic wall or beyond normal anatomic borders and have fuzzy and indistinct boundaries. When applying color Doppler, artifacts usually do not produce interruption in the pattern of blood flow as would be seen with the presence of a true and false lumen.

3. ANSWER: D. There is in vivo and in vitro evidence to support that linear artifacts within the ascending aorta are caused by ultrasound reflection. In their classic experiment, Appelbe and collaborators introduced an ultrasound probe in a water tank containing two balloons placed in series: a posterior "left atrial balloon" and an anterior "aortic balloon." They observed that a linear image was consistently present within the aortic balloon when its diameter exceeded the diameter of the left atrial balloon, and since these contained only water, the image was by definition an artifact. Artifacts are more likely to appear when the aortic diameter exceeds the left atrial diameter. Evangelista et al described the utility of M-Mode applied during transesophageal echocardiography in recognizing artifacts as they evaluated 132 patients with suspected aortic dissection. A type A artifact within the ascending aorta was defined as that located twice as far from the transducer as from the posterior aortic wall as seen Figure 2-11A. (T = transducer; LA = left atrium; AA = ascending aorta.) By using M-mode echocardiography they were also able to show the unrelated motion of intimal flaps to the posterior aortic wall. Artifacts usually move parallel to the posterior aortic wall.

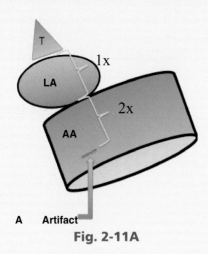

Fig. 2-11A

A type B artifact is located at twice the distance from the right pulmonary artery posterior wall as from the posterior aortic wall (Fig. 2-11B). (RPA = right pulmonary artery; AA = ascending aorta.)

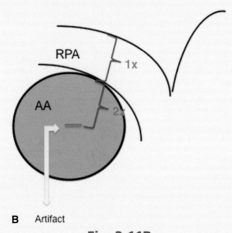

Fig. 2-11B

4. ANSWER: B. When an ultrasound beam meets the interface between two different media, part of it is reflected and part of it continues into the second medium. The amount of energy reflected is proportional to the difference in acoustic impedance of the two media: the larger the impedance mismatch between the media (myocardium-air) the higher the chance that multiple reflections will develop. This is also more likely to occur when the interface is oriented perpendicular to the direction of propagation. When this strongly reflected echo created at the interface returns to the transducer, some of its energy is redirected back into the patient and it can be

reflected again at the same interface. This second echo returns to the transducer at a later time, and the image will be displayed farther away from the real structure since it is assumed to have arisen from a greater depth. Multiple reflections may occur when several interfaces are present for reflection, such as is the case of a mechanical valve disc. The intensity of the reverberation lines decreases as the distance from the transducer increases. M-mode echocardiography can help recognize the lack of independent motion of reverberation artifacts. Reverberations can be reduced or eliminated by changing the frequency or depth of the transducer. See Figure 2-12 with two examples of how reverberation artifacts are created. (T = transmitted pulse; R = reflected pulse; L = returned pulse.)

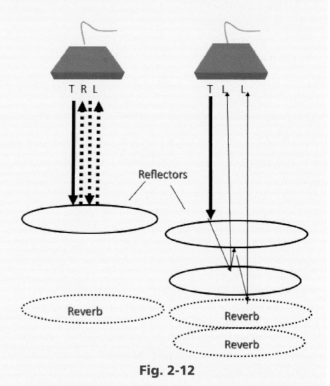

Fig. 2-12

5. ANSWER: C. Tissue harmonic signals pass through the body wall only one time. In fundamental imaging, the ultrasound beam passes through the body wall first when emitted from the transducer and a second time upon its return. Harmonic signals are generated in the tissue from within the body, beyond the body wall, which leads to a reduction in distortion and scattering. The transmitted wave is a fundamental ultrasound signal and the return ultrasound wave is a harmonic signal. Side lobes are weaker pulses when compared to the main ultrasound beam. These weaker pulses generated by fundamental imaging produce little or no harmonics. Side lobe artifacts and reverberations are less likely to develop with harmonic imaging.

6. ANSWER: B. A focused ultrasound beam emitted by a transducer has a near field (proximal area to the transducer), focal zone, and far field (distal area to the transducer). In the focal zone (not the far field), the beam width of the ultrasound is decreased as it reaches its minimum diameter. In the far zone, the beam width becomes wider, and the lateral resolution degrades (lateral resolution diminishes as the depth increases). When the lateral resolution from a specific region is reduced, a beam-width type of artifact can appear, leading to an alteration in the size or shape of a structure. For example, struts on a prosthetic valve can look longer than the actual size. Beam-width artifacts can also simulate valvular vegetations. Focusing narrows the beam width and the lateral resolution improves, hence reducing the possibility of developing a beam-width artifact.

7. ANSWER: E. Losi and collaborators found that an ascending aorta diameter of >5 cm was a determinant of artifact appearance (sensitivity of 91%, specificity of 86%). However, some patients with a normal aorta diameter can have artifacts and some with a dilated aorta may not. By adding an atrial/aortic ratio of ≤0.6 to an aortic size of >5 cm, the specificity and positive predictive value for the diagnosis of an aortic artifact when an aortic dissection was suspected became 100%. M-mode echocardiography can reduce the false-positive diagnosis of an ascending aorta dissection. In vitro and in vivo evidence has shown that linear artifacts within the ascending aorta are usually found at twice the distance between the transducer and the atrial-aortic interface and are more likely to appear when the aortic diameter is twice the atrial diameter. Not only are these artifacts seen at twice the distance but also move with twice the amplitude as the interface.

8. ANSWER: B. The ultrasound waves emitted by the transducer travel in straight lines. Most of the energy is concentrated along a main or central beam. However, not all the energy remains within this central beam. Some of the energy is also directed to the sides of the central beam, which can produce echoes that will return to the transducer. The machine assumes that these echoes originate from points along the central or main beam axis, and the image will be displayed within this central beam. In a side lobe artifact, an image will appear in the wrong location but in the same direction of the main beam. In essence, this is a form of beam-width artifact.

9. ANSWER: C. Refraction is produced when the transmitted ultrasound beam is deviated from its straight path line (change in the angle of incidence) as it crosses the boundary between two media with different propagation velocities. In other words, the soundbeam bends and causes an artifact displaying a "duplicated" structure. The refracted beam is reflected back to the transducer, and this signal is assumed to be along the original scan line, leading to an image being displayed in the wrong location. In essence, refraction leads to the lateral displacement of structures from their correct location. See Figure 2-13. (T = transmitted pulse; L = returned pulse; T' = transmitted and refracted pulse; L' = returned refracted pulse.)

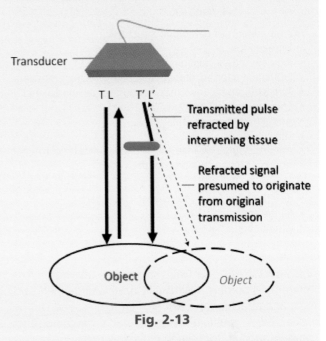

Fig. 2-13

10. ANSWER: B. The correct imaging of deep structures is determined by the pulse repetition frequency (PRF). PRF is related to the depth of view. As imaging depth increases, PRF decreases. In order to avoid range ambiguity, the PRF is reduced when scanning deeper structures, allowing the impulse to return to the transducer on time before the next pulse is emitted. Range ambiguity can lead to the incorrect placement of structures closer to the transducer than their actual location.

11. ANSWER B. The mirror-image artifact (also known as cross talk) in spectral Doppler echocardiography appears as a symmetric signal of usually less intensity than the true flow signal in the opposite side of the baseline. The spectral mirror image occurs when the Doppler gains are set too high and it can be reduced by decreasing the power output or gain.

12. ANSWER: B. Left ventricular thrombus develops almost exclusively in the region of a wall motion abnormality, most commonly seen in an akinetic, dyskinetic, or aneurysmal segment, usually at the apex. It is usually laminar, with discrete shape and borders and may appear as protruding or mobile. Its motion is concordant with the left ventricular wall. Increasing the transducer frequency, decreasing the depth, using multiple views, or utilizing the contrast agents can all help distinguish a left ventricular thrombus from an artifact (Table 2-1). The mechanical index should be decreased when using contrast to avoid excessive destruction of the bubbles.

TABLE 2-1   Differential of Structures/Artifacts in the Left Ventricle

Normal variants or pathologic structures:
- False tendons
- Prominent trabeculations/hypertrabeculation syndrome
- Prominent papillary muscles (accessory papillary muscle)
- Tumors (fibroma, myxoma, rhabdomyoma, lipoma, etc)
- Endomyocardial fibrosis (EMF)
- Apical hypertrophy (Yamaguchi's)
- Thrombus
- Aneurysms/pseudoaneurysms/congenital diverticuli
- Noncompaction cardiomyopathy

Artifact types:
- Reverberation (near-field clutter, comet tail)
- Range ambiguity
- Attenuation (shadowing)

---

13. ANSWER: C. True structures do not cross anatomical borders, will usually have well-defined borders and attachments to nearby structures, and can be visualized in multiple views. Artifacts have indistinct borders and are not seen in multiple views.

14. ANSWER: B. Mirror-image artifacts are produced when a structure is located in front of a strong reflector, or highly reflective surface, causing a near total reflection of the ultrasound beam. The transducer assumes a single reflection from the strong reflector to the transducer, though on its path back to the transducer, the ultrasound is instead reflected back again to the strong reflector and then finally back to the transducer. Given this delay in time to return to the transducer, the image is assumed to be similar but at a greater depth. Refraction is produced by deflection of the ultrasound beam from its expected straight line, as it crosses the interface between two media with different propagation velocities. When structures located outside the main ultrasound beam are interrogated, a side lobe type of artifact can develop, as explained previously.

15. ANSWER: B. Ring-down artifact is caused when a central fluid collection is trapped by a ring of air bubbles. The pocket of fluid and air continuously resonates reflecting back ultrasound and creating a region of a bright reflector. Posterior to this bright reflector of vibrating fluid and air is a linear beam of ultrasound

referred to as a ring-down artifact. This is different from a comet tail artifact that is caused by reverberation of bright reflectors. Ring-down artifact is most common in any organ where there are air bubbles and water, such as the gastrointestinal system, but may be seen in cardiac imaging.

16. ANSWER: D. The arrow in Figure 2-1 is pointing to an image created by range-ambiguity echoes, which generate an apparent "mass" within the left ventricle. This can be better visualized in Video 2-6A. Changing the depth can help eliminate this type of artifact as shown in Video 2-6B. After increasing the depth, the artifact disappears. The range ambiguity artifact can cause echoes from distant structures to appear closer to the transducer (see Figure 2-14; below; T = transmitted pulse; L = returned pulse; L' = returned pulse during next listen cycle). As stated before, PRF is automatically reduced when imaging deeper structures. Side lobes develop when echoes returning from reflecting surfaces on the sides of the main beam create images that appear to be in the wrong location. They correspond to a form of beam-width artifact. Refraction is due to a distortion of the ultrasound beam by tissue, resulting in side-by-side double image.

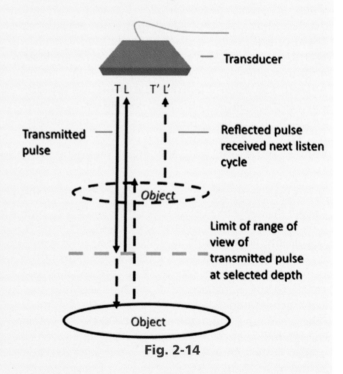

Fig. 2-14

17. ANSWER: C. This type of artifact is known as near-field clutter. It is created from high-amplitude reflections from the transducer and affects the near field of the ultrasound beam. The appearance of additional echoes in the near field can mask weaker echoes of true anatomic structures or mimic a mass or thrombus. It is often misinterpreted as a left ventricular thrombus. Improving the near-field resolution with higher frequency transducers, changing the views, and using contrast agents and harmonic imaging can all help reduce or eliminate this type of artifact (Fig. 2-15; T = transmitted pulse; L = returned pulse).

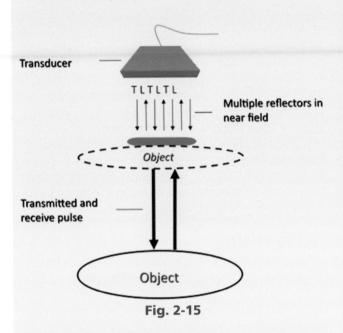

Transducer

T L T L T L

Multiple reflectors in near field

Object

Transmitted and receive pulse

Object

Fig. 2-15

18. *ANSWER: E.* This is an example of a beam-width artifact, which can cause an image to appear in the wrong location. All flow signals encountered at any point along the main beam are displayed as if they originate from that same beam axis. For this reason, strong flow signals at the margins of the beam (at the sides) create echoes that will be interpreted by the machine as arising from a point along the central beam, and the image will be displayed in the wrong location. This is commonly seen in apical views when trying to visualize structures in the far field, where the beam is the widest. In Figure 2-3, the arrow is pointing to a beam-width artifact (better appreciated in Video 2-7A), secondary to a calcified aortic valve/ascending aorta which is out of plane. Video 2-7B shows absence of turbulence and the color going "through" the image, consistent with an artifact.

19. *ANSWER: B.* This is an example of a beam-width artifact. The ultrasound beam is wide enough to detect both antegrade (ascending aorta) and retrograde (proximal descending aorta) flows. The resulting spectral tracing shows the superimposition of the adjacent flows. Near-field clutter, ghosting, and shadowing type of artifacts are covered elsewhere in this chapter.

20. *ANSWER: D.* This is an example of a side lobe artifact, which is generated from the warfarin (Coumadin) ridge. It is assumed that the ultrasound waves travel in straight lines and most of the energy is concentrated along a main or central beam. However, not all the energy remains within this central beam and some is directed to the side lobes. This ultrasound energy can encounter a reflector (Coumadin ridge in this case) which can produce echoes that will return to the transducer. The machine assumes that these originate from points along the main beam axis, and displays the image in the wrong location (within the left atrium). This is a form of beam-width artifact. This is better appreciated in Video 2-8.

21. *ANSWER: C.* Figure 2-6 is an M-mode image in the parasternal long-axis view at the level of the mitral valve showing attenuation of the mitral valve. Attenuation of ultrasound is a product of scattering, absorption, or reflection of sound waves in this case due to increased lung tissue during inspiration.

22. *ANSWER: D.* Figure 2-7 shows shielding of the left atrium caused by a mechanical aortic valve. Shielding refers to the presence of a bright beam of ultrasound artifact that obscures the visualization of tissue beyond this point. Shadowing refers to the attenuation of ultrasound beyond a bright reflector that similarly obscures the visualization of ultrasound. Ghosting refers to color Doppler that is distorted beyond anatomic borders because of multiple reflections. As described earlier, attenuation is due to scattering, absorption, or reflection. Refraction is due to bending of the ultrasound beam that results in an appearance of side-to-side images.

23. *ANSWER: B.* The arrow in Figure 2-8 is pointing to echoes that appear beyond a prosthetic mitral valve, extending into the left atrium. These are called reverberations. They are characterized as multiple horizontal lines that are equidistant with decreasing intensity and increasing depth.

24. *ANSWER: C.* Figure 2-9 shows an example of ghosting, which is a type of artifact that can develop with color Doppler. Ghosting refers to color Doppler that is distorted beyond anatomic borders because of multiple reflections.

25. *ANSWER: C.* This is an example of a reverberation type of artifact within the left atrial appendage, caused by a prominent Coumadin ridge. This can be easily mistaken for a thrombus within the left atrial appendage. There are several findings that can help differentiate this artifact from an actual thrombus. Its motion is synchronous with the Coumadin ridge and it has an intensity that is less than the ridge but similar in dimension. It also does not appear to have a typical attachment for thrombus. The absence of spontaneous echo contrast and the left atrial appendage velocities can also be helpful to determine the likelihood of a thrombus. Finally, when intravenous contrast is used, this should fill in the area in question.

26. ANSWER: C. Shadowing is an attenuation type of artifact and it refers to the reduction in echo amplitude from reflectors that lie behind a strongly reflecting or attenuating structure, which weakens the sound distal to it and the area is displayed as a darker region. This can be seen in patients with mechanical valve prosthesis such as the one shown in Video 2-1, pacemaker wires, and other intracardiac devices. The video also shows significant reverberations caused by a mechanical valve that can cause a shadowing effect potentially obscuring the presence of valvular regurgitation. When this type of artifact appears, an alternate acoustic window is needed for evaluation of the area that lies behind the strongly reflecting object. In the case presented, a subcostal view could provide a better visualization of the left atrium. Reverberations or multiple reflections from an interface can make an artifact appear in the far field of the image. These reflections between the interface and the transducer create linear artifacts that do not correspond to anatomic structures.

KEY POINTS:

- Shadowing is an attenuation type of artifact that consists in the weakening of echoes distal to a strong reflector, most commonly mechanical valves.
- An alternate window is useful in the evaluation of the area that lies behind the strong specular reflector.

27. ANSWER: C. This is an example of a refraction type of artifact that can create the appearance of a double image, which in this case is the aortic valve. Refraction is produced when the transmitted ultrasound beam is deviated from its straight path line (change in the angle of incidence) as it crosses the boundary between two media with different propagation velocities.

KEY POINTS:

- Refraction of the ultrasound beam causes displacement of structures laterally from their true location.
- Refraction is produced when the transmitted ultrasound beam is deviated from its straight path line (change in the angle of incidence) as it crosses the boundary between two media with different propagation velocities.

28. ANSWER: B. The image in Video 2-3 shows an artifact secondary to breast implants. The types of artifacts caused by breast implants either silicone or saline are not well described. Breast implants, particularly saline type, may cause attenuation of ultrasound. Other band-like artifacts and shadows occur in the field of view that obscure the visualization of cardiac structure. Artifacts from breast implants can appear in both the parasternal and apical views resulting in the need to acquire the images from off axis positions. This often leads to suboptimal image quality and challenging interpretations. This study demonstrates a broad band of ultrasound artifacts extending around the heart in the parasternal long-axis view.

KEY POINT:

- Breast implants may cause multiple artifacts that result in off-axis images and difficult image interpretation.

29. ANSWER: D. The image in Video 2-4 shows an example of a color Doppler artifact known as ghosting. This is a color Doppler artifact that creates brief (transient) flashes of color painted over true anatomic structures and does not correspond to true flow patterns. These "ghosts" usually appear as either red or blue patterns and bleed into areas of tissue and they are produced by the motion of strong reflectors.

KEY POINT:

- Transient flashes of color over true anatomic structures do not correspond to true flow patterns.

30. ANSWER: C. This is an example of a mirror-image artifact. Another structure that appears identical to the mitral valve appears to be present in the far field. The real mitral valve exists on one side of a strong reflector (specular reflector), which in this case is predominantly formed by the posterior pericardium (pericardium, pleura, and the lung). The sound emitted by the ultrasound probe is reflected by the posterior pericardium, at an angle that equals the angle of incidence, traveling then toward the mitral valve. From here, it gets reflected again toward the strong reflector (posterior pericardium, which is acting as a "mirror") and then back to the transducer. Since sound is assumed to travel along a straight-line path to and from the transducer, this reflected mitral valve will appear in the same direction in which the sound was initially transmitted. However, it took some "extra" time for the sound wave to travel between the posterior pericardium, mitral valve, posterior pericardium again, and then to the transducer, and for this reason the reflected structure will appear "deeper" than the specular reflector.

KEY POINTS:

- The ultrasonic wave emitted by the ultrasound probe travels along a straight-line path to and from the transducer.
- The amount of energy reflected is proportional to the difference in acoustic impedance of two media: the larger the impedance mismatch between the media (myocardium-air) the higher the chance that multiple reflections will develop.

SUGGESTED READINGS

Appelbe AF, Walker PG, Yeoh JK, et al. Clinical significance and origin of artifacts in transesophageal echocardiography of the thoracic aorta. *J Am Coll Cardiol.* 1993;21:754–760.

Ballal RS, Nanda NC, Gatewood R, et al. Usefulness of transesophageal echocardiography in assessment of aortic dissection. *Circulation.* 1991;84:1903–1914.

Erbel R, Engberding R, Daniel W, et al. Echocardiography in diagnosis of aortic dissection. *Lancet.* 1989;1:457–461.

Evangelista A, Garcia-del-Castillo H, Gonzalez-Alujas T, et al. Diagnosis of ascending aortic dissection by transesophageal echocardiography: utility of M-Mode in recognizing artifacts. *J Am Coll Cardiol.* 1996;27:102–107.

Feigenbaum H, Armstrong WF, Ryan T, eds. *Feigenbaum's Echocardiography.* 6th ed. Philadelphia: Lippincott Williams & Wilkins; 2005.

Hedrick WR, Peterson CL. Image artifacts in real-time ultrasound. *J Diag Med Sonog.* 1995;11:300–308.

Kremkau FW. *Diagnostic Ultrasound Principles and Instruments.* St. Louis: Saunders Elsevier; 2006.

Losi MA, Betocchi S, Briguori C, et al. Determinants of aortic artifacts during transesophageal echocardiography of the ascending aorta. *Am Heart J.* 1999;137:967–972.

Nienaber CA, Spielmann RP, von Kodolitsch Y, et al. Diagnosis of thoracic aortic dissection: magnetic resonance imaging versus ransesophageal echocardiography. *Circulation.* 1992;992;85:434–447.

Otto CM. *Textbook of Clinical Echocardiography.* Philadelphia: Elsevier Saunders; 2004.

Vignon P, Spencer KT, Rambaud G, et al. Differential transesophageal echocardiographic diagnosis between linear artifacts and intraluminal flap of aortic dissection or disruption. *Chest.* 2001;119:1778–1790.

Weyman AE. *Principles and Practice of Echocardiography.* Lea & Febiger; 1994.

Transthoracic Echocardiography: M-Mode and Two-Dimensional

Gerard P. Aurigemma and Dennis A. Tighe

1. Which leaflets of the tricuspid valve are visualized on the apical four-chamber view?
   A. Septal and anterior.
   B. Septal and posterior.
   C. Anterior and posterior.
   D. None of above.

2. Calculation of left ventricular (LV) mass on the basis of M-mode echocardiography assumes that the geometry of the LV is:
   A. Spherical.
   B. Ellipsoid.
   C. Cylindrical.
   D. None of the above.

3. Which parameter of systolic function is independent of ventricular preload?
   A. Ejection fraction (EF).
   B. Peak rate of change in pressure (dP/dT).
   C. End systolic volume.
   D. Fractional shortening.
   E. Velocity of circumferential fiber shortening (Vcf).

4. In which of the following conditions would auscultation reveal a soft first heart sound?
   A. Mitral stenosis.
   B. Calcific aortic stenosis.
   C. Right bundle branch block.
   D. First degree atrioventricular (AV) block.

5. According to the American Society of Echocardiography's most recent guidelines, chamber dimensions on 2D (two- dimensional) echocardiography should be measured:
   A. Leading edge to leading edge.
   B. Trailing edge to leading edge.
   C. Trailing edge to trailing edge.
   D. None of the above.

6. Which statement concerning quantitation of LV volumes is true?
   A. Echo. LV volumes are usually similar to contrast angiographic volumes.
   B. Echo. LV volumes are usually smaller than contrast angiographic volumes.
   C. Echo. LV volumes are usually greater than contrast angiographic volumes.
   D. Echo. LV volumes are usually much greater than contrast angiographic volumes.

7. In which condition would you expect to see normal motion of the interventricular septum on M-mode?
   A. Right ventricular pacing.
   B. Severe tricuspid regurgitation.
   C. Atrial septal defect.
   D. Aortic valve replacement.
   E. Aortic insufficiency.

8. The biplane method of disks shows an EF of 60% in a 40-year-old woman with palpitations. Systolic strains are also measured using speckle-tracking software. What would be expected values for systolic strains in the longitudinal and radial directions?
   A. 10% and 20%.
   B. 20% and 40%.
   C. 40% and 60%.
   D. None of the above.

9. The American Society of Echocardiography's recommended method to calculate LV EF on the basis of 2D echocardiography is:
   A. Area length.
   B. The truncated ellipse.
   C. Automated boundary detection.
   D. Teichholz method.
   E. Biplane method of disks.

10. The principal determinant of the first component of the pulmonary vein systolic velocity (S1) is:
    A. RV systolic pressure.
    B. Left atrial pressure.
    C. LV systolic function.
    D. Atrial relaxation.

11. Of the following conditions, which is most likely to be characterized by an improvement in LV EF following valve replacement:
    A. Acute severe mitral regurgitation due to flail leaflet.
    B. Chronic severe aortic stenosis.
    C. Severe mitral stenosis.
    D. Acute aortic regurgitation due to bacterial endocarditis.

12. In which condition is LV mass index expected to be lowest?
    A. Mitral stenosis.
    B. Ventriculoseptal defect with a significant left-to-right shunt.
    C. Chronic severe aortic regurgitation.
    D. Chronic severe mitral regurgitation due to mitral valve prolapse.

13. Which of the following is most helpful in preventing foreshortening of the apex in standard 2D imaging:
    A. Placing the transducer at the site of the most forceful apical impulse.
    B. Use of perflutren contrast.
    C. Use of a cut out mattress.
    D. Shifting to a shallow left lateral decubitus position.

14. When comparing 2D with M-mode echocardiography, which of the following statements is true?
    A. The axial resolution of M-mode echocardiography is superior to that of 2D echocardiography.
    B. The temporal resolution of M-mode echocardiography is superior to that of 2D echocardiography.
    C. The axial resolution of M-mode echocardiography is inferior to that of 2D echocardiography.
    D. The lateral resolution of M-mode echocardiography is superior to that of 2D echocardiography.

15. Of the following M-mode signs, which is most specific to suggest the presence of cardiac tamponade?
    A. Right atrial inversion for less than one-third of the cardiac cycle.
    B. Plethora of the inferior vena cava (IVC).
    C. Rapid mitral EF slope.
    D. Right ventricular diastolic collapse.

16. This M-mode echocardiogram was taken from the study of a 48-year-old man with dyspnea (Fig. 3-1). His blood pressure is 120/90 mm Hg. What may be said about this patient's hemodynamic state?

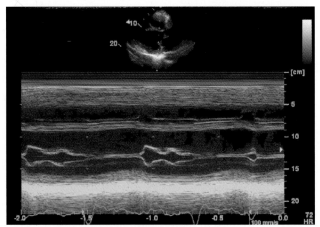

Fig. 3-1

A. There is severe aortic regurgitation.
B. The LV end-diastolic pressure is high.
C. The stroke volume is normal.
D. The stroke volume is low.
E. The cardiac output is normal.

17. A 54-year-old man undergoes echocardiography. He has severe hypertension, refractory to three drugs. He has no history of coronary or valvular heart disease. His septal and posterior wall thickness is 12 mm and his end-diastolic dimension is 44 mm. His LV mass index is 92 g/m². Which statement regarding this patient is most accurate (Fig. 3-2)?

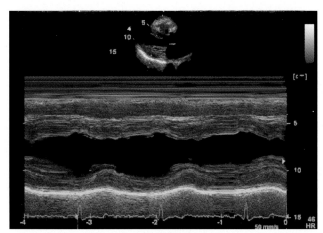

Fig. 3-2

A. He has concentric remodeling.
B. He likely has normal diastolic function.
C. Left ventricular function is likely abnormal.
D. He has LV hypertrophy.

18. The tracings in Figure 3-3A and B are tissue Doppler tracings taken from the study of an asymptomatic 62-year-old woman undergoing echocardiography for the evaluation of a systolic murmur. Which of the following is correct?

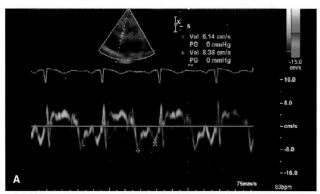

Fig. 3-3A

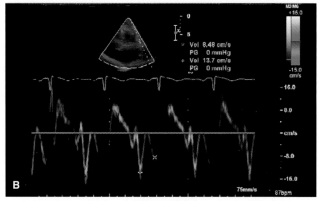

Fig. 3-3B

A. Figure 3-3A is taken from the septal annulus.
B. The patient likely has an infiltrative cardiomyopathy.
C. The patient likely has constrictive pericarditis.

19. A 43-year-old man is seen in your office for exercise-induced dyspnea. He has no history of heart failure symptoms or prior coronary heart disease. On a standard Bruce protocol exercise treadmill test (ETT), he is only able to complete 5 minutes before stopping due to dyspnea. His resting blood pressure is 150/90 mm Hg. His study showed normal LV size, mildly increased wall thickness, and an EF of 50%. As part of his echocardiographic evaluation, longitudinal strain imaging (A) and tissue Doppler imaging (B) are completed. An image from this study is shown in Figure 3-4. What is the least likely conclusion, given the data presented? See Video 3-1.

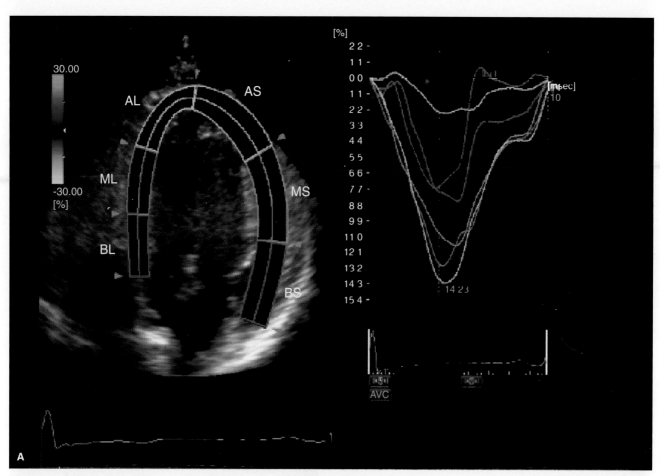

Fig. 3-4A

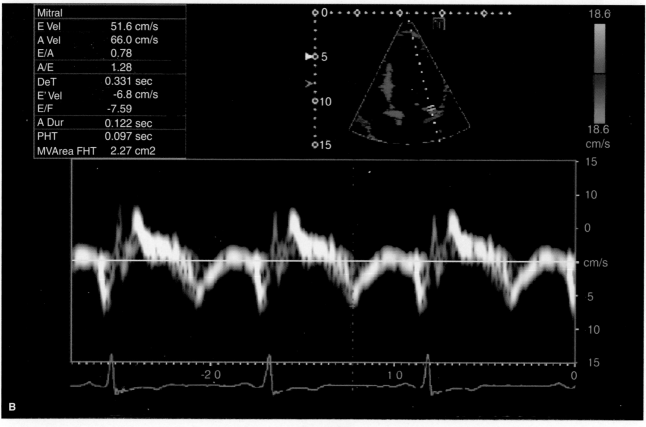

Mitral	
E Vel	51.6 cm/s
A Vel	66.0 cm/s
E/A	0.78
A/E	1.28
DeT	0.331 sec
E' Vel	-6.8 cm/s
E/F	-7.59
A Dur	0.122 sec
PHT	0.097 sec
MVArea FHT	2.27 cm2

Fig. 3-4B

A. He has normal heart.

B. He has hypertrophic cardiomyopathy.

C. He has an infiltrative cardiomyopathy.

D. He has hypertensive heart disease.

20. This M-mode is taken from the study of a 59-year-old man who presents with severe heart failure symptoms (Fig. 3-5). You would expect his exam to show:

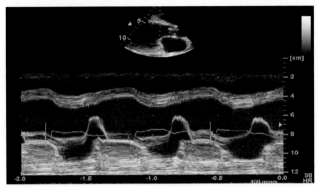

Fig. 3-5

A. An opening snap.

B. Rales.

C. An apical systolic murmur.

D. A holodiastolic murmur.

21. A 56-year-old man presents to the hospital with progressive shortness of breath. Based on the results of the recorded M-mode echocardiogram (Fig. 3-6), the following conclusions can be drawn:

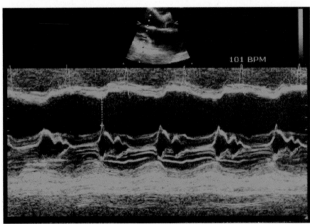

Fig. 3-6

A. The LV cavity size is normal, stroke volume is increased, and LV end-diastolic pressure is normal.

B. The LV cavity is dilated, stroke volume is reduced, and the LV end-diastolic pressure is increased.

C. The LV cavity is dilated, stroke volume is reduced, and LV end-diastolic pressure is normal.

D. The LV cavity size is normal, stroke volume is increased, and mean left atrial pressure is increased.

22. The structures depicted on the RV inflow view in Figure 3-7 include:

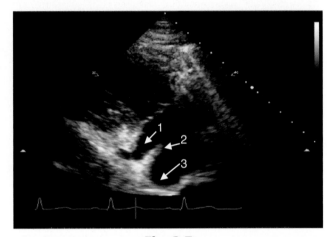

Fig. 3-7

A:
1) The orifice of the IVC.
2) The eustachian valve.
3) The superior vena cava.

B:
1) The coronary sinus.
2) The crista terminalis.
3) The orifice of the superior vena cava.

C:
1) The coronary sinus.
2) The eustachian valve.
3) The orifice of the IVC.

D:
1) The coronary sinus.
2) A prominent Chiari network.
3) The orifice of the IVC.

23. The condition most commonly associated with the M-mode finding in Figure 3-8 is:

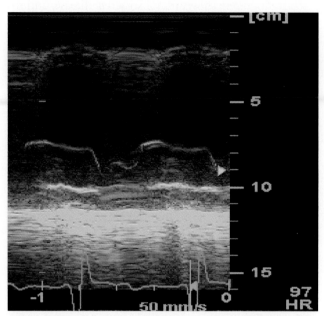

Fig. 3-8

A. Chronic severe pulmonary arterial hypertension.
B. Severe pulmonary valve stenosis.
C. Primary tricuspid valve regurgitation.
D. Acute pulmonary emboli.

24. A 55-year-old woman is admitted to the hospital with syncope. Based on the M-mode shown in Figure 3-9, what is your diagnosis?

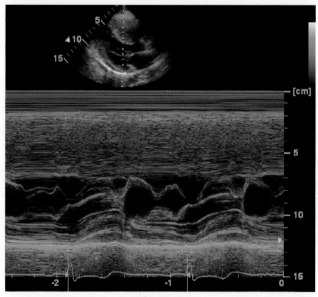

Fig. 3-9

A. Hypertrophic obstructive cardiomyopathy.
B. Acute severe mitral regurgitation due to flail mitral leaflet.
C. Constrictive pericarditis.
D. Aortic regurgitation, unknown severity.

25. The M-mode in Figure 3-10 is most consistent with what abnormality?

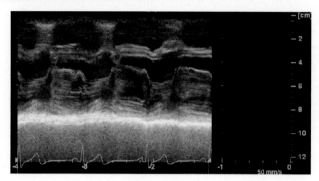

Fig. 3-10

A. Acute severe aortic regurgitation.
B. Rheumatic mitral stenosis.
C. Left atrial myxoma.
D. Hypertrophic cardiomyopathy.

CASE 1:

26. A 30-year-old woman presents for evaluation of shortness of breath. As part of that evaluation, a 2D echocardiogram is requested. A highly mobile echodensity was noted in the right atrium (Video 3-2). Based on this image, the most likely diagnosis is:

A. The moderator band.
B. A mobile thrombus.
C. The eustachian valve.
D. A pacing catheter.
E. A Chiari complex.

CASE 2:

27. A 60-year-old man presents to hospital with 2 weeks of fever and shortness of breath. As part of his diagnostic evaluation, a 2D echocardiogram is obtained. The image in Video 3-3 is representative of the findings on the complete echocardiogram. Based on this image, the following conclusions can be drawn:

A. A vegetation involving the mitral valve is present.
B. A left pleural effusion and pericardial effusion are present.
C. A large pericardial effusion with evidence of tamponade is present.
D. A large left pleural effusion is present.

CASE 3:

A 75-year-old woman undergoes echocardiography for the evaluation of chest pain. Video 3-4 shows a parasternal long axis view.

28. The image shown demonstrates:
    A. Marked left atrial enlargement.
    B. A large thoracic mass.
    C. A dissection involving the descending aorta.
    D. Both a pericardial and pleural effusion.

29. Of the following, the maneuver that would most likely clarify the diagnosis would be:
    A. Ingestion of a carbonated beverage.
    B. Injection of agitated saline contrast through the left antecubital vein.
    C. Administration of a perflutren contrast agent.
    D. Valsalva maneuver.

CASE 4:

A 73-year-old woman develops profound dyspnea and chest pressure after an emotional encounter with her parish priest. She has a history of hypertension and depression but is otherwise well. The history is negative for prior symptoms of coronary artery disease and there is no history of any cardiovascular disease beyond the hypertension.

The initial electrocardiogram, obtained within 1 hour of the development of symptoms, is interpreted as normal. Initial biomarkers determinations are likewise normal. See Videos 3-5 A, B, and C.

Troponin I at 6 hours, however, is abnormal and continues to rise, whereas the creatine phosphokinase (CPK) remains within the normal range, with positive myocardial band (MB) determination.

30. Based on the data you have, the most likely diagnosis is:
    A. An acute left anterior descending artery (LAD) territory infarction.
    B. Apical hypertrophic cardiomyopathy.
    C. Stress cardiomyopathy.
    D. None of the above.

31. The patient continues to have symptoms and is taken to the catheterization suite, where the ventriculogram in Video 3-6 is obtained. Coronary arteriography shows nonobstructive disease, and the filling pressures are at the upper limits of normal. The patient remains symptomatic. The evening of admission, approximately 12 hours after presentation and 4 hours after the catheterization is completed, she is noted to be severely hypotensive, with systolic pressure in the 70 to 80 mm Hg range. See Video 3-6 and Figure 3-11.

Likely explanations for hypotension in this case include:

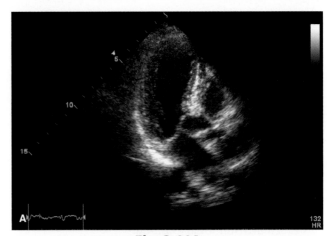

Fig. 3-11A

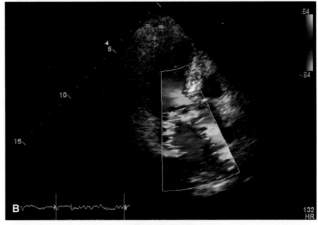

Fig. 3-11B

A. Myocardial rupture.
B. Mitral regurgitation due to papillary muscle dysfunction.
C. LV outflow tract obstruction.
D. Ventriculoseptal rupture.

CASE 5:

A 46-year-old man is seen by you to evaluate dyspnea on exertion. He complains of being "winded" easily and notes that these symptoms have progressed over the past few months. Nevertheless, he belongs to a local gym and is able to exercise on various "cardio" machines, such as the treadmill and stationary bicycle, for 1 hour. He also lifts weights. He denies recreational drug use, drinks 2–5 beers per week, and takes no supplements.

He has a history of hypertension and is being treated with amlodipine and hydrochlorothiazide; treatment with an angiotensin-converting enzyme inhibitor was unsuccessful, and he was unable to tolerate β-blocker therapy. His blood pressure is 150/100 mm Hg. His physical examination shows nonpitting edema of both ankles, the aforementioned hypertension, but is otherwise unremarkable. See Videos 3-7 A, B, and C.

You interpret the echo as showing left ventricular hypertrophy (LVH), no significant valvular heart disease. Biplane method of disks shows an end-diastolic volume of 200 cm^3 and an end-diastolic volume of 120 cm^3.

32. How would you report the LV function?
    A. Normal EF.
    B. Low normal EF.
    C. Reduced EF.

33. Longitudinal strain is performed and is shown in Video 3-8. Do these data support your conclusion from question 32?
    A. Support.
    B. Do not support.

34. Tissue Doppler tracings obtained from the septal (Fig. 3-12A) and lateral (Fig. 3-12B) annulus. Given these data and the 2D echocardiographic data already shown, of the following choices, which is the least likely diagnosis for the LV structure and functional findings?

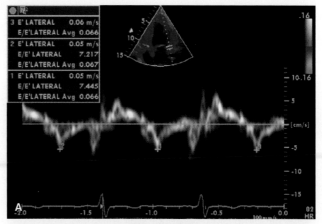

Fig. 3-12A

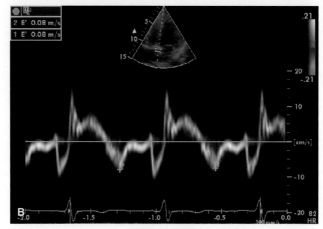

Fig. 3-12B

A. Hypertrophic cardiomyopathy.
B. Athletic heart syndrome.
C. Cardiac sarcoidosis.
D. Coronary artery disease.

ANSWERS

1. ANSWER: A. On transthoracic imaging, the posterior leaflet of the tricuspid valve is only visualized on the RV inflow view. The septal and anterior leaflets are visualized on the apical four-chamber view.

2. ANSWER: B. LV mass and LV volume measurements from M-mode and 2D echo are based on the geometric assumptions that the ventricle is an ellipsoid with a 2:1 long-axis to short-axis ratio. The mass formula, LV mass $(g) = 0.8 (1.04 [(LVIDd + PWTd + SWTd)^3 − LVIDd^3]) + 0.6$ (where LVIDd, PWTd, and SWTd are diastolic LV internal dimension, posterior wall thickness, and septal thickness, respectively) calculates the volumes of an inner and outer ellipsoid and subtracts the inner volume from the outer volume. The resulting volume is that of a "shell" of myocardium. The volume of this shell of myocardium is then multiplied by the specific gravity of myocardium, $1.04 g/m^2$, to yield LV mass. This geometric assumption limits the applicability of the formula to normally shaped hearts.

3. ANSWER: C. Virtually all parameters of systolic function (EF, dP/dT, fractional shortening, and Vcf shortening) depend on loading conditions. Preload is the force that acts to stretch the myocardial fibers at end diastole, and is related to end-diastolic volume. By Starling's law of the heart, increased preload will be associated with increased fiber stretch and increased force of contraction. Afterload is the force that opposes LV ejection.

End-systolic volume is also a parameter of systolic function. A related concept is that at any given contractile state, the LV will contract to the same end-systolic volume even as the LV diastolic volume increases.

4. ANSWER: D. The degree to which the mitral valve leaflets are separated when ventricular activation closes the mitral valve is an important determinant of the loudness of the mitral component of the S1. Accordingly, in a patient with a long PR interval (choice D), the mitral and tricuspid leaflets float into a semi-closed position because of the long period between atrial contraction and ventricular activation. Mitral stenosis is characterized by a loud first sound, if the leaflets are pliable, because the transmitral gradient at end diastole prevents the leaflets from drifting close together. Calcific aortic stenosis (by itself) or right bundle branch block do not have much of an impact on the loudness of the S1.

5. ANSWER: D. According to the most recent echocardiographic quantification guidelines, "Use of 2D echocardiographically derived linear dimensions overcomes the common problem of oblique parasternal images resulting in overestimation of cavity and wall dimensions from M-mode. Consequently, it is now possible to measure the actual visualized thickness of the ventricular septum and other chamber dimensions as defined by the actual tissue–blood interface, rather than the distance between the leading edge echoes, which had previously been recommended."

6. ANSWER: B. Numerous comparison studies have shown that LV volumes derived from echocardiography are systematically smaller than those derived from contrast angiography. The two reasons for this discrepancy are that echocardiographic algorithms that utilize apical views (e.g. biplane method of disks) underestimate the true length of the LV, when compared with angiography; and second, angiographic contrast fills the recesses between trabeculations, yielding a larger area.

7. ANSWER: E. The interventricular septum normally moves posterior (leftward) in early ventricular systole. Paradoxical septal motion is an early systolic anterior (rightward) motion of the septum. Thickening of the septum still occurs. Paradoxical septal motion is associated with conditions in which there is RV volume overload, or left bundle branch block, either developed or due to RV pacing. After aortic valve replacement, or indeed any cardiac surgery, there is prominent translation of the heart that can give the appearance of paradoxical septal motion. Aortic insufficiency, a situation in which there is LV volume overload, would not be expected to be associated with paradoxical septal motion and is, therefore, the correct answer.

8. ANSWER: B. Left ventricular systolic function involves the coordinated contraction of longitudinal and circumferential fibers. In the normal LV, subendocardial and subepicardial fibers are oriented longitudinally. In the midwall, fibers are oriented circumferentially. Descriptors of systolic function include the percentage shortening of the LV along the long-axis (apex-to-base) orientation. This percentage shortening of the long axis in normal patients ranges from 15%–25%. This percent longitudinal shortening is also known as longitudinal strain. This means that if the LV is 10 cm in length at end diastole, its end-systolic length would be about 8 cm. The "compression" or "shortening" of the length is 2 cm and as a percentage of initial length, it would be 20%. This in essence is longitudinal systolic strain.

Circumferential fiber shortening leads to wall thickening and reduction of the radius of the LV. This wall thickening, in the normal ventricle, averages approximately 30% to 40%, and is known as radial strain, the percent change in the thickness of the ventricular wall going from end diastole to end systole. As an example, a normal LV wall might have a wall thickness of 1.0 cm in diastole and, if the wall thickens 40%, a wall thickness of 1.4 cm at end systole.

9. ANSWER: E. Numerous 2D echocardiographic methods have been utilized to assess EF. Limitations for each method should be expected because all of these methods are based on geometric assumptions. Using apical longitudinal views, the modified Simpson's method, also known as the biplane method of disks, has been endorsed by the American Society of Echocardiography to calculate EF on the basis of 2D echocardiography in most instances.

10. ANSWER: D. Many variables affect pulmonary vein flow. These include age, preload, LV systolic function, AV conduction, and heart rate. In patients with normal systolic function, S2 velocity is related to LA pressure. By contrast, S1 is more closely related to atrial relaxation.

11. ANSWER: B. This question requires some understanding of LV function in valvular heart disease. LV EF is inversely related to afterload and directly related to preload and inotropic state. Afterload, or wall stress, is directly related to systolic pressure and heart size, and inversely related to wall thickness. In acute severe regurgitation of either mitral or aortic valve, catecholamine tone is high, which supports the pump function despite severe regurgitation. Thus, of the following choices, chronic severe aortic stenosis (AS) is the most likely condition to have high afterload; in mitral stenosis, afterload is low, as is the case in acute mitral regurgitation (MR), where the LV ejects into the "low impedance" left atrium. In both acute severe MR and AR, catecholamine tone is likely to be high and EF is often normal if not above normal. Thus, LV EF in the latter two conditions would not be expected to rise significantly. Furthermore, LV EF would not be expected to decrease significantly after mitral valve replacement (MVR) for mitral stenosis (MS), as the afterload in that condition is usually normal. By contrast, in severe AS, systolic loads are often quite high, due to very high intracavitary pressures and, in later stages, cavity dilation. Hypertrophy may be inadequate to normalize afterload. However, following aortic valve replacement (AVR), systolic pressure comes down, heart size usually decreases (if there is dilation), and these factors lead to lower afterload and improved EF.

12. ANSWER: A. Choices B–D will feature LV dilation, but choice A does not. Since the LV mass formula (see question 2) depends on chamber size, a large LV will usually be associated with a large LV mass index.

13. ANSWER: C. In general, foreshortening of the apex will be minimized by use of a steep left lateral decubitus position, a cut out mattress, and avoiding the most forceful apical impulse.

14. ANSWER: B. The high temporal resolution of M-mode echocardiography is due to the fact that this technique has a much higher sampling rate compared with 2D echocardiography. For both techniques, the axial resolution is similar because the same transducer frequency is used. Lateral resolution is superior with 2D echocardiography because sampling occurs only along a single scan line with the M-mode technique.

15. ANSWER: D. Right atrial inversion and plethora of the IVC are sensitive signs suggesting increased intraperi-

cardial pressures but they are not the most specific signs suggesting cardiac tamponade. When right atrial inversion extends for more than one-third of the cardiac cycle, the reported specificity is high. Plethora of the IVC is a nonspecific marker associated with increased right atrial pressures; plethora can be observed even when the right atrial pressure is not increased as is seen with certain highly trained athletes. With inspiration, the mitral EF slope has been observed to diminish and, thus, is not rapid in the presence of cardiac tamponade. Of the choices available, right ventricular diastolic collapse is the most specific sign of cardiac tamponade.

16. ANSWER: D. This study was obtained in a patient with an idiopathic dilated cardiomyopathy. The M-mode echocardiogram shows marked dilation, with an end-diastolic dimension approaching 6 cm, and an end-systolic dimension of 5.5 cm. The fractional shortening is therefore quite low. There is a large separation between the anterior leaflet of the mitral valve and the septum (the "e-point septal separation," because the peak anterior position of the anterior leaflet is known as the e point in M-mode parlance). This sign is associated with a low forward stroke volume. It is important to realize that LV dilation by itself does not lead to an abnormal e-point septal separation. An individual with severe aortic regurgitation might have a dilated LV but normal fractional shortening. In that case, the e-point septal separation would be normal.

As for the incorrect choices, while this patient might have high left ventricular end diastolic pressure (LVEDP), there is no definite evidence thereof. The pathognomonic M-mode sign of this physiology, the so-called a-c shoulder or b-bump is not present. (Figure 3-13 shows a prominent b-bump.)

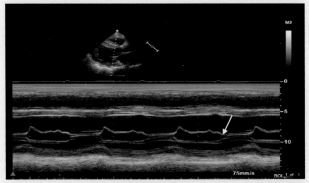

Fig. 3-13

As far as cardiac output is concerned, recall that it can be normal despite a low stroke volume, if there is compensatory tachycardia. Finally, the etiology of the LV dysfunction shown in this case could have been chronic aortic regurgitation, with the development of contractile failure, but this M-mode tracing is not specific for such a cardiomyopathy. The lack of fluttering of the mitral leaflets provides some evidence against significant aortic regurgitation.

17. ANSWER: A. This patient's LV mass index is normal, by the partition values in the ASE quantitation guidelines, so he does not have LV hypertrophy, by definition. According to the pioneering work of Ganau et al., and as recommended by the ASE quantitation guidelines, the combination of a high relative wall thickness with a normal LV mass index is termed concentric remodeling. This individual clearly has an elevated relative wall thickness, defined as (2 × PWTd)/LVIDd with the upper limit of normal 0.42. The term concentric hypertrophy refers to an elevated LV mass index (i.e., 95 g/M^2 in women, greater than 115 g/M^2 in men) and a high relative wall thickness.

According to work by Wachtell and coworkers, most individuals with hypertension and evidence of remodeling, as the case with this individual, have abnormalities in diastolic filling.

The M-mode clearly shows normal fractional shortening; although this is not necessarily the same as a normal EF. The absence of coronary heart disease by history argues that global EF is normal.

18. ANSWER: A. Tissue Doppler tracings give insight into systolic and diastolic function and can be used to estimate LV filling pressures in many instances. Some basic facts about tissue Doppler imaging tracings are that the septal annulus diastolic velocity is less than the lateral annulus velocity in the absence of coronary heart disease/myocardial infarction. A notable exception to this generalization is constrictive pericarditis (annulus paradoxus).

There are data concerning normal values for tissue Doppler diastolic velocities, which vary inversely with age; according to data from Tighe et al., the mean tissue Doppler E, obtained from the lateral annulus, in normal individuals aged 60–70 years is 12 ± 3 cm/sec. At the age of 62 years, the velocity shown (13.7 cm/sec) is within the expected range.

19. ANSWER: A. These data show significant systolic and diastolic dysfunction in this patient with symptoms of exertional dyspnea. The strain image demonstrates longitudinal strain. Longitudinal strain can be thought of as the degree of compression of 6 segments of myocardium along the long axis. Normal data from our laboratory indicate that longitudinal strain averages 22% ± 3%. There is regional variation in strain values, with higher values seen in the apical segments. In this example, however, the highest strain values are approximately 14%, which are low and indicative of systolic dysfunction. The values demonstrate the usual apex-to-base gradient, though the values are consistently lower than normal. In addition, what secures the diagnosis of abnormal LV function is the tissue Doppler diastolic findings. The average diastolic velocities for a 43-year-old normal individual should be in the range of 16 ± 4 cm/sec, more than twice as high as what is shown. Thus, the systolic and diastolic data shown indicate abnormalities of systolic and diastolic function. Given that there are no focal wall motion abnormalities, one must suspect a global process, such as infiltrative cardiomyopathy (e.g., amyloidosis), hypertrophic cardiomyopathy, or severe hypertensive heart disease, where some of the dysfunction may be related to high afterload.

20. ANSWER: D. The M-mode shows a classic example of early mitral valve closure which is pathognomonic of acute severe AR. There is also LV dilation and a generous e-point septal separation. The early closure of the mitral valve is caused by the rapid equilibration of LV diastolic pressure and aortic diastolic pressure. Patients with acute severe aortic regurgitation are likely to have evidence of elevated filling pressure and rales. An opening snap is heard in patients with rheumatic mitral stenosis with pliable leaflets. This is not the echocardiogram of such a patient. An apical systolic murmur implies mitral regurgitation and there is no suggestion that this patient has coexisting MR.

21. ANSWER: B. This 56-year-old man presented with symptoms and signs of heart failure. This M-mode echocardiogram is recorded through the mitral leaflet tips (Fig. 3-14). This recording shows significantly increased LV cavitary dimensions in systole and diastole (stippled arrows), a significantly increased e-point septal separation distance (stippled lines), and interrupted AC closure of the mitral valve echo. The findings of this M-mode echocardiogram suggest that very poor systolic performance is present. The LV cavity is dilated and the LV EF is severely reduced. Stroke volume is severely reduced as indicated by the increased e-point septal separation distance (normal <7 mm). The LV end-diastolic pressure is elevated as indicated by the presence of the interrupted AC closure or "b-bump." The mean left atrial pressure, although likely elevated, cannot be derived from the information presented.

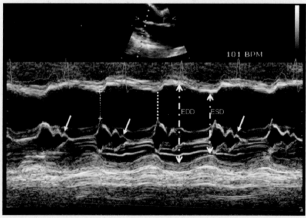

Fig. 3-14

22. ANSWER: C. The right ventricular inflow view in Figure 3-15 illustrates the origin of the coronary sinus in the posterior septal space adjacent to the tricuspid valve leaflet. The eustachian valve, also known as the right sinus valve or the valve of the IVC, is somewhat prominent in this example. Adjacent to the eustachian valve is the orifice of the IVC. Also well illustrated in this view are the posterior and anterior leaflets of the tricuspid valve (small stippled arrows). A Chiari complex is derived embryologically from the same structures as the eustachian valve; however, it would appear as a highly mobile thin filamentous structure. The orifice of the superior vena cava cannot normally be seen in this tomographic imaging plane.

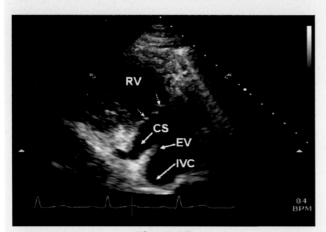

Fig. 3-15

23. ANSWER: A. This M-mode recording of the pulmonary valve illustrates the "flying-W sign" (Fig. 3-16). The normal pulmonary valve M-mode is characterized by presystolic a-wave with motion away from the transducer followed by further posterior motion of the valve leaflet during systole. With chronic severe pulmonary hypertension, a characteristic appearance to the M-mode tracing, termed "the flying-W sign," may be generated. This tracing is characterized by the loss of the a-wave (solid arrow) and mid-systolic notching (stippled arrow). With pulmonary valve stenosis, the a-wave is characteristically preserved, or even accentuated, and mid-systolic notching is not observed. In a pure right heart volume load state, such as occurs with primary tricuspid regurgitation, one would not expect pulmonary hypertension to be present and thus the pulmonary valve M-mode tracing should not be altered significantly. Among patients with acute pulmonary embolism, the level of elevation of the pulmonary artery pressure does not usually exceed 50 mm Hg and thus the M-mode findings of chronic severe pulmonary arterial hypertension would not be expected to be observed.

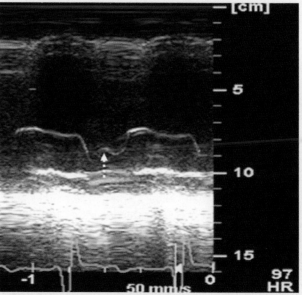

Fig. 3-16

24. ANSWER: A. This M-mode shows evidence of systolic anterior motion of the mitral valve, a sign that is pathognomonic for hypertrophic obstructive cardiomyopathy (Fig. 3-17). Recent work has shown that 70% of patients with hypertrophic cardiomyopathy have obstruction either at rest or provoked by exercise. In hypertrophic obstructive cardiomyopathy, there is hyperdynamic systolic function, with low levels of wall stress; the LV outflow tract is narrowed by septal hypertrophy and, in some patients, by anterior displacement of the mitral valve. The posterior systolic motion of the interventricular septum further narrows the LV outflow tract; this results in high LV outflow tract blood velocities, which pull the mitral valve leaflet toward the interventricular septum (Venturi effect). The arrow points to systolic anterior motion of the mitral valve with septal–mitral contact (see Video 3-9).

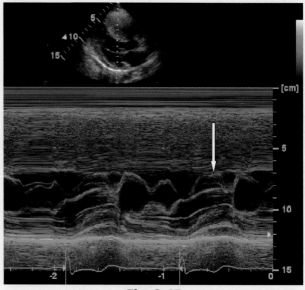

Fig. 3-17

25. ANSWER: C. This M-mode recording illustrates a classic case of a left atrial myxoma prolapsing into the mitral orifice with valve opening (Fig. 3-10, shown in real time on the accompanying Video 3-10). The tumor (Myx) appears as a mass of echoes behind the mitral valve during diastole. Note the echo free space behind the anterior leaflet at the onset of diastole (thin arrows). This occurs because a time lag exists between the early diastolic opening of the valve and when the tumor mass subsequently moves into the mitral orifice. Although the mitral EF slope is diminished significantly (thick white arrow), this recording is not consistent with rheumatic mitral stenosis. The mitral leaflets are not thickened and the posterior leaflet moves normally (black arrow). Findings consistent with the presence of acute severe aortic insufficiency, such as high-frequency diastolic fluttering of the mitral valve or, possibly, the interventricular septum (depending upon jet direction) and premature mitral valve closure, are not demonstrated. With hypertrophic obstructive cardiomyopathy, increased thickness of the interventricular septum and systolic anterior motion of the mitral apparatus would be expected; these findings are not demonstrated on this M-mode recording (Fig. 3-18).

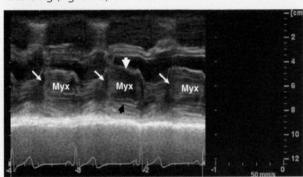

Fig. 3-18

26. ANSWER: E. This ultrasound exhibits normal biventricular size and function. The structure in question is a filamentous thin mobile structure in the right atrium extending from the area of the eustachian valve toward the interatrial septum. This finding is most consistent with the presence of a Chiari complex, a remnant of the right venous valve. The appearance here is quite typical in that this filamentous structure has an undulating appearance when viewed in real time. The moderator band is a structure noted within the right ventricle. The eustachian valve would appear as a more solid, protuberant, and nonmobile structure arising along the posterior margin of the IVC and coronary sinus. A pacing catheter would also present as a linear structure traversing the cavity of the right atrium. However, it would not be expected to appear as mobile nor be filamentous in nature as the structure demonstrated in this example. An intracavitary thrombus may appear as a mobile structure within the right atrium. Most often, however, right atrial thrombus has a multilobulated appearance and exhibits a worm-

like shape often reflecting its origin from the deep veins. Some authors have described such a thrombus as having "popcorn" appearance. The thin, filamentous, and mobile nature of this structure and its typical anatomical location make a thrombus very unlikely in this situation.

KEY POINTS:
- One should be familiar with normal anatomic variants in the right atrium.
- Chiari network is a thin, filamentous structure in the right atrium.

27. ANSWER: B. This patient with fever and shortness of breath has both a large left pleural effusion and a small-to-moderate sized pericardial effusion. No evidence of right ventricular diastolic collapse or left atrial collapse is noted to suggest the diagnosis of a pericardial effusion under significant pressure. The limited images of the mitral valve do not show a mobile or oscillating echodensity that would be diagnostic of vegetation involving the mitral valve. While a large left pleural effusion is present, the most precise answer also should describe the presence of the pericardial effusion. In Panel A, the pericardial effusion (Pericard Eff) and pleural effusion (PL Eff) are illustrated. As shown in this still frame, the descending thoracic aorta (*) serves as a useful marker to help differentiate left pleural effusions from pericardial effusions. Typically pleural effusions lie posterior to the descending thoracic aorta while pericardial effusions lie in a more anterior location. In this example the pericardial reflection is well visualized (black arrow) and helps to clearly differentiate

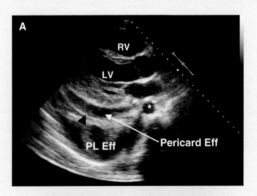

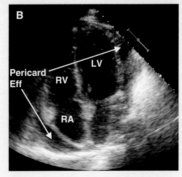

the pleural from pericardial spaces. In panel B, pericardial effusion (Pericard Eff) adjacent to the lateral borders of the right atrium (RA) and left ventricle (LV) is visualized (arrows). No evidence for right heart compression is evident. RV, right ventricle.

KEY POINTS:

■ Pleural and pericardial effusion often coexist.

■ The descending aorta demarcates pericardial from pleural fluid collections.

28 and 29. ANSWERS: B and A. In Fig. 3-19A, the echocardiogram shows that the patient has a large hiatal hernia. The accompanying CT scan in Fig. 3-19B demonstrates a hiatal hernia (large white arrow) that is clearly encroaching on the left atrium (smaller white arrow). Hiatal hernias are commonly encountered in clinical echocardiography and are seen as cystic masses. These masses may be mistaken for an atrial space-occupying structure. With transthoracic echocardiography, the administration of a carbonated beverage can produce a contrast effect within the hiatal hernia and can be used as a diagnostic maneuver to demonstrate its true nature as a pseudomass. Although perflutren contrast would certainly demonstrate whether this structure is cardiac or vascular, it would not be as likely to unambiguously make the diagnosis. Agitated saline injected through the left antecubital vein is useful for many indications, including helping to diagnosis an anomalous left superior vena cava draining into the coronary sinus. In general, the structure shown is too large to be a dilated coronary sinus. Finally, a Valsalva maneuver might be helpful in the diagnosis of a hiatal hernia, in that it might provoke a "disparate degree of encroachment on the left atrium attributable to respiratory motion." However, ingestion of a carbonated beverage would likely make the diagnosis clearer.

KEY POINTS:

■ A carbonated beverage can help with the diagnosis of a hiatal hernia by showing contrast in this mediastinal structure.

■ Hiatal hernia is a benign condition which can masquerade as a mass compressing the LA.

30. ANSWER: C. This patient's syndrome is consistent with the syndrome of stress cardiomyopathy, apical variety. Thanks to the widespread availability of echocardiography, this is a syndrome that is now widely recognized. The initial reports of this syndrome came from Japanese investigators, who have given it the name "takotsubo" because the shape of the ventricle in systole is reminiscent of an octopus trap, with a narrow neck and wide bottom. Biomarker release is different than acute myocardial infarction (MI), with peak CPK determinations much lower, and it can even be normal. Resolution of the wall motion abnormality can be seen as early as 48 hours following symptom onset.

At present, stress cardiomyopathy is a clinical diagnosis, even one of exclusion, in patients presenting with a chest pain syndrome. Criteria have been published by Tsuchihashi et al. These include chest symptoms or electrocardiographic changes suggestive of acute myocardial infarction, reversible apical dysfunction demonstrated by ventriculography, and absence of significant coronary artery narrowing on coronary arteriography performed within 48 hours of symptom onset.

More recently, investigators in western countries, including the United States, have described an identical clinical syndrome. The typical patient is a woman in the seventh decade who experiences chest symptoms triggered by, or in association with, severe emotional distress or a medical procedure. At initial presentation, transient

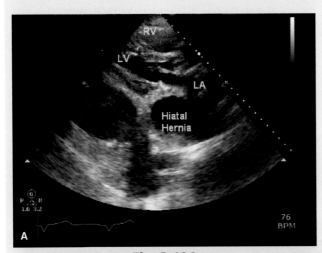

Fig. 3-19A

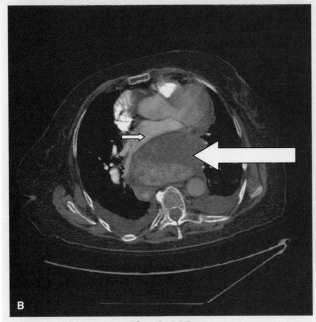

Fig. 3-19B

apical ballooning is difficult, if not impossible to distinguish from acute LAD territory MI. The extent of wall motion abnormality on echocardiography, in our experience, tends to exceed that seen in LAD territory infarction, in that the akinetic areas tend to involve more than one coronary perfusion territory; this has been confirmed by more recent series. However, the diagnosis is made by the return of function.

The ubiquity of emotional stress or preceding medical illness (often a respiratory crisis) is suggestive of catecholamine toxicity. The distribution of wall motion abnormalities far exceeds the usual territory of the LAD coronary artery because it involves so much of the inferior wall. Nevertheless, a cardiac catheterization should still be strongly considered to exclude CAD.

There is really no significant evidence for apical hypertrophic cardiomyopathy. In apical hypertrophic cardiomyopathy, there is significant hypertrophy confined to the apex of the LV.

31. ANSWER: C. This patient has developed LV outflow tract (LVOT) obstruction with significant mitral regurgitation as shown in Figure 3-11 and Video 3-6. Figure 3-20A highlights systolic anterior motion of the mitral valve in this systolic frame. Figure 3-20B demonstrates turbulent LVOT flow as well as MR.

It is likely that the hyperdynamic function at the base of the heart, along with unfavorable geometry in this region, has led to conditions which promote obstruction. The mechanism is similar to what is observed in hypertrophic cardiomyopathy or even in individuals with large LAD territory MI.

KEY POINTS:
- Stress cardiomyopathy is in the differential diagnosis of patients presenting with echocardiographic findings of an acute LAD territory MI.
- Stress cardiomyopathy can be complicated by LVOT obstruction.

32. ANSWER: C. The calculated EF would be 40%, (200–120)/200 × 100%. This would place this EF in the reduced or abnormal range.

33. ANSWER: A. The strain values are low, which implies systolic dysfunction in the longitudinal plane.

34. ANSWER: B. To summarize, the data demonstrate a reduced EF, without significant focal wall motion abnormalities or focal areas of necrosis. The tissue Doppler e' is low for an individual of this age group. The data shown point to a diffuse myopathic disease and point away from the diagnosis of athletic hypertrophy. This is because, while global function (e.g., EF) may be reduced in athletes, it is highly unlikely that tissue Doppler velocities would be low. Cardiac sarcoidosis is unlikely because this tends to create focal wall motion abnormalities because of focal infiltration and inflammation. Finally, ischemic heart disease is possible but would tend to be associated with focal wall motion abnormalities, as opposed to more global dysfunction.

It can be challenging to distinguish hypertrophic cardiomyopathy from secondary causes of hypertrophy, the most commonly encountered of which, of course, is

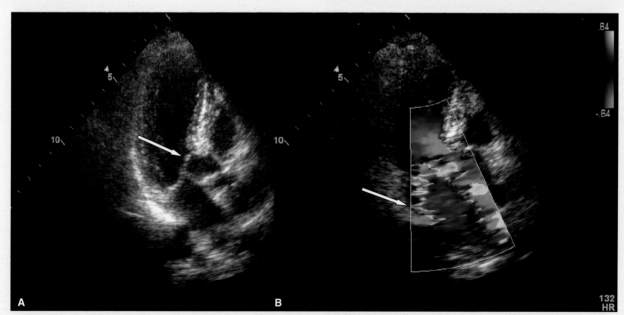

Fig. 3-20A-B

hypertension. However, given the patient's history, coronary artery disease is the more likely of the two, statistically.

This patient underwent an extensive evaluation which included cardiac MR and coronary arteriography. The arteriography showed no evidence of obstructive CAD and the MR showed patchy late enhancement using gadolinium. The calculated volumetric EF was 42%. Subsequent myocardial biopsy was interpreted as showing evidence of hypertensive heart disease.

KEY POINTS:

- Tissue Doppler can help detect subtle abnormalities in function, which give clues to a diffuse myopathic process.
- Speckle tracking values for normal individuals have been established.

SUGGESTED READINGS

D'Cruz IA, Hancock HL. Echocardiographic characteristics of diaphragmatic hiatus hernia. *Am J Cardiol.* 1995;75:308–310.

Dec GW. Recognition of the apical ballooning syndrome in the United States. *Circulation.* 2005;111:388–390.

Ganau A, Devereux RB, Roman MJ, et al. Patterns of left ventricular hypertrophy and geometric remodeling in essential hypertension. *J Am Coll Cardiol.* 1992;19:1550–1558.

Hurlburt HM, Aurigemma GP, Hill JC, et al. Direct ultrasound measurement of longitudinal, circumferential and radial strain using 2-dimensional strain imaging in normal adults. *Echocardiography.* 2007;24:723–731.

Koskinas K, Oikonomou K, Karapatsoudi E, et al. Echocardiographic manifestation of hiatus hernia simulating a left atrial mass: case report. *Cardiovasc Ultrasound.* 2008;6:46.

Lang RM, Bierig M, Devereux RB, et al. Chamber Quantification Writing Group; American Society of Echocardiography's Guidelines and Standards Committee; European Association of Echocardiography. Recommendations for chamber quantification: a report from the American Society of Echocardiography's Guidelines and Standards Committee and the Chamber Quantification Writing Group, developed in conjunction with the European Association of Echocardiography, a branch of the European Society of Cardiology. *J Am Soc Echocardiogr.* 2005;18:1440–1463.

Maron MS, Olivotto I, Zenovich AG, et al. Hypertrophic cardiomyopathy is predominantly a disease of left ventricular outflow tract obstruction. *Circulation.* 2006;114:2232–2239.

Narayanan A, Aurigemma G, Chinali M, et al. Cardiac mechanics in mild hypertensive heart disease: a speckle-strain imaging study. *Cir Cardiovasc Imaging* 2009;2:382–390.

Seth PS, Aurigemma GP, Krasnow JM, et al. A syndrome of transient left ventricular apical wall motion abnormality in the absence of coronary disease: a perspective from the United States. *Cardiology.* 2003;100:61–66.

Sharkey SW, Lesser JR, Zenovich AG, et al. Acute and reversible cardiomyopathy provoked by stress in women from the United States. *Circulation.* 2005;111:472–479.

Tabata T, Thomas JD, Klein AL. Pulmonary venous flow by Doppler echocardiography: revisited 12 years later. *J Am Coll Cardiol.* 2003;41:1243–1250.

Tighe DA, Vinch CS, Hill JC, et al. Influence of age on assessment of diastolic function by Doppler tissue imaging. *Am J Cardiol.* 2003; 91:254–257.

Tsuchihashi K, Ueshima K, Uchida T, et al. Transient left ventricular apical ballooning without coronary artery stenosis: a novel heart syndrome mimicking acute myocardial infarction. Angina Pectoris-Myocardial Infarction Investigations in Japan. *J Am Coll Cardiol.* 2001;38:11–18.

Wachtell K, Smith G, Gerdts E, et al. Left ventricular filling patterns in patients with systemic hypertension and left ventricular hypertrophy (the LIFE study). Losartan intervention for endpoint. *Am J Cardiol.* 2000;85:466–472.

Wittstein IS, Thiemann DR, Lima JA, et al. Neurohumoral features of myocardial stunning due to sudden emotional stress. *N Engl J Med.* 2005;352:539–548.

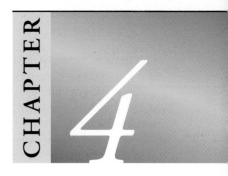

Three-dimensional Echocardiography

Lissa Sugeng, Sonal Chandra, and Lynn Weinert

1. Early efforts in three-dimensional (3D) imaging required a series of two-dimensional (2D) images. Which method(s) use this approach?
   A. Sparse matrix array.
   B. Fully sampled matrix array.
   C. Freehand and mechanically driven scanning.
   D. Phased array.
   E. Pyramidal array.

2. Which factors affect the quality of 3D reconstructions derived from 2D images?
   A. 2D image quality, motion artifact, and electrocardiogram (ECG) and respiratory gating.
   B. 2D image quality.
   C. Image density.
   D. ECG and respiratory gating.
   E. Image density, gain, persistence, and frame rate.

3. Which of the following is currently utilized in 3D imaging?
   A. Sparse matrix array transducer and ECG and respiratory gating.
   B. Sparse matrix array transducer and ECG gating.
   C. Fully sampled matrix array transducer and ECG and respiratory gating.
   D. Fully sampled matrix array transducer, ECG gating, and a breath hold.
   E. B. and C.

4. Assessment of left ventricular (LV) function is pivotal in clinical decision making. Which of the following imaging modes should be used to obtain a 3D volume data set for assessment of LV volume and function?
   A. Live 3D mode (narrow-angled acquisition).
   B. 3D zoom mode.
   C. Full-volume mode (wide-angled acquisition).
   D. Biplane imaging mode.
   E. Triplane imaging mode.

5. Which of the following statements is true regarding the accuracy and reproducibility of 2D echocardiography (2DE) versus 3D echocardiography (3DE) in regard to assessment of LV volumes?
   A. 3DE has superior accuracy and reproducibility compared with 2DE.
   B. 2DE has better accuracy and reproducibility compared with 3DE.
   C. Both 2DE and 3DE have similar accuracy and reproducibility.
   D. Both 2DE and 3DE have similar accuracy and but differ in reproducibility.
   E. All of the above are incorrect.

6. What is the primary reason influencing the difference in accuracy observed between 2DE and 3DE?
   A. Image quality is better with 3DE.
   B. Frame rate is higher with 3DE.
   C. Quantitative methods used result in improved accuracy with 3DE.
   D. Less artifacts with 3DE.
   E. Ability to obtain a true long-axis in a 3D volume data set.

7. Left atrial volume reflects the long-term effects of high left atrial pressure, severity of diastolic dysfunction, and is a predictor of mortality and outcome. Which quantitative method has the best test-retest variability?
   A. M-mode echocardiography.
   B. Prolate ellipsoid.
   C. Biplane Simpson's.
   D. Area-length method.
   E. 3DE.

8. Which statement pertaining to 3D assessment of the right ventricle (RV) is correct?
   A. Quantitation of RV function by 3DE is an online program using method of discs.
   B. Quantitation of RV volumes is accurate and reproducible using method of discs.
   C. Quantitation of RV volumes is a widespread application since it is most accurate and reproducible.
   D. Quantitation of RV volumes involves geometric modeling and mathematical equations easily performed off-line.
   E. Quantitation of RV volumes is similar to LV assessment using a bullet-shaped geometric model.

9. What factor is primarily responsible for making quantitative assessment of the RV so challenging?
   A. The shape of the tricuspid valve annulus.
   B. The presence of the moderator band.
   C. The shape of the right ventricular cavity.
   D. The interdependence of the LV and RV.
   E. Heavy trabeculation of the RV.

10. Why is the diagnosis of mitral valve prolapse established only in the long-axis view?
    A. Based on 2DE studies, the long-axis view is most sensitive in visualizing prolapse.
    B. Based on 2DE studies, the four-chamber and two-chamber views are less sensitive but more specific in visualizing prolapse.
    C. Based on 3DE studies, since the mitral valve annulus is planar, the mitral leaflets ascend above the annulus the most in a long-axis view.
    D. Based on 3DE studies, since the mitral valve annulus is nonplanar, the mitral leaflets can ascend above the annulus in a four-chamber view.
    E. The mitral valve annulus, leaflets, and papillary muscles are best seen from a long-axis view.

11. What is the mechanism of mitral regurgitation in patients with chronic ischemia?
    A. Typically, there is anterior mitral leaflet displacement.
    B. There is elongation of chordae tendineae.
    C. There is tethering of the posterior leaflet due to displacement of the posteromedial papillary muscle and an increase in the anterior-posterior annular perimeter.
    D. There is equal mitral annular dilatation due to increased interventricular pressure.
    E. There is bilateral displacement of the papillary muscle.

12. 3DE has been recommended as the new standard for measurement of mitral valve area in patients with mitral stenosis. Which statement pertaining to measurements (quantification) of mitral valve area is correct?
    A. 3DE has more accurate and reproducible measurements because the 2D cut plane can be obtained and placed en-face to the mitral valve orifice.
    B. 3DE is accurate but not as reproducible as 2D planimetry because of plane angulations.
    C. 3DE is not as accurate but reproducible compared with 2D planimetry because of the effect of thresholding and opacification used.
    D. 3DE is as accurate as 2D planimetry but not as reproducible compared to the flow convergence method.
    E. 3DE is as accurate as 2D planimetry but not as reproducible as the pressure half-time method.

13. Which modality is most accurate and reliable to use for measuring the mitral valve orifice area after balloon mitral valvuloplasty for mitral stenosis?
    A. Pressure half-time.
    B. Flow convergence method.
    C. 2D planimetry.
    D. 3D planimetry.
    E. Continuity equation.

14. Advantages of 3D echocardiographic assessment of an atrial septal defect (ASD) include:

A. En-face view of the ASD and accurate assessment of the size, shape, and location of the defect and surrounding rim.

B. En-face view of the ASD and assessment of only the size and shape of the defect.

C. En-face view of the ASD and the relationship to other structures.

D. Ability to observe the ASD from different orientations.

E. Ability to measure the defect from both right and left atrial perspectives.

15. Which statement is correct pertaining to contrast 3DE?

A. Contrast 3DE has been extensively used to evaluate myocardial perfusion.

B. Contrast 3DE is easily performed with or without triggered imaging.

C. Contrast 3DE can be used to evaluate the volume of left atrial masses.

D. Contrast 3DE is performed using only agitated saline.

E. Contrast 3DE has been used to improve LV volume and ejection fraction quantitation.

16. A 52-year-old man presents with a history of tricuspid valve endocarditis due to intravenous drug use. He is status post treatment 3 months ago and now presents with fevers and congestive heart failure. On presentation, he was noted to have a 3/6 holosystolic murmur at the left sternal border radiating to the axilla. See Figure 4-1.

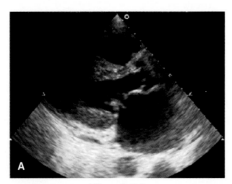

Fig. 4-1A

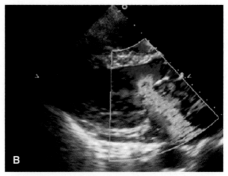

Fig. 4-1B

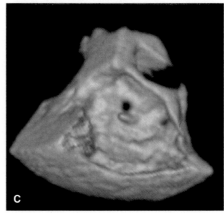

Fig. 4-1C

Based on this finding you conclude:

A. There is a posterior leaflet vegetation with mitral regurgitation.

B. There is an anterior leaflet perforation with significant mitral regurgitation.

C. There is a posterior leaflet perforation with significant mitral regurgitation.

D. There is a ruptured chordae with mitral regurgitation.

E. There is a flail mitral leaflet with significant regurgitation.

17. What would you do next?

A. Continue with medical management and follow-up with serial echocardiograms.

B. Continue antibiotic therapy and follow-up with serial transesophageal echocardiograms.

C. Ask your interventionalist to close this percutaneously.

D. Ask for a surgical consultation for mitral valve repair.

E. Discharge to drug rehabilitation, continue medical therapy, and arrange for follow-up in clinic.

18. A 35-year-old woman from Guatemala has a history of rheumatic fever as a child, had balloon valvuloplasty when she was a teenager, and has not had follow-up since her arrival to the United States. She does not complain of shortness of breath with housework.

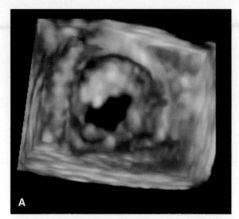

Fig. 4-2A

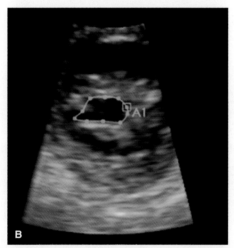

Fig. 4-2B

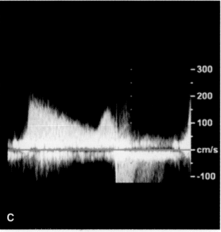

Fig. 4-2C

Her echocardiogram shows the following (Fig. 4-2):

A. Mitral valve prolapse and significant mitral regurgitation.

B. Normal opening of the mitral valve consistent with successful balloon valvuloplasty.

C. Decreased opening of the mitral valve leaflets due to low flow.

D. Decreased mitral valve opening due to restenosis.

E. Severe mitral stenosis with atrial fibrillation.

19. The mitral valve orifice area measured by 3D planimetry demonstrated a mitral valve area of 1.4 cm^2 with a mean mitral valve gradient of 5 mm Hg. The right ventricular systolic pressure was 40 mm Hg. Since she does not complain of dyspnea with housework but typically tries not to exert herself, what is your next choice of management?

A. Start amiodarone since she probably has atrial fibrillation as a cause of shortness of breath.

B. Place her on warfarin (Coumadin) since she probably has atrial fibrillation.

C. Inform her that she needs another balloon mitral valvuloplasty.

D. Inform her that she will need a mitral valve repair.

E. Schedule a stress echo to demonstrate an increase in mitral valve gradient and right ventricular systolic pressure during exercise.

20. A 60-year-old man with a history of hypertension and hypercholesterolemia has a routine follow-up with a new primary care physician who hears a holosystolic murmur at the apex radiating to the axilla on examination. The patient did not have a history of fever, weight loss, recent trauma to the chest, or rheumatologic illness. He noted difficulty working in his garden because of fatigue. At the end of the visit, he remembered that on a previous health physical for the Army he was told that he had a murmur. A transthoracic echocardiogram revealed severe mitral regurgitation but was unable to elucidate the mechanism of mitral regurgitation. After being referred to a cardiologist, a 2D and 3D TEE (transesophageal echocardiogram) was performed.

Figure 4-3 is a view from a left atrial perspective demonstrating the mitral valve from a surgeon's view. (Ao = Aorta; LAA = left atrial appendage.)

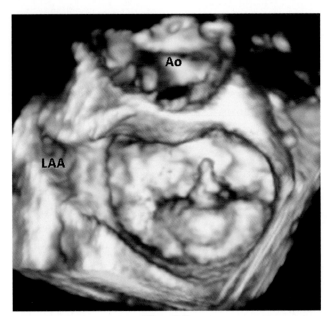

Fig. 4-3

Which segment of the mitral valve is the cause of the mitral regurgitation?

A. A1
B. A2
C. P1
D. P2
E. P3

21. What is the mechanism of mitral regurgitation in this patient?
    A. Bacterial endocarditis with a vegetation on the P2 scallop.
    B. Barlow disease.
    C. Rheumatic heart disease.
    D. SLE (systemic lupus erythematosis) with P2 Libman-Sacks lesion.
    E. Flail P2 scallop.

22. A 75-year-old woman with a history of a mitral valve replacement, hypertension, and hypercholesterolemia presents with progressive shortness of breath, lower extremity edema, and palpitations. She has been faithfully taking all her medications including Coumadin. Her blood pressure is 180/100 mm Hg, heart rate is 100 bpm, and on auscultation, she has loud mechanical heart sounds and a 2/6 murmur that is nonradiating at the apex.

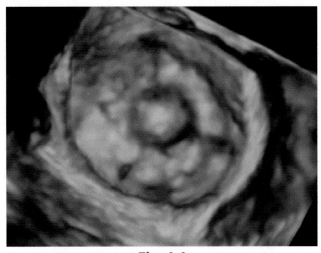

Fig. 4-4

From the TEE demonstrated in Figure 4-4, what type of mechanical valve does she have?

A. Bioprosthetic valve.
B. Homograft.
C. Ball-Cage valve.
D. Single tilting disc valve.
E. Bileaflet tilting disc valve.

23. After giving her furosemide, a beta-blocker, and angiotensin-converting enzyme inhibitor, her blood pressure is 120/80 mm Hg and heart rate is 65 bpm. She still has lower extremity edema and feels breathless vacuuming. Reviewing her echocardiogram again, she has a mean mitral valve gradient of 4 mm Hg and mitral regurgitation (Fig. 4-5).

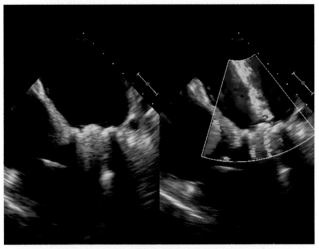

Fig. 4-5

What do you decide to do next?
A. Increase her doses of diuretics and beta-blocker.
B. Increase anticoagulation and consider heparin therapy.
C. Add high-dose statin therapy.
D. Thrombolytics.
E. Mitral valve replacement.

24. A 60-year-old man has a history of mitral valve prolapse and severe mitral regurgitation. He does not admit to having symptoms and tells you that his wife told him to go to the physician's office. She notices that he is more sedentary and does not walk as fast as he used to. On auscultation, he has a 3/6 murmur at the apex radiating to his axilla and back with an absent S1 and loud P2 component. He has severe mitral regurgitation by transthoracic echocardiogram. Because of poor acoustic windows on TTE study, he agrees to a TEE. A 3D image of the mitral valve as visualized from a left atrial perspective is shown in Figure 4-6. (AV = aortic valve.)

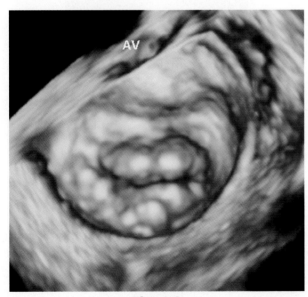

Fig. 4-6

What are your findings?
A. There is mitral stenosis.
B. There is a P2 scallop flail.
C. There is A2 and P2 prolapse.
D. There is multiscallop prolapse including A2, A3, P2, P3 and the medial commissure.
E. There is multiscallop prolapse including A1, A2, P2, P1 and the lateral commissure.

25. A 40-year-old man with a dilated cardiomyopathy had improvement in his symptoms after undergoing mitral valve surgery 6 months ago. He had improved exercise tolerance after the surgery but now presents with breathlessness going up a flight of stairs, lower extremity edema, and coughing that wakes him during the night. On echocardiogram, you find that he has severe mitral regurgitation and a vague echodensity that appears like calcification. A 3D TEE is shown from a left atrial perspective in Figure 4-7. (Ao = aorta.)

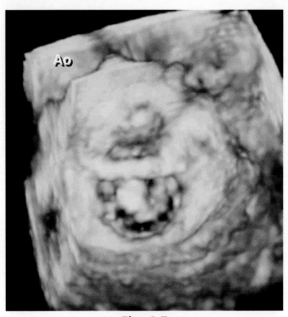

Fig. 4-7

What are your findings?
A. There is a complete dehiscence of the mitral valve annuloplasty ring from the posterior mitral annulus.
B. There is endocarditis of the mitral valve ring.
C. There is a single tilting disc valve.
D. There is a bileaflet tilting disc valve.
E. There is a bileaflet tilting disc valve with significant mitral valve dehiscence.

CASE 1:

A 45-year-old woman with mitral valve prolapse and severe mitral regurgitation has complained of fatigue when riding her bicycle, particularly going up a hill. Prior to surgery, a TEE was performed to determine the extent of the lesion (Videos 4-1 A and B). (AV = aortic valve.)

26. Which scallop is involved in causing mitral regurgitation? Please review Videos 4-1 A and B and Figure 4-8.

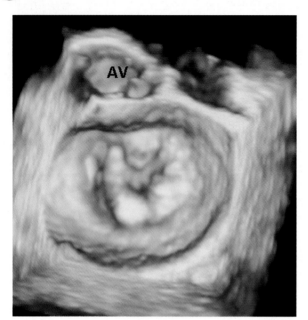

Fig. 4-8

A. P1
B. P2
C. P3
D. P2–P3
E. P1–P2

27. The surgeon would like to know the possibility of systolic anterior motion (SAM) in this patient. After reviewing these images, which parameter obtained from the images in Figure 4-9 predicts a risk of SAM after mitral valve repair?

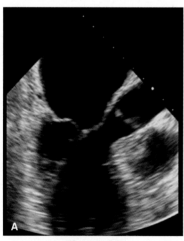

Fig. 4-9A

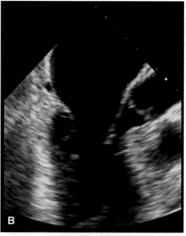

Fig. 4-9B

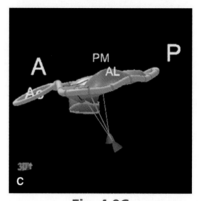

Fig. 4-9C

A. The C-septal distance is 2.2 cm and a posterior leaflet length of 1.9 cm.
B. The anterior length to posterior leaflet length ratio is 1.3 cm.
C. The aortic mitral angle is 160 degrees.
D. The LV internal dimension is less than 4 cm.
E. The mitral annulus is 4 cm.

CASE 2:

A 63-year-old gentleman with a history of a mitral valve replacement presented with chest discomfort. On physical examination, an audible click is heard with a diastolic murmur. He was evaluated with a cardiac catheterization and was found to have no significant coronary obstruction. On further investigation, he admits that he has not been taking Coumadin regularly over many months but has not noticed change in his physical activity. A TEE was performed revealing the 3D image in diastole from a left atrial perspective (Fig. 4-10); please review Videos 4-2A and B. (Ao = Aorta; LAA = left atrial appendage.)

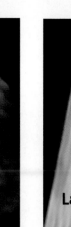

Fig. 4-10

28. What are the findings seen in Figure 4-10 and Video 4-2A?
- A. This is a normal bileaflet mechanical mitral valve.
- B. This is a single tilting disc valve.
- C. There is valve vegetation.
- D. There is a valvular dehiscence and an immobile mitral valve disc.
- E. There is thrombosed mitral valve leaflet.

CASE 3:

A 66-year-old man is referred to you because his primary physician noted a murmur during his first office visit. He tells you that he has known about the murmur since he was a teenager but has never gone to a physician for follow-up. He still works taking care of school maintenance. He walks on the treadmill for exercise at 4 mph and a 10% incline on occasion for half an hour 4 days a week. He fervently denies shortness of breath with this activity. On transthoracic echo, you find severe mitral regurgitation based on flow convergence calculation (Effective Regurgitant Orifice [ERO] = 0.4 cm^2) with normal LV function (Ejection fraction [EF] = 65%). Since the mechanism of regurgitation was difficult to discern on transthoracic imaging, a TEE was performed revealing the abnormality in Figure 4-11. (Ao = Aorta; Lat= lateral)

29. What is the mechanism of mitral seen in Figure 4-11 and Video 4-3?
- A. P1 flail.
- B. P2 flail.
- C. P3 prolapse.
- D. Severe prolapse of P2 and P3 flail.
- E. Severe prolapse of P2–P3.

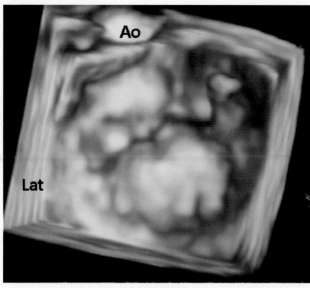

Fig. 4-11

CASE 4:

A 45-year-old Hispanic woman has a history of rheumatic fever as a child and had balloon mitral valvuloplasty as young adult. She now feels fatigued doing housework such as vacuuming her living room and has been unable to walk up a hill to get to the market. She is currently on a beta-blocker with a heart rate of 55 bpm. On transthoracic echocardiogram, she has a mean mitral valve gradient of 5.4 mm Hg, moderate mitral regurgitation, and moderate aortic stenosis. On TEE, 3D imaging of the mitral valve, a 3D mitral valve area planimetry demonstrates an orifice area of 0.6 cm^2, as shown in Figure 4-12A. The mitral valve anatomy is shown from a left atrial (Fig. 4-12B) and LV (Fig. 4-12C) perspective (also see Video 4-4). (Ao = aorta; LC = left commissure; MC = medial commissure; LVOT = LV outflow tract.)

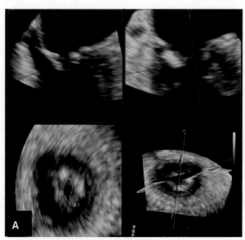

Fig. 4-12A

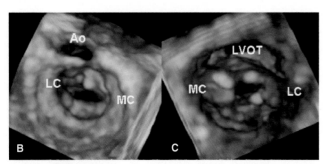

Fig. 4-12B   **Fig. 4-12C**

30. What findings are seen in Figure 4-12?
    A. There is symmetric fusion of the medial and lateral commissures, with more fibrosis/thickening of the subvalvular apparatus, and calcification of the A2 segment.
    B. There is asymmetric fusion of the medial commissure with severe subvalvular fibrosis.
    C. There is asymmetric fusion of the lateral commissure with severe subvalvular fibrosis.
    D. There is asymmetric fusion of the medial commissure with mild subvalvular fibrosis.
    E. There is mild mitral stenosis with equal fusion of medial and lateral commissures.

31. With these findings, what would you recommend?
    A. Increasing beta-blockers to achieve a heart rate in the 40s.
    B. Perform a bicycle stress test to measure an increase in right ventricular systolic pressure.
    C. Coumadin for stroke prevention.
    D. Balloon mitral valvuloplasty.
    E. Mitral valve replacement and aortic valve replacement.

CASE 5:

A 40-year-old man has a history of a dilated cardiomyopathy. He had a VSD (Ventricular septal defect), and ASD repaired in childhood who now presents with congestive heart failure. He recently had his teeth extracted and had fevers and chills about a month before. His cardiologist noted that his murmur was more noticeable. A transthoracic echo could not delineate the mechanism of his regurgitation, so he underwent a TEE. (LA = left atrium; RA = right atrium; RV = right ventricle.)

32. On live 3D echo imaging shown in Figure 4-13 and in Video 4-5, you notice that he has:

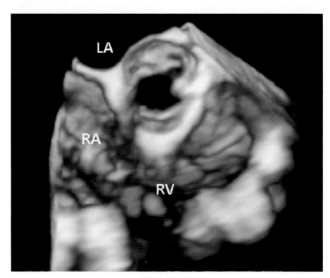

Fig. 4-13

    A. A normal aortic valve.
    B. A bicuspid aortic valve.
    C. Severe aortic stenosis.
    D. Rheumatic aortic stenosis with doming of the leaflets.
    E. A supravalvar membrane.

---

the location in time and space. Hence, patients with atrial fibrillation or irregular heartbeats were usually excluded in studies. The data integrity in such patients could not be ensured.

3. ANSWER D. The first volumetric scanner was introduced by von Ramm. This scanner was a sparse array transducer consisting of 256 elements firing non-simultaneously. The resolution was poor, frame rates were low, and the sector angle was narrow (60 degrees) and resulted in 2D cut-planes in a 3D volume. The current volumetric transducer called the fully sampled matrix array transducer has a smaller footprint, improved image quality, higher frame rates, better penetration, and harmonic capabilities. It is able to display 2D images, perform bi- or triplane imaging, acquire true "real-time" 3D images; and in some probes, pulse and continuous wave Doppler.

4. ANSWER C. The real-time three-dimensional (RT3D) imaging modes are (1) live 3D or narrow-angle acquisition, (2) zoom mode, and (3) full-volume mode or wide-angle mode. If the region of interest is small, such as valves, small cardiac masses or the interatrial septum, a zoom mode of acquisition should be used. For cardiac chambers, a full-volume or wide-angle acquisition mode is the preferred method since it will allow inclusion of the entire chamber.

5. ANSWER A. Three-dimensional echocardiography has repeatedly been shown to be superior to two-dimensional echocardiography (2DE) when compared with cardiac magnetic resonance imaging as a gold standard. Specifically, real-time three-dimensional echocardiographic studies have demonstrated less variability in repeated measurements (intra- and interobserver variability), which is explained by the ease of obtaining a common long-axis in 3D volume data. Image alignment is pivotal in the accuracy of 2D quantitation of LV volumes. Although both 2DE and 3DE underestimate LV volumes, underestimation occurs mostly when using 2DE methods for quantitation (Biplane Simpson's Method or method of discs).

6. ANSWER E. The primary difference in accuracy between 2DE and 3DE is the ability to obtain a true long-axis in two orthogonal planes from a 3D volume data set. Foreshortening is a ubiquitous problem in traditional 2DE, frequently occurring in a two-chamber view. This difference in long-axis length leads to underestimation seen in both LV mass and LV volume measurements. Certainly, quantitative methods may also influence the accuracy; however, this is not well established. When the 3DE biplane use of method of discs was compared to online automated border detection software, there was higher accuracy and less underestimation with automated border detection. However, in another study comparing online and off-line 3D software, there was higher accuracy with off-line 3D software due to greater user interaction in drawing endocardial borders and less interpolation.

7. ANSWER E. Three-dimensional echocardiography has the lowest test-retest variability compared with other methods, making it the best modality to use for serial follow-up of patients long term.

8. ANSWER B. The right ventricle (RV) has been described as a crescent-shaped ventricle not easily conforming to any geometric shape. Therefore, its quantitative assessment is very difficult. Right ventricle imaging has previously required a reconstructive 3D method using either rotation or a freehand approach, but currently real-time 3DE is the method of choice. Most efforts in quantitation of the RV have utilized the method of discs. This method results in accurate and reproducible assessment. Off-line assessment using a rotational approach and automated border detection has also been proven to be accurate but does not have widespread use.

9. ANSWER C. The shape of the RV does not conform to any known geometric shape. The tricuspid annulus is not on the same level with the pulmonary valve which also makes it challenging when determining the last basal slice.

10. ANSWER D. The true structure of the mitral valve annulus was revealed in large part on the basis of 3D studies. With this in-depth analysis of the mitral valve, we now understand that the anterior and posterior mitral valve annular points are higher than the medial and lateral mitral annulus. Hence, leaflets in the four-chamber view appear to rise above the mitral annulus even in absence of prolapse. This seminal study changed the diagnosis of mitral valve prolapse.

11. ANSWER C. Chronic ischemia leads to distortion of the left ventricle, particularly, displacement of the posteromedial papillary muscle that leads to tethering of the posterior mitral leaflet. There is also evidence of an increase in the anterior-posterior annular perimeter. Three-dimensional reconstructions performed in animal studies have led to a better understanding of the mechanism of ischemic mitral regurgitation.

12. ANSWER A. Measurement of mitral valve area in patients with rheumatic mitral stenosis is more accurate and has less variability with 3DE compared with conventional 2D methods using the invasive Gorlin equation as the reference standard. Generally, 3DE underestimates the valve area whereas 2DE overestimates the valve area. The advantage of 3DE is that the cut-plane can be angulated, adjusted, and placed at the tips of the mitral leaflets en-face to the mitral orifice. Two-dimensional valve area planimetry is highly dependent on the imaging plane obtained by the operator.

13. *ANSWER D.* In patients post–balloon mitral valvuloplasty, 3DE measurements of the mitral valve orifice are more accurate and reliable compared with the pressure half-time method and 2D planimetry. A continuity equation should not be used in the setting of coexisting aortic or mitral regurgitation, as the latter is usually a complication of valvuloplasty.

14. *ANSWER A.* Three-dimensional echocardiography has clear advantages over 2DE since it provides unique en-face views of the atrial septal defect (ASD), accurate measurements of size and surrounding rim, and location of defect. Studies have shown, ASD shape varied from being round, to oval, and racquet-shaped with a variation of 68% in size during the cardiac cycle. Three-dimensional echocardiography has also played a role in sizing of ASDs for closure. It has been demonstrated that 3D measurements are more accurate than 2D measurements and there is less underestimation of size when compared to balloon stretched diameters.

15. *ANSWER E.* A triggered acquisition seems to increase the signal-to-noise ratio and a continuous infusion of contrast is probably better than an injection. Its use is not widespread probably due to the cost and difficulty with administration of continuous infusion of contrast during 3D acquisition. The detection of perfusion abnormalities using 3DE and contrast has been limited to animal studies and has been used only in a limited number of cases.

16. *ANSWER B.* This patient has an anterior leaflet perforation with severe mitral regurgitation through the perforated leaflet. In the parasternal long-axis view, there is a discontinuity of the anterior leaflet with a mobile echodensity in proximity to the perforation, which could be part of the leaflet or vegetation. On the reconstructed 3D image, there is a large area of perforation of the anterior leaflet seen from a left atrial perspective.

17. *ANSWER D.* The class I indications for mitral valve surgery in the setting of endocarditis include severe mitral regurgitation resulting in heart failure, mitral regurgitation with evidence of elevated LV end-diastolic or left atrial pressure, or moderate/severe pulmonary hypertension, fungal or highly resistant organisms causing endocarditis, or those complicated by heart block, abscess, or destructive lesions (e.g., sinus of Valsalva to right atrium, RV or left atrium fistula; mitral leaflet perforation; or infection in the annulus fibrosa). Severe mitral

regurgitation with heart failure and a perforated leaflet were indications for surgery in this patient. Three-dimensional echocardiographic findings were confirmed with intraoperative surgical pathology (Fig. 4-14).

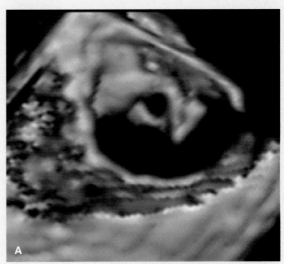

Fig. 4-14A

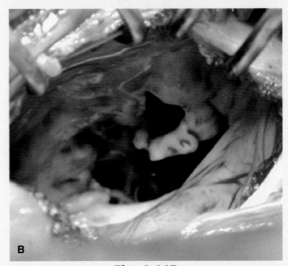

Fig. 4-14B

18. *ANSWER D.* This patient has moderate mitral stenosis with a moderate transmitral gradient. Figure 4-15D is a view of the mitral valve from a LV perspective. There is doming of the anterior mitral leaflet with medial and lateral commissural fusion. Using multiplanar reconstruction, a 2D cut-plane can be placed at the tips of the mitral leaflet en-face to the valve opening to derive a mitral valve area. In this case, the mitral valve orifice area was 1.4 cm^2.

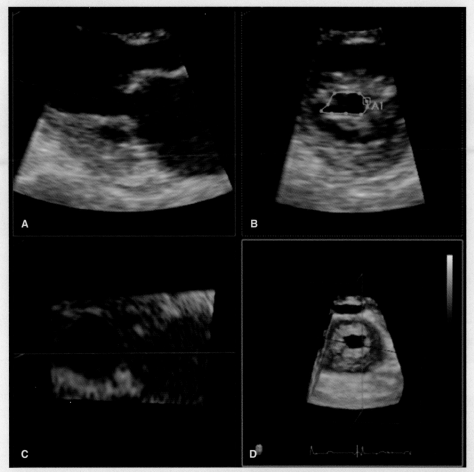

Fig. 4-15

19. ANSWER E. This patient with mitral stenosis has a valve area of ≤1.5 cm² with a gradient of 5 mm Hg and mild pulmonary hypertension. In asymptomatic moderate mitral stenosis, there is an indication to perform stress echo testing to evaluate a rise in mean mitral valve gradients or an increase in pulmonary pressures of >15 mm Hg or >60 mm Hg. If patients have valve morphology amenable to valvuloplasty and meet these criteria then there is an indication for percutaneous balloon mitral valvuloplasty.

20. ANSWER D. The abnormal scallop in this case is the P2 scallop. The P2 scallop is most frequently affected and is typically across from the aorta (Fig. 4-16). (Ao = Aorta; LAA = left atrial appendage.)

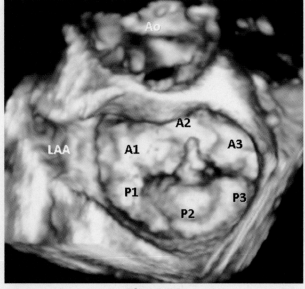

Fig. 4-16

21. ANSWER E. This is a P2 scallop that is flail (Fig. 4-17). The tip of the ruptured chordae can be seen from this left atrial perspective, noted by the arrows.

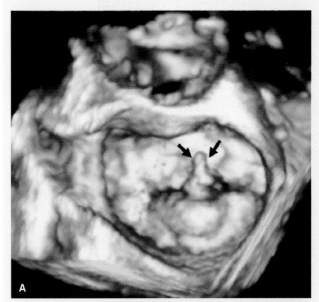

Fig. 4-17A

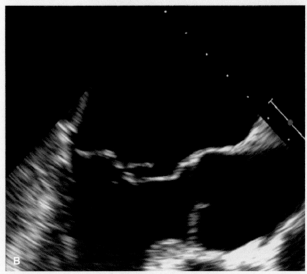

Fig. 4-17B

22. ANSWER C. This is a Ball-Cage valve. Figure 4-18 demonstrates the ball moving up above the annulus in systole.

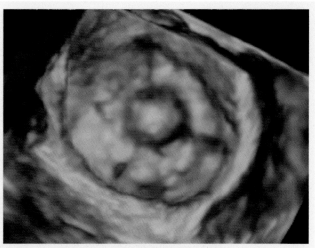

Fig. 4-18

23. ANSWER E. Since the patient's symptoms persist even with maximum medical therapy, mitral valve replacement is advised. The patient takes Coumadin regularly with a therapeutic INR and her symptoms are progressive which indicates that this is probably not an acute event such as valve thrombosis. The most likely problem since she has had this valve for many years is pannus. On echocardiogram, she has mitral regurgitation that is significant. Typically, there is only a small amount of physiologic mitral regurgitation with a Ball-Cage valve due to the movement of the ball upward toward the left atrium.

24. ANSWER D. Besides the multisegmental prolapse and the medial commissural involvement, there is calcification over the P2 scallop noted by the arrow (Fig. 4-19). (AV = aortic valve; C = commissure.)

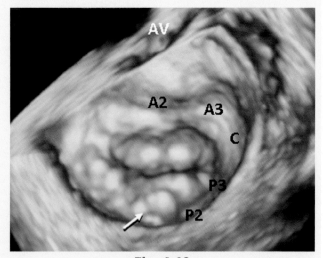

Fig. 4-19

25. ANSWER A. There is complete dehiscence of the mitral valve ring from the posterior mitral annulus, but the ring is still attached at the fibrous trigone from this left atrial view.

26. ANSWER B. Figure 4-20 is a view of the mitral valve leaflets from a left atrial perspective. The scallop involved in this case is P2 as shown by the arrow. The P3 scallop is also evident in the left atrial view; however, the P1 segment is small and is probably under the P2 segment during this systolic phase. In Video 4-1A, this P2 scallop is seen to flail into the left atrium. In Video 4-1B, a series of images during 2D TEE imaging demonstrates the flail P2 scallop with severe eccentric anteriorly directed mitral regurgitation. (AV = aortic valve.)

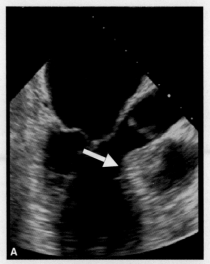

Fig. 4-21A

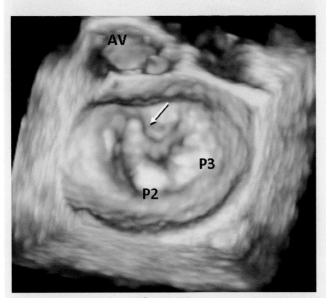

Fig. 4-20

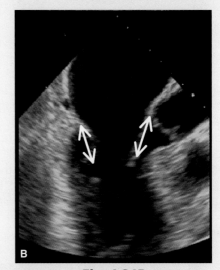

Fig. 4-21B

27. ANSWER A. There are several 2DE parameters that predict the risk of systolic anterior motion (SAM) after mitral valve repair. The predictors of SAM post–mitral valve repair are (1) coaptation to septal distance (C-Sept) <2.6 cm, (2) posterior mitral valve leaflet height >1.5 cm, (3) the anterior leaflet/posterior leaflet height ratio (AL/PL) of <1, and (4) aortic mitral angle <130 degrees. Figure 4-21A demonstrates the C-Sept (coaptation to septal) distance that measured 2.2 cm. Figure 4-21B shows the length of the posterior and anterior leaflet which were 1.9 and 2.6 cm with a AL/PL ratio of 1.3. Lastly, Figure 4-21C is a mitral valve analysis that provides the aortic mitral angle measurement of 160 degrees. There is a higher likelihood of SAM post repair when the C-Sept distance is <2.6 cm, the posterior leaflet length is >1.5 cm, the AL/PL ratio is <1, and the aortic mitral angle is <130 degrees.

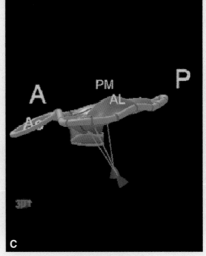

Fig. 4-21C

KEY POINTS:

■ Three-dimensional echocardiography is able to determine the involved mitral valve scallop, particularly, P1-A1 and P3-A3 segments.

■ The predictors of SAM post–mitral valve repair are (1) coaptation to septal distance (C-Sept) <2.6 cm, (2) posterior mitral valve leaflet height >1.5 cm, (3) the anterior leaflet/posterior leaflet height ratio (AL/PL) of <1, and (4) aortic mitral angle <130 degrees.

28. ANSWER D. From this left atrial view of the mitral valve in diastole, only one leaflet appears to open (Fig. 4-22). The opened leaflet (arrow) reveals a darker background since the ventricle is segmented during a zoom acquisition, whereas the thrombosed leaflet is the same appearance as the surrounding structure. This can be better appreciated in Video 4-2A. Two-dimensional TEE images in Video 4-2B (a four-chamber and long axis view) are shown. In the midesophageal four-chamber view, there is an immobile mitral valve leaflet also confirmed in a long-axis view. With color flow Doppler imaging, there is a laterally directed eccentric jet and color flow through the mitral valve leaflet that is not thrombosed. Three-dimensional color Doppler imaging reconfirms this finding demonstrating flow through the mobile leaflet and also the area of dehiscence (indicated by the double white arrows)—please review Video 4-2C. Hence, there is a thrombosed leaflet and a paravalvular leak due to dehiscence. (Ao = Aorta; LAA = left atrial appendage.)

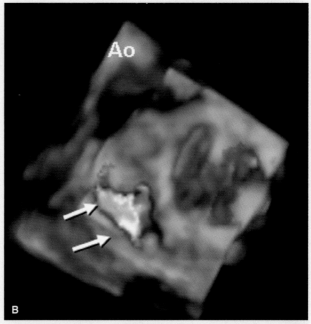

Fig. 4-22B

KEY POINTS:

■ Three-dimensional echocardiography may aid in demonstrating a thrombosed mechanical leaflet.

■ Three-dimensional echocardiography is able to demonstrate the exact site of valvular dehiscence for paravalvular regurgitation allowing for precise presurgical planning.

29. ANSWER D. In this systolic phase, the mitral valve is seen from a left atrial orientation. Most of the P2 leaflet appears myxomatous prolapsing into the left atrium. The P3 scallop tip is flail since the tip of the leaflet is directed superiorly to the left atrium.

KEY POINT:

■ Three-dimensional echocardiography is able to determine the involved mitral valve scallop and the presence of prolapse or flail.

30. ANSWER A. Figure 4-12A shows a multiplanar reconstruction from a zoomed acquisition of the mitral valve. There are two orthogonal views on the top panels and in the bottom left panel, there is a short-axis plane that is placed at the tips of the mitral leaflets. This ability to place this plane at the tips of the mitral leaflets allows better accuracy and reproducibility of the mitral valve orifice area. From a left atrial perspective (Fig. 4-12B), the posterior leaflet appears smooth

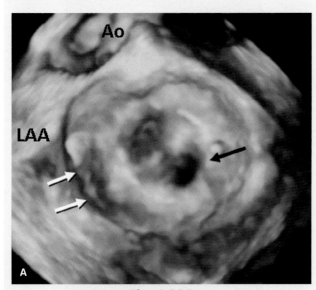

Fig. 4-22A

and short. There is a calcific nodule on the A2 scallop. The lateral and medial commissures are sometimes seen from this left atrial view. Typically the LV orientation (Fig. 4-12C) demonstrates the nature of the commissures best. Here the medial commissure appears thickened with significant fusion compared with the lateral commissure which has less thickening.

31. ANSWER E. This patient who is symptomatic with severe mitral stenosis, moderate mitral regurgitation, and moderate aortic stenosis does not need further stress testing. This patient has maximum medical therapy with beta-blockers and so further aortic valve nodal blocking is not warranted. There is no mention of whether this patient had atrial fibrillation, a previous embolic event, or evidence of left atrial thrombus which are all class I indications for Coumadin therapy. An enlarged left atrial diameter of >55 cm or presence of left atrial spontaneous echo contrast is a class IIb indication with level B and C evidence. Since she has moderate mitral regurgitation, there are no indications for balloon mitral valvuloplasty and the patient should have a mitral valve and aortic valve replacement due to the concomitant aortic stenosis.

KEY POINT:

■ Mitral valve area determined by 3DE allows for improved accuracy and reproducibility due to confirmation of assessment done at the tips of the leaflets.

32. ANSWER B. A narrow-angled acquisition (live 3D imaging mode) is performed on a short-axis view of the aortic valve. There are two distinct leaflets without a raphe. There is calcification noted by the arrow (Fig. 4-23). (LA = left atrium; RA = right atrium; RV = right ventricle.)

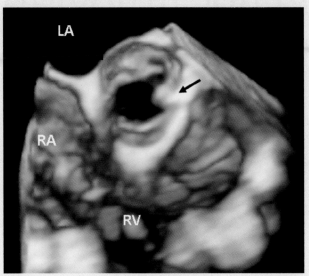

Fig. 4-23

KEY POINT:

■ The anatomy of the aortic valve is well seen by 3DE.

SUGGESTED READINGS

Bonow RO, Carabello BA, Chatterjee K, et al. 2008 Focused update incorporated into the ACC/AHA 2006 guidelines for the management of patients with valvular heart disease a report of the American College of Cardiology/American Heart Association Task Force on Practice Guidelines (Writing Committee to Revise the 1998 Guidelines for the Management of Patients With Valvular Heart Disease): endorsed by the Society of Cardiovascular Anesthesiologists, Society for Cardiovascular Angiography and Interventions, and Society of Thoracic Surgeons. *Circulation.* 2008;118:e523–e661.

Gillinov AM, Cosgrove DM III. Modified sliding leaflet technique for repair of the mitral valve. *Ann Thorac Surg.* 1999;68:2356–2357.

Jenkins C, Bricknell K, Marwick TH. Use of real-time three-dimensional echocardiography to measure left atrial volume comparison with other echocardiographic techniques. *J Am Soc Echocardiogr.* 2005;18:991–997.

Lee KS, Stewart WJ, Lever HM, et al. Mechanism of outflow tract obstruction causing failed mitral valve repair. Anterior displacement of leaflet coaptation. *Circulation.* 1993;88:II24–II29.

Maslow AD, Regan MM, Haering JM, et al. Echocardiographic predictors of left ventricular outflow tract obstruction and systolic anterior motion of the mitral valve after mitral valve reconstruction for myxomatous valve disease. *J Am Coll Cardiol.* 1999;34:2096–2104.

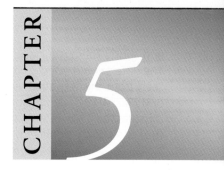

Transesophageal Echocardiography

L. Leonardo Rodriguez

1. Which of the following left atrial appendage (LAA) emptying velocities are associated with stroke in patients with atrial fibrillation?
   A. >50 cm/sec.
   B. <2 m/sec.
   C. 20 mm/sec.
   D. <20 cm/sec.
   E. None of the above.

2. The sensitivity of transesophageal echocardiography (TEE) for acute ascending aortic dissection is:
   A. 100%.
   B. 80%–89%.
   C. >95%.
   D. 75%–80%.
   E. Better compared to descending thoracic dissections.

3. The specificity of TEE for all aortic dissections is:
   A. 100%.
   B. 50%.
   C. ≥75%.
   D. >90%.
   E. As good as transthoracic echocardiography (TTE).

4. The most consistent method to visualize the right pulmonary veins by TEE is:
   A. Transducer array set at 0–30 degrees and rotate probe to the right.
   B. Transducer array set at 90–130 degrees and rotate probe to the right.
   C. Transducer array set at 0–30 degrees and rotate probe to the extreme left.
   D. Transducer array set at 45–60 degrees with clockwise probe rotation.

5. The most consistent method to visualize the left pulmonary veins by TEE is:
   A. Transducer array set at 90–100 degrees and rotate probe to the right.
   B. Transducer array set at 110–140 degrees and counterclockwise rotation.
   C. Transducer array set at 0–30 degrees and rotate probe to the extreme left.
   D. Transducer array set at 45–60 degrees and rotate probe to the extreme right.

6. The transverse sinus is:
   A. A pericardial reflection between the posterolateral left ventricular wall, the left atrium, and the right pulmonary vein.
   B. A pericardial reflection between the left atrium and great vessels.
   C. A pericardial reflection between the right atrium and right ventricle.
   D. The posterior sinus in bicuspid aortic valves.
   E. The proximal portion of the coronary sinus.

7. Aortic valvular gradients are best obtained using TEE in which view?
   A. Midesophageal window with anterior flexion.
   B. Midesophageal window with retroflexion.
   C. Deep transgastric window at 30 degrees with retroflexion.
   D. Deep transgastric window at 0 degree with anteflexion.

8. Which of the following is considered an *inappropriate* use of TEE?
   A. Evaluation of a patient with atrial fibrillation/flutter for left atrial thrombus or spontaneous contrast when a decision has been made to anticoagulate and not to perform cardioversion.
   B. Evaluation of a patient with atrial fibrillation/flutter to facilitate clinical decision making with regards to anticoagulation and/or cardioversion and/or radiofrequency ablation.
   C. Guidance during percutaneous noncoronary cardiac interventions including septal ablation in patients with hypertrophic cardiomyopathy, mitral valvuloplasty, Patent foramen ovale/atrial septal defect (PFO/ASD) closure, and radiofrequency ablation.
   D. Persistent fever in a patient with an intracardiac device.

9. Which of the following statements is correct about TEE findings in patients with atrial fibrillation?
   A. Cardioversion can be safely performed off anticoagulation if TEE is negative for thrombus.
   B. Spontaneous echo contrast is common and does not offer independent prognostic value.
   C. Spontaneous echo contrast is highly associated with previous stroke or peripheral embolism in patients with atrial fibrillation.
   D. Surgical ligation excludes flow into the left atrial appendage in >90% of the cases.

10. The differential diagnosis in patients with suspected aortic valve endocarditis includes:
    A. Lambl's excrescences, Arantius nodules, fibroelastoma, and Tebessian nodules.
    B. Chiari strands, unicuspid raphe, fibroelastomas, and fibromas.
    C. Lambl's excrescences, Arantius nodules, and fibroelastomas.
    D. Ruptured chordi, Arantius nodules, and eustachian valve.

11. The relative risk of stroke in patients with aortic arch atheroma >4 mm is:
    A. >2.0 times even after correction for other risk factors.
    B. Not significant after adjusting for atrial fibrillation and carotid disease.
    C. <2 times if you correct for atrial fibrillation, carotid disease, and peripheral artery disease.
    D. Only significant in patients with coronary artery disease.

12. The distal ascending aorta is difficult to be visualized by TEE for what reason?
    A. The esophagus is to the right of the distal ascending aorta.
    B. Interference from the trachea.
    C. The esophagus is too close to the ascending aorta.
    D. None of the above.

13. Which of the following statements is correct regarding methemoglobinemia occurring after benzocaine topical anesthetic for TEE?
    A. Oxygen saturation is low, arterial PO_2 is normal and there is no cyanosis.
    B. There is no cyanosis, low oxygen saturation, and low arterial PO_2.
    C. There is cyanosis, low oxygen saturation, and normal arterial PO_2.
    D. The treatment of choice is 100% oxygen.

14. When encountering resistance to insertion of the TEE probe in the midesophagus, which of the following maneuvers is recommended?
    A. Withdraw the probe to the mouth and reinsert.
    B. Withdraw the probe slightly, anteflex, and try again to advance the probe forward.
    C. Withdraw the probe slightly, retroflex, and try again to advance the probe forward.
    D. Withdraw the probe and recommend an endoscopy.

15. Which of the following is an absolute contraindication for TEE
    A. Prothrombin time/International normalized ratio PT INR level of 4.9.
    B. Cervical arthritis.
    C. Hiatal hernia.
    D. Esophageal varices.
    E. Uncooperative patient.

16. What is the main pathologic finding in this midesophageal view (Fig. 5-1)?

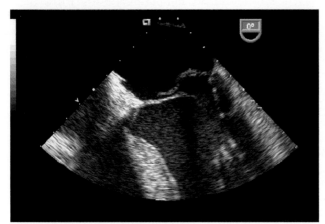

Fig. 5-1

A. Bileaflet mitral valve (MV) prolapsed.
B. Large vegetation.
C. Systolic anterior motion of the mitral valve.
D. Flail posterior mitral valve leaflet.

17. The pulmonary vein flow from the prior patient is consistent with (Fig. 5-2):

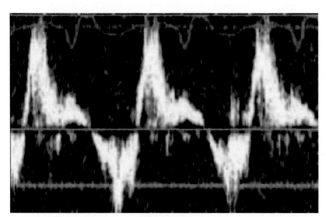

Fig. 5-2

A. Large atrial reversal secondary to increased left ventricular end diastolic pressure (LVEDP).
B. Mild mitral regurgitation.
C. Severe mitral regurgitation.
D. Mitral stenosis.

18. This short axis of the aortic valve shows (Fig. 5-3):

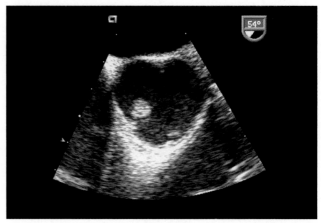

Fig. 5-3

A. Bicuspid aortic valve.
B. Lambl's excrescence.
C. Fibroelastoma of the left coronary cusp.
D. Fibroelastoma of the noncoronary cusp.

19. What is the finding in this patient with back pain (Fig. 5-4)?

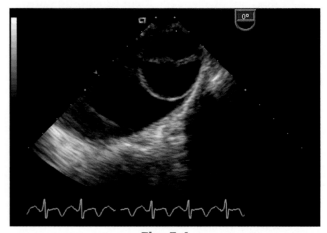

Fig. 5-4

A. Ascending aorta with intramural hematoma.
B. Descending aorta with intramural hematoma.
C. Descending aorta dissection with pericardial effusion.
D. Descending aorta dissection with left pleural effusion.

20. What is the main finding in this biplane view of the LAA in Figure 5-5?

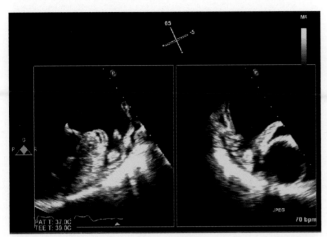

Fig. 5-5

A. Spontaneous echo contrast.
B. Spontaneous echo contrast with prominent pectinate muscles.
C. Normal left atrial appendage.
D. Multiple left atrial thrombi.

21. Which of the following statements is correct regarding the findings seen in Figure 5-6?

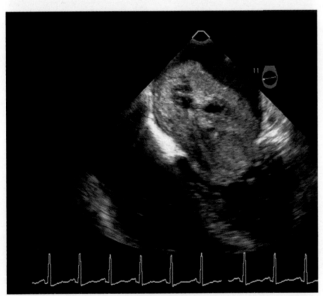

Fig. 5-6A

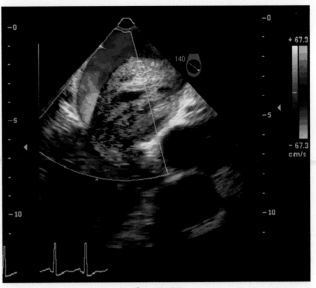

Fig. 5-6B

A. It is the most common benign tumor of the heart.
B. It is usually attached to the interatrial septum.
C. Surgery is the treatment of choice.
D. All of the above.

22. Which of the following structures is visualized in Figure 5-7?

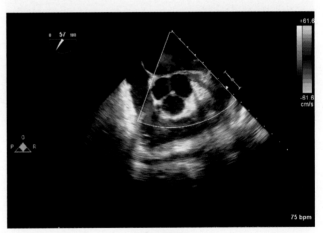

Fig. 5-7

A. Right coronary artery.
B. Periaortic abscess.
C. Anomalous origin of the left main coronary artery.
D. Normal left main trunk.

23. The abnormality of the aortic valve seen in Figure 5-8 is consistent with:

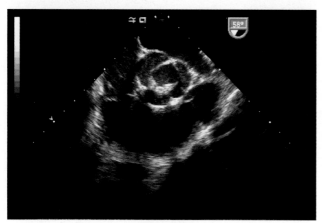

Fig. 5-8

A. Rheumatic aortic valve disease.
B. Normal bioprosthetic valve.
C. Bicuspid aortic valve.
D. Unicuspid aortic valve.

24. This color Doppler image of the pulmonary vein bifurcation (angle - 110 degrees) most likely represents Figure 5-9:

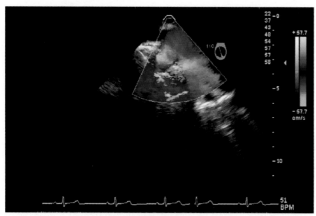

Fig. 5-9

A. The left pulmonary veins.
B. The right pulmonary veins.
C. The right upper and left upper pulmonary veins.
D. The right lower and left lower pulmonary veins.

25. Figure 5-10A and B were acquired minutes apart. What is the most likely explanation for the difference?

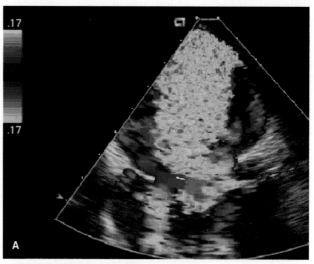

Fig. 5-10A

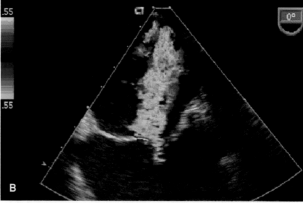

Fig. 5-10B

A. Phenylephrine infusion.
B. Change in equipment settings.
C. Failed mitral valve repair.
D. Systolic anterior motion of the mitral valve.

CASE 1:

The patient is a 65-year-old man who was operated on in 2000 and underwent coronary revascularization as well as a mitral valve repair with an annuloplasty band. Following surgery, he never recuperated well.

26. The findings seen on the echocardiogram in Figure 5-11 are most consistent with: (See also Videos 5-1 A–C):

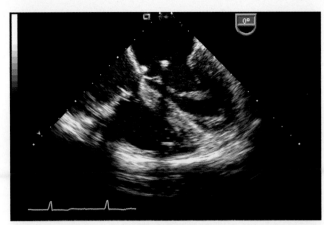

Fig. 5-11

A. Ring dehiscence.
B. Flail mitral leaflet.
C. Perimitral ring abscess.
D. Restrictive posterior leaflet.

27. The best treatment for this patient is:
    A. 6 weeks of antibiotics.
    B. Initiate antibiotics and operate within 1 week.
    C. Redo mitral valve surgery.
    D. Vasodilators and diuretics.

CASE 2:

This patient is a 50-year-old female being evaluated for right ventricular dilatation (see Videos 5-2A and B).

28. The finding shown in Figure 5-12 is frequently associated with:

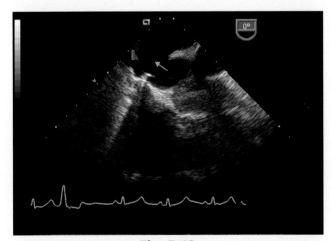

Fig. 5-12

A. Cleft anterior mitral valve.
B. A normal variant.
C. Anomalous pulmonary drainage.
D. Continuous murmur.

29. This pathology often requires:
    A. Medical management.
    B. Surgical closure.
    C. Percutaneous closure.
    D. No treatment.

CASE 3:

This is a 65-year-old patient with atrial fibrillation. A TEE is performed prior to cardioversion.

30. The structure incidentally found and marked with the arrow in Figure 5-13 represents (see also Video 5-3):
    A. Descending aorta.
    B. Aneurysm of the circumflex artery.
    C. Left lower pulmonary vein.
    D. Dilated coronary sinus.

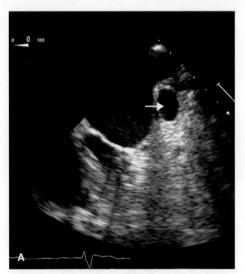

Fig. 5-13A

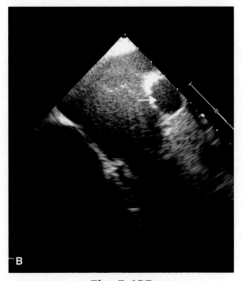

Fig. 5-13B

31. The best way to corroborate your diagnosis is:
  A. Coronary angiogram.
  B. Agitated saline through left arm.
  C. Transthoracic echocardiogram with microbubles (contrast).
  D. Posterior rotation of the probe and longitudinal view of the aorta.

CASE 4:

A 79-year-old female has undergone surgery for mitral regurgitation.

32. This echocardiogram shows (see Figure 5-14 and Videos 5-4A–C):

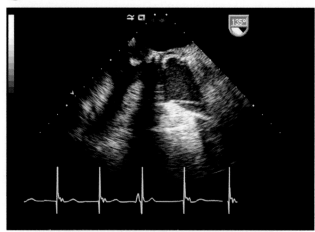

Fig. 5-14

  A. Periaortic fluid.
  B. Aortic dissection.
  C. Artifact from Swan-Ganz Catheter.
  D. Normal intraoperative findings.

CASE 5:

This echocardiogram was done in a 46-year-old man with exertional chest pain (see Videos 5-5A and B).

33. The short-axis view in Figure 5-15 shows:

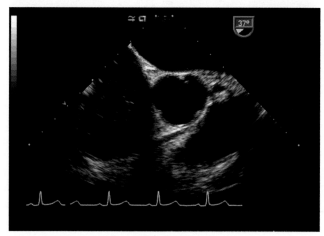

Fig. 5-15

  A. Aortic dissection.
  B. Anomalous origin of the left coronary artery.
  C. Pulmonary embolism.
  D. Anomalous origin of the right coronary artery.

ANSWERS

1. ANSWER: D. In patients with nonvalvular atrial fibrillation, low left atrial emptying velocities (<20 cm/sec) have been associated with severe spontaneous echocardiographic contrast, appendage thrombus, and subsequent cardioembolic events. Data also suggest that patients with severe echo contrast have a poor prognosis with increased mortality.

2. ANSWER: C. TEE is a sensitive and highly specific technique for the diagnosis of aortic dissection. Intimal flaps are easily visualized when present in the proximal ascending aorta, distal arch, and descending thoracic aorta. Studies comparing TEE with computer tomography (CT) and magnetic resonance imaging (MRI) have shown that its sensitivity is >95%.

3. ANSWER: C. The specificity of TEE for aortic dissection detection is approximately 75%. The reduced specificity is the result of false positive findings in the ascending aorta due to reverberation artifacts.

4. ANSWER: D. Pulmonary veins evaluation is part of a comprehensive TEE evaluation. Pulmonary vein flow may add important information in patients with mitral regurgitation, anomalous pulmonary vein drainage, and in patients after pulmonary vein isolation procedures. Visualization of the right pulmonary vein is most challenging but can usually be seen from a 45–60 degree transducer position with clockwise rotation.

5. ANSWER: B. The left upper pulmonary vein is the easiest to visualize because of its close proximity to the left atrial appendage. Left pulmonary veins are usually seen at 110–140 degrees with counterclockwise rotation.

6. ANSWER: B. The transverse pericardial sinus is important for the cardiac surgeon because it is through this sinus where they usually place the aortic clamp. During routine TEE, it is important to remember that the pericardial reflection may contain small amounts of fluid. Operators without experience may misinterpret this finding as aortic dissection or periaortic abscess.

7. ANSWER: D. The evaluation of patients with aortic stenosis using TEE includes visualization of the aortic valve anatomy and planimetry of the aortic valve area. When possible, transvalvular gradients are obtained. However, obtaining accurate transaortic gradients can be technically challenging. It requires a deep transgastric view at 0 degree with anteflexion of the probe's tip. The objective is alignment of the aortic valve and proximal ascending aorta as parallel as possible with the CW Doppler cursor. Alternatively, the transducer position can be set at 90–100 degrees and the probe slowly pulled back keeping the anteflexion and the tip adjusted with the lateral knob. These maneuvers are important not only in patients with valvular aortic stenosis but also in patients with hypertrophic obstructive cardiomyopathy.

8. ANSWER: A. In 2007, the criteria for appropriateness for echocardiography were published. A group of experts were asked to assess whether the use of the test for each indication was appropriate, uncertain, or inappropriate. Of the options offered in question 8, answer (A) was considered an inappropriate indication for TEE. In patients with atrial fibrillation that are already anticoagulated and are *not going* to undergo electrical or pharmacological cardioversion, it is not necessary to evaluate for the presence of left atrial thrombus. TEE remains a useful tool in patients undergoing cardioversion or pulmonary vein isolation to rule out left atrial thrombus. TEE is also widely used in the guidance of noncoronary interventions and is important in assessing for the presence of vegetations in patients with suspected infection of an intracardiac device.

9. ANSWER: C. In patients with permanent atrial fibrillation, the presence of severe spontaneous contrast or smoke is a marker of increased risk of thromboembolic events. Electrical cardioversion causes left atrial appendage stunning with increased severity of echocontrast immediately after the procedure. There have been published series of cases of embolic stroke after cardioversion in patients with a negative TEE for left atrial thrombus who are not anticoagulated. For that reason, patients should have therapeutic levels of anticoagulation before proceeding with cardioversion. A recent series of patients with surgical LAA ligation showed a high incidence of residual flow between the left atrium (LA) and LAA.

10. ANSWER: C. TEE is highly sensitive for vegetations; however, other valvular structures should be considered in the differential diagnosis. In the aortic valve, these structures include Lambl's excrescences, thickened Arantius

nodules, and fibroelastomas. Lambl's excrescences are filamentous structures attached to the ventricular side of the valve. Arantius nodules are present at the center of the free margin of each of the three cusps of the aortic valve. Fibroelastomas are benign tumors often attached to the aortic side of the valve.

11. ANSWER: A. Evaluation for source of embolism is one of the most common indications for TEE. Atrial fibrillation, PFO, valvular heart disease, and diseases of the aorta are frequent sources of stroke. Severe atheroma of the ascending aorta and/or arch carries a high risk of subsequent stroke. This finding is also important in patients undergoing open heart surgery because clamping of the aorta may dislodge the atheroma and cause a stroke or embolism to other organs. Identification of ascending atheroma may be difficult using TEE and in the operating room TEE is usually complemented with epicardial echocardiography. Large, protruding atheromas in the aortic arch are associated with an increase risk of stroke, >2 times even after correcting for carotid stenosis, atrial fibrillation, and other risk factors.

12. ANSWER: B. TEE is an excellent technique to visualize the ascending aorta, distal arch, and the descending thoracic aorta. However, the distal aorta and proximal arch constitute a blind spot for TEE visualization. The blind spot is caused by the interposition of air, located in the trachea and main bronchi, between the echo-transducer and the aorta.

13. ANSWER: C. Methemoglobinemia related to benzocaine topical anesthetic given during TEE is a rare reaction occurring in ~0.1% of patients. Methemoglobin levels are elevated due to conversion of iron from a reduced to oxidized form of hemoglobin which results in poor oxygen carrying capacity. This results in cyanosis, low oxygen saturation levels, and normal arterial PO_2 levels. The treatment of choice is intravenous methylene blue.

14. ANSWER: C. Sometimes the TEE probe will become coiled in the esophagus with the tip pointed toward the mouth. Often this can be remedied by withdrawing the probe to a slight extent, retroflexion of the probe, and then attempting to advance the probe forward. However, it is always true that if simple maneuvers such as this do not work then the TEE should not be continued and an endoscopy should be performed to rule out stricture or obstructing lesions.

15. ANSWER: E. Absolute contraindications to TEE include esophageal or pharyngeal obstruction, instability of the cervical vertebrae, active gastrointestinal bleeding from an unknown source or severe bleeding diathesis or overanticoagulation, or an uncooperative patient. Relative contraindications include esophageal varices, PT INR >3.5 < 5.0, or platelet count <50,000.

16. ANSWER: D. Degenerative mitral valve disease is the most common cause of severe mitral regurgitation requiring surgery. Echocardiography is the main diagnostic modality to assess mitral valve disease. Although TTE often offers enough diagnostic information, TEE is the gold standard for anatomical definition. Posterior mitral prolapse and/or flail are more common than anterior mitral pathology. A flail leaflet is diagnosed when ruptured chordae are visualized and the tip of the leaflet points superiorly into the left atrium in systole. In cases of posterior leaflet flail, the regurgitant jet is anteriorly directed.

17. ANSWER: C. Pulmonary vein flow assessment is part of a comprehensive evaluation in patients with mitral regurgitation. Figure 5-2 shows holosystolic flow reversal consistent with severe mitral regurgitation. In patients with mild mitral regurgitation, usually the pulmonary vein flow is normal with predominant or mildly blunted systolic flow. A large atrial reversal is seen in patients with increased end diastolic pressure. In patients with mitral stenosis, the typical finding is a slow deceleration slope in the diastolic wave of the pulmonary vein flow.

18. ANSWER: D. Papillary fibroelastomas are benign tumors that can be seen on the aortic valve. These tumors are described as small, well-delineated, pedunculated masses with a predilection for valvular endocardium. These tumors can be highly mobile and carry an embolic risk. The diagnoses are usually incidental or during investigation for an embolic source. Sun et al. have summarized the echocardiographic characteristics of fibroelastomas:
- The tumor is round or oval, irregular in appearance, with well-demarcated borders and a homogeneous texture.
- Most are relatively small <20 mm.
- Nearly half have small stalks, and those with stalks are mobile.
- They may be single or multiple and are often associated with valvular disease.
- They more commonly appear on the aortic valve followed by the mitral valve.

19. ANSWER: D. This is an example of an aortic dissection flap of the descending thoracic aorta with associated pleural effusion. Note the characteristic intimal flap that separates the true from the false lumen. The presence of a pleural effusion may represent a contained rupture but more often this represents an inflammatory pleural reaction. In patients with associated ascending aortic dissection with involvement of the aortic valve, pleural effusion may also indicate congestive heart failure.

20. ANSWER: D. This example shows two left atrial appendage thrombi. They are usually related to stagnant flow that can be seen in patients with atrial fibrillation or mitral valve disease, in particular stenotic lesions. These thrombi are more often seen at the tip of the appendage. Although usually they are single, they can be multilobulated. Differential diagnoses include prominent pectinate muscles and severe spontaneous echo contrast. Pectinate muscles are usually easy to identify using a multiplane TEE probe and can be seen as finger-like structures at 100–110 degrees rotation. Severe spontaneous echo contrast (sludge) can be challenging to differentiate from a true clot. In some cases, the use of commercially available echo contrast agents may be helpful.

21. ANSWER: D. Myxomas are the most common benign tumors of the heart. They can be found in any of the heart cavities but most often in the left atrium. Typically, these tumors are attached by a stalk to the interatrial septum. Surgery is usually indicated due to the potential for embolism or obstruction of the mitral valve orifice. In most cases, these are single tumors; although in their familial form, they can be multiple and recurrent. Carney's syndrome is an autosomal dominantly transmitted multisystem tumorous disorder characterized by myxomas (heart, skin, and breast), spotty skin pigmentation (lentigines and blue nevi), endocrine tumors (adrenal, testicular, thyroid, and pituitary), and peripheral nerve tumors (schwannomas). In Carney's syndrome, the cardiac myxomas are also multiple and contribute to the mortality of this disease.

22. ANSWER: D. The proximal coronary arteries can be visualized using TEE. In patients with normal origin of the coronaries, the left main can be visualized as shown in the example. The right coronary artery can be more challenging due to its anterior origin and can be masked by aortic calcification.

23. ANSWER: D. This is an example of a unicuspid aortic valve. This is a relative rare entity accounting for less than 5% of the adult population with aortic stenosis requiring surgery. Unicuspid valves can be unicommissural (most common) or acommissural.

24. ANSWER: A. Visualization of the pulmonary veins is important in a variety of situations: postpulmonary vein ablation, in patients with sinus venosus ASD, and in the assessment of mitral regurgitation. The easiest vein to visualize is the left upper pulmonary vein that runs next to the left atrial appendage. It is possible to visualize the bifurcation of the left and right pulmonary veins. The left pulmonary veins are typically seen from 110 to 140 degrees with counterclockwise rotation. In the example, the bifurcation can be easily seen with a transducer position at 110 degrees, and Figure 5-16 corresponds to the left upper (A) and left lower (B) pulmonary veins. The right pulmonary veins are usually

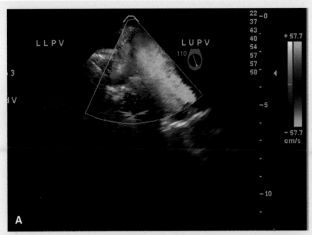

Fig. 5-16A

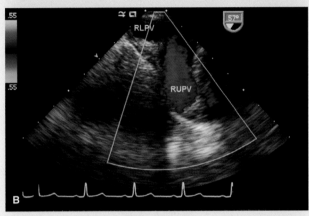

Fig. 5-16B

visualized from 45 to 60 degrees transducer position with clockwise rotation. (RLPV: right lower pulmonary vein; RUPV: right upper pulmonary vein).

25. ANSWER: B. The answer is a change in the echo settings, in particular the Nyquist limit. This is a frequent mistake in evaluating regurgitant lesions. The appearance of a jet by color Doppler depends on jet momentum (flow × velocity). In addition, changes in gain, pulse repetition frequency, and Nyquist limit may markedly change the size of the jet. The standard Nyquist limit to evaluate a regurgitant lesion is around 45–60 cm/sec. In this particular example, the Nyquist limit was lowered to interrogate the interatrial septum (low-velocity PFO flow) and then was not changed back to assess the degree of mitral regurgitation.

26. ANSWER: A. This case shows a typical dehiscence of the posterior aspect of the mitral annuloplasty ring. By two-dimensional (2D) echocardiography, it should be suspected when a bright echodensity is seen "floating" in the middle of the mitral annular orifice (See Video 5.1A). Color flow can be seen around the ring in systole and diastole (Video 5-1B). Three-dimensional echocardiography is the gold standard for the evaluation of these patients as it allows confirmation of the diagnosis and visualization of the extent of the ring detachment

from the annulus (Video 5-1C). Ring dehiscence occurs more often when undersized rings are used (Fig. 5-17).

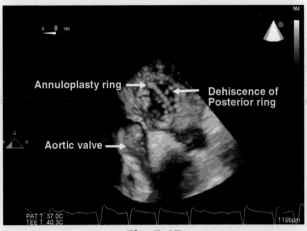

Fig. 5-17

27. ANSWER: C. The patient requires a reoperation. Often, a second repair can be performed using a slightly larger annuloplasty ring.

KEY POINTS:

■ Dehiscence of an annuloplasty ring should be suspected when the a portion of the ring appears "floating" in the middle of the mitral annular orifice and there is associated mitral regurgitation.

■ Three-dimensional echocardiography is the gold standard for confirmation of mitral annuloplasty dehiscence.

■ Reoperation and repeat repair are often required for dehiscence and significant mitral regurgitation.

28. ANSWER: C. Atrial septal defects can occur in multiple locations of the interatrial septum. This case shows a sinus venosus defect. This defect is commonly associated with anomalous drainages of the right pulmonary veins and frequently requires surgical treatment. The diagnosis can be missed unless it is suspected and appropriate images obtained (Fig. 5-18A).

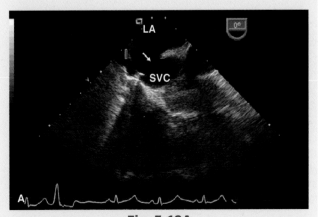

Fig. 5-18A

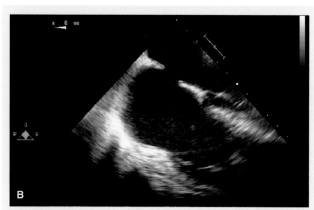

Fig. 5-18B

This figure shows a 0 degree view at the level of the great vessels with slight counterclockwise rotation. The objective of this view is to visualize the superior vena cava that normally appears as a closed circle. In the case of a sinus venosus ASD, a defect in the SVC can be seen (see arrow) (seen also in Videos 5-6A and 5-2A). This should be confirmed in a bicaval view (90–120 degrees) (Video 5-2B). Careful interrogation of all pulmonary veins is mandatory. The most common ASD is the ostium secundum type as shown in Figure 5-18B and biplane view in Video 5-6B. This defect is located in the fossa ovalis and occurs when there is an inadequate septum primum. Another type of interatrial septal defect is ostium primum (a type of endocardial cushion defect) that is usually accompanied by a mitral leaflet cleft.

29. *ANSWER: B.* A sinus venosous defect is not amenable to percutaneous closure.

KEY POINTS:

■ Sinus venosus defects are associated with right ventricular enlargement and anomalous drainage of the right pulmonary veins.

■ Detection of a sinus venosus defect requires that appropriate views are obtained to visualize the superior vena cava.

■ Sinus venosus type ASD requires surgical closure.

30. *ANSWER: D.* This structure represents a severely dilated coronary sinus (CS). The most common cause of CS dilatation is right atrial hypertension due to right-sided heart failure, tricuspid regurgitation, or pulmonary hypertension. However, the degree of dilatation as seen in this example almost always is caused by a persistent left superior vena cava draining into the CS. Another more rare cause of significant dilatation of the CS is anomalous pulmonary vein drainage in the CS. Additional imaging at 0 degree by advancing the probe deeper will also show the CS draining into the RA (Fig. 5-19A).

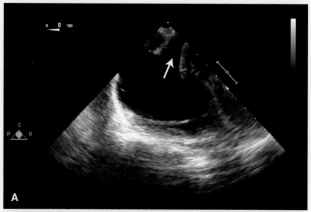

Fig. 5-19A

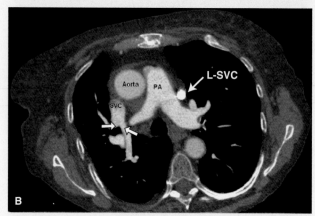

Fig. 5-19B

Persistent left SVC is a benign variant and usually does not require other diagnostic tests. Incidentally, the case shown had anomalous right pulmonary vein drainage in the right SVC found on a CT scan (Fig. 5-19B). (PA: pulmonary artery; SVC: superior vena cava; L-SVC: persistent left superior vena cava)

31. *ANSWER: B.* Confirmation of the suspected persistent left SVC is done by injecting agitated saline into the left arm and showing early appearance of the bubbles in the coronary sinus before the right atrium (Video 5-7).

KEY POINTS:

■ A dilated CS is most often due to right atrial hypertension but other causes include fistula to the CS, anomalous pulmonary vein drainage to the CS, or a left SVC to the CS.

■ A left SVC is almost always a benign anatomic variant.

■ Confirmation of a left SVC to CS connection can be obtained by demonstrating bubbles injected into the left arm vein appearing in the CS prior to the right atrium.

32. ANSWER: B. This case shows an aortic dissection that is a rare complication from cardiac surgery. Type A aortic dissection is a surgical emergency with high early mortality if left untreated. Noninvasive diagnostic techniques include CT, MRI, and TEE. All of them have high sensitivity and specificity. The diagnosis by TEE is based on the demonstration of an intimal flap. This appears as a linear echodensity with independent motion. Color flow Doppler is also helpful and demonstrates no or very low flow in the false lumen. It is always important to corroborate the findings in orthogonal views (Videos 5-4A and B). The origin of the coronaries and their relationship to the intimal flap should be imaged when possible (Video 5-4C). Fluid in the pericardial recesses can be confusing in inexperienced hands, but it can be clarified by its contour and the lack of flow as seen in Figure 5-20, and in Video 5-8.

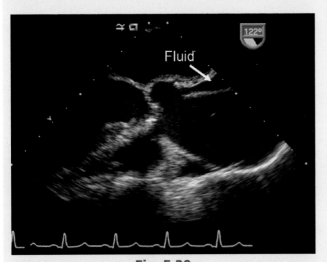

Fig. 5-20

Certain ultrasound artifacts can make the diagnosis of dissection challenging. These artifacts are also linear densities but they do not respect anatomic boundaries and usually move in parallel to the source of the artifact (usually a high reflective surface such as a catheter or calcified wall).

KEY POINTS:

■ Aortic dissection is a rare complication of cardiac surgery.

■ Demonstration of aortic dissection requires imaging in orthogonal views to demonstrate an intimal flap with true and false lumens or an intramural hematoma.

■ Important ancillary information that is useful to the surgeon includes the presence or absence of flow in the coronary ostia and involvement of the aortic valve with significant aortic regurgitation.

33. ANSWER: D. This case illustrates an anomalous origin of the right coronary artery from the left sinus of Valsalva. Real time images show this finding in better detail (Videos 5-5A and B). An anomalous origin of the RCA from the left coronary sinus has important implications because usually the initial segment has a transmural course and then runs between the aorta and the pulmonary artery (see 3D rendering of a CT scan in Figure 5-21) often compressing the lumen. (LMC: left main coronary artery; RVOT: right ventricular outflow tract).

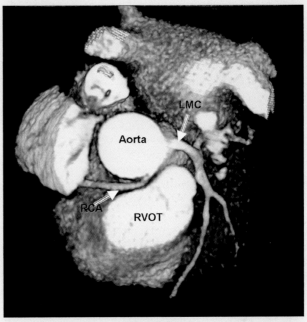

Fig. 5-21

The incidence of an anomalous right coronary from the left coronary sinus is around 0.1%–0.2% in an angiographic series. Angina, syncope, sudden death, and myocardial infarction have been associated with this abnormality.

KEY POINTS:

■ Anomalous origin of the right coronary artery from the left sinus of Valsalva is a rare congenital anomaly associated with angina, myocardial infarction, and sudden cardiac death

■ With careful imaging, it can be visualized using TEE but requires confirmation with CTA or cardiac catheterization.

SUGGESTED READINGS

Amarenco P, Cohen A, Tzourio C, et al. Atherosclerotic disease of the aortic arch and the risk of ischemic stroke. *N Engl J Med*. 1994;331: 1474–1479.

Brown RD Jr, Khandheria BK, Edwards WD. Cardiac papillary fibroelastoma: a treatable cause of transient ischemic attack and ischemic stroke detected by transesophageal echocardiography. *Mayo Clin Proc*. 1995;70:863–868.

Douglas PS, Khandheria B, Stainback RF, et al. ACCF/ASE/ACEP/ASNC/SCAI/SCCT/SCMR 2007 appropriateness criteria for transthoracic and transesophageal echocardiography: a report of the American College of Cardiology Foundation Quality Strategic Directions Committee Appropriateness Criteria Working Group, American Society of Echocardiography, American College of Emergency Physicians, American Society of Nuclear Cardiology, Society for Cardiovascular Angiography and Interventions, Society of Cardiovascular Computed Tomography, and the Society for Cardiovascular Magnetic Resonance endorsed by the American College of Chest Physicians and the Society of Critical Care Medicine. *J Am Coll Cardiol*. 2007;50:187–204.

Fehske W, Grayburn PA, Omran H, et al. Morphology of the mitral valve as displayed by multiplane transesophageal echocardiography. *J Am Soc Echocardiogr*. 1994;7:472–479.

Garduno C, Chew S, Forbess J, Smith PK, Grocott HP. Persistent left superior vena cava and partial anomalous pulmonary venous connection: incidental diagnosis by transesophageal echocardiography during coronary artery bypass surgery. *J Am Soc Echocardiogr*. 1999;12:682–685.

Goldman ME, Pearce LA, Hart RG, et al. Pathophysiologic correlates of thromboembolism in nonvalvular atrial fibrillation: I. Reduced flow velocity in the left atrial appendage (The Stroke Prevention in Atrial Fibrillation [SPAF-III] Study). *J Am Soc Echocardiogr*. 1999;12:1080–1087.

Goldstein SA, Campbell A, Mintz GS, Pichard A, Leon M, Lindsay J Jr. Feasibility of on-line transesophageal echocardiography during balloon mitral valvulotomy: experience with 93 patients. *J Heart Valve Dis*. 1994;3:136–148.

Grimm RA, Stewart WJ, Maloney JD, et al. Impact of electrical cardioversion for atrial fibrillation on left atrial appendage function and spontaneous echo contrast: characterization by simultaneous transesophageal echocardiography. *J Am Coll Cardiol*. 1993;22: 1359–1366.

Hurle JM, Garcia-Martinez V, Sanchez-Quintana D. Morphologic characteristics and structure of surface excrescences (Lambl's excrescences) in the normal aortic valve. *Am J Cardiol*. 1986;58: 1223–1227.

Katz ES, Tunick PA, Colvin SB, Culliford AT, Kronzon I. Aortic dissection complicating cardiac surgery: diagnosis by intraoperative biplane transesophageal echocardiography. *J Am Soc Echocardiogr*. 1993;6:217–222.

Kronzon I, Tunick PA. Transesophageal echocardiography as a tool in the evaluation of patients with embolic disorders. *Prog Cardiovasc Dis*. 1993;36:39–60.

Kronzon I, Sugeng L, Perk G, et al. Real-time 3-dimensional transesophageal echocardiography in the evaluation of post-operative mitral annuloplasty ring and prosthetic valve dehiscence. *J Am Coll Cardiol*. 2009;53: 1543–1547.

Kronzon I, Tunick PA, Freedberg RS, et al. Transesophageal echocardiography is superior to transthoracic echocardiography in the diagnosis of sinus venosus atrial septal defect. *J Am Coll Cardiol*. 1991;17: 537–542.

Muller S, Feuchtner G, Bonatti J, et al. Value of transesophageal 3D echocardiography as an adjunct to conventional 2D imaging in preoperative evaluation of cardiac masses. *Echocardiography*. 2008; 25:624–631.

Nienaber CA, von Kodolitsch Y, Nicolas V, et al. The diagnosis of thoracic aortic dissection by noninvasive imaging procedures. *N Engl J Med*. 1993;328:1–9.

Nienaber CA, Kische S, Skriabina V, Ince H. Noninvasive imaging approaches to evaluate the patient with known or suspected aortic disease. *Circ Cardiovasc Imaging*. 2009;2:499–506.

Novaro GM, Mishra M, Griffin BP. Incidence and echocardiographic features of congenital unicuspid aortic valve in an adult population. *J Heart Valve Dis*. 2003;12:674–678.

O'Gara P, Sugeng L, Lang R, et al. The role of imaging in chronic degenerative mitral regurgitation. *JACC Cardiovasc Imaging*. 2008; 1:221–237.

Ohta Y, Ohta T, Kobayashi S, Izumi S, Shimada T. Anomalous origin of the right coronary artery from the left sinus of valsalva: diagnosis by multiplane transesophageal echocardiography. *Echocardiography*. 2002;19:161–163.

Perez de Isla L, de Castro R, Zamorano JL, et al. Diagnosis and treatment of cardiac myxomas by transesophageal echocardiography. *Am J Cardiol*. 2002;90: 1419–1421.

Reeder GS, Khandheria BK, Seward JB, Tajik AJ. Transesophageal echocardiography and cardiac masses. *Mayo Clin Proc*. 1991;66: 1101–1109.

Salcedo EE, Quaife RA, Seres T, Carroll JD. A framework for systematic characterization of the mitral valve by real-time three-dimensional transesophageal echocardiography. *J Am Soc Echocardiogr*. 2009; 22:1087–1099.

Sun JP, Asher CR, Yang XS, et al. Clinical and echocardiographic characteristics of papillary fibroelastomas: a retrospective and prospective study in 162 patients. *Circulation*. 2001;103:2687–2693.

Verhorst PM, Kamp O, Visser CA, Verheugt FW. Left atrial appendage flow velocity assessment using transesophageal echocardiography in nonrheumatic atrial fibrillation and systemic embolism. *Am J Cardiol*. 1993;71:192–196.

Zabalgoitia M, Halperin JL, Pearce LA, Blackshear JL, Asinger RW, Hart RG. Transesophageal echocardiographic correlates of clinical risk of thromboembolism in nonvalvular atrial fibrillation. Stroke Prevention in Atrial Fibrillation III Investigators. *J Am Coll Cardiol*. 1998;31:1622–1626.

Sonographer Goal Oriented Technique

Annitta J. Morehead

1. For most parasternal views, posing the patient in which of the following positions will most likely yield improved images?
   A. Trendelenburg position with arm extended up.
   B. Ventral decubitus position with left arm extended up.
   C. Dorsal decubitus position with left arm extended up.
   D. Steep right lateral decubitus position with left arm extended up.
   E. Steep left lateral decubitus position with left arm extended up.

2. The sonographer must be able to distinguish image artifact from anatomic findings. To rule out image artifact and demonstrate true anatomic findings, which of the following rules should be applied?
   A. The finding in question must be visualized by both a high frequency and a low frequency transducer.
   B. The finding in question must be visualized in all parasternal and apical views.
   C. The finding in question must be visualized in at least two image views.
   D. The finding in question must be visualized in at least three image views.
   E. The finding in question must be ruled out using contrast for chamber opacification.

3. In patients with technically difficult parasternal images, which of the following views can be substituted for the parasternal long-axis view?
   A. Apical two-chamber.
   B. Apical long-axis.
   C. Apical four-chamber.
   D. Apical five-chamber.
   E. Subcostal four-chamber.

4. Which views can be obtained from the left parasternal long-axis view by including a medial angulation as well as a lateral angulation of the transducer?
   A. Right ventricular (RV) inflow and RV outflow.
   B. Left ventricular (LV) inflow and LV outflow.
   C. RV outflow and pulmonary vein inflow.
   D. Inferior vena cava and hepatic vein.
   E. Ascending aorta and descending aorta.

5. Which of the following transthoracic imaging windows is best for assessing the LV apex?
   A. Parasternal.
   B. Apical.
   C. Subcostal.
   D. Supraclavicular.
   E. Suprasternal.

6. Which of the following series of images constitutes the parasternal short-axis two-dimensional (2D) examination?
   A. Left ventricle, right ventricle, left atrium (LA), and right atrium (RA).
   B. LV apical level, LV papillary muscles level, LV basal level, mitral valve view, and the aortic, pulmonic, and tricuspid valves view.
   C. LA, mitral valve, LV, aortic valve, and RV.
   D. LV, mitral valve, and LA.
   E. RV, tricuspid valve, and RA.

7. Decreased wall motion is referred to as which of the following terms?
   A. Normal wall motion.
   B. Hyperkinetic wall motion.
   C. Hypokinetic wall motion.
   D. Akinetic wall motion.
   E. Dyskinetic wall motion.

8. The LA is accurately planimetered for volume estimation at which stage of the cardiac cycle?
   A. End ventricular diastole.
   B. End ventricular systole.
   C. Mid ventricular systole.
   D. Onset of ventricular diastole.
   E. Onset of ventricular systole.

9. Subcostal views can be significantly improved by which of the following maneuvers?
   A. The Valsalva maneuver.
   B. Held exhalation.
   C. Several quick deep sniffs.
   D. Held inhalation.
   E. Supine position with 45 degrees leg elevation.

10. Mitral valve prolapse (MVP) is best demonstrated in which of the following imaging modes and views?
    A. 2D parasternal short-axis view.
    B. 2D apical four-chamber view.
    C. 2D derived M-mode parasternal long-axis view.
    D. 2D apical long-axis view.
    E. 2D parasternal long-axis view.

11. The sonographer can verify that maximum peak E wave Doppler velocity of LV inflow has been acquired by performing which of the following as a comparative?
    A. Pulsed wave Doppler (PWD) of LV inflow with sample volume placed 1 cm distal to mitral annulus.
    B. PWD of RV inflow.
    C. Continuous wave Doppler of LV inflow.
    D. Continuous wave Doppler of RV inflow.
    E. PWD of pulmonary vein.

12. A diastolic Doppler examination includes tissue Doppler imaging (TDI) of the lateral and septal mitral annuli. A common operator error is careless sample volume placement at which location?
    A. LV apical segment.
    B. LV mid ventricular segment.
    C. LV basal segment.
    D. RV septal annulus.
    E. RV basal segment.

13. If left atrial enlargement is observed with no evidence of valvular disease, the sonographer should perform which of the following to further evaluate the etiology?
    A. Agitated saline contrast injection.
    B. LV opacification contrast injection.
    C. Diastolic function assessment.
    D. Stress echocardiography.
    E. Valsalva maneuver.

14. The sonographer should do which of the following to more accurately locate the mitral regurgitant orifice when collecting image data to calculate the proximal isovelocity surface area (PISA)?
    A. Decrease the depth resulting in better resolution of the mitral valve.
    B. Shift the color Doppler velocity baseline to approximately 80 cm/s.
    C. Shift the color Doppler velocity baseline to approximately 40 cm/s.
    D. Decrease the mechanical index (MI) to the range of 0.1–0.8.
    E. Freeze the color Doppler image, toggle color Doppler on and off revealing the 2D image to locate the orifice.

15. In which of the following scenarios should the sonographer use the fundamental image mode instead of the harmonic image mode?
    A. Thin patient with technically difficult images.
    B. Obese patient with technically difficult images.
    C. Chronic obstructive pulmonary disease patient.
    D. Patient with pectus excavatum.
    E. There is no specific condition to exclusively use fundamental mode.

16. The parasternal images in Figure 6-1 were obtained in diastole and systole. From which intercostal space should standard images ideally be obtained?

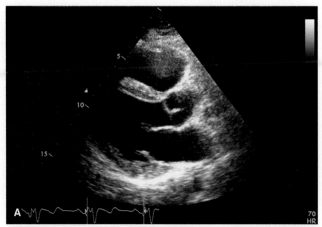

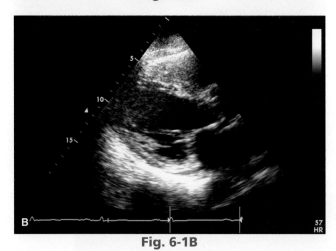

Fig. 6-1A

Fig. 6-1B

A. The third intercostal space.
B. The fourth intercostal space.
C. The fifth intercostal space.
D. The sixth intercostal space.
E. The highest intercostal space possible.

17. What technical difference is seen in these apical images between Figure 6-2A and B versus Figure 6-2C and D that will result in differing determination of the ejection fraction.

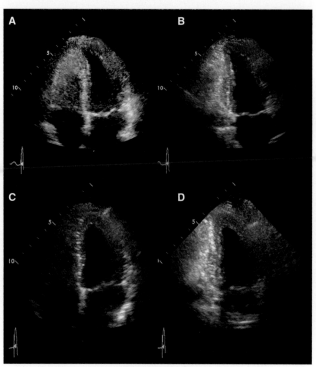

Fig. 6-2A–D

A. Poor visualization of endocardial borders in the sector near field.
B. Foreshortening of the LV apex in A and B.
C. Foreshortening of the LV apex in C and D.
D. Too much depth.
E. Image sector too narrow.

18. During which stage of the cardiac cycle were the apical images in Figure 6-3 obtained to measure left atrial volume?

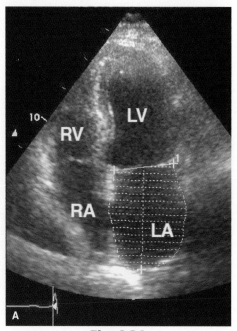

Fig. 6-3A

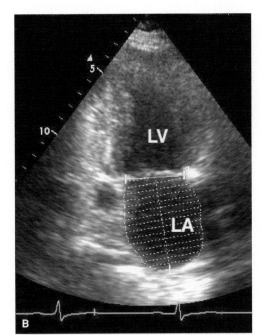

Fig. 6-3B

A. Ventricular end systole.
B. Ventricular mid systole.
C. Ventricular end diastole.
D. Ventricular mid diastole.
E. Atrial end systole.

19. Which of the following PWD images in Figure 6-4 demonstrates the most accurate technique?

A. Panel A.
B. Panel B.
C. Panel C.

20. What common mistake is made acquiring Doppler data of RV inflow in the apical four-chamber image, as in Figure 6-5?

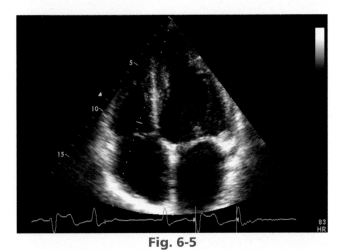

Fig. 6-5

A. Doppler sample volume size is too small.
B. Color Doppler gain setting is too high.
C. Doppler sweep speed is too fast.
D. Misaligned Doppler cursor.
E. 2D image depth is too deep.

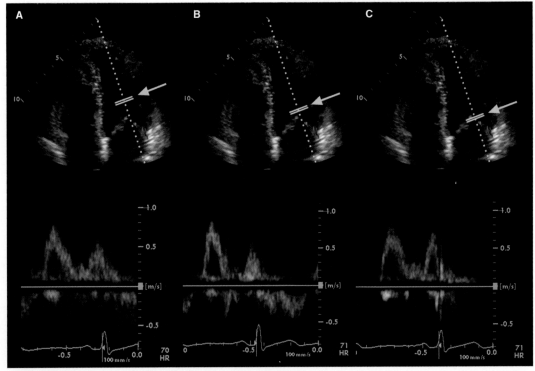

Fig. 6-4A–C

21. Which of the following maneuvers best explains the difference in mitral inflow pattern between Figure 6-6A and Figure 6-6B?

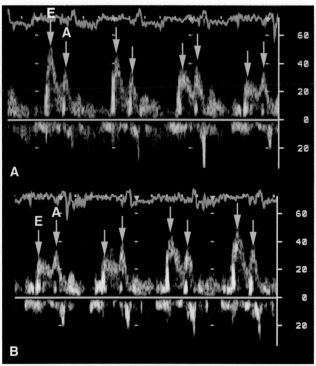

Fig. 6-6A–B

A. Figure 6-6A is performed with leg elevation and Figure 6-6B with lowering of the legs to the supine position.

B. Figure 6-6A is performed while giving fluids and Figure 6-6B while giving a diuretic.

C. Figure 6-6A is the baseline and Figure 6-6B is performed with the Valsalva maneuver.

D. Figure 6-6A is performed with the Valsalva maneuver and Figure 6-6B after reversal from Valsalva.

22. Which of the following statements best describes the most optimal technique for pulmonary vein flow, explaining the difference between Figure 6-7A and Figure 6-7B?

A. Figure 6-7A, sample volume size was 1–2 mm, placed at the junction of the LA and pulmonary vein.

B. Figure 6-7B, sample volume size was 3–4 mm, placed at the junction of the LA and pulmonary vein.

C. Figure 6-7A, sample volume size was 1–2 mm, placed 1 cm into the pulmonary vein.

D. Figure 6-7B, sample volume size was 3–4 mm, placed 1 cm into the pulmonary vein.

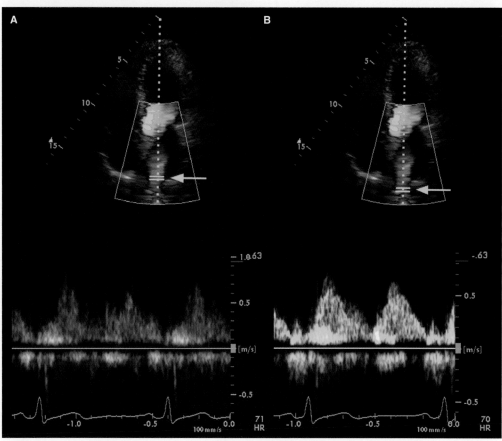

Fig. 6-7A–B

23. What images are obtained in this patient with aortic regurgitation (Fig. 6-8)?

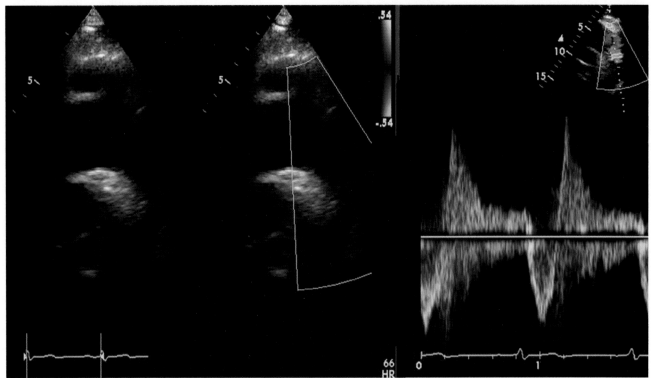

Fig. 6-8

A. High right parasternal 2D and pulsed Doppler.
B. High right parasternal 2D and continuous wave Doppler.
C. Suprasternal notch 2D and continuous wave Doppler.
D. Suprasternal notch 2D and PWD.

24. Which of the following Doppler tissue images of the lateral and septal mitral annulus are correct (Fig. 6-9)?
A. A and C are correct.
B. B and D are correct.
C. A and C and B and D are correct and should be averaged.

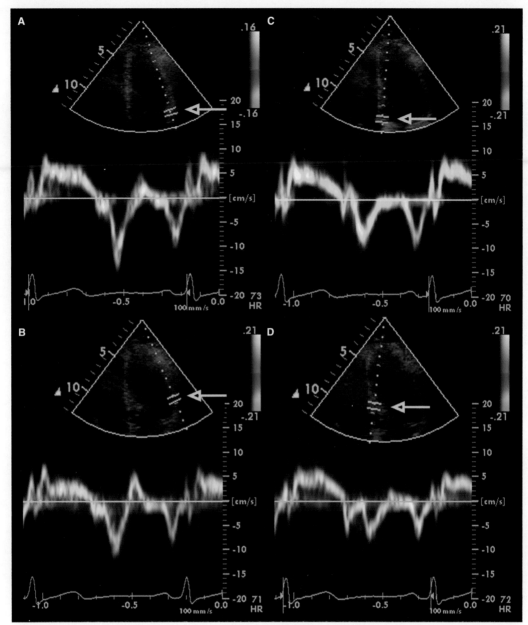

Fig. 6-9A–D

25. What is the cause of poor echo contrast effect in the apical region of this four-chamber view (Fig. 6-10)?
    A. Image artifact.
    B. Papillary muscle.
    C. Large trabeculation.
    D. Time gain settings are too low.
    E. MI setting is too high.

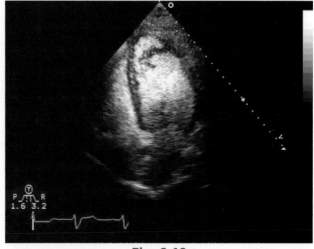

Fig. 6-10

ANSWERS

1. ANSWER: E. Patient positioning can significantly impact image quality helping to place the heart closer to the chest wall and stretching the intercostal spaces. The sonographer should position the patient in a steep left lateral decubitus position with the left arm extended up. This position helps bring the heart closer to the chest wall and subsequently closer to the transducer. The sonographer will then attempt to image the parasternal long- and short-axis views from the highest possible intercostal space. Depending on the patient's chest configuration, the third, fourth, or fifth intercostal space may be the highest and most appropriate. Patients with pectus excavatum are likely to a have lower left parasternal window. The goal is to obtain the tomographically correct view where cardiac structures are perpendicular or 90 degrees in relationship to the ultrasound beam. The sonographer should always attempt imaging from a high parasternal view and moving down an intercostal space at a time until the correct intercostal space is achieved.

2. ANSWER: C. Imaging artifacts commonly result from acoustic shadowing, reverberations, and a low signal-to-noise ratio as well as other contributors. The finding in question must be visualized in at least two image views to rule out image artifact as well as to demonstrate accurate anatomy.

3. ANSWER: B. Some patients are technically difficult to image from the parasternal long- and short-axis windows. This can limit interpretation due to the lack of parasternal image data. The apical long-axis is an acceptable alternative view to the parasternal long-axis view because anatomy in the apical long-axis view is identical to the parasternal long-axis view with the added "bonus" of visualization of the apical segments. This view might be difficult to obtain in tall thin patients.

4. ANSWER: A. The sonographer can easily obtain image data of the RV inflow (tricuspid inflow) and RV outflow (pulmonic outflow). The RV inflow is obtained by tilting the transducer inferiorly and medially from the original parasternal long-axis view. The sonographer may image the RV inflow from the same intercostal space, as the parasternal long-axis view of the LV or the sonographer might be required to move one intercostal space lower to optimize the RV inflow view.

The RV outflow view from the parasternal long-axis position is obtained by simply tilting the transducer in the opposite, lateral direction to visualize the RV outflow.

These two views are often forgotten; however, they are particularly helpful for adding valuable information about the right heart.

5. ANSWER: B. The transthoracic apical window is best for evaluating the true apical region of the LV. The apical region is mostly likely to develop an aneurysm after a myocardial infarction as well as apical thrombi formation. Interrogation of the apical region from the apical four-chamber, apical two-chamber and apical long-axis views places the ventricular apex in the ultrasound near field, further enhancing visualization of the apical region. The sonographer can gain additional information by including parasternal apical short-axis images. This view is achieved by aiming the transducer toward the apex while panning the apical segments. This is particularly helpful in further assessing or ruling out apical thrombi.

6. ANSWER: B. The parasternal short-axis view includes this series of images (1) LV apical level; (2) LV papillary muscles level; (3) LV basal level; (4) mitral valve view; and (5) the aortic, pulmonic, and tricuspid valves view.

7. ANSWER: C. Decreased wall motion is described as hypokinesis, which is seen as reduced muscle thickening relative to normal segments. This may contribute to LV remodeling and/or a reduced EF. Akinetic wall motion describes the absence of significant wall motion and dyskinetic wall motion means that the segment is moving outward during systole.

8. ANSWER: B. Assessment of left atrial function includes a measure of left atrial volume. The sonographer should collect apical four-chamber and two-chamber views maximizing the left atrial size. Accurate assessment of the left atrial volume requires tracing the maximum size of the LA in both the four- and two-chamber views at end ventricular systole. At this point in time, the LA will be at its maximum size.

9. ANSWER: D. Subcostal views add additional information especially when parasternal views are technically difficult. The sonographer can obtain images from beneath the rib cage resulting in the four-chamber plane. This is an excellent window for evaluating the atrial septum because the septum is perpendicular to the ultrasound beam. The sonographer can rotate the transducer counterclockwise approximately 90 degrees resulting in short-axis views. To improve visualization of the heart in the subcostal views, the sonographer can instruct the patient to "inhale and hold" for as long as the patient can tolerate. This held inhalation maneuver lowers the diaphragm and pulls the heart toward the transducer bringing the heart closer to the transducer resulting in improved images.

10. ANSWER: E. MVP is a common valvular abnormality observed on echocardiographic examination and is defined as displacement of the mitral valve leaflet(s) breaking the annulus plane into the LA. The parasternal long-axis view places the mitral leaflets perpendicular to the ultrasound beam and therefore best reveals mitral valve leaflet motion. It also visualizes the superior portion of the annulus which has a saddle-shaped geometry. The apical four-chamber view should not be used as a sole image to diagnose MVP because the inferior portion of the annulus is seen. This can lead to over diagnosis of MVP.

11. *ANSWER: C.* Accurate Doppler data is critical to diagnosing diastolic dysfunction. PWD velocity of LV inflow (peak E wave) is routinely measured in a diastolic Doppler evaluation. Diastolic filling of the LV is obtained most accurately by placing the PWD sample volume at the tips of the mitral valve leaflets. The goal is to obtain the highest or maximum peak E velocity measurement of the LV filling. To verify that peak E wave velocity has been acquired, the sonographer can juxtapose the PWD peak E wave to the continuous wave Doppler peak E wave of LV inflow. The sonographer should search for the maximum velocity and can use continuous wave Doppler as an aid in determining the maximum velocity.

12. *ANSWER: C.* TDI must be collected from the mitral annulus when assessing diastolic function. The LV lateral and septal basal segments are sometimes sampled in error. The sonographer must take care to ensure that the sample volume is appropriately placed in the annulus region as opposed to the basal segment which is commonly used for assessing LV dyssynchrony.

13. *ANSWER: C.* Chronically elevated LV end diastolic and left atrial pressures eventually lead to atrial enlargement. The sonographer should be suspicious of diastolic dysfunction when left atrial or bi-atrial enlargement is observed with no evidence for valve disease. The left and right atria should be appropriately planimetered to report maximum volume measurements and a complete diastolic echocardiographic assessment.

14. *ANSWER: E.* Quantification of mitral regurgitation includes obtaining the PISA. A component of PISA is the aliasing radius diameter. The sonographer must accurately locate the regurgitant orifice to correctly measure the color Doppler aliasing radius. It is often easy to observe the color Doppler contour; however, it may be difficult to observe the orifice itself. The sonographer can freeze the optimal color Doppler contour image then simply remove the color display from the image. The sonographer should locate the regurgitant orifice and place the first cursor, then return the color display and place the second cursor at the first aliasing velocity.

15. *ANSWER: E.* There is no specific condition to exclusively use the fundamental mode. Resolution is critical to collecting high-quality images. Using higher-frequency transducers will provide better axial, and lateral resolution, however, may result in increased attenuation during tissue propagation. There is a trade-off between high spatial resolution and sensitivity for interrogating structures in the far field or deeper in the body. The sonographer should tailor each exam specific to each patient's requirements. Depending on pathology, an exam may include both harmonic and fundamental imaging and keeping in mind that high-resolution results in a loss of penetration and low-resolution results in greater penetration.

16. *ANSWER: E.* A standard transthoracic echocardiographic exam traditionally begins with the left parasternal long-axis view. The goal is to place the transducer in such a way that the ultrasound transects the long-axis of the heart where resulting images yield accurate tomographic planes for analysis. In most cases, the highest intercostal space possible will yield the accurate imaging plane. The sonographer should sample the image from several intercostal spaces using the highest space, potentially up to the third intercostal space.

17. *ANSWER: C.* Echocardiographic assessment of LV function typically includes a measure of EF% acquired from the apical four- and two-chamber views. A common scanning error is foreshortening of the LV apex resulting in under reporting the volume measurements. An accurate apical image plane reveals a somewhat "pointed" appearance as demonstrated in Figure 6-2A and B rather than a "rounded" appearance with the apical segments contracting toward each other as demonstrated in Figure 6-2C and D. In a foreshortened plane, the apex will appear rounded with apical segments contracting toward the mitral valve. The sonographer should attempt imaging from a lower apical intercostal space and move the transducer to a slightly more lateral position. As well, the sonographer may reposition the patient to either a steeper or lower lateral decubitus position depending on individual results.

Figure 6-11 demonstrates an accurate EF measurement resulting from accurate apical image planes.

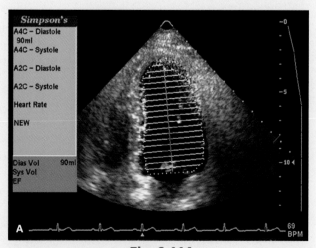

Fig. 6-11A

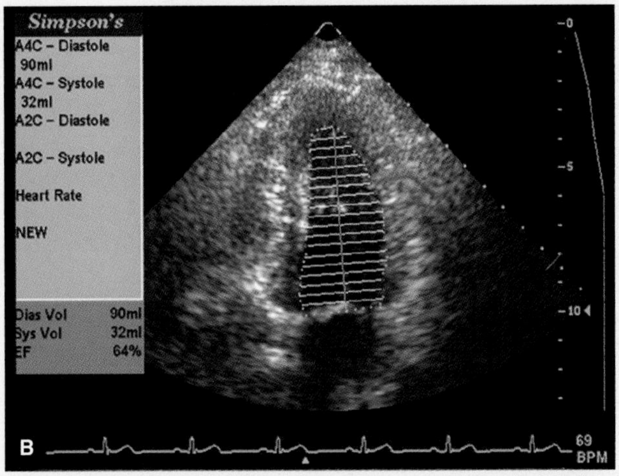

Fig. 6-11B

18. ANSWER: A. Measurement of left atrial volume is performed by tracing the LA in the apical four- and two-chamber views. The sonographer should scroll through the cardiac cycle locating ventricular end systole where the LA is largest. The left atrial chamber is traced starting at one mitral annulus and tracing along the internal atrial border until reaching the opposing mitral annulus. Allow the automatic volume-tracing feature to "close" the loop completing the volume measure by connecting both annuli with a straight line. Note that the tenting areas of the mitral valve as well as pulmonary veins are not included in the left atrial volume measurements. Attention to these details is critical in reporting accurate atrial volumes.

19. ANSWER: B. LV inflow Doppler assessment is a main stay of a diastolic function examination. The sonographer should place a 1–3 mm PWD sample volume at the tips of the mitral valve and using slight manipulations moving the sample volume placement until the maximum peak E wave velocity is located.

The goal is to obtain the highest E velocity profile as demonstrated in Figure 6-4B. Note that in Figure 6-4C, the A wave increases in size and the sample volume is placed closer to the mitral annulus. This sample volume placement is only appropriate and correct for the timing measurement of the A-wave duration.

Figure 6-4A demonstrates PWD sample volume too far from the mitral leaflet tips. Figure 6-4B demonstrates PWD sample volume appropriately placed at the mitral leaflet tips. Figure 6-4C demonstrates PWD sample volume too close to the mitral annulus.

See Table 6-1 for a listing of Diastolic Function Exam System Settings.

20. ANSWER: D. Collection of RV inflow Doppler and tricuspid regurgitation Doppler data requires accurate alignment of the Doppler cursor. Consistent with Doppler

TABLE 6-1 Diastolic Function Exam System Settings

Observation	View	Modality	Sample Volume Placement or Cursor Placement	Sample Volume Size (mm)	Velocity Filter (Hz)	Sweep Speed (mm/sec)
Left heart						
LA size (volume/area)	A4Ch or A2Ch	2D				
LV inflow	A4Ch	PWD	SV between mitral valve leaflet tips	1–3	200	50 or 100
A-wave duration	A4Ch	PWD	SV 5 mm nearer to mitral annulus than where sampled for LV inflow	1–3	200	50 or 100
PV flow	A4Ch	PWD	SV 1 cm into pulmonary vein	3–4	200	50 or 100
LV inflow CMM	A4Ch	CMM	Activate color Doppler in LV. Cursor placement in highest velocity color signal. Activate M-mode			100
IVRT	Between A4Ch and A5Ch	PWD or CWD	Cursor placement intermediate between LV inflow and LV outflow		200–400	100
MV lateral annulus	A4Ch	TDI	SV lateral mitral annulus	5	100	50 or 100
MV medial annulus	A4Ch	TDI	SV medial mitral annulus	5	100	50 or 100

A2Ch, apical two chamber; A4Ch, apical four chamber; A5Ch, apical five chamber; CMM, color M-mode; CWD, continuous wave Doppler; Hz, Hertz; IVRT, isovolumic relaxation time; LA, left atrium; LV, left ventricle; mm, millimeter; MV, mitral valve; PV, pulmonary vein; PWD, pulsed wave Doppler; sec, second; SV, sample volume; 2D, two dimensional.

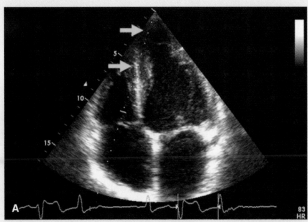

Fig. 6-12A

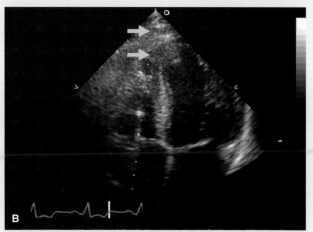

Fig. 6-12B

principles, the Doppler cursor must be as parallel to RV inflow as possible. Correct Doppler cursor alignment, both continuous and pulsed wave, will yield a clean spectral display as well as the maximum peak Doppler velocities. Figure 6-12A shows misalignment of the Doppler cursor and Figure 6-12B shows more optimal alignment.

21. ANSWER: D. To differentiate normal diastolic function from pseudonormal diastolic dysfunction, the sonographer can perform a Valsalva maneuver. The purpose of the Valsalva maneuver is to reveal the true A wave velocity or atrial contribution. Pseudonormal pattern is reflective of an E wave velocity greater than A wave velocity and indicative of elevated LV filling pressures and prolonged relaxation. The E wave has a deceleration time that is similar to normal. During Valsalva, the preload and LV filling pressures are reduced and the E wave gradually reduces velocity, whereas the A wave increases velocity signaling a pseudonormal filling pattern. Note in Figure 6-6 the E and A wave reversal during Valsalva in Panel A that reverses after recovery from Valsalva in Panel B.

22. ANSWER: D. Assessing pulmonary vein data correctly requires that the sample volume be 3–4 mm

in size and placed at least 1 cm into the pulmonary vein.

Figure 6-7 demonstrates the use of color Doppler to guide placement of the PWD sample volume. Search for the red "flame" appearance that represents left atrial filling from the pulmonary vein.

Panel A demonstrates the incorrect placement of the sample volume at the junction of the LA and the pulmonary vein which results in poor Doppler profile that is contaminated by flow within the LA. Panel B demonstrates a high quality Doppler profile that resulted from placing the 3–4 mm sample volume at minimum 1 cm into the pulmonary vein.

23. ANSWER: D. Aortic regurgitation can be quantified by evidence of LV volume overload, color flow Doppler, continuous wave Doppler, as well as PWD of blood flow in the descending aorta from the suprasternal notch. The sonographer adds valuable supporting information by interrogating the descending aorta for holodiastolic flow reversal using pulsed Doppler, which would indicate signification aortic regurgitation (Fig. 6-13).

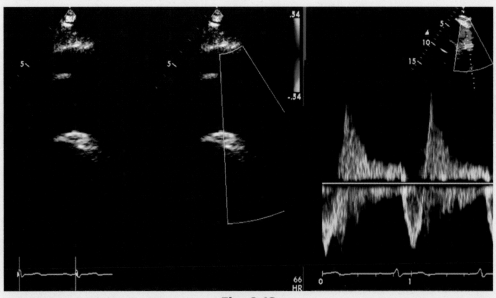

Fig. 6-13

24. ANSWER A. TDI is an integral component of a diastolic echocardiographic assessment. In the apical four-chamber or two-chamber view, the sonographer should place the TDI sample volume on the mitral annulus of interest avoiding the basal segment of the LV. When the TDI sample volume is appropriately placed on the annulus, the e' and a' profiles will reflect peak annular velocities below the zero baseline. The velocity profile is below the baseline reflective of annular tissue velocity away from the transducer in the apical views. If the TDI sample volume is erroneously placed on the basal segment, the velocity profile will continue to be displayed below the baseline; however, the É and Á velocity profiles will be blunted not representing the peak velocity.

Note in Figure 6-9 B and D the blunted é peak velocity as compared with the true é peak velocity in Figure 6-9A and C.

Figure 6-9A demonstrates a TDI sample volume that is correctly placed at basal lateral annulus.

Figure 6-9B demonstrates a TDI sample volume that is incorrectly placed at the basal lateral annulus.

Figure 6-9C demonstrates a TDI sample volume that is correctly placed at the basal septal segment.

Figure 6-9D demonstrates a TDI sample volume that is incorrectly placed at the basal septal segment.

25. ANSWER E. Echo contrast is an effective tool when used correctly to improve visualization of cardiac structures as well as improve reader confidence in technically difficult images. In this apical four-chamber example of LV opacification, the apical portion of the LV chamber is poorly opacified. Poor LV opacification in the apical region is most likely attributed to a high MI setting and has been described as a "swirling effect." The contrast microspheres are rapidly destroyed when the MI is too high while imaging the apical views. The destruction occurs primarily in the apical region of the LV chamber because it is closest to the transducer thus resulting in microsphere destruction. Contrast replenishment in the apical region is not fast enough which results in a contrast/noncontrast "swirling" appearance. In general, the recommended range settings for MI during LV opacification is between 0.1 and 0.8.

Note in Figure 6-10 that the MI setting is 0.7 resulting in a contrast/noncontrast "swirling" appearance. In this case, the sonographer should have continued to decrease the MI until the "swirling effect" is no longer visualized.

SUGGESTED READINGS

Anderson RH, Ho SY, Brecker SJ. Anatomic basis of cross-sectional echocardiography. *Heart.* 2001;85:716–720.

Baumgartner H, Hung J, Bermejo J, et al. Echocardiographic assessment of valve stenosis EAE/ASE recommendations for clinical practice. *J Am Soc Echocardiogr.* 2009;22:1–23.

Bierig SM, Ehler D, Knoll ML, et al. Minimum standards for the cardiac sonographer: a position paper. ASECHO.ORG, November 2005 http//www.asefiles.org/sonographerminimumstandards.pdf. Accessed July 14, 2009.

Gorcsan J III, Abraham T, Agler DA, et al. Echocardiography for cardiac resynchronization therapy recommendations for performance and reporting: a report from the American Society of Echocardiography Dyssynchrony Writing Group endorsed by the Heart Rhythm Society. *J Am Soc Echocardiogr.* 2008;21:191–213.

Lang RM, Bierig M, Devereux RB, et al. Recommendations for chamber quantification: a report from the American Society of Echocardiography's Guidelines and Standards Committee and the Chamber Quantification Writing Group, developed in conjunction with the European Association of Echocardiography, a branch of the European Society of Cardiology. *J Am Soc Echocardiogr.* 2005;18:1440–1463.

Mulvagh SL, Rakowski CH, Vannan MA, et al. American Society of Echocardiography Consensus Statement on the Clinical Applications of Ultrasonic Contrast Agents in Echocardiography. *J Am Soc Echocardiogr.* 2008;21:1179–1201.

Nagueh SF, Appleton CP, Gillebert TC, et al. Recommendations for the evaluation of left ventricular diastolic function by echocardiography. *J Am Soc Echocardiogr.* 2009;22:107–133.

Quiñones MA, Otto CM, Stoddard M, et al. Recommendations for quantification of Doppler echocardiography: a report from the Doppler quantification task force of the nomenclature and standards committee of the American Society of Echocardiography. *J Am Soc Echocardiogr.* 2002;15:167–184.

Waggoner AD, Ehler D, Adams D, et al. Guidelines for the cardiac sonographer in the performance of contrast echocardiography recommendations of the American Society of Echocardiography Council on Cardiac Sonography. *J Am Soc Echocardiogr.* 2001;14:417–420.

Zoghbi WA, Enriquez-Sarano M, Foster E, et al. Recommendations for evaluation of the severity of native valvular regurgitation with two-dimensional and Doppler echocardiography. *J Am Soc Echocardiogr.* 2003;16:777–802.

Doppler and Hemodynamics

Muhamed Saric and Itzhak Kronzon

1. On echocardiography, the diameter of the inferior vena cava is measured at 1.6 cm during expiration and 0.6 cm after the patient is asked to sniff. The right atrial pressure is estimated at:
   A. 0–5 mm Hg.
   B. 5–10 mm Hg.
   C. 10–20 mm Hg.
   D. Indeterminate.

2. A 32-year-old woman is referred for evaluation of rheumatic mitral valve stenosis. No mitral regurgitation was noted. The following values were obtained by Doppler echocardiography:

TABLE 7-1

E-wave deceleration time	910 msec
Mean diastolic mitral gradient	17 mm Hg
Diastolic mitral inflow velocity-time integral	66 cm
Heart rate	85 bpm

   The following statement is TRUE:
   A. Mitral valve area can be calculated by dividing 220 into deceleration time.
   B. Stroke volume across the mitral valve is 72 ml per beat.
   C. Pressure half-time is 355 msec.
   D. Mitral valve area is 0.8 cm^2.

E. During exertion, her mean gradient is expected to decrease.

3. A 21-year-old man with dyspnea on exertion and enlarged pulmonary artery on chest X-ray underwent transthoracic echocardiography. The study revealed patent ductus arteriosus (PDA) and the following:

TABLE 7-2

Left ventricular outflow tract (LVOT) diameter	2.0 cm
LVOT velocity-time integral	31 cm
Right ventricular outflow tract (RVOT) diameter	2.5 cm
RVOT velocity-time integral	12 cm
Heart rate	80 bpm

   The following statement is TRUE:
   A. Systemic blood flow (*Qs*) is 7.8 l/minute.
   B. The ratio of pulmonic to systemic blood flow (*Qp:Qs*) is less than one.
   C. Stroke volume entering the lungs is 38 ml per beat.
   D. Patient is cyanotic in the lower parts of the body.
   E. The ratio of stroke volume through the left ventricular outflow tract (LVOT) and the stroke volume through the right ventricular outflow tract (RVOT) is equal to the *Qp:Qs* ratio in this patient.

4. A 39-year-old woman was admitted for severe shortness of breath on exertion. On transthoracic echocardiogram, there was mild pulmonic regurgitation. Continuous-wave spectral Doppler tracings of the pulmonic regurgitant jet reveal the following:

TABLE 7-3

Early diastolic peak velocity	3.0 m/sec
End-diastolic velocity	2.0 m/sec

Examination of the inferior vena cava by M-mode echocardiography demonstrated the following:

TABLE 7-4

IVC diameter during expiration	2.6 cm
IVC diameter during inspiration	2.6 cm

The following statement is TRUE:
A. Right atrial pressure is estimated at 6 mm Hg.
B. Pulmonary artery diastolic pressure is approximately 31 mm Hg.
C. Pulmonary artery diastolic pressure is 36 mm Hg minus the right atrial pressure.
D. Pulmonary artery diastolic pressure cannot be assessed if the pulmonic regurgitation is only mild.
E. Pulmonary artery diastolic pressure is normal.

5. A 42-year-old man was admitted to the hospital after a 1-month history of intermittent fever and progressive shortness of breath. Blood cultures grew *Streptococcus viridans*. On transesophageal echocardiogram, perforation of the anterior mitral leaflet and mitral regurgitation were seen. On color Doppler imaging, a well-formed flow convergence proximal isovelocity surface area (PISA) shell was visualized on the ventricular side of the mitral valve in systole. In addition, the following was noted:

TABLE 7-5

Maximal mitral regurgitation PISA radius	1.0 cm
Aliasing velocity at which PISA radius measured	45 cm/sec
Peak velocity of mitral regurgitation jet	500 cm/sec
Velocity-time integral of mitral regurgitation	140 cm

The following statement is TRUE:
A. Vena contracta of the mitral regurgitant flow is expected to be less than 0.3 cm.
B. Effective regurgitant orifice area of mitral regurgitation is approximately 0.6 cm^2.
C. Instantaneous flow rate across the mitral valve using the PISA method is 70 ml per second.
D. Mitral regurgitation is moderate (2+).
E. Regurgitant volume is 40 ml/beat.

6. An 84-year-old obese woman with a history of hypertension and chronic renal insufficiency became very short of breath at a rehabilitation facility 2 weeks after elective hip replacement. Transthoracic echocardiogram revealed normal left ventricular systolic function, no mitral or aortic valve disease, and the following:

TABLE 7-6

Peak velocity of the mitral E wave	125 cm/sec
Flow propagation velocity of mitral inflow on color M mode	31 cm/sec
Peak velocity of tricuspid regurgitant jet	4 m/sec
Estimated right atrial pressure	15 mm Hg

The following statement is TRUE:
A. Mean pulmonary artery wedge pressure is markedly elevated.
B. On mitral inflow, E to A ratio is expected to be less than 1.
C. Pulmonary artery systolic pressure is 64 mm Hg.
D. The ratio of peak E-wave velocity to the peak medial mitral annular tissue Doppler velocity is expected to be less than 8.
E. Flow propagation velocity of mitral inflow on color M mode is normal for her age.

7. A 44-year-old man with a trileaflet aortic valve and a dilated aortic root measuring 5.5 cm at the level of sinuses of Valsalva is being evaluated for aortic regurgitation.
The following statement is TRUE:
A. Regurgitant fraction of 65% would indicate that the aortic regurgitation is severe.
B. Like the size of flow convergence (PISA) radius, the size of vena contracta is strongly influenced by Nyquist limit setting.

C. Vena contracta of at least 0.2 cm would indicate that the aortic regurgitation is severe.

D. Regurgitant volume of 30 ml per beat is consistent with severe aortic regurgitation.

E. Vena contracta obtained by 2D echocardiography can be used to calculate regurgitant volume.

8. A 62-year-old man with a history of treated hypertension, chronic atrial fibrillation, and bicuspid aortic valve had a transthoracic echocardiogram done. The study showed the following:

TABLE 7-7

Peak velocity of mitral regurgitant jet	6.0 m/sec
dP/dt of mitral regurgitant jet	1,900 mm Hg/sec
Ratio of peak mitral E wave to peak velocity of medial mitral annulus (E/e')	16
Vena contracta of mitral regurgitation	0.2 cm

Systemic blood pressure at the time of the study was 120/70 mm Hg.

The following statement is TRUE:

A. Peak-to-peak aortic gradient is 90 mm Hg.

B. Patient is in cardiogenic shock due to left ventricular systolic dysfunction.

C. Mean left atrial pressure is approximately 20 mm Hg.

D. The size of vena contracta is diagnostic of severe mitral regurgitation.

E. Left atrial pressure cannot be estimated by the E/e' method in patients with atrial fibrillation.

9. A 67-year-old man with aortic regurgitation underwent transthoracic echocardiographic examination. There was no mitral stenosis or regurgitation. The following values were obtained:

TABLE 7-8

Peak diastolic velocity of aortic regurgitant jet	5.0 m/sec
End-diastolic velocity of aortic regurgitant jet	3.7 m/sec
Pressure half-time of aortic regurgitant jet	656 msec
Peak aortic antegrade flow velocity	2.2 m/sec
Blood pressure	130/65 mm Hg

Based on the above data, one can conclude:

A. Pressure half-time is consistent with severe aortic regurgitation.

B. Aortic valve area can be estimated as 220 divided by pressure half-time.

C. Peak left ventricular systolic pressure is lower than the systolic blood pressure.

D. Left ventricular end-diastolic pressure is estimated at 10 mm Hg.

E. Aortic valve area cannot be calculated using continuity equation because there is aortic regurgitation.

10. A 25-year-old woman is being evaluated for percutaneous closure of her secundum atrial septal defect (ASD). Transthoracic echocardiography demonstrated mild tricuspid regurgitation, no pulmonic stenosis, and the following:

TABLE 7-9

Pulmonary artery systolic pressure	65 mm Hg
Pulmonary artery diastolic pressure	35 mm Hg
Left atrial pressure	10 mm Hg
Right ventricular outflow tract (RVOT) diameter	2.6 cm
RVOT velocity-time integral	30 cm
Left ventricular outflow tract (LVOT) diameter	2.0 cm
LVOT velocity-time integral	20 cm
Heart rate	75 bpm

Based on the above data, one can conclude:

A. Patient should be advised against ASD closure because pulmonary hypertension is present.

B. Pulmonary vascular resistance is approximately 16 Wood units.

C. The ratio of pulmonary to systemic blood flow (Qp:Qs) is approximately 2.5:1.

D. Shunt flow is larger than the pulmonic flow (Qp).

E. Patient is cyanotic.

11. A 35-year-old woman was noted on clinical exam to have a systolic murmur and was referred for transthoracic echocardiography. The exam revealed perimembranous ventricular septal defect (VSD), mild tricuspid regurgitation, pulmonic stenosis, intact aortic valve, and the following:

TABLE 7-10

Blood pressure	120/80 mm Hg
Peak systolic velocity across the VSD	3.0 m/sec
End-diastolic velocity across the VSD	1.0 m/sec
Estimated right atrial pressure	10 mm Hg
Peak systolic gradient across pulmonic valve	55 mm Hg
Left ventricular end-diastolic pressure	12 mm Hg

The following statement is TRUE:
A. Right ventricular systolic pressure is 46 mm Hg.
B. Pulmonary artery systolic pressure is 29 mm Hg.
C. Right ventricular systolic pressure is 84 mm Hg above the right atrial pressure.
D. Pulmonary artery systolic pressure is 45 mm Hg higher than the right ventricular systolic pressure.
E. Right ventricular end-diastolic pressure is 28 mm Hg.

12. A 21-year-old college student is noted to have fixed splitting of the second heart sound and right bundle branch block.

Real-time three-dimensional transesophageal echocardiogram revealed a 1.2 cm secundum ASD that was circular in shape. On color Doppler, a well-formed hemispheric flow convergence (PISA) shell is seen on the left atrial side of the ASD. The following data were also obtained:

TABLE 7-11

Blood pressure	120/80 mm Hg
Heart rate	100 bpm
PISA radius	0.7 cm
Velocity-time integral of left-to-right flow across ASD	80 cm
Left ventricular outflow tract (LVOT) diameter	2.0 cm
LVOT velocity-time integral	19 cm

The following statement is true:
A. Ratio of pulmonic to systemic flow (Qp:Qs) is 1.8:1.0.
B. Shunt flow across the ASD is approximately 9.0 l/minute.
C. The difference between the pulmonic and systemic stroke volume is 180 ml.
D. Systemic stroke volume is 150 ml.
E. Pulmonic blood flow (Qp) is approximately 7.0 l/min.

13. A 35-year-old woman presented with sudden onset of dyspnea and pulmonary edema. She underwent bedside transthoracic echocardiography which revealed hyperdynamic left ventricular systolic function, normal aortic valve, and mitral regurgitation.

The following data were obtained at the time of transthoracic echocardiogram:

TABLE 7-12

Blood pressure	95/50 mm Hg
Heart rate	120 bpm
Peak velocity of mitral regurgitant jet	4.0 m/sec
Time interval from onset of mitral regurgitation to jet velocity of 1 m/sec	5 msec
Time interval from onset of mitral regurgitation to jet velocity of 3 m/sec	25 msec
Vena contracta of mitral regurgitation	0.8 cm

The following statement is TRUE:
A. Peak velocity of the mitral inflow E wave is expected to be low.
B. Left atrial pressure is low.
C. Pulmonary venous flow velocity pattern on spectral Doppler is likely to reveal flow reversal during early diastole.
D. Rate of pressure rise (*dP/dt*) in the left ventricle is 1,600 mm Hg per second.
E. Left ventricular systolic function is markedly diminished.

14. A 29-year-old Bangladeshi woman with rheumatic mitral stenosis is referred to the cardiac catheterization lab for percutaneous mitral balloon valvuloplasty. Upon placement of the pigtail catheter in the left ventricle, the following values were obtained:

TABLE 7-13

Left ventricular peak systolic pressure	124 mm Hg
Early left ventricular diastolic pressure	7 mm Hg
Left ventricular end-diastolic pressure	10 mm Hg

Transesophageal echocardiogram prior to valvuloplasty revealed the absence of both mitral and aortic regurgitation, as well as the following:

TABLE 7-14

Heart rate	104 bpm
Time-velocity integral of diastolic mitral flow	65 cm
Mean mitral valve gradient in diastole	21 mm Hg
Mitral pressure half-time	270 msec

The following statement is TRUE:
A. Mean left atrial pressure is expected to be lower than the mean left ventricular diastolic pressure.
B. Peak velocity of the mitral inflow E wave is expected to be low.
C. Pressure half-time may be unreliable in patients prior to valvuloplasty.
D. Mitral valve area is 0.6 cm^2.
E. Mean left atrial pressure is approximately 28 mm Hg.

15. An 81-year-old woman with a systolic heart murmur was referred for an echocardiogram. A heavily calcified aortic valve and normal mitral valve were noted on 2D imaging. Doppler echocardiography of the aortic valve revealed:

TABLE 7-15

Left ventricular outflow tract (LVOT) diameter	1.9 cm
Peak velocity across the aortic valve	5.0 m/sec
Peak LVOT velocity	1.0 m/sec
LVOT velocity-time integral (VTI)	20 cm

The following statement is TRUE:
A. Aortic valve area cannot be calculated because aortic valve velocity-time integral is not stated.
B. Aortic valve stenosis is subvalvular.

C. Aortic valve area is likely to be less than 1 cm^2.
D. Left ventricular stroke volume is 80 ml per beat.
E. Systolic blood pressure is approximately 100 mm Hg above the left ventricular systolic pressure.

16. This continuous-wave spectral Doppler tracing of the tricuspid regurgitant jet comes from an 18-year-old woman with pulmonic valve stenosis (Fig. 7-1). The peak pulmonic valve gradient is 24 mm Hg. Right atrial pressure is estimated at 10 mm Hg. The following is TRUE about this patient:

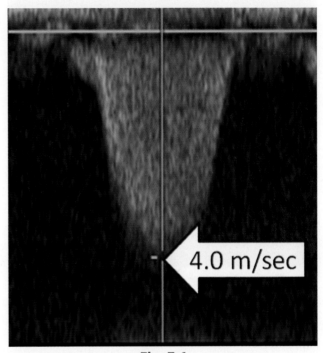

4.0 m/sec

Fig. 7-1

A. Peak pulmonary artery systolic pressure is higher than the right ventricular peak systolic pressure.
B. Right ventricular peak systolic pressure is 64 mm Hg above than the pulmonary artery peak systolic pressure.
C. Pulmonary artery peak systolic pressure is 50 mm Hg.
D. Right ventricular peak systolic pressure is 24 mm Hg less than the peak pulmonary artery systolic pressure.
E. Right ventricular peak systolic pressure is 108 mm Hg.

17. An 82-year-old man was referred for evaluation of a systolic ejection murmur. On parasternal long-axis view, the left ventricular outflow tract diameter was measured at 2.0 cm.

Spectral Doppler tracings were obtained in or through the left ventricular outflow tract in the apical 5-chamber view (Fig. 7-2).

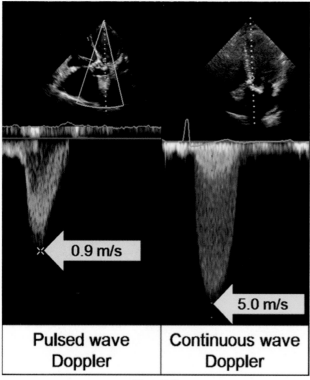

Fig. 7-2

The following statement is TRUE:
A. Increased cardiac output alone may explain the elevated gradient across the aortic valve.
B. Marked difference between the subvalvular and valvular velocities in this patient may also be seen in severe aortic regurgitation.
C. Patient has a very severe aortic valve stenosis with a mean gradient of approximately 60 mm Hg.
D. Aortic valve area is greater than 1.0 cm^2.
E. Patient has hypertrophic obstructive cardiomyopathy (HOCM).

18. The continuous-wave spectral Doppler tracing in Figure 7-3, from a 21-year-old woman represents the flow velocity profile in the main pulmonary artery. Based on this tracing, the following is TRUE about this patient:

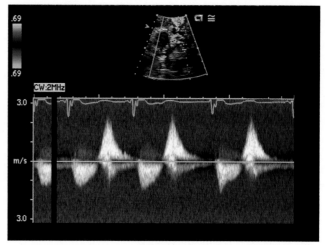

Fig. 7-3

A. End-diastolic gradient across the pulmonic valve is high.
B. There is severe pulmonic valve stenosis.
C. Pulmonary artery systolic pressure is 9 mm Hg above the right ventricular pressure.
D. Pulmonic valve regurgitation is severe.
E. The velocity profile is diagnostic of PDA.

19. The tracings in Figure 7-4 were obtained from an 82-year-old woman with a normal left ventricular ejection fraction of 65%. Figure 7-4A represents

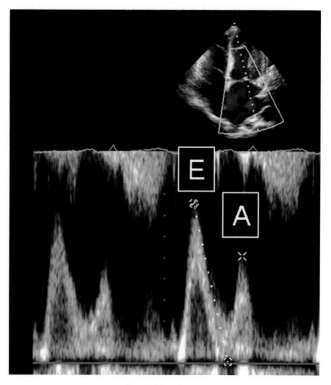

MITRAL INFLOW
Peak E wave velocity = 142 cm/s
E wave deceleration time = 148 msec
Fig. 7-4A

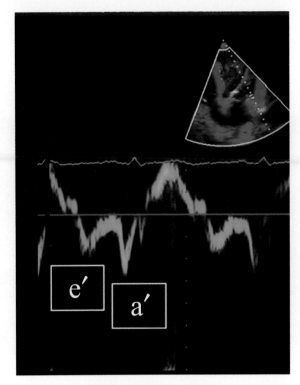

LATERAL MITRAL ANNULUS
Peak e′ velocity = 8 cm/sec
Peak a′ velocity = 10 cm/sec
Fig. 7-4B

MITRAL INFLOW

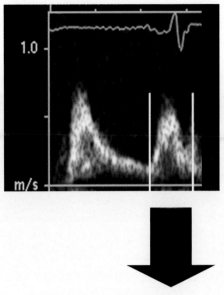

Mitral A wave duration = 170 msec
Fig. 7-5A

PULMONARY VENOUS FLOW

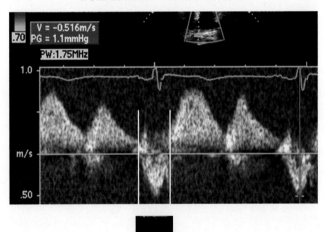

Atrial reversal wave
Duration = 210 msec; peak velocity 50 cm/sec
Fig. 7-5B

blood flow velocity pattern obtained by placing a pulsed Doppler sample volume at the mitral leaflet tips. Figure 7-4B represents tissue Doppler of the lateral mitral annulus.

Based on these two tracings, the following is TRUE:

A. The patient has excellent exercise capacity.
B. Abnormal left ventricular relaxation alone explains the mitral inflow pattern.
C. Left atrial pressure is elevated.
D. Patient has normal left ventricular diastolic function.
E. Mitral E-wave velocity is expected to increase following the Valsalva maneuver.

---

20. Figure 7-5A and B were obtained from the same patient at the same heart rate.

The following statement is TRUE:

A. Mitral inflow pattern is diagnostic of restrictive filling.
B. Left ventricular end-diastolic pressure is elevated.
C. The higher the peak velocity of the atrial reversal wave in pulmonary veins, the lower the left ventricular pressure.
D. The absence of atrial reversal wave in pulmonary vein tracings indicates pulmonary hypertension due to left ventricular dysfunction.
E. Ratio of peak systolic to peak diastolic velocity in pulmonary veins of more than 1 is indicative of elevated left atrial pressure.

21. Upward deflection in respirometry recordings indicates inspiration while the downward deflection indicates expiration (Fig. 7-6).

M Mode Recording in Short Axis at Papillary Muscle Level

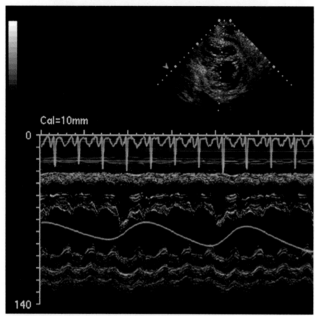

Fig. 7-6A

Hepatic Vein Pulsed Doppler

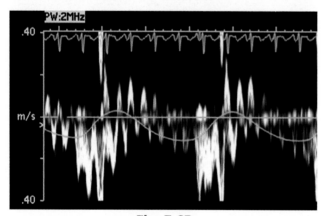

Fig. 7-6B

The following statement is TRUE:
A. There is no ventricular interdependence.
B. Expiratory increase in diastolic flow reversal in hepatic veins suggests constriction.
C. Abnormal interventricular septal motion is due to right ventricular volume overload.
D. Inspiratory increase in forward hepatic vein flow velocities is abnormal.
E. Above M-mode recordings are diagnostic of a large pericardial effusion and tamponade.

22. A 33-year-old man has had a murmur since childhood. The transthoracic spectral Doppler tracings in Figure 7-7 are obtained from the suprasternal view.

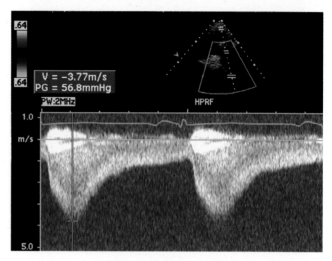

Peak systolic velocity 3.77 m/sec
End-diastolic velocity 1.0 msec
Fig. 7-7

The following statement is TRUE:
A. The pattern of diastolic flow is indicative of severe aortic regurgitation.
B. The tracings are diagnostic of aortic coarctation.
C. Quadricuspid aortic valve is the most common cause of aortic stenosis associated with the above flow velocity pattern.
D. The recordings are obtained from the ascending aorta and represent severe aortic stenosis.
E. Patient's blood pressure in the legs is markedly higher than in the arms.

23. A 91-year-old woman presents with severe shortness of breath. The two spectral Doppler recordings in Figure 7-8 were obtained from two different valves. The vertical line in each tracing marks the onset of QRS.

The following statement is TRUE:
A. Figure 7-8B represents a tricuspid regurgitant jet and the patient has severely elevated right ventricular systolic pressure.
B. Figure 7-8A represents severe aortic stenosis because the jet starts during the isovolumic contraction period.
C. The jet with the shorter duration represents aortic stenosis.

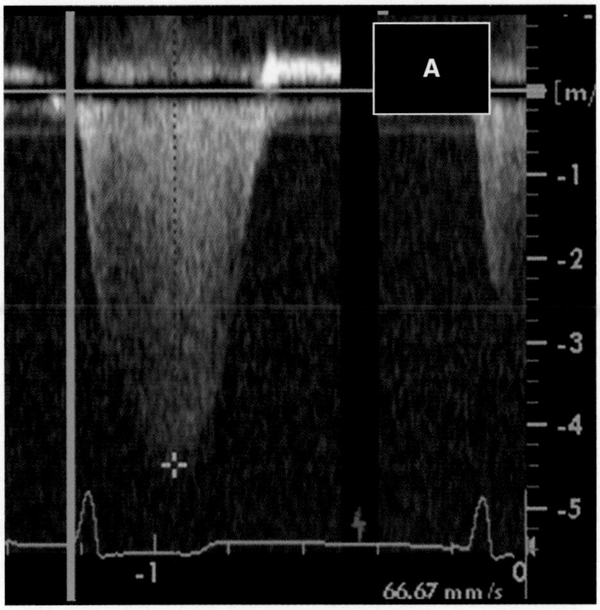

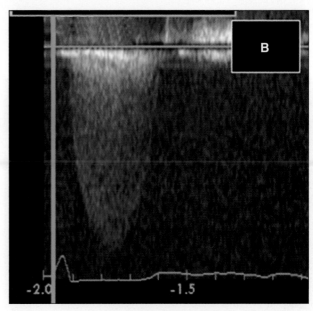

Peak velocity = 4.5 m/sec
Jet duration = 515 msec
Fig. 7-8A

Peak velocity = 5.0 m/sec
Jet duration = 345 msec
Fig. 7-8B

D. Peak velocity of 5.0 m/sec in Figure 7-8B is not compatible with a tricuspid regurgitant jet.

E. Systolic function of both ventricles is severely diminished.

---

24. A 55-year-old man with hypertension treated with a beta blocker, and advanced gastric carcinoma presents with sudden onset of severe shortness of breath. The spectral pulsed Doppler recordings in Figure 7-9 were obtained at the mitral leaflet tips. Upward deflection in respirometry recordings indicates inspiration while the downward deflection indicates expiration.

The following statement is TRUE:

A. Respiratory variations in peak velocity of late diastolic flow (A wave) of more than 25% favor constriction over tamponade.

B. Marked decrease in peak E-wave velocity seen at the onset of inspiration is consistent with the diagnosis of tamponade.

C. Findings are characteristic of restrictive cardiomyopathy.

D. The ratio of early to late diastolic peak mitral velocity (E/A ratio) of less than 1 favors the diagnosis of constrictive pericarditis.

E. Treatment with diuretics would markedly improve patient's shortness of breath.

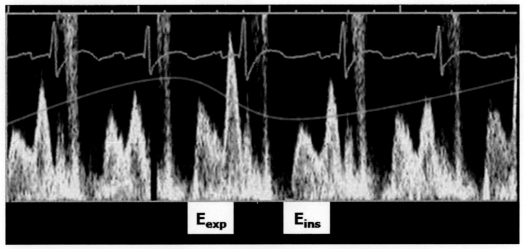

Expiratory peak E wave velocity (E_{exp}) = 170 cm/sec
Inspiratory peak E wave velocity (E_{ins}) = 110 cm/sec
E wave deceleration time = 260 msec
Fig. 7-9

25. 28-year-old man with liver disease presents with jugular venous distensions (Fig. 7-10).

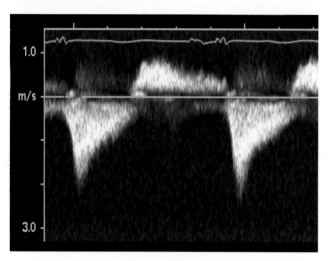

Peak velocity of tricuspid regurgitant jet = 2.2 m/sec

Fig. 7-10

The following statement is TRUE:

A. Right atrial pressure rises progressively towards the end of ventricular systole.

B. Right ventricular systolic function is markedly diminished.

C. Peak velocity of 2.2 m/sec excludes the diagnosis of pulmonary hypertension.

D. Tricuspid regurgitation is likely mild.

E. There is right ventricular midcavitary gradient during systole.

CASE 1:

A 78-year-old obese woman with a history of hypertension and poorly controlled diabetes mellitus developed progressive chest pain and shortness of breath for the past 2 days. She had no prior history of coronary revascularization or heart surgery. Her son brought her to the emergency department where she was noted to be diaphoretic and tachypneic.

Electrocardiogram in the emergency department revealed normal sinus rhythm, right bundle branch block, and ST elevations in anteroseptal leads.

Blood pressure 90/50 mm Hg; heart rate 100 beats per minute; oral temperature 98.7 degrees. On auscultation of the lungs, rales were noted bilaterally throughout the lung fields. The heart exam revealed prominent

S3 and no murmur. Serum troponin was elevated at 40 ng/ml (normal <5 ng/ml). There was marked pulmonary edema on chest X-ray.

Transthoracic echocardiogram at the time of presentation revealed hypokinesis of six left ventricular segments supplied by the left anterior descending artery; ejection fraction was estimated at 40%. There was mild regurgitation of a structurally normal native mitral valve.

26. The patient was transferred to the intensive care unit where a Swan-Ganz catheter was placed. Pulmonary artery wedge pressure was 38 mm Hg. Tissue Doppler of the medial mitral annulus and pulsed Doppler recordings with the sample volume at the tips of the mitral valve leaflets were obtained at that time. Patient was in normal sinus rhythm. Peak velocity of the early annular tissue Doppler wave (e′) was 5 cm/sec. Which of the following mitral flow velocity patterns is the most likely at this time?

A. Figure 7-11A.

B. Figure 7-11B.

C. Figure 7-11C.

D. Figure 7-11D.

E. Figure 7-11E.

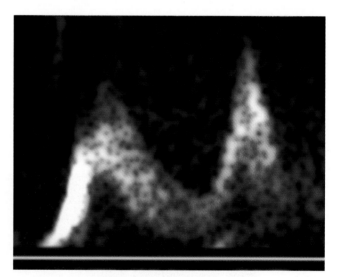

Peak E wave velocity = 45 cm/sec

Fig. 7-11A

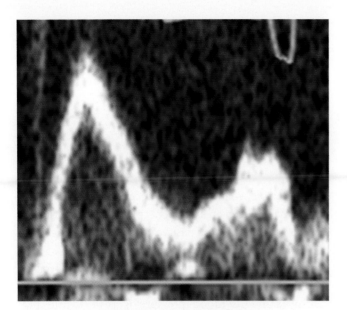

Peak E wave velocity = 60 cm/sec

Fig. 7-11B

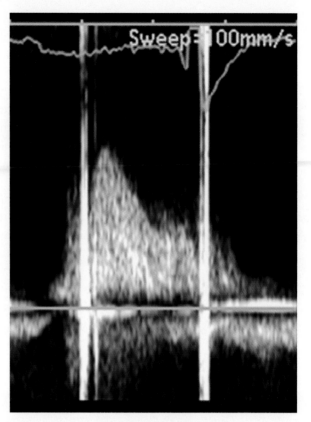

Peak E wave velocity = 200 cm/sec

Fig. 7-11D

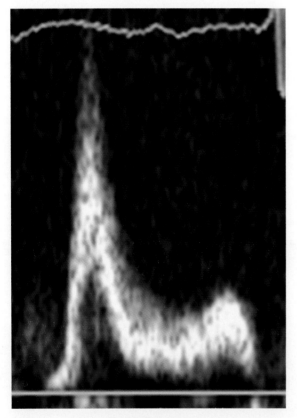

Peak E wave velocity = 150 cm/sec

Fig. 7-11C

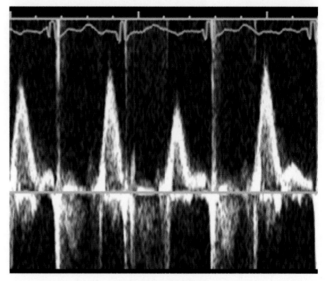

Peak E wave velocity varies from beat to beat (between 60 and 80 cm/sec)

Fig. 7-11E

27. From the emergency department, she was taken for coronary angiogram which revealed total occlusion of the proximal anterior descending artery and diffuse atherosclerosis in the left circumflex artery. Percutanous coronary intervention was attempted but the stent could not be deployed in the left anterior descending artery. She was then transferred to the intensive care unit. After appropriate medical therapy, she was discharged home free of symptoms on hospital day five.

Three days later, she collapsed. Her neighbor called 911 and the patient was intubated in the field for severe hypoxemia. On admission, she was afebrile. Laboratory data revealed normal white blood cell count. Chest X-ray in the emergency department demonstrated massive bilateral pulmonary edema. The following data were obtained by echocardiography the same day. (Fig. 7-12 and Video 7-1.)

TEE image of mitral valve in systole in midesophageal view

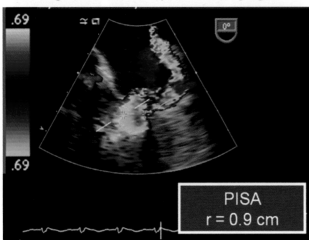

Color Doppler demonstrating PISA on the left ventricular side of the mitral valve; radius is 0.9 cm
Peak systolic velocity of mitral regurgitant jet is 4.2 m/sec

Fig. 7-12

The degree of mitral regurgitation is:
A. Trivial.
B. Mild (1+).
C. Moderate (2+).
D. Moderate to severe (3+).
E. Severe (4+).

28. The most likely etiology of mitral regurgitation in this patient is:
A. Papillary muscle rupture.
B. Bacterial endocarditis.
C. Mitral annular dilatation.
D. Rheumatic heart disease.
E. Mitral valve prolapse.

CASE 2:

A 56-year-old man who is a recent immigrant from Argentina has been an avid soccer player since childhood. He reports that over the past year or so, he no longer can run around the soccer field as he used to because of exertional dyspnea. He initially saw a pulmonary specialist who ruled out exercise-induced asthma.

On exam, his blood pressure is 170/70 mm Hg; heart rate 72 beats per minute with a regular rhythm; and room air oxygen saturation by pulse oxymetry 98%. He has no central or peripheral cyanosis. His lungs are clear. First heart sound (S1) is normal while the second heart sound (S2) is obscured by the continuous, machinery-type murmur best heard in the left upper chest. There is no peripheral edema.

Echocardiography revealed PDA, normal left ventricular systolic function, no valvular disease, and no hypertrophic cardiomyopathy. Right atrial pressure is estimated at 10 mm Hg.

29. The spectral Doppler tracing in Figure 7-13 represents flow across the PDA obtained by transthoracic echocardiography.

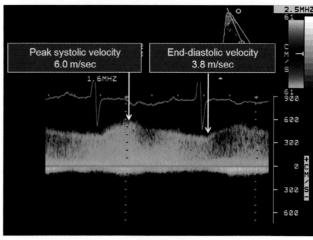

Fig. 7-13

The following statement is TRUE:

A. Pulmonary artery diastolic pressure is 21 mm Hg above the right atrial pressure.

B. The tracing was obtained by pulsed wave Doppler technique.

C. Pulmonary artery pressure is estimated at 26/12 mm Hg.

D. Pulmonary artery systolic pressure is 110 mm Hg.

E. PDA is very large because the flow occurs throughout the cardiac cycle.

30. This transthoracic echocardiographic color Doppler image in the parasternal short-axis view at the level of the PDA comes from the same study as the spectral tracing in previous question (Fig. 7-14).

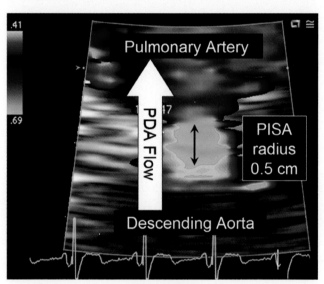

Fig. 7-14

Using the PISA method, the cross-sectional area of the PDA at its aortic end during maximum flow is:

A. 0.01 cm².

B. 0.13 cm².

C. 0.22 cm².

D. 1.3 cm².

E. 2.2 cm².

CASE 3:

A 24-year-old college athlete collapsed on the basketball court. The coach promptly used the automatic external defibrillator which delivered an apporopriate shock and revived the patient. The patient was then brought to the emergency department.

On physical examination, he was lying comfortably in bed, fully awake, and alert and oriented. Blood pressure 144/72 mm Hg; heart rate 64 beats per minute. Lungs were clear on auscultation. Cardiac exam revealed a crescendo-decrescendo systolic ejection murmur along the left sternal border which increased with Valsalva maneuver. The carotid upstroke was brisk and there was bisferient pulse.

31. Transthoracic echocardiogram performed in the emergency department demonstrated hypertrophic cardiomyopathy with asymmetric septal hypertrophy, systolic anterior motion, and normal left ventricular systolic function. Aortic valve was normal. Left atrial pressure was estimated at 10 mm Hg. There was eccentric mitral regurgitation; and the spectral Doppler of the mitral regurgitant jet is depicted in Figure 7-15.

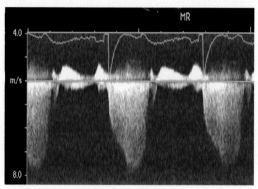

Peak velocity of mitral regurgitant jet = 8 m/sec
Fig. 7-15

The following statement is TRUE:

A. Envelope of the mitral regurgitant jet is not fully recorded because the early systolic portion of the jet is missing.

B. Left ventricular systolic pressure is low.

C. Maximal instantaneous left ventricular outflow gradient is 122 mm Hg.

D. Mitral regurgitation is partly diastolic.

E. Peak left ventricular systolic pressure is 246 mm Hg.

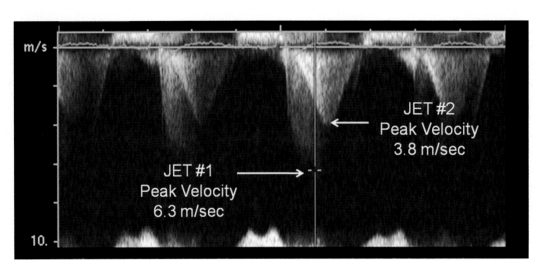

Fig. 7-16

32. The patient was started on oral disopyramide. Repeat echocardiogram was obtained and the spectral tracing in Figure 7-16 was obtained. Left atrial pressure was again estimated at 10 mm Hg. Otherwise, there were no significant changes on his echocardiogram.

    The following statement is TRUE:

    A. The shape of the mitral regurgitant jet is now suggestive of mitral valve prolapse with click and systolic murmur.

    B. Flow velocity pattern of jet #2 is typical of valvular aortic stenosis.

    C. Left ventricular outflow gradient has dropped by about 50% compared to the initial echocardiogram.

    D. Patient has developed intracavitary gradient as demonstrated by jet #1.

    E. Peak left ventricular systolic pressure is now 159 mm Hg minus the left atrial pressure.

CASE 4:

A 66-year-old man with a longstanding history of ethanol abuse complains of orthopnea, paroxysmal nocturnal dyspnea, and lower extremity edema.

He is tachypneic and tachycardic. Blood pressure 90/50 mm Hg, heart rate 110 bpm; weight 80 kg; height 175 cm; and body surface area 2.0 m². Auscultation of the lungs reveals bibasilar rales. Cardiac exam demonstrate S3 gallop and no murmur. There is bilateral lower extremity pitting edema pretibially.

Transthoracic echocardiogram revealed global left ventricular hypokinesis with an estimated ejection fraction of 25%.

33. To calculate the left atrial volume, the data in Figure 7-17 were obtained:

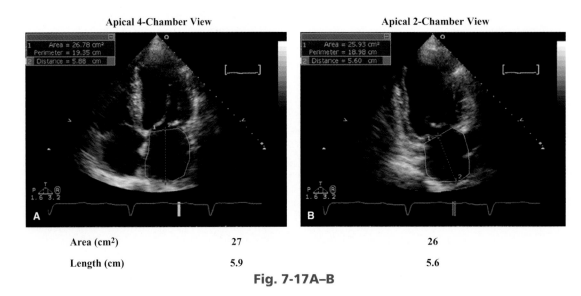

	Apical 4-Chamber View	Apical 2-Chamber View
Area (cm²)	27	26
Length (cm)	5.9	5.6

Fig. 7-17A–B

The left atrial volume index is approximately:

A. 20 ml/m^2.
B. 30 ml/m^2.
C. 40 ml/m^2.
D. 50 ml/m^2.
E. 60 ml/m^2.

34. Mitral inflow and pulmonary venous flow velocity spectral Doppler tracings were obtained on admission and after 5 days of appropriate medical therapy including intravenous diuretics (Fig. 7-18).

The following was the result of the appropriate medical therapy:

A. Left ventricular preload has increased.
B. Left atrial pressure has decreased.
C. Normal mitral filling pattern was replaced with the pattern of abnormal relaxation.
D. Patient has developed atrial flutter.
E. The change in mitral filling pattern seen in this patient portends grave long-term prognosis.

CASE 5:

A 23-year-old college student came back to the United States from an extended trip to rural areas of the Indian subcontinent complaining of dyspnea on exertion and chest pain on deep inspiration.

INITIAL STUDY

Mitral Inflow

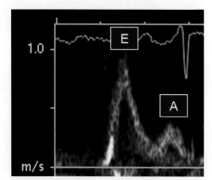

Mitral E wave deceleration time 140 msec
Fig. 7-18A

FOLLOW-UP STUDY

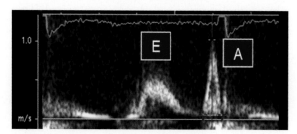

Mitral E wave deceleration time 270 msec
Fig. 7-18B

Pulmonary Vein

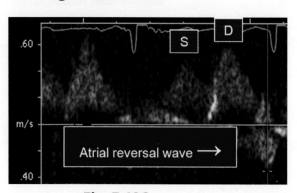

Fig. 7-18C

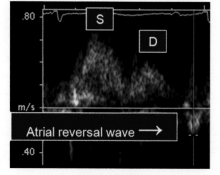

Fig. 7-18D

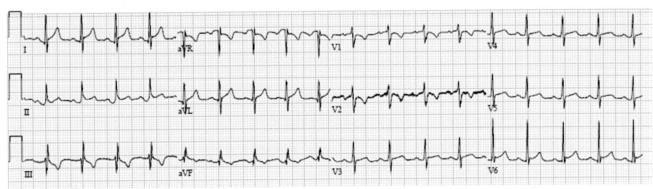

Fig. 7-19

On initial outpatient exam, he was afebrile. His lungs were clear on auscultation. There was a friction rub throughout the precordium. The electrocardiogram was suggestive of pericarditis (Fig. 7-19).

He was prescribed an oral course of a nonsteroidal anti-inflammatory agent (NSAID) and was sent home; however, despite taking the NSAID for 2 weeks, there was worsening of his chest pain. Computed tomography of the chest revealed a large pericardial and left pleural effusion with clinical and echocardiographic signs of tamponade. Purified protein derivative (PPD) skin test for tuberculosis was positive. The pericardial effusion was drained percutaneously and the patient was started on appropriate antituberculosis medical therapy.

His chest pain resolved completely but his shortness of breath persisted and he started developing bilateral ankle edema. Transthoracic echocardiogram was ordered.

35. Figure 7-20 was also obtained on the echocardiogram.

   In these recordings, the upstroke of the respirometry curve denotes inspiration, and the downstroke indicates expiration. The following is true:
   A. Restrictive cardiomyopathy of the left ventricle is present.
   B. Right atrial pressure is low.
   C. Left ventricular flow propagation velocity (Vp) is abnormal.
   D. Patient has constrictive pericarditis.
   E. Degree of respiratory variations in the mitral inflow is normal.

Mitral inflow spectral Doppler

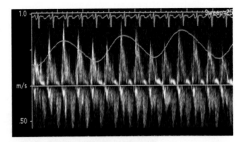

Fig. 7-20A

Left ventricular color M mode

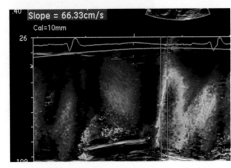

Fig. 7-20B

Inferior vena cava

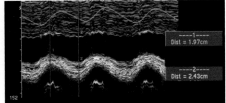

Fig. 7-20C

36. Video 7-2, obtained in the apical 4-chamber view demonstrates abnormal septal motion which is due to:
   A. Right ventricular pressure overload.
   B. Right ventricular volume overload.
   C. Left bundle branch block.
   D. Ventricular interdependence.
   E. Cardiac surgery.

ANSWERS

1. ANSWER: A. During expiration, the inferior vena cava (IVC) has a normal diameter of 2.1 cm or less. The measurement should be obtained perpendicular to the long axis of the IVC just proximal to the junction of the hepatic veins which lie approximately 0.5 to 3 cm proximal to the IVC-right atrial junction. During spontaneous (negative pressure) inspiration, the diameter of a normal IVC decreases by more than 50%. The patient should be asked to sniff during evaluation for inspiratory diameter change; normal resting inspiration may not be sufficient to induce proper response.

The expiratory diameter of the IVC and the percent diameter decrease during inspiration are dependent on the magnitude of the right atrial pressure (RAP). Table 7-16 demonstrates how RAP can be estimated from IVC diameter and percent change in diameter during the sniff maneuver.

TABLE 7-16

IVC Diameter (cm)	IVC Diameter Change with Inspiration	Mean RAP (mm Hg)	RAP Range (mm Hg)	Hepatic Vein	Tricuspid E/e′
≤2.1	>50%	3	0–5	S wave dominant pattern	E/e′ ≤ 6
Indeterminate Pattern		8	5–10		
>2.1	<50%	15	10–20	D wave dominant pattern	E/e′ > 6

In our patient, the expiratory diameter was 1.6 cm and there was >50% decrease in IVC diameter with inspiration:

Percent change with inspiration = (1.6 cm – 0.6 cm)/ 1.6 cm = 63%.

It is important to emphasize that the above methodology may not apply to athletes (who have physiologic enlargement of IVC) or intubated patients receiving positive-pressure ventilation.

2. ANSWER: D. Mitral valve area (MVA) can be calculated using the pressure half-time (PHT) method:

$$MVA = \frac{220}{PHT} \qquad \text{(Eq. 1)}$$

In this question, PHT was not given. However, PHT can be calculated from the stated mitral deceleration time (DT) using the following formula:

$$PHT = 0.29 \times DT \qquad \text{(Eq. 2)}$$

Thus in our patient:

$$PHT = 0.29 \times DT = 0.29 \times 910$$
$$= 264 \text{ msec}$$

$$MVA = 220/PHT = 220/264 = 0.8 \text{ cm}^2$$

Alternatively, Eqs. 1 and 2 can be combined into the following one:

$$MVA = \frac{759}{DT} \qquad \text{(Eq. 3)}$$

In our patient then:

$$MVA = 759/DT = 759/910 = 0.8 \text{ cm}^2$$

Therefore, answer (D) is correct.

Answer (A) is incorrect because the MVA is calculated by dividing 220 into PHT (Eq. 1) and not DT.

Answer (B) is incorrect because the stroke volume (SV) across the mitral valve in this patient is 53 ml per beat. Once the MVA is calculated, SV and cardiac output (CO) can be derived using the following formulas:

$$SV = MVA \times VTI$$
$$CO = SV \times HR$$

where VTI is the mitral velocity-time integral during diastole, and HR is the heart rate.

In our patient, mitral VTI during diastole was 66 cm and the heart rate was 85 bpm:

$$SV = 0.8 \text{ cm}^2 \times 66 \text{ cm} = 53 \text{ ml}$$
$$CO = 53 \text{ mL} \times 85 \text{ bpm} = 4.5 \text{ l/min}$$

Answer (C) is incorrect because as shown above, PHT in this patient was 264 msec and not 355 msec.

Answer (E) is incorrect because the resting gradient of mitral stenosis is expected to increase with augmentation of CO such as during exercise, fever, or pregnancy.

3. ANSWER: E. Patient has patent ductus arteriosus (PDA), which is an extracardiac shunt resulting from a communication between the descending thoracic aorta (DTA) and the proximal left pulmonary artery.

In utero, the blood that reaches the pulmonary artery from the right ventricle cannot enter the collapsed lungs; instead, it is diverted across the ductus arteriosus into the DTA. Soon after birth, the pressure in the pulmonary artery falls below the pressure in DTA and the blood flow in the ductus arteriosus reverses its direction. It now flows from the DTA into the pulmonary artery. High oxygen content of the ductal blood triggers the closure of ductus arteriosus in most newborns. In rare instances, the communication persists in the postneonatal period giving rise to PDA.

In individuals with PDA, the systemic blood flow (Qs) reaches the right heart through systemic veins and continues through the right ventricular outflow tract (RVOT) into the main pulmonary artery. At that level, Qs is joined by the shunt flow (SF) entering the pulmonary artery through the PDA. The sum of Q_s and SF represents the amount of blood flow that enters the pulmonary circulation (Q_p).

After passing through the lungs, Q_p enters the left heart through the pulmonary veins and exits through the left ventricular outflow tract (LVOT) into the aorta. At the level of the descending aorta, Q_p divides into SF which enters the PDA, and Q_s which continues into the peripheral systemic circulation to ultimately reach the right heart through systemic veins.

Note that in individuals with PDA, the flow across the RVOT represents Q_s and the flow across the LVOT represents Q_p. Therefore, answer (E) is correct.

This is in contrast to atrial and ventricular septal defects where LVOT flow represents Q_s and the RVOT flow represent Q_p. Since in most individuals with PDA, $Q_p > Q_s$, it is the left heart and not the right heart that dilates to accommodate the excess blood flow.

The general echocardiographic formula to calculate volumetric flow (Q) is:

$$Q = CSA \times VTI \times HR \qquad \text{(Eq. 1)}$$

where CSA is the cross-sectional area, VTI is the velocity-time integral, and HR is the heart rate.

One can use right and left ventricular outflow tracts to calculate volumetric flow. Since both tracts are assumed to be circular in shape, the CSA can be expressed in the equations as:

$$CSA = \left(\frac{1}{2} \times D \right)^2 \times \pi \qquad \text{(Eq. 2)}$$

where D is the diameter of the outflow tract. Equation 1 after expressing CSA in terms of Eq. 2 becomes:

$$Q = \left(\frac{1}{2} \times D \right)^2 \times \pi \times VTI \times HR \text{ seconds}$$

Calculations for our patient are summarized in this table:

TABLE 7-17

	LVOT	RVOT	Shunt Across PDA
Diameter (cm)	2.0	2.5	
Area (cm²)	3.1	4.9	
VTI (cm)	31	12	
SV (ml)	97	59	97 − 59 = 38
HR	80	80	
	Qp	**Qs**	
Flow (l/min)	7.8	4.7	
Qp:Qs	1.7	1	

Answer (A) is incorrect because the flow rate of 7.8 l/minute across the LVOT represents Q_p and not Q_s in patients with PDA.

Answer (B) is incorrect because $Q_p:Q_s$ in this patient is greater than 1 (it is 1.7:1).

Answer (C) is incorrect because the SV that enters the lungs (97 ml per beat) is the sum of the systemic SV (59 ml per beat) that entered the main pulmonary artery through the RVOT and the shunt flow (38 ml per beat) that came into the pulmonary artery through the PDA.

Answer (D) is incorrect because Q_p is much greater than Q_s, the shunt flow is in the left-to-right direction, and the patient is unlikely to be cyanotic. In patients with PDA who develop Eisenmenger physiology, there is a right-to-left shunt. Such patients are cyanotic in the lower parts of the body because the deoxygenated blood from the pulmonary artery crosses the PDA and enters the descending thoracic aorta past the origins of the aortic arch vessels, which supply fully oxygenated blood to the head and the arms.

4. ANSWER: B. This patient with severe shortness of breath has elevated pulmonary artery diastolic pressure (PADP). Using the end-diastolic velocity (V) of the pulmonic regurgitant jet and the $4V^2$ formula, one can calculate the pressure gradient (ΔP) between the PADP and the end-diastolic right ventricular pressure (RVDP).

$$\Delta P = PADP - RVDP = 4 \times V^2 \qquad \text{(Eq. 1)}$$

In the absence of tricuspid stenosis, RVDP is the same as the RAP. Thus, the pressure gradient can also be expressed as:

$$\Delta P = PADP - RAP = 4 \times V^2 \qquad \text{(Eq. 2)}$$

Rearranging Eq. 2, PADP can be calculated in the following manner:

$$PADP = 4 \times V^2 + RAP \qquad \text{(Eq. 3)}$$

where V is the end-diastolic velocity of the pulmonic regurgitant jet, and RAP is the right atrial pressure.

As explained in the answer to question 1, RAP can be estimated from the expiratory size of the IVC and the percent decrease in diameter change with inspiration. In our patient, the IVC is dilated (>2.1 cm) and the IVC diameter does not change with inspiration. The estimated RAP is thus approximately 15 mm Hg.

Once RAP is known, we can then calculate PADP:

$$PADP = 4 \times (2 \text{ m/sec})^2 + 15, \text{ or } 31 \text{ mm Hg}$$

Therefore, answer (B) is correct.

Answer (A) is incorrect because RAP in this patient is approximately 15 mm Hg as demonstrated above.

Answer (C) is incorrect for two reasons: (1) Pressure gradient between PADP and RVDP is 16 mm Hg and not 36 mm Hg; and (2) PADP is calculated by adding RAP to the gradient between PADP and RVDP, and not subtracting from it.

Answer (D) is incorrect because even in mild pulmonic regurgitation, appropriate spectral Doppler tracings of the regurgitant jet can be obtained.

Answer (E) is incorrect because normal PADP ranges typically between 5 and 16 mm Hg.

5. ANSWER: B. Severe mitral regurgitation (grades 3+ and 4+) is defined by the following criteria:

TABLE 7-18

	Severe MR
Regurgitant orifice (cm^2)	≥0.4
Regurgitant fraction	≥50%
Regurgitant volume (ml)	≥60
Vena contracta (cm)	≥0.7

Regurgitant orifice area (ROA) can be calculated using the following formula:

$$ROA_{MR} = 2 \times \pi \times r^2 \times \frac{Valias}{Vmax} \quad \text{(Eq. 1)}$$

where r is the PISA radius, $Valias$ is the aliasing velocity at which PISA radius is measured, and $Vmax$ is the maximum velocity of the mitral regurgitant jet on spectral Doppler.

In Eq. 1, the expression $2 \times \pi \times r^2 \times Valias$ represents instantaneous flow rate (IFR):

$$IFR = 2 \times \pi \times r^2 \times Valias \quad \text{(Eq. 2)}$$

Now Eq. 1 can be expressed as:

$$ROA_{MR} = \frac{IFR}{Vmax} \quad \text{(Eq. 3)}$$

In our patient, IFR is calculated as:

$$IFR = 2 \times 3.14 \times (1.0 \text{ cm})^2 \times 45 \text{ cm/sec}$$
$$= 283 \text{ ml/sec}$$

and ROA as:

$$ROA_{MR} = 283/500 \text{ cm/sec} = 0.6 \text{ cm}^2$$

Therefore, answer (B) is correct.

Answer (A) is incorrect because the vena contracta in severe mitral regurgitation is > 0.7 cm.

Answer (C) is incorrect because the IFR of the mitral regurgitant jet in this patient is 283 ml per second as calculated above.

Answer (D) is incorrect because mitral regurgitation is severe since ROA > 0.4 cm^2 (it is 0.6 cm^2).

Answer (E) is incorrect because the regurgitant volume (RegV) in this patient is 79 ml per beat. RV can be calculated as:

$$RegV = ROA_{MR} \times VTI_{MR} \quad \text{(Eq. 4)}$$

where VTI_{MR} is the velocity-time integral of the mitral regurgitant jet.

In our patient, RV equals 0.6 cm^2 × 140 cm, or 79 ml per beat. This is again consistent with severe mitral regurgitation (RV > 60 ml per beat).

6. ANSWER: A. The patient presents with shortness of breath due to elevated pulmonary artery wedge pressure (PAWP). In most instances, PAWP elevation is the result of high left atrial pressure (LAP) elevation.

PAWP can be estimated from the following formula:

$$PAWP = 4.6 + 5.27 \times \frac{E}{Vp}$$

where E is the peak blood flow velocity of the mitral inflow in cm/sec, and Vp is the flow propagation velocity of the mitral inflow (in cm/sec) obtained by color M mode. The Vp recording of this patient is demonstrated in Figure 7-21.

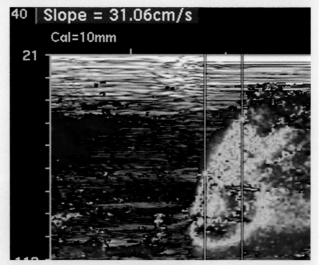

Fig. 7-21

Vp measures the rate at which red blood cells reach the LV apex from the mitral valve level during early diastole. The rate of blood flow from the mitral valve to the LV apex is determined by the rate of LV relaxation during early diastole. Therefore, Vp is an indirect measure of the rate of LV relaxation; the lower the Vp, the slower the LV relaxation and higher the left ventricular diastolic pressure (LVDP) are.

In our patient:

$$PAWP = 4.6 + 5.27 \times \frac{125}{31} = 26$$

With the value of 26 mm Hg, PAWP is elevated; normal PAWP is <12 mm Hg. Therefore, answer (A) is correct.

Answer (B) is incorrect because in patients with markedly elevated LAP and PAWP, the peak velocity of the mitral E wave is typically higher than that of the mitral A wave. The patients have either the pseudonormal filling pattern (E/A is between 1.0 and 2.0; E-wave DT >160 msec) or the restrictive filling pattern (E/A > 2 and E-wave DT <160 msec).

Answer (C) is incorrect because the pulmonary artery systolic pressure (PASP) is 64 mm Hg plus the RAP, or 64 + 15 = 79 mm Hg. In the absence of pulmonic stenosis (PS), PASP is the same as the right ventricular systolic pressure (RVSP). Peak velocity (V) of the tricuspid regurgitant flow can be used to estimated the RV-to-RA pressure gradient (ΔP) at peak systole:

$$\Delta P = 4 \times V^2 = (4 \text{ m/sec})^2 = 64 \text{ mm Hg}$$

By adding the RAP to ΔP, RVSP (and, by extension, PASP) can be calculated:

$$RVSP = PASP = \Delta P + RAP$$
$$= 64 + 15 = 79 \text{ mm Hg}$$

Answer (D) is incorrect because the ratio of mitral E wave to mitral annular tissue Doppler e' wave is expected to be greater than 15 in patients with markedly elevated LAP and PAWP. The E/e' ratio is further discussed in the answer to question 8.

Answer (E) is incorrect because the normal Vp velocity is >55 cm/sec in young individuals and >45 cm/sec in middle-aged and elderly individuals.

7. ANSWER: A. Severe aortic regurgitation (grades 3+ and 4+) is defined by the following criteria:

TABLE 7-19

	Severe AR
Regurgitant orifice (cm²)	≥0.3
Regurgitant fraction	≥50%
Regurgitant volume (ml)	≥60
Vena contracta (cm)	≥0.6

Therefore, answer A is correct; the regurgitant fraction of 65% indicates a severe aortic regurgitation.

Answer (B) is incorrect because vena contracta is not strongly influenced by Nyquist limit color Doppler settings. This is in contrast to PISA radius. By changing the color Doppler Nyquist limit, one also automatically changes the velocity filter. The role of the velocity filter is to prevent color encoding of low velocities. By lowering the color Doppler Nyquist limit, one lowers the velocity filter allowing for inclusion of lower velocities and an increase in the color area. Because vena contracta contains predominantly high velocities, altering the Nyquist limit will not change significantly the size of vena contracta diameter. This is in contrast to PISA radius, which becomes progressively larger with lower Nyquist limits.

The impact of changes in color Doppler Nyquist limit on vena contracta is demonstrated in Figure 7-22.

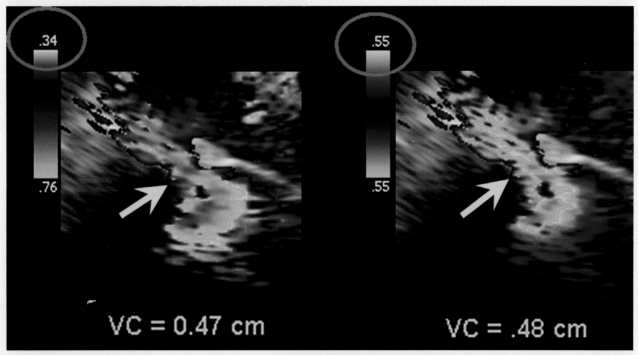

Fig. 7-22

Answer (C) is incorrect because in severe aortic regurgitation, vena contracta is >0.3 cm.

Answer (D) is incorrect because in severe aortic regurgitation, regurgitant volume is >60 ml per beat.

Answer (E) is incorrect because the diameter of vena contracta obtained by 2D echocardiography should not be used to calculate the regurgitant volume. Instead, the 2D diameter of vena contracta should be used for semiquantitative assessment of the degree of aortic regurgitation.

8. *ANSWER: C.* The E/e' ratio is directly proportional to the LAP. The peak velocity of the mitral annular tissue Doppler e' wave is directly proportional to the rate of LV relaxation during early diastole. The slower the LV relaxation, the higher the left ventricular diastolic pressure (LVDP). Once LVDP rises, there is a concomitant rise in the LAP and PAWP to allow for better filling of a stiff LV. The higher the LAP, the taller the mitral E wave becomes. In summary, as the LV diastolic dysfunction worsens, the peak velocity of the annular tissue e' wave gets smaller, the mitral E wave gets higher, and the E/e' ratio becomes progressively larger reflecting the rising LAP and PAWP.

The E/e' ratio can be used to estimate LAP in two ways. One approach is to use it semiquantitatively as shown in the table.

TABLE 7-20

	Left Atrial Pressure		
	Normal	Indeterminate	Elevated
E/e' using medial e'	<8	8–15	>15
E/e' using lateral e'	<8	8–12	>12

Thus, by E/e' ratio of 16 alone, our patient has an elevated LAP. The other approach is to estimate LAP numerically using the following equation:

$$LAP = 1.9 + 1.24 \times \frac{E}{e'} \qquad (Eq.\ 1)$$

In our patient:

$$LAP = 1.9 + 1.24 \times 16 = 22$$

An LAP of 22 mm Hg is significantly elevated; normal LAP is <12 mm Hg.

A simplified form of Eq. 1 is:

$$LAP = 4 + \frac{E}{e'} \qquad (Eq.\ 2)$$

A comparison between LAP estimates using Eq. 1 and Eq. 2 is given in Figure 7-23A.

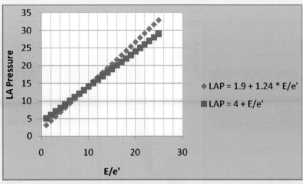

Fig. 7-23A

In our patient, LAP can be estimated by Eq. 2 as 4 + 16, or 20 mm Hg.

Therefore, answer (C) is correct.

Answer (A) is incorrect because the peak-to-peak gradient of aortic stenosis in this patient is 44 mm Hg.

To calculate the peak-to-peak gradient of aortic stenosis, we first need to calculate the peak left ventricular systolic pressure (LVSP) using the following formula:

$$LVSP = \Delta P_{MR} + LAP \qquad (Eq.\ 3)$$

where ΔP_{MR} is the peak systolic gradient of the mitral regurgitant jet, and LAP is the left atrial pressure. After expressing ΔP_{MR} in terms of the peak velocity (V) of the mitral regurgitant jet, Eq. 1 becomes:

$$LVSP = 4 \times V^2 + LAP \qquad (Eq.\ 4)$$

In our patient:

$$LVSP = 4 \times (6.0\ m/sec)^2 + 20$$
$$= 164\ mm\ Hg$$

Once LVSP is known, the peak-to-peak aortic gradient (P2P) can be calculated as:

$$P2P = LVSP - SBP \qquad (Eq.\ 5)$$

where SBP is the systolic blood pressure.

In our patient:

$$P2P = 164 - 120 = 44\ mm\ Hg$$

It is important to emphasize that this pressure gradient, which is commonly measured on cardiac catheterization, is not a physiologic one because it represents a pressure difference at separate points in time as demonstrated in Figure 7-23B. P2P is lower than the peak instantaneous gradient (PIP) obtained by continuous-wave Doppler across the aortic valve.

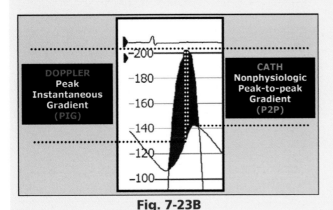

Fig. 7-23B

Answer (B) is incorrect because left ventricular *dP/dt* is normal. Patients with cardiogenic shock have low *dP/dt* values. Normal *dP/dt* = 1,661 +/− 323 mm Hg/sec. In this case, dP/dt is 1,900 mm Hg/sec.

Answer (D) is incorrect because in severe mitral regurgitation vena contracta is >0.7 cm.

Answer (E) is incorrect because either Eq. 1 or Eq. 2 is applicable irrespective of the atrial rhythm (normal sinus rhythm, atrial fibrillation, etc).

9. ANSWER: D. Figure 7-24 shows the continuous-wave spectral Doppler tracings of our patient.

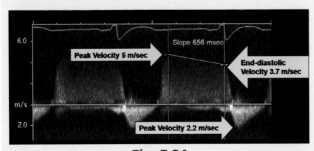

Fig. 7-24

Using the end-diastolic velocity (*V*) of the aortic regurgitant jet, one can calculate the pressure gradient (Δ*P*) between the diastolic blood pressure (DBP) and the left ventricular end-diastolic pressure (LVEDP).

$$\Delta P = DBP - LVEDP = 4 \times V^2 \qquad \text{(Eq. 1)}$$

Rearranging Eq. 1, LVEDP can be calculated in the following manner if the DBP is known:

$$LVEDP = DBP - 4 \times V^2 \qquad \text{(Eq. 2)}$$

In our patient:

$$LVEDP = 65 \text{ mm Hg} - 4 \times (3.7 \text{ m/sec})^2 = 10 \text{ mm Hg}$$

Therefore, answer (D) is correct.

Answer (A) is incorrect because in severe aortic regurgitation, PHT is <300 msec.

Answer (B) is incorrect because the aortic valve area cannot be calculated by 220 into PHT; i.e., the formula for calculating the MVA.

Answer (C) is incorrect because the peak LVSP is always higher than the systolic blood pressure in patients with aortic stenosis. LVSP becomes progressively higher than SBP as the aortic stenosis becomes more severe. The LVSP-to-SBP pressure gradient is referred to as the peak-to-peak aortic gradient as discussed in the answer to question 8.

Answer (E) is incorrect because the continuity equation can be used to calculate the aortic valve area in patients with or without aortic regurgitation. The continuity principle states that the SV across the LVOT is the same as the SV across the aortic valve (AV):

$$LVOT\ SV = AV\ SV \qquad \text{(Eq. 3)}$$

Since the SV can be expressed as the product of the cross-sectional area (CSA) and the flow velocity integral (VTI), Eq. 3 becomes:

$$CSA_{LVOT} \times VTI_{LVOT} = CSA_{AV} \times VTI_{AV} \qquad \text{(Eq. 4)}$$

In patients with aortic regurgitation, there is an increase in antegrade flow from the left ventricle into the aorta due to augmentation of the true left ventricular SV by the aortic regurgitant volume. However, this increase equally affects the flow through the left ventricular outflow tract and the aortic valve in systole. In Eq. 5, this will be reflected in a proportional increase in VTI_{LVOT} and VTI_{AV}.

By continuity equation, the AV area (CSA_{AV}) can be calculated as follows:

$$CSA_{AV} = CSA_{LVOT} \times \frac{VTI_{LVOT}}{VTI_{AV}} \qquad \text{(Eq. 5)}$$

In aortic regurgitation, there is augmentation of VTI_{LVOT} and VTI_{AV}. However, the ratio of the two VTIs remains the same; therefore, the calculated value of CSA_{AV} is not affected by the presence of aortic regurgitation.

10. ANSWER: C. The patient has an atrial septal defect (ASD) with a left-to-right shunt. An ASD is an intracardiac shunt at the atrial level. Systemic blood flow (*Q*s) reaches the right atrium through systemic veins. At the level of the right atrium, it is joined by the shunt flow which enters the right atrium from the left atrium across the ASD. The sum of *Q*s and the shunt flow then passes through the RVOT into the pulmonary circulation. Therefore, the sum of *Q*s and the shunt flow represents the pulmonary blood flow (Qp). This Qp reaches the left atrium through the pulmonary veins. At the left atrial level, Qp divides into shunt flow (which traverses ASD to reach the right atrium), and Qs which enters the left ventricle. Qs then passes through the LVOT into the aorta and eventually reaches the right atrium through systemic veins.

In summary, flow through LVOT represents Qs, while the flow through RVOT represents Qp in patients with ASD.

Shunt calculations for this patient are summarized in the following table:

TABLE 7-21

	RVOT	LVOT	Comment
Diameter (cm)	2.6	2.0	
Area (cm²)	5.3	3.1	Calculated using formula Area = (0.5 × Diameter)² × π
VTI (cm)	30	20	
SV (ml)	159	63	Calculated using formula SV = Area × VTI
Heart rate (beats per minute)	75	75	Calculated using formula Flow = SV × Heart rate
Flow (l/min)	11.9	4.7	Shunt flow is the difference between Qp and Qs, or 7.2 l/min.
	Pulmonic flow (Qp)	Systemic flow (Qs)	
Qp:Qs	2.5:1		

Because Qp:Qs = 2.5:1, the answer (C) is correct.

Answer (A) is incorrect because the presence of pulmonary hypertension per se does not preclude ASD closure. It is the degree of pulmonary vascular resistance (PVR) that determines whether a patient is a candidate for ASD closure or not, as discussed below.

Answer (B) is incorrect because the patient's PVR is essentially normal. Using the Ohm's law, PVR can be calculated as:

$$PVR = \frac{\Delta P}{Qp} \quad \text{(Eq. 1)}$$

where Qp is the pulmonary blood flow (in l/minute), and ΔP is the pressure gradient across the pulmonary circulation. ΔP is the difference between the mean pulmonary artery pressure (MPP) and the mean LAP. Equation 1 then becomes:

$$PVR = \frac{MPP - LAP}{Qp} \quad \text{(Eq. 2)}$$

MPP can be calculated from PASP and the PADP using the following equation:

$$MPP = PADP + \frac{1}{2} \times (PASP - PADP) \quad \text{(Eq. 3)}$$

In this patient:

$$MPP = 25 + \frac{1}{2} \times (55 - 25) = 40 \text{ mm Hg}$$

Once MPP is known, we can use Eq. 2 to calculated PVR:

$$PVR = \frac{40 - 10}{11.9} = \frac{30}{11.9} = 3.4 \text{ Wood units}$$

Normal PVR is 1–2 Wood units (80–160 dyne × sec × cm⁻⁵). In this patient, PVR is only modestly elevated. In principle, ASD closure should not be performed if PVR is 2/3 or more of the systemic vascular resistance (SVR). Since normal SVR is approximately 13 Wood units (range 11–16 Wood units, or 900–1300 dyne × sec × cm⁻⁵), PVR > 9 Wood units usually precludes ASD closure.

Answer (D) is incorrect because the shunt flow in this patient is 7.2 l/min. Shunt flow is the difference between Qp and Qs. In this patient:

$$SF = Qp - Qs = 11.9 - 4.7 = 7.2 \text{ l/min}$$

Answer (E) is incorrect because Qp is much larger than Qs, the shunt flow is in the left-to-right direction, and thus the patient is not expected to be cyanotic.

11. *ANSWER: B.* The presence of ventricular septal defect (VSD) allows for calculation of the RVSP and, by extension, the PASP if the SBP is known.

RVSP in a patient with VSD and no left ventricular outflow obstruction can be calculated as:

$$RVSP = SBP - \text{Peak systolic VSD gradient} \quad \text{(Eq. 1)}$$

Using the peak systolic velocity (V) across the VSD, peak systolic VSD gradient can be calculated as:

$$\text{Peak systolic VSD gradient} = 4 \times V^2 \qquad \text{(Eq. 2)}$$

By combining Eqs. 1 and 2, RVSP is then calculated as:

$$\text{RVSP} = \text{SBP} - 4 \times V^2 \qquad \text{(Eq. 3)}$$

Thus, in this patient, RVSP = $120 - 4 \times (3.0 \text{ m/sec})^2$ = 84 mm Hg.

When there is no PS, PASP = RVSP. However, this patient has PS with a peak systolic gradient of 55 mm Hg across the pulmonic valve. In the presence of PS, the relationship between RVSP and PASP is as follows:

$$\text{PASP} = \text{RVSP} - \text{Peak PS Gradient} \qquad \text{(Eq. 4)}$$

In our patient, PASP = $84 - 55 = 29$ mm Hg. Therefore, the answer (B) is correct.

Answer (A) is incorrect because RVSP in this patient is 84 mm Hg as calculated above.

Answer (C) is incorrect because the RAP is not required for RVSP estimation using the VSD method.

Answer (D) is incorrect because PASP is lower than RVSP due to the presence of PS. RVSP exceeds PASP by 55 mm Hg, which is the peak gradient across the stenosed pulmonic valve.

Answer (E) is incorrect because the right ventricular end-diastolic pressure (RVEDP) in this patient is not 28 mmHg but is 8 mmHg as shown below.

If the LVEDP is known, the RVEDP can be calculated as:

$$\text{RVEDP} = \text{LVEDP} - \text{End-diastolic VSD gradient} \qquad \text{(Eq. 5)}$$

Using the end-diastolic velocity (V) across the VSD, the end-diastolic VSD gradient can be calculated as:

$$\text{End-diastolic VSD gradient} = 4 \times V^2 \qquad \text{(Eq. 6)}$$

By combining Eqs. 5 and 6, RVEDP is then calculated as:

$$\text{RVEDP} = \text{LVEDP} - 4 \times V^2 \qquad \text{(Eq. 7)}$$

where V is the end-diastolic velocity across the VSD. In our patient:

$$\text{RVEDP} = 12 - 4 \times (1 \text{ m/sec})^2 = 12 - 4 = 8 \text{ mm Hg}$$

12. ANSWER: B. The pulmonic flow (Qp) in patients with an atrial septal defect (ASD) is the sum of the shunt flow (SF) across the ASD and the systemic flow (Qs). SF can be calculated either directly or as the difference between Qp and Qs.

One method for direct calculation of SF is the standard echocardiographic formula for determining flow through an orifice:

$$\text{Flow} = \text{CSA} \times \text{VTI} \times \text{HR}$$

where CSA is the cross-sectional area of the orifice, VTI is the velocity-time integral at the level of the orifice, and HR is the heart rate.

In the first step, we will calculate the CSA of the atrial septal defect with a diameter of 1.2 cm. Since the ASD is circular in shape, the ASD area can be calculated as:

$$\text{CSA}_{\text{ASD}} = (\tfrac{1}{2} \times \text{ASD diameter})^2 \times \pi$$

In our patient:

$$\text{CSA}_{\text{ASD}} = (\tfrac{1}{2} \times 1.2 \text{ cm})^2 \times 3.14$$
$$= 0.36 \times 3.14 = 1.13 \text{ cm}^2$$

Next, we can calculate the SV across the ASD as:

$$\text{ASD shunt SV} = \text{CSA}_{\text{ASD}} \times \text{VTI}_{\text{ASD}}$$

In our patient:

$$\text{ASD shunt SV} = 1.13 \text{ cm}^2 \times 80 \text{ cm}$$
$$= 90 \text{ ml per beat}$$

In the final step, by multiplying the ASD shunt SV by the heart rate, one can calculated the shunt flow across the ASD. In our patient:

$$\text{ASD shunt flow} = 90 \text{ ml} \times 100 \text{ bpm} = 9.0 \text{ l/min}$$

Therefore, the answer (B) is correct.

Answer (A) is incorrect because the Qp:Qs in this patient is 2.5:1. In this patient, Qs is calculated at the level of the LVOT using the formula:

$$Qs = \text{CSA}_{\text{LVOT}} \times \text{VTI}_{\text{LVOT}} \times \text{HR}$$

where CSA_{LVOT} is the cross-sectional area of LVOT, VTI_{LVOT} is the velocity-time integral at the LVOT level, and HR is the heart rate. In our patient:

$$Qs = (\tfrac{1}{2} \times 2.0 \text{ cm})^2 \times \pi \times 19 \text{ cm} \times 100 \text{ bpm}$$
$$= 60 \text{ ml} \times 100 \text{ bpm} = 6.0 \text{ l/minute}$$

In the next step, we can calculate Qp as:

$$Qp = Qs + \text{ASD shunt flow}$$

In our patient:

$$Qp = 6.0 \text{ l/minute} + 9.0 \text{ l/minute} = 15.0 \text{ l/minute}.$$

Once Qp and Qs are known, we can calculate the $Qp:Qs$ ratio:

$$Qp:Qs = 15.0 \text{ l/minute} : 6.0 \text{ l/minute} = 2.5:1$$

Answer (C) is incorrect because the difference between systemic and SV in this patient is 90 ml/ beat. This value represents the ASD shunt SV calculated above.

Answer (D) is incorrect because the systemic SV in this patient is 60 ml per beat as calculated above.

Answer (E) is incorrect because the Qp in this patient is 15.0 l/minute as calculated above. Calculations related to this question are summarized in this table.

TABLE 7-22

	LVOT	ASD	RVOT	Comments
Diameter (cm)	2.0	1.2		
Area (cm²)	3.10	1.13		
VTI (cm)	19	80		
SV (ml)	60	90	150	RVOT SV is the sum of LVOT and ASD SV
Heart rate (beats per minute)	100	100		
Flow (l/min)	6.0	9.0	15.0	Qp is the sum of Qp and ASD shunt flow.
	Systemic flow (Qs)	Shunt flow	Pulmonic flow (Qp)	Qp:Qs = 2.5

13. ANSWER: D. Continuous Doppler spectral tracing of the mitral regurgitant jet can be used to estimate the rate of pressure rise (*dP*) in the left ventricle over time (*dt*), a measure of left ventricular systolic function, using the following formula:

$$dP/dt = \frac{\Delta P}{RTI} \qquad \text{(Eq. 1)}$$

where RTI is the relative time interval, measured in seconds, between mitral regurgitant jet velocities of 1 m/sec (*V1*) and 3 m/sec (*V2*). ΔP represents the pressure difference between the left ventricular

to left atrial pressure gradients at *V2* and *V1* (Figure 7-25A).

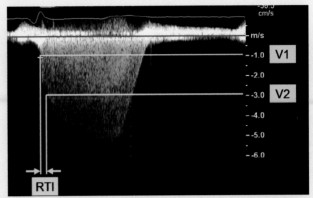

Fig. 7-25A

This pressure difference can be calculated as:

$$\Delta P = 4 \times (V_2)^2 - 4 \times (V_1)^2$$
$$\Delta P = 4 \times (3 \text{ m/sec})^2 - 4 \times (1 \text{ m/sec})^2$$
$$= 4 \times 9 - 4 \times 1 = 36 - 4$$
$$\Delta P = 32 \text{ mm Hg}$$

Now, Eq. 1 can be expressed as:

$$dP/dt = \frac{32}{RTI} \qquad \text{(Eq. 2)}$$

In the next step, we will calculate RTI in our patient:

$$RTI = \text{Time at } V2 - \text{Time at } V1 = 25 \text{ msec}$$
$$- 5 \text{ msec} = 20 \text{ msec}$$

Since Eq. 2 RTI is expressed in seconds, we have to convert our patient's RTI from milliseconds to seconds:

$$RTI = 20 \text{ msec} = 0.02 \text{ seconds}$$

Once RTI is known, we can calculate *dP/dt* in our patient:

$$dP/dt = \text{to } 32/0.02 = 1,600 \text{ mm Hg/sec}$$

Therefore, answer (D) is correct.

Answer (A) is incorrect because the peak velocity of mitral E wave in severe mitral regurgitation is expected to be high. Peak velocity across an orifice is directly related to flow across that orifice. Since the flow is the product of SV and heart rate, peak velocity is then a direct function (*f*) of SV:

$$dP/dt = 32 / RVI \qquad \text{(Eq. 3)}$$

In mitral regurgitation, SV that crosses the mitral valve in diastole is the sum of the systemic stroke volume (SV$_{LVOT}$) and the RegV. Thus, Eq. 3 can be expressed as:

$$E\text{-wave velocity} = f(SV_{LVOT} + RegV) \quad \text{(Eq. 4)}$$

The more severe the mitral regurgitation is, the larger the RegV, and therefore, the higher the peak velocity of the mitral inflow E wave. When native mitral regurgitation is severe (as is the case in this patient as judged by the vena contracta >0.7 cm), peak E velocity is expected to be >1.5 m/sec. In severe prosthetic mitral regurgitation, the peak E velocity is usually >2.0 m/sec.

Answer (B) is incorrect because LAP in this patient is elevated. The patient presents with severe mitral regurgitation (vena contracta > 0.7 cm) and pulmonary edema due to elevated left atrial pressure (LAP).

Using the peak velocity (Vmax) of the mitral regurgitant jet, one can calculate the pressure gradient (ΔP) between the peak left ventricular systolic pressure (LVSP) and the LAP:

$$\Delta P = 4 \times Vmax^2 \quad \text{(Eq. 5)}$$

In our patient:

$$\Delta P = 4 \times (4.0 \text{ m/sec})^2 = 4 \times 16 = 64 \text{ mm Hg}$$

The sum of this pressure gradient and LAP during systole represents the peak LVSP:

$$LVSP = \Delta P + LAP \quad \text{(Eq. 6)}$$

By rearranging Eq. 6, we can solve for LAP:

$$LAP = LVSP - \Delta P \quad \text{(Eq. 7)}$$

The LAP calculated by this method represents a value on the CV wave portion of the left atrial pressure tracing.

LVSP is not given in the question. In this patient who does not have aortic stenosis or left ventricular outflow obstruction, LVSP is equal to systolic blood pressure (SBP). Thus, we can express Eq. 7 as:

$$LAP = SBP - \Delta P \quad \text{(Eq. 8)}$$

In our patient, whose SBP was 95 mm Hg and whose ΔP was calculated above at 64 mm Hg, LAP is then calculated as:

$$LAP = 95 \text{ mm Hg} - 64 \text{ mm Hg} = 31 \text{ mm Hg}$$

This LAP of 31 mm Hg is highly elevated (normal LAP is <12 mm Hg).

Answer (C) is incorrect because in severe mitral regurgitation there may be a flow reversal in systolic (S) but not diastolic (D) wave on pulmonary venous flow

velocity tracings. An example of S-wave reversal due to severe mitral regurgitation is shown in Figure 7-25B.

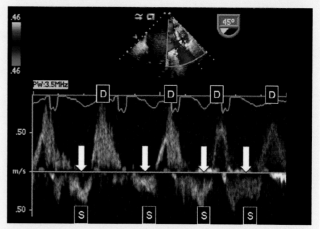

Systolic wave reversal (*arrows*) in the left upper pulmonary vein due to severe mitral regurgitation is seen on spectral Doppler recordings on a transesophageal echocardiography. S, systolic wave; D, diastolic wave.

Fig. 7-25B

Answer (E) is incorrect because *dP/dt* in this patient is estimated at 1,600 mm Hg/sec, which is normal. (Normal *dP/dt* = 1661 +/− 323 mm Hg/sec). The value of 800 mm Hg/sec would indicate a markedly diminished LV systolic function as seen in cardiogenic shock, for example.

14. ANSWER: E. In mitral stenosis, there is a pressure gradient between the left atrium and the left ventricle during diastole. In this patient, the mean diastolic pressure gradient is markedly elevated (21 mm Hg). Mean diastolic pressure gradient of >10 mm Hg is consistent with severe mitral stenosis as shown in this table.

TABLE 7-23

	Mild MS	Moderate MS	Severe MS
MVA (cm²)	>1.5	1.0–1.5	<1.0
Mean diastolic gradient (mm Hg)	<5	5–10	>10

In this young patient, left ventricular diastolic pressures are normal. Mean LAP can be calculated as:

$$LAP = \text{Mean mitral gradient in diastole} + \text{Early LV diastolic pressure}$$

In our patient:

$$LAP \text{ is } 21 \text{ mm Hg} + 7 \text{ mm Hg} = 28 \text{ mm Hg}$$

Therefore, answer (E) is correct.

Answer (A) is incorrect because in mitral stenosis, there is an antegrade flow driven by a pressure gradient between the left atrium and the left ventricle in diastole. Therefore, the mean left atrial pressure is higher than the mean left ventricular diastolic pressure.

Answer (B) is incorrect because in mitral stenosis, the peak velocity of the mitral E wave is expected to be high. Velocity (V) across an orifice is inversely related to the CSA of the orifice:

$$V \approx \frac{1}{CSA} \qquad \text{(Eq. 1)}$$

For mitral stenosis, CSA equals the MVA and Eq. 1 becomes:

$$V \approx \frac{1}{MVA} \qquad \text{(Eq. 2)}$$

Therefore, the smaller the MVA (i.e., the more severe the mitral stenosis), the higher the peak velocity of the mitral E wave.

Answer (C) is incorrect because the pressure-half time method may be unreliable immediately after but not before the mitral valvuloplasty. Pressure-half time method assumes that the left ventricular pressure and compliance are normal, and therefore that the deceleration slope of the mitral E wave on spectral Doppler tracings in diastole is the function of the MVA alone.

Immediately after valvuloplasty, there is a sudden increase in the mitral orifice area leading to an increase in the SV delivered to the left ventricle in early diastole. Since the left ventricle compliance cannot change acutely, the left ventricular diastolic pressure increases. With the rise in the left ventricular diastolic pressure, the diastolic gradient between the left atrium and the left ventricle decreases and the mitral PHT shortens above and beyond what would be expected by an increase in the MVA alone after valvuloplasty. Therefore, the pressure-half time method may lead to calculation of an erroneously large MVA.

Answer (D) is incorrect because the MVA by pressure-half time (PHT) method in this patient is 0.8 cm²:

$$MVA = \frac{220}{PHT} = \frac{220}{270} = 0.8$$

15. *ANSWER: C.* When velocity-time integrals are not available, aortic valve area (AVA) can be calculated using the following modified continuity equation:

$$AVA = CSA_{LVOT} \times \frac{V_{LVOT}}{V_{AV}} \qquad \text{(Eq. 1)}$$

where CSA_{LVOT} is the CSA of the LVOT, V_{LVOT} is the peak systolic LVOT velocity, and V_{AV} is the peak systolic AV velocity.

The V_{LVOT}/V_{AV} ratio of the two velocities is referred to as the dimensionless index (DI). Thus, Eq. 1 can be expressed as:

$$AVA = CSA_{LVOT} \times DI \qquad \text{(Eq. 2)}$$

After expressing the LVOT area in terms of LVOT diameter (D), Eq. 2 becomes:

$$AVA = \pi \times \left(\frac{1}{2} \times D\right)^2 \times DI \qquad \text{(Eq. 3)}$$

In our patient:

AVA = 3.14 × (½ × 1.9 cm)² × (1 m/sec) / (5 m/sec)
AVA = 2.84 cm² × 0.2
AVA = 0.6 cm²

Therefore, answer (C) is correct.

As a rule, when the dimensionless index (DI) is <0.25, the AVA is <1.0 cm² across the range of LVOT diameters commonly encountered in adults as demonstrated in this table:

TABLE 7-24

LVOT Diameter (cm)	LVOT Area (cm²)	AVA (cm²) if DI = 0.25
1.8	2.54	0.64
1.9	2.84	0.71
2.0	3.14	0.79
2.1	3.46	0.87
2.2	3.80	0.95

Answer (A) is incorrect because the modified continuity equation using the dimensionless index, as explained above, can be used to calculate the AVA when velocity-time integrals are unavailable.

Answer (B) is incorrect because the subvalvular (LVOT) velocity is normal (1.0 m/sec).

Answer (D) is incorrect because the left ventricular SV in this patient is 57 ml per beat. Left ventricular SV can be calculated as follows:

SV = π × (½ × LVOT diameter)² × VTI$_{LVOT}$
SV = 3.14 × (½ × 1.9 cm)² × 20 cm
SV = 57 ml per beat

Answer (E) is incorrect because in aortic stenosis, the left ventricular peak systolic pressure exceeds the systolic blood pressure. The magnitude of this pressure difference (peak-to-peak gradient) is proportional to the severity of aortic stenosis.

16. ANSWER: C. Peak RVSP in a patient with or without PS can be calculated as:

$$RVSP = \text{Peak RV-to-RA systolic gradient} + RAP \quad \text{(Eq. 1)}$$

Since RV-to-RA systolic gradient can be estimated from the peak systolic velocity of the tricuspid regurgitant (V), Eq. 1 can be expressed as:

$$RVSP = 4 \times V^2 + RAP \quad \text{(Eq. 2)}$$

In the absence of PS, RVSP is equal to PASP. In PS, however, peak RVSP exceeds PASP. The difference between the two pressures represents the peak gradient of PS. Therefore, in patients with PS, PASP is estimated as:

$$PASP = RVSP - PS\ Gradient \quad \text{(Eq. 3)}$$

In our patient:

$$RVSP = 4 \times (4.0\ \text{m/sec})^2 + 10 = 74\ \text{mm Hg}$$
$$PASP = 74 - 24 = 50\ \text{mm Hg}$$

Therefore, answer (C) is correct.

All calculations are graphically summarized in Figure 7-26; RVP, right ventricular pressure; RAP, right atrial pressure; PAP, pulmonary artery pressure.

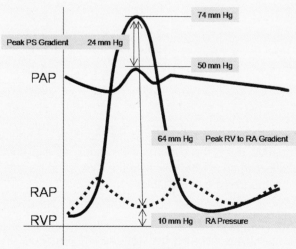

Fig. 7-26

Answer (A) is incorrect because in the presence of pulmonic valve stenosis, RVSP exceeds PASP as shown in this figure above.

Answer (B) is incorrect because RVSP exceeds PASP by 24 mm Hg, the value of the peak systolic gradient across the pulmonic valve.

Answer (D) is incorrect because RVSP is 24 mm Hg more than PASP.

Answer (E) is incorrect because RVSP is 74 mm Hg as calculated above.

17. ANSWER: C. Peak gradient ($\Delta Pmax$) of aortic stenosis can be calculated from the peak systolic velocity (V) across the aortic valve obtained by continuous-wave Doppler using the modified Bernoulli equation:

$$\Delta Pmax = 4 \times V^2 \quad \text{(Eq. 1)}$$

The mean aortic valve gradient ($\Delta Pmean$) is approximately 60% of the peak gradient ($\Delta Pmax$):

$$\Delta Pmean = 0.6 \times \Delta Pmax \quad \text{(Eq. 2)}$$

In our patient:

$$\Delta Pmax = 4 \times (5.0\ \text{m/sec})^2 = 100\ \text{mm Hg}$$
$$\Delta Pmean = 0.6 \times 100\ \text{mm Hg} = 60\ \text{mm Hg}$$

Therefore, answer (C) is correct.

Answer (A) is incorrect because increased CO (as during pregnancy, for instance) leads to a proportional increase in both LVOT and aortic velocities. In this patient, there is a marked difference between the peak systolic LVOT velocity (0.9 m/sec) and the peak systolic aortic velocity (5.0 m/sec) indicative of aortic stenosis.

Answer (B) is incorrect because in aortic regurgitation there is a proportional increase in both LVOT and aortic velocities in systole due to augmentation of the left ventricular SV by the recirculating regurgitant volume. A wide discrepancy in the peak LVOT and aortic velocities in systole is not expected in severe aortic regurgitation.

Answer (D) is incorrect because the aortic valve area in this patient is less than 1.0 cm². AVA in this patient can be estimated using the modified continuity equation:

$$AVA = CSA_{LVOT} \times \frac{V_{LVOT}}{V_{AV}} \quad \text{(Eq. 3)}$$

After expressing the LVOT area in terms of LVOT diameter (D), Eq. 3 becomes:

$$AVA = \pi \times \left(\frac{1}{2} \times D\right)^2 \times \frac{V_{LVOT}}{V_{AV}} \quad \text{(Eq. 4)}$$

where CSA_{LVOT} is the cross-sectional area of the LVOT, V_{LVOT} is the peak systolic LVOT velocity, and V_{AV} is the peak aortic velocity in systole.

In this patient:

$$AVA = 3.14 \times \left(\frac{1}{2} \times 2.0\right)^2 \times \frac{0.9}{5.0} = 0.6\ \text{cm}^2$$

Answer (E) is incorrect because the subvalvular (LVOT) velocity of 0.9 m/sec is normal.

18. *ANSWER: D.* The patient has severe pulmonic valve regurgitation, a common long-term complication of tetralogy of Fallot repair.

Because of a large regurgitant orifice, the pressure gradient between the pulmonary artery and the right ventricle equalizes rapidly. Equalization is achieved by middiastole and there is no measurable end-diastolic gradient as demonstrated in Figure 7-27.

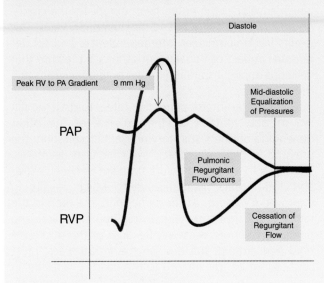

Fig. 7-27

This rapid deceleration and premature cessation of the pulmonic regurgitant jet is a characteristic finding of severe pulmonic regurgitation. Therefore, answer (D) is correct.

Answer (A) is incorrect because the end-diastolic gradient in severe pulmonic regurgitation is approaching zero.

Answer (B) is incorrect because the peak antegrade velocity across the pulmonic valve in systole is only elevated to about 1.5 m/sec (peak systolic gradient = 4 × 1.5^2 = 9 mm Hg). This is consistent with pulmonic regurgitation alone. During systole, SV is augmented by the recirculating regurgitant volume. This flow augmentation leads to higher systolic velocities across the pulmonic valve based on the fundamental equation of fluid dynamics:

$$V = \frac{Q}{PVA} = \frac{SV \times HR}{PVA}$$

where V is the antegrade velocity across the pulmonic valve, Q is the volumetric flow across the pulmonic valve in systole, SV is the stroke volume, HR is the heart rate, and PVA is the pulmonic valve area. Thus, when PVA remains constant, any increase in SV leads to elevation in the transvalvular velocity.

Answer (C) is incorrect as it is the right ventricular systolic pressure that exceeds the pulmonary artery pressure by only 9 mm Hg.

Answer (E) is incorrect because in uncomplicated PDA, antegrade flow occurs during both systole and diastole. In the patient's tracing, there is antegrade flow in systole and retrograde flow in diastole.

19. *ANSWER: C.* The tracings were obtained from an elderly woman presenting with acutely decompensated heart failure.

Mean left atrial pressure can be estimated semi-quantitatively from the ratio of peak flow velocity of mitral E wave and the peak velocity of mitral annular tissue Doppler e' wave according to this chart:

TABLE 7-25

	Left Atrial Pressure		
	Normal	Indeterminate	Elevated
E/e' using medial e'	<8	8–15	>15
E/e' using lateral e'	<8	8–12	>12

In our patient, E/lateral e' is 142/8, or 18. This ratio is consistent with elevated left atrial pressure. Therefore, answer C is correct.

Answer (A) is incorrect because the patient is likely to have poor exercise capacity with exertional dyspnea given the elevation of left atrial pressure even at rest. With exertion, left atrial pressure is expected to rise even further.

Answer (B) is incorrect because the patient's mitral inflow pattern is a combination of abnormal left ventricular relaxation and elevated left atrial pressure. The mitral E/A ratio that is greater than 2 in conjunction with a rapid E-wave DT (<160 msec) indicates a restrictive filling pattern. The features of different filling patterns in individuals older than 60 years are summarized in this table.

TABLE 7-26

Filling Pattern	Diastolic Dysfunction	Mitral Inflow E/A	Deceleration Time (msec)	Pulmonary Vein S/D	Mitral Annular e' (cm/s)
Normal	None	0.6–1.3	≤258	>1	>8
Abnormal relaxation	Mild	<0.8	>258	>1	<8
Pseudonormal	Moderate	0.8–2	160–258	<1	<8
Restrictive filling	Severe	>2	<160	<1	<8

Answer (D) is incorrect because the patient has a restrictive filling pattern. This is an abnormal finding and consistent with severe left ventricular diastolic dysfunction.

Answer (E) is incorrect because with the Valsalva maneuver, the peak velocity of the mitral E wave is expected to decrease. Valsalva maneuver decreases preload and leads to a lower early diastolic pressure gradient between the left atrium and left ventricle. This leads to a lower peak velocity of the mitral E wave and a lower mitral E/A ratio.

20. ANSWER: B. In sinus rhythm, the left atrium contracts following the P wave on EKG and the blood is propelled both forward into the left ventricle across the mitral valve, as well as backward into the pulmonary veins, which lack valves. The velocity profile of the forward flow is responsible for the mitral inflow A wave, while the retrograde flow into the pulmonary veins is responsible for the atrial reversal (AR) wave.

When the left ventricular diastolic pressure is elevated at the time of atrial contraction, both the peak velocity and the duration of the AR wave are increased. A peak AR velocity of >35 cm/sec is indicative of elevated LV end-diastolic pressure.

Elevation of LV end-diastolic pressure can also be inferred when the duration of the AR wave is >30 msec more than the duration of the mitral inflow A wave. In our patient, the peak velocity of AR was 50 cm/sec, and AR outlasted mitral A wave by 40 msec (210−170 msec); both are indicative of an elevated LV diastolic pressure. Therefore, answer (B) is correct.

For further explanation, the reader is referred to Figure 13 in the Canadian Consensus Recommendations for the Measurement and Reporting of Diastolic Dysfunction by Echocardiography (*J Am Soc Echocardiogr* 1996;9:736−760).

Answer (A) is incorrect because a restrictive filling pattern is characterized by a mitral inflow E/A ratio > 2; in this patient peak E-wave velocity is barely higher than the peak A-wave velocity.

Answer (C) is incorrect because the higher the peak velocity of the atrial reversal wave in the pulmonary vein spectral tracing, the higher the left ventricular diastolic pressure.

Answer (D) is incorrect because with left ventricular dysfunction, there is an increase in the left ventricular diastolic pressure leading to secondary pulmonary hypertension. Because of LV diastolic pressure elevation, the pulmonary vein atrial reversal wave is likely to be prominent (as explained above) rather than absent. Atrial reversal wave is absent in atrial arrhythmias, such as atrial fibrillation.

Answer (E) is incorrect because when left atrial pressure is elevated in older patients, the peak velocity of the systolic wave (S wave) in the pulmonary vein tracings is generally lower than the peak velocity of the diastolic wave (D wave). The higher the left atrial pressure, the lower the S/D ratio is.

21. ANSWER: B. In constrictive pericarditis, ventricular filling is constrained by an inelastic pericardial sac which envelopes the entire heart except for the cranial portion of the left atrium and the pulmonary veins. This results in (1) ventricular interdependence, and (2) differential impact of negative intrathoracic pressure that develops during inspiration on the pulmonary veins and the heart.

Ventricular interdependence refers to diastolic filling of one ventricle at the expense of the other depending on the respiratory phase. In inspiration, the pressure in the intrathoracic systemic vein decreases. This leads to a larger pressure gradient between extra- and intrathoracic systemic veins which results in improved RV filling. At the same time, the drop in the intrathoracic pressure with inspiration decreases the pulmonary venous pressure. Because of the thickened rigid pericardium, the drop in the intrathoracic pressure cannot be transmitted to the heart; this results in a decreased pressure gradient between the pulmonary veins and the left atrium, and decreased LV filling in diastole.

The net effect of inspiration is such that the right ventricle fills at the expense of the left ventricle, and the interventricular septum moves toward the left ventricle. The opposite occurs in expiration. This is illustrated in the M-mode recordings of our patient. The recordings also demonstrate no pericardial effusion.

With inspiration, the drop in intrathoracic pressure enhances forward flow in the hepatic veins in normal individuals; in constrictive pericarditis, there is an exaggeration of this inspiratory forward flow enhancement. During expiration, the rightward shift impedes RV filling; the rise in the the RV diastolic pressure then leads to an expiratory increase in hepatic vein flow reversal. Therefore, answer (B) is correct.

Answer (A) is incorrect because the presence of marked reciprocal changes in the right and left ventricular filling that are phasic with respiration are indicative of ventricular interdependence.

Answer (C) is incorrect because the abnormal septal motion due to right ventricular overload (as in atrial septal defect or severe tricuspid regurgitation) is characterized by flattening of the interventricular septum with each diastole rather than being phasic with respiration.

Answer (D) is incorrect because inspiratory increase in antegrade velocities is a normal finding. During inspiration, the drop in intrathoracic pressures enhances systemic venous return. This increased flow into the right heart elevates antegrade velocities in the hepatic veins.

Answer (E) is incorrect because the M mode reveals no echo lucency posterior to the left ventricle that would be diagnostic of a large pericardial effusion. Instead, it shows pericardial thickening. It is important to emphasize, however, that the abnormal interventricular septal motion phasic with respiration is encountered in both tamponade and constrictive pericarditis.

22. ANSWER: B. In a normal descending aorta, antegrade flow occurs only in systole and there is a small flow reversal in early diastole as depicted in the pulsed wave Doppler tracing in Figure 7-28A:

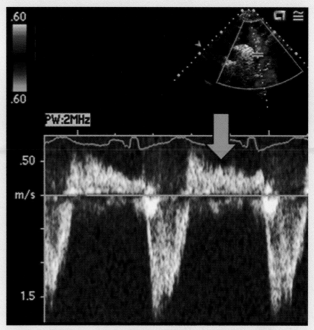

Fig. 7-28B

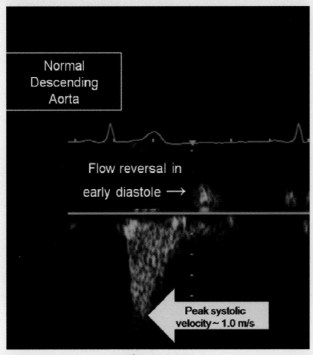

Fig. 7-28A

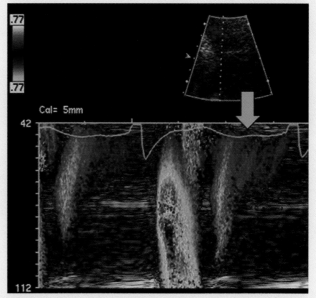

Fig. 7-28C

The pulsed-wave Doppler tracing in Figure 7-7 is abnormal as it demonstrates antegrade flow is through the cardiac cycle. In addition, there is a large peak systolic gradient across the coarctation of almost 60 mm Hg. The presence of a holodiastolic antegrade flow in conjunction with a large systolic gradient is indicative of severe aortic coarctation. Therefore, answer B is correct.

Answer (A) is incorrect because in severe aortic regurgitation, there is a retrograde flow throughout diastole (holodiastolic flow reversal) as demonstrated in Figure 7-28B and C.

Answer (C) is incorrect because it is the bicuspid and not quadricuspid aortic valve that is typically associated with aortic coarctation. It is estimated that between 25% and 46% of all individuals with coarctation have a bicuspid aortic valve.

Answer (D) is incorrect for two reasons. First, if this were a recording from the ascending aorta, forward velocities would have been recorded above the baseline and not below it. Second, aortic stenosis is not characterized by an antegrade diastolic gradient across the aortic valve.

Answer (E) is incorrect because coarctation usually occurs distal to the origin of the neck arteries, and the blood pressure in the arms is higher than in the legs.

23. *ANSWER: C.* Normal systole consist of isovolumic contraction time and ejection period. Flow across the aortic valve, whether the valve is normal or stenotic, occurs only during the ejection period of systole. In contrast, tricuspid regurgitant jet extends throughout the systole. Thus, on a spectral Doppler tracing, the aortic stenosis jet is of a shorter duration and has a later onset compared to the tricuspid regurgitant as demonstrated in these figures. Therefore, answer C is correct.

Answer (A) is incorrect because Figure 7-8B represents the flow velocity pattern across the aortic valve. Note the short time interval (isovolumic contraction time) between the QRS and the onset of flow in Figure 7-8B. In contrast, the onset of the tricuspid regurgitant jet in Figure 7-8A coincides with the QRS on EKG.

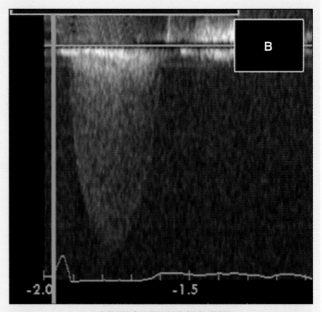

AORTIC STENOSIS JET
Peak velocity = 5.0 m/sec
Jet duration = 345 msec

Answer (B) is incorrect because the aortic jet starts after the isovolumic contraction period.

Answer (D) is incorrect because a peak velocity of 5 m/sec does not exclude a tricuspid regurgitant jet; such a tricuspid jet velocity can be recorded in a patient with a very severe pulmonary hypertension (pulmonary systolic pressure >100 mm Hg).

Answer (E) is incorrect because the systolic function of both ventricles appears normal given the rapid rise in velocities from their baseline to their peak values. This rapid flow acceleration is consistent with a normal *dP/dt*, a measure of systolic function.

24. *ANSWER: B.* In both tamponade and constrictive pericarditis, there is impairment in ventricular filling during the diastole. In tamponade, the impediment is caused by the pericardial fluid around the heart; while in constrictive pericarditis, the impediment is caused by a thickened, rigid, and sometimes calcified pericardium.

In tamponade, the left ventricular filling is impaired from the onset of diastole. On spectral Doppler tracings of mitral inflow, this is manifested by the pattern of abnormal relaxation (peak velocity of the mitral E wave is lower than that of the A wave, and the DT of the E wave is prolonged).

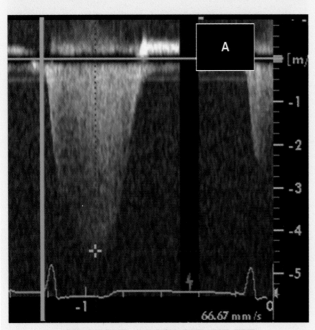

TRICUSPID REGURGITANT JET
Peak velocity = 4.5 m/sec
Jet duration = 515 msec

In contrast, in constrictive pericarditis, early diastolic filling is rapid but then abruptly decreases in late diastole when the expanding myocardium reaches the rigid pericardium. This can be demonstrated by either cardiac catheterization or Doppler echocardiography. On cardiac catheterization, there is a rapid y descent in RAP tracings, and a dip-and-plateau pattern on right ventricular pressure tracings. On spectral Doppler recordings of mitral inflow, there is a restrictive filling pattern (the ratio of peak E wave to peak A wave velocity >2; DT of E wave <160 msec).

Both in tamponade and constrictive pericarditis, there is ventricular interdependence, which was discussed in the answer to question 21. Because of ventricular interdependence, there is marked decrease in left ventricular filling during inspiration. The magnitude of inspiratory drop in early diastolic filling (as measured by peak velocity of mitral E wave) is directly proportional to the severity of either tamponade or constrictive pericarditis. In normal individuals, inspiratory drop in peak E wave velocity with inspiration is small; in tamponade and constrictive pericarditis, the inspiratory drop is >25%. One uses the following formula to calculate percent respiratory variation in the peak velocity of mitral E wave (ΔE):

$$\Delta E = \frac{E_{\text{Expiration}} - E_{\text{Inspiration}}}{E_{\text{Expiration}}}$$

Bear in mind that marked respiratory variations are not unique to tamponade and constrictive pericarditis; they also occur with labored breathing, asthma, chronic obstructive lung disease, pulmonary embolism, and obesity.

In our patient:

$$\Delta E = \frac{170 - 110}{170} = \frac{60}{170} = 35\%$$

In summary, the combination of the abnormal relaxation mitral inflow pattern and the marked respiratory variations in the peak velocity of the mitral inflow E wave are consistent with the diagnosis of cardiac tamponade. Therefore, answer (E) is correct.

Answer (A) is incorrect because in both tamponade and constrictive pericarditis, the respiratory variations are measured in the peak velocity of the E wave, not the A wave.

Answer (C) is incorrect for two reasons. First, the mitral inflow filling pattern in this patient demonstrates abnormal relaxation (E/A < 1) rather than restrictive fill-

ing (E/A > 2 and E-wave DT <160 msec). Second, there are no significant respiratory variations in mitral inflow in patients with restrictive cardiomyopathy. An additional distinction between restrictive cardiomyopathy and constrictive pericarditis is the peak velocity of the mitral annular tissue Doppler early diastolic e' wave. The e' velocity is normal or increased in constrictive pericarditis and diminished in restrictive cardiomyopathy.

Answer (D) is incorrect because an E/A < 1 favors tamponade over constrictive pericarditis as discussed above.

Answer (E) is incorrect because diuretics should not be administered to patients with tamponade physiology since the decrease in preload caused by diuretics would further impair ventricular filling.

25. ANSWER: A. The spectral recordings were obtained from a patient with very severe tricuspid regurgitation. When the tricuspid regurgitant orifice is large, there is ventricularization of the RAP which results in a very rapid pressure equilibration between right ventricular pressure (RVP) and the RAP as demonstrated in the pressure tracings in Figure 7-29A.

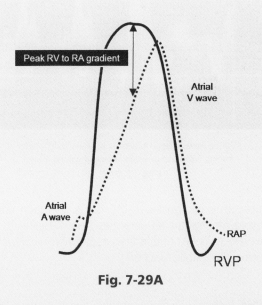

Fig. 7-29A

The rapid rise in the RAP results in rapid deceleration slope of the tricuspid regurgitant jet (arrow in the continuous Doppler tracing of the tricuspid regurgitant jet, Fig. 7-29B). Therefore, answer (A) is correct.

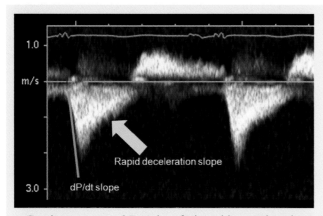

Continuous spectral Doppler of tricuspid regurgitant jet
Fig. 7-29B

Clinically, a patient with this type of tricuspid regurgitation typically has a pulsatile liver. An echocardiographic correlate of pulsatile liver is the systolic wave reversal in these hepatic vein spectral Doppler tracings (Fig. 7-29C).

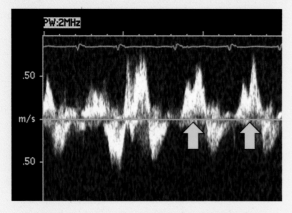

Systolic wave reversal in hepatic vein spectral Doppler tracing indicative of severe tricuspid regurgitation.
Fig. 7-29C

Answer (B) is incorrect because the acceleration rate in tricuspid regurgitant jet velocities from baseline to the peak velocity is fast and indicative of a normal *dP/dt* and a normal RV systolic function.

Answer (C) is incorrect because of the rapid pressure equilibration between the RV and RA due to rapid rise in the RA pressure; the peak velocity of the tricuspid regurgitant jet is often low even in the presence of significant pulmonary hypertension.

Answer (D) is incorrect because the flow velocity profile of this patient's tricuspid regurgitant jet is typical of severe tricuspid regurgitation (low peak velocity; rapid deceleration slope due to rapid pressure equilibration between RV and RA).

Answer (E) is incorrect because the spectral Doppler tracing of a midcavitary right ventricular gradient has its peak in late systole. In this patient, the jet peaks in early systole.

26. ANSWER: C. The patient initially presents with acutely decompensated heart failure due to acute coronary syndrome (non-ST elevation myocardial infarction) in the distribution of the left anterior descending coronary artery.

The five mitral inflow patterns presented in question 26 were as follows:

TABLE 7-27

A	Abnormal relaxation pattern (Grade I diastolic dysfunction)
B	Pseudonormal pattern (Grade II diastolic dysfunction)
C	Restrictive filling pattern (Grade III diastolic dysfunction)
D	Mitral inflow in a patient with a mechanical mitral valve (note the vertical line artifact due to opening and closing of the prosthetic leaflets).
E	Mitral inflow in a patient with atrial fibrillation.

Since the patient has normal native mitral valve and was in normal sinus rhythm at the time of study, patterns D and E do not belong to this patient.

Using the E/e' ratio concept (discussed in the answer to question 8), we can estimate the mean pulmonary artery wedge pressure (PAWP) for the remaining three patterns:

TABLE 7-28

Pattern	Peak E Velocity (cm/sec)	Peak e' Velocity (cm/sec)	PAWP = 1.9 + 1.24 × (E/e') (mm Hg)	PAWP = 4 + E/e' (mm Hg)
A	45	5	13	13
B	60	5	17	16
C	150	5	39	34

Of the three remaining patterns, only the restrictive filling (pattern C) predicts a PAWP that is in general agreement with the 38 mm Hg value obtained invasively by Swan-Ganz catheter. Therefore, answer (C) is correct.

KEY POINTS:

- In normal sinus rhythm, the mitral inflow pattern is characterized by two antegrade waves: E wave in early diastole, and A wave in late diastole following atrial contraction. In atrial fibrillation, the A wave is abolished.
- In elderly patients, the ratio of peak E and A velocities is usually <1 and the DT of the mitral E wave is prolonged.
- Elevation in left atrial pressure in elderly individuals leads to a progressive increase in the E/A ratio and a progressive shortening of the mitral E-wave DT. With progressive increase in left atrial pressure, the abnormal relaxation pattern gradually becomes pseudonormal. With further increase in the left atrial pressures, the mitral filling pattern becomes restrictive.

27. ANSWER: E. The severity of mitral regurgitation can be assessed using the PISA method to calculate the effective regurgitant orifice area (EROA):

$$EROA = 2 \times \pi \times r^2 \times \frac{Valias}{Vmax}$$

In our patient, radius was 0.9 cm, $Valias$ was 69 cm/sec, and $Vmax$ was 420 cm/sec:

$$EROA = 2 \times 3.14 \times (0.9)^2 \times (69/420) = 0.8 \text{ cm}^2$$

This EROA is very large (Table 7-29) and indicative of severe mitral regurgitation.

Therefore, answer (E) is correct.

KEY POINTS:

- Proximal isovelocity surface area (PISA) method can be used to calculate the effective regurgitant orifice (ROA) of mitral regurgitation.
- To calculate ROA, the following three parameters are required: the PISA radius, the aliasing velocity at which PISA radius is measured, and the peak velocity of the mitral regurgitant flow.
- In severe mitral regurgitation, ROA is usually ≥ 0.4 cm^2 (≥ 40 mm^2).

28. ANSWER: A. The patient presented with severe acute mitral regurgitation 8 days after a myocardial infarction in the territory of the left anterior descending artery that resulted in the rupture of the anterolateral papillary muscle. The course of events is consistent with the timeframe in which papillary muscle rupture, a mechanical complication of myocardial infarction, typically occurs.

The additional TEE images in Figure 7-30 further illustrate the case.

TABLE 7-29

	Mild (1+)	Moderate (2+)	Moderate-Severe (3+)	Severe (4+)
EROA (cm^2)	<0.2	0.20–0.29	0.30–0.39	$\geq$0.4
Regurgitant fraction	<30%	30–39%	40–49%	$\geq$50%
Regurgitant volume (mL)	30	30–44	45–59	$\geq$60
Vena contracta (cm)	<0.3			$\geq$0.7

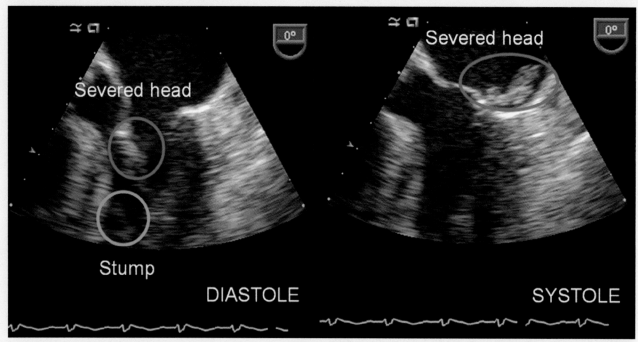

Fig. 7-30

(See also Video 7-3, ruptured anterolateral papillary muscle; TEE image at 0 degree.)

Rupture of the anterolateral papillary muscle is less common than the rupture of the posteromedial one. The anterolateral papillary muscle usually has a dual blood supply from both the left anterior descending and left circumflex arteries. In contrast, the posteromedial papillary muscle has a solitary blood supply from either the right coronary or left circumflex artery. Our patient had total proximal occlusion of the left anterior descending artery and diffuse disease in the left circumflex artery.

Answer (B) is incorrect because the clinical findings are inconsistent with bacteremia: the patient is afebrile and has a normal white blood count. In addition, a vegetation would appear as a shaggy, independently mobile echo density attached typically to the atrial side of the mitral valve. The mass seen in this patient is attached to the mitral chordae and represents a severed head of the anterolateral papillary muscle.

Answer (C) is incorrect because mitral annular dilatation typically leads to mitral regurgitation with a central jet. In this patient, the jet is highly eccentric which is consistent with papillary muscle rupture.

Answer (D) is incorrect because rheumatic mitral valve disease is a chronic disorder that typically begins in childhood and progresses over many years. In our patient, the mitral valve was normal on initial admission and became severely regurgitant only days later. In addition, TEE imaging of the mitral valve in this patient lacks typical findings of rheumatic valve disease, such as leaflet thickening and calcification, chordal fusion and shortening, etc.

Answer (E) is incorrect because mitral valve prolapse due to myxomatous generation is a chronic valvulopathy that would have been recognized on the initial echocardiogram at the time of first hospitalization. Mitral valve prolapse is characterized by floppy mitral leaflets that protrude into the left atrium above the mitral annular plane in systole due to leaflet and chordal elongation. Papillary muscle rupture is not a typical complication of mitral valve prolapse.

KEY POINTS:

- Common causes of severe acute mitral regurgitation include papillary muscle rupture, myxomatous degeneration of the mitral valve (which may lead to prolapsed and flail mitral leaflets), and mitral valve endocarditis.
- Papillary muscle rupture is a subacute complication of a myocardial infarction occurring usually 2–7 days after myocardial infarction.
- Rupture of the posterior papillary muscle is more common than the rupture of the anterior papillary muscle in survivors of myocardial infarction.

29. ANSWER: C. This patient has a PDA with a left-to-right shunt from the descending thoracic aorta to the left pulmonary artery throughout the cardiac cycle.

Using the spectral Doppler tracings of the PDA flow, one can calculate the peak systolic gradient (PSG) and end-diastolic gradient (EDG) across the PDA.

$$PSG = 4 \times PSV^2$$
$$EDG = 4 \times EDV^2$$

where PSV is the peak systolic velocity and EDV is the end-diastolic velocity across the PDA.

In our patient:

$$PSG = 4 \times (6.0 \text{ m/sec})^2 = 4 \times 36 = 144 \text{ mm Hg}$$
$$EDG = 4 \times (3.8 \text{ m/sec})^2 = 4 \times 14.4 = 58 \text{ mm Hg}$$

By subtracting PSG and EDG from systolic and diastolic blood pressures, respectively, one can estimate pulmonary artery systolic blood pressure (SBP) and diastolic blood pressure (DBP)

$$PASP = SBP - PSG$$
$$PADP = DBP - EDG$$

In our patient:

$$PASP = 170 - 144 = 26 \text{ mm Hg}$$
$$PADP = 70 - 58 = 12 \text{ mm Hg}$$

Therefore, answer B is correct. This patient's calculations are summarized in Table 7-30.

TABLE 7-30

	Velocity (m/sec)	PDA Gradient (mm Hg)	Blood Pressure (mm Hg)	Estimated Pulmonary Artery Pressure (mm Hg)
Systole	6.0	144	170	26
Diastole	3.8	58	70	12

Answer (A) is incorrect because the RAP is not needed to calculate PADP in a patient with PDA when DBP and EDG are known.

Answer (B) is incorrect because a pulsed wave Doppler technique would not have been able to record such high velocities (including a peak velocity of 6 m/sec) without aliasing in an adult.

Answer (D) is incorrect because PASP in this patient is 30 mm Hg as calculated above.

Answer (E) is incorrect because flow across an uncomplicated PDA occurs throughout the cardiac cycle irrespective of a PDA size. This is because in uncomplicated PDA, the pressures in the descending aorta are higher than the pressures in the pulmonary artery throughout the cardiac cycle.

KEY POINTS:

- In uncomplicated PDA, there is a continuous flow from the descending thoracic aorta into the pulmonary artery.
- Maximum flow velocity of PDA occurs at peak systole while the minimum velocity occurs at end diastole.
- If the blood pressure of a patient with PDA is measured at the time of PDA flow velocity recordings, one can calculate both the pulmonary artery systolic and pulmonary artery diastolic pressures using the peak systolic and end diastolic velocities of PDA flow.

30. *ANSWER: B.* The PISA method can be used to estimate the effective orifice area (EOA) of the PDA at its aortic end:

$$EOA = 2 \times \pi \times r^2 \times \frac{Valias}{Vmax}$$

where r is the PISA radius, $Valias$ is the PISA aliasing velocity, and $Vmax$ is the peak systolic velocity across the PDA.

In our patient:

$$EOA = 2 \times 3.14 \times (0.5 \text{ cm})^2 \times 41/500 = 0.13 \text{ cm}^2$$

Note that the color bar baseline was shifted upward. Of the two Nyquist limits (41 cm/sec for antegrade flow and 69 cm/sec for retrograde flow), one should use the one in the direction of PDA flow, which is 41 cm/sec.

Assuming a circular shape, the PDA orifice in this patient would then have a diameter of approximately 4 mm. The area (A) of a circle is calculated as:

$$A = \left(\frac{d}{2}\right)^2 \times \pi$$

where d is the PDA diameter. In our patient:

$$0.13 = \left(\frac{d}{2}\right)^2 \times 3.14 = \frac{0.13}{3.14} = \left(\frac{d}{2}\right)^2$$

Solving for diameter (d):

$$d = 2 \times \sqrt{\frac{0.13}{3.14}} = 0.4 \text{ cm} = 4 \text{ mm}$$

The diameter of a PDA usually ranges between 0.9 and 11.2 mm (median 2.6 mm).

KEY POINTS:

▓ The PISA method can be used to calculate the size of the aortic orifice of a PDA.

▓ The following three parameters are needed to calculate the PDA orifice area: PISA radius, aliasing velocity at which PISA is measured, and the peak velocity of the PDA flow.

▓ The diameter of a PDA usually ranges between 0.9 and 11.2 mm (median 2.6 mm).

31. ANSWER: C. This patient has hypertrophic obstructive cardiomyopathy (HOCM) with asymmetric septal hypertrophy. Systolic anterior motion of the mitral leaflets in HOCM leads to (1) dynamic LVOT obstruction, and (2) mitral regurgitation. Both the gradient across the LVOT and the gradient across the mitral valve peak late in systole.

One can calculate the peak systolic LVOT gradient from the following three parameters: peak gradient of mitral regurgitant jet, left atrial pressure, and systolic blood pressure.

Step 1: Calculate the peak systolic LV-to-LA gradient.

Using the peak velocity of the mitral regurgitant jet, one can calculated the peak systolic pressure gradient (ΔP_{MR}) between the left ventricle (LV) and the left atrium (LA):

$$\Delta P_{MR} = 4 \times V^2$$

where V is the peak velocity of the mitral regurgitant jet.

In our patient:

$$\Delta P_{MR} = 4 \times (8 \text{ m/sec})^2 = 4 \times 64 = 256 \text{ mm Hg}$$

Step 2: Calculate the peak LVSP.

By definition, ΔP_{MR} is the difference between the peak LVSP and the LA pressure (LAP):

$$\Delta P_{MR} = LVSP - LAP$$

Solving for LVSP:

$$LVSP = \Delta P_{MR} + LAP$$

In our patient:

$$LVSP = 256 \text{ mm Hg} + 10 \text{ mm Hg} = 266 \text{ mm Hg}$$

Step 3: Calculate maximal instantaneous left ventricular outflow gradient (ΔP_{LVOT}).

ΔP_{LVOT} is the pressure difference between the LVSP and the systolic blood pressure (SBP):

$$\Delta P_{LVOT} = LVSP - SBP$$

In our patient:

$$\Delta P_{LVOT} = 266 \text{ mm Hg} - 144 \text{ mm Hg} = 122 \text{ mm Hg}$$

Therefore, answer (C) is correct. All these calculations are summarized in Figure 7-31A.

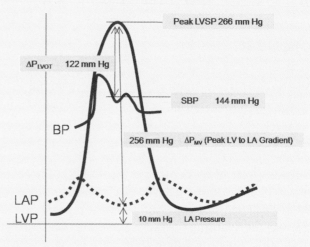

Fig. 7-31A

Answer (A) is incorrect because in HOCM, mitral regurgitation increases progressively toward mid to late systole. MR in HOCM is the result of systolic anterior motion (SAM); the anterior leaflet moves progressively toward the interventricular septum and away from the coaptation line with the posterior leaflet. This results in an MR velocity profile that peaks late in systole. Therefore, in our patient, the initial portion of the mitral regurgitant jet is not missing from the Doppler tracing; the Doppler velocity profile is typical for HOCM-related MR.

Answer (B) is incorrect because LVSP is very high. It is calculated above at 266 mm Hg. Normal LVSP is the same as the normal SBP, which is around 120 mm Hg.

Answer (D) is incorrect because there is no diastolic MR in this patient. Typically, MR is a systolic phenomenon. In rare instances, MR can start in late diastole (diastolic MR) and continue into systole. Diastolic MR may occur in severe LV systolic dysfunction or with complete heart block.

Different MR velocity profiles are summarized in Figure 7-31B.

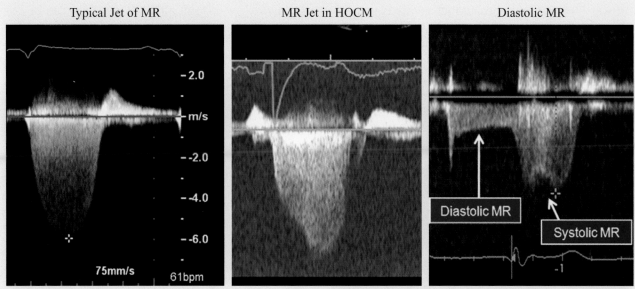

Typical Jet of MR | MR Jet in HOCM | Diastolic MR

Diastolic MR

Systolic MR

75mm/s 61bpm

Fig. 7-31B

Answer (E) is incorrect because the peak LV systolic pressure in this patient is 266 mm Hg as calculated above.

KEY POINTS:

■ In a patient with hypertrophic cardiomyopathy and a left ventricular outflow gradient, the flow velocity pattern of a mitral regurgitant jet typically peaks late in systole.

■ Using the peak velocity of the mitral regurgitant flow and the systolic blood pressure, one can indirectly calculate the peak instantaneous left ventricular outflow gradient.

■ Diastolic mitral regurgitation is not typically associated with hypertrophic obstructive cardiomyopathy.

32. ANSWER: C. In this patient with HOCM, jet #1 represents the systolic flow velocity pattern across the LVOT, and jet #2 represents the flow velocity pattern of the mitral regurgitant (MR) jet.

Jet #1 has a sawtooth appearance because the gradient characteristically peaks late in systole. The systolic anterior motion of the mitral valve in HOCM progressively narrows the LVOT toward the end of systole. This, in turn, results in ever-increasing systolic blood velocities through the LVOT and the late peaking velocity profile typical of HOCM.

Using the $\Delta P = 4V^2$ formula, we can calculate the peak systolic instantaneous gradient (ΔP_{LVOT}) across the LVOT, where V represents the peak velocity of jet #1.

$$\Delta P_{LVOT} = 4 \times (3.8 \text{ m/sec})^2 = 4 \times 14.4$$
$$= 58 \text{ mm Hg}$$

Since the pretreatment ΔP_{LVOT} was 120 mm Hg, there was an approximately 50% drop in the gradient on the repeat echocardiogram:

$$\text{Percent drop in } \Delta P_{LVOT} = (122 - 58)/122$$
$$= 64/122 \approx 50\%$$

Therefore, answer (C) is correct.

Answer (A) is incorrect because in mitral valve prolapse with click and systolic murmur, mitral regurgitation characteristically does not occur in early systole. The prolapse usually does not create a regurgitant orifice until midsystole. Once the regurgitant orifice is created, mitral regurgitation continues until the end of systole. The difference in the shape of the mitral regurgitant spectral jet between mitral valve prolapse and HOCM is depicted in Figure 7-32A.

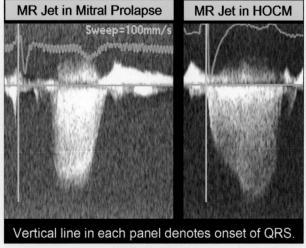

MR Jet in Mitral Prolapse | MR Jet in HOCM

Sweep=100mm/s

Vertical line in each panel denotes onset of QRS.

Fig. 7-32A

Answer (B) is incorrect because jet #2 starts immediately after the QRS complex on the EKG. Therefore, the jet encompasses the isovolumic contraction time. Aortic stenosis flow does not occur in that early portion of systole. For further discussion of this topic, please see the answer to question 23.

Answer (D) is incorrect because an intracavitary left ventricular gradient tapers off and peaks even later in systole than the LVOT gradient as shown in Figure 7-32B.

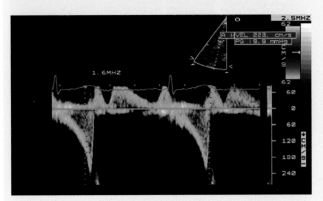

Pulsed wave spectral Doppler tracing of a left ventricular intracavitary gradient.

Fig. 7-32B

Answer (E) is incorrect because the peak LVSP is calculated as:

$$LVSP = \Delta P_{MR} + LAP \qquad \text{(Eq. 1)}$$

where ΔPMR is the peak systolic gradient of the mitral regurgitant jet, and LAP is the left atrial pressure. After expressing ΔPMR in terms of the peak systolic velocity (V) of the mitral regurgitant jet, Eq. 1 becomes:

$$LVSP = 4 \times V^2 + LAP \qquad \text{(Eq. 2)}$$

In our patient:

$$LVSP = 4 \times (6.3 \text{ m/sec})^2 + 10$$
$$LVSP = 159 + 10 = 169 \text{ mm Hg}$$

KEY POINTS:

■ In a patient with HOCM, the left ventricular outflow gradient characteristically peaks late in systole.

■ Using the peak velocity (V) of the flow velocity pattern across the left ventricular gradient, one can calculate the peak instantaneous pressure gradient (ΔP) as $\Delta P = 4 \times V^2$.

■ Intracavitary left ventricular gradient peaks even later in systole compared to the left ventricular outflow gradient.

33. ANSWER: D. Left atrial volume (LAV) can be calculated using the area-length method. The mathematical formula requires three parameters: left atrial area in the apical 4-chamber view (A1), left atrial area in the apical 2-chamber view (A2), and the shorter of the two atrial lengths (L) whether it be in the apical 4- or apical 2-chamber view.

$$LAV = \frac{8 \times A1 \times A2}{3 \times \pi \times L}$$

The formula can be simplified by calculating the $8/3\pi$ ratio as 0.85:

$$LAV = 0.85 \times \frac{A1 \times A2}{L}$$

In our patient:

$$LAV = 0.85 \times \frac{27 \times 26}{5.6} = 107 \text{ ml}$$

LAV index (LAVI) is calculating by dividing LAV into the body surface area (BSA):

$$LAVI = \frac{LAV}{BSA}$$

In our patient:

$$LAVI = 107 \text{ ml}/2.1 \text{ m}^2 \approx 50 \text{ ml/m}^2$$

Therefore, answer (D) is correct. This is a severely elevated LAVI (see reference table here).

TABLE 7-31

	LA Volume Index (ml/m^2)
Normal	≤28
Mild dilatation	29–33
Moderate dilatation	34–39
Severe dilatation	≥40

KEY POINTS:

■ Area-length method is the recommended method for calculating the LAV. Once calculated, the volume should be indexed for patient's body surface area.

■ LAV should be calculated as an average of atrial volumes obtained in the apical 4-chamber and apical 2-chamber views.

■ Chronic elevation of LAP leads to progressive increase in LAVI.

34. ANSWER: B. The initial echocardiogram, which was obtained at the time of acutely decompensated heart failure, demonstrates the restrictive filling pattern. Because of the high left atrial pressures, the early diastolic gradient across the mitral valve is high. This results in a tall mitral E wave and the ratio of peak mitral E to peak mitral A wave that is usually >2. In addition, the mitral E wave has rapid deceleration (DT <160 msec). In the pulmonary venous spectral Doppler tracings, the peak of the systolic (S) wave is lower than the peak of the diastolic (D) wave. The height of the S wave is inversely related to the left atrial pressure. All these findings in mitral and pulmonary vein pulsed wave Doppler tracings are consistent with the restrictive filling pattern.

With appropriate medical treatment, including diuretics, left atrial pressure decreases and the mitral inflow reverts to the pattern of abnormal relaxation common in the patient's age group. The pattern is characterized by an E < A pattern in the mitral inflow and a prolonged DT of the mitral E wave. In the pulmonary veins, the peak velocity of the S wave now exceeds the peak velocity of the D wave (S > D), reflective of lower left atrial pressures.

Therefore, answer B is correct.

Different mitral and pulmonary vein filling patterns as well as their relationship to mean left atrial pressure are summarized in Figure 7-33.

Answer (A) is incorrect because the preload has decreased from the initial to the subsequent study as judged by the decrease in the mean left atrial pressure.

Answer (C) is incorrect because the initial filling pattern was not normal; it was restrictive. A normal pattern cannot be distinguished from a pseudonormal pattern by mitral and pulmonary flow patterns alone. Ancillary data, such as the peak velocity of the mitral annular tissue Doppler e' wave, are required to distinguish a normal (e' > 8 cm/sec) from pseudonormal pattern (e' < 8 cm/sec).

Answer (D) is incorrect because the presence of a prominent and normally timed A wave in mitral inflow and the S wave in the pulmonary vein argue against atrial arrhythmias, such as atrial flutter or atrial fibrillation. In these atrial arrhythmias, the peak velocities of the mitral A wave and the pulmonary vein S wave are greatly diminished.

Answer (E) is incorrect because it is the persistence of the restrictive pattern despite appropriate medical therapy that portends a grave prognosis with a 2-year mortality estimated at 50% in patients with a left ventricular ejection fraction of <40%. In this patient, the change from the restrictive filling to the abnormal relaxation pattern actually portends a better prognosis.

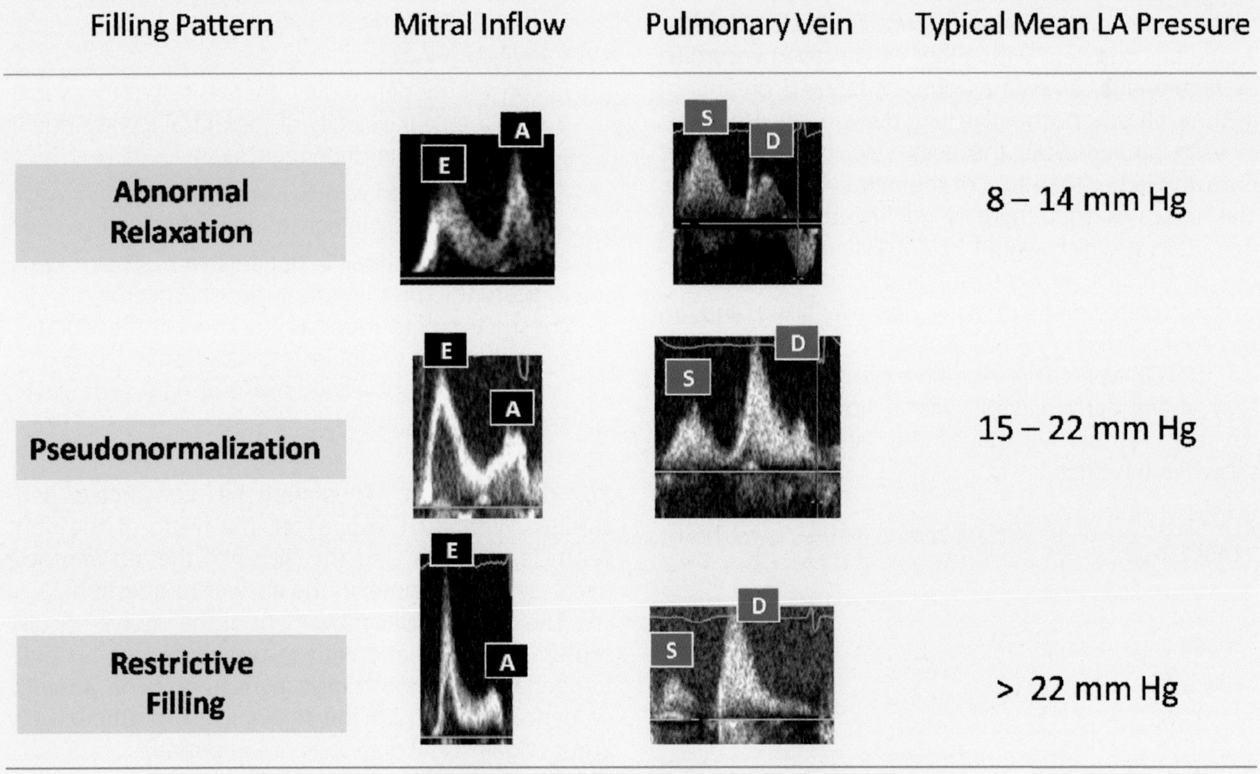

Filling Pattern	Mitral Inflow	Pulmonary Vein	Typical Mean LA Pressure
Abnormal Relaxation			8 – 14 mm Hg
Pseudonormalization			15 – 22 mm Hg
Restrictive Filling			> 22 mm Hg

Fig. 7-33

KEY POINTS:

▨ In a healthy elderly individual, mitral inflow E wave has a lower peak velocity than the A wave (E < A) and there is prolonged E-wave DT. In the pulmonary venous flow velocity recordings, the peak velocity of the systolic (S) wave is typically higher than the peak velocity of the diastolic (D) wave (S > D) in that age group.

▨ With left atrial pressure elevation, there is a progressive increase in the velocity of the mitral E wave, shortening of its DT, and an increase in the E/A ratio. In addition, there is an inverse relationship between the left atrial pressure and the peak velocity of the pulmonary vein S wave; the higher the left atrial pressure, the lower the peak velocity of the S wave and lower the S/D ratio.

▨ Therapy with diuretics in patients with elevated left atrial pressure typically leads to lowering of the peak velocity of the mitral E wave and an increase in the peak velocity of the pulmonary vein S wave.

35. ANSWER: D. The three recordings from this patient are consistent with the diagnosis of constrictive pericarditis.

MITRAL INFLOW—The mitral inflow spectral Doppler tracings demonstrate marked respiratory variations in the mitral E-wave velocities. Such a finding would be consistent with either constrictive pericarditis or tamponade, as well as obesity, labored breathing, asthma, chronic obstructive lung disease, etc. However, in each cardiac cycle, the peak velocity of the mitral E wave is larger than that of the mitral A wave (E > A). This indicates that there is no impediment to early mitral filling which would be consistent with constrictive pericarditis. In contrast, tamponade is characterized by impediment in early diastolic filling and an E < A.

COLOR M MODE—The flow propagation velocity (Vp) of the early diastolic mitral flow is normal (66 cm/sec). Normal Vp values are age dependent as shown in this table.

TABLE 7-32

	Normal Vp (cm/sec)
Young	>55
Elderly	>45

Vp measures the rate of left ventricular myocardial relaxation. The faster the rate of myocardial relaxation, the higher the Vp. Typically, there is no significant myocardial involvement in constrictive pericarditis, Vp is

normal. This is in contrast to restrictive cardiomyopathy which is a myocardial disorder characterized by impaired relaxation and compliance. In restrictive cardiomyopathy, Vp is low.

IVC—In constrictive pericarditis, there is plethora of the IVC as demonstrated by the M-mode recordings in this patient. The IVC is dilated (2.43 cm in expiration), and collapses less than 50% with inspiration (inspiratory diameter of IVC = 1.97 cm). The finding is indicative of an elevated RAP (10–20 mm Hg) as discussed in answer to question 1. Such a finding is consistent with the diagnosis with constrictive pericarditis. However, IVC plethora is also found in other conditions of elevated RAP, such as tricuspid stenosis, severe tricuspid regurgitation, right ventricular infarct, etc.

Therefore, answer D is correct.

Answer (A) is incorrect because in restrictive cardiomyopathy there are no marked respiratory variations in the mitral E-wave velocities. In addition, Vp is low in restrictive cardiomyopathy.

Answer (B) is incorrect because the IVC plethora is indicative of an elevated RAP.

Answer (C) is incorrect because Vp in this patient is normal (>55 cm/sec).

Answer (E) is incorrect because there are marker respiratory variations (>30%) in the peak velocity of the mitral E wave.

KEY POINTS:

▨ In constrictive pericarditis, there is respiratory variation in the peak velocity of the mitral E wave due to ventricular interdependence.

▨ Flow propagation velocity (Vp) of the mitral E wave is typically normal in constrictive pericarditis.

▨ IVC is often plethoric in patients with constrictive pericarditis. This plethora is not specific for constrictive pericarditis as it occurs in other conditions that lead to significant elevation in the RAP (such as tricuspid valve stenosis or right ventricular systolic dysfunction).

36. ANSWER: D. The patient has constrictive pericarditis. With each inspiration, the filling of the right ventricle increases and the filling of the left ventricle decreases as explained in the answer to question 21.

The characteristic movement of the interventricular septum that is phasic with respiration occurs in both tamponade and constrictive pericarditis. The absence of pericardial effusion on the apical 4-chamber view argues against the diagnosis of tamponade.

The abnormal septal motions stated in the remaining four answers are not phasic with respiration. Their characteristics are summarized in this table.

TABLE 7-33

Right ventricular pressure overload	Interventricular septum flattens in systole and diastole. In the short axis, left ventricular contour becomes D-shaped rather than circular in both systole and diastole.
Right ventricular volume overload	Interventricular septum flattens in diastole. In the short axis, left ventricular contour becomes D-shaped rather than circular during diastole.
Left bundle branch block	Interventricular septum moves posteriorly in the pre-ejection period, and then moves anteriorly (away from the posterior left ventricular wall) during the ejection phase of systole.
Cardiac surgery	Movement of the interventricular septum toward the right ventricle rather than the left ventricle in systole, with normal thickening.

KEY POINTS:

- Paradoxical interventricular septal motion can occur with each cardiac beat or may be phasic with respiration.
- Examples of paradoxical septal motion with each beat include right ventricular pressure or volume overload, left bundle branch block, and status post pericardiotomy.
- Paradoxical septal motion that is phasic with respiration is encountered in constrictive pericarditis, tamponade, labored breathing, obesity, pulmonary embolism, etc.

SUGGESTED READINGS

Abbasi AS, Eber LM, MacAlpin RN, et al. Paradoxical motion of interventricular septum in left bundle branch block. *Circulation*. 1974;49:423–427.

Abdalla I, Murray RD, Lee JC, et al. Duration of pulmonary venous atrial reversal flow velocity and mitral inflow A wave: new measure of severity of cardiac amyloidosis. *J Am Soc Echocardiogr*. 1998;11:1125–1133.

Bargiggia GS, Bertucci C, Recusani F, et al. A new method for estimating left ventricular dP/dt by continuous wave Doppler-echocardiography. Validation studies at cardiac catheterization. *Circulation*. 1990;82:316–317.

Bonow RO, Carabello BA, Chatterjee K, et al. ACC/AHA 2006 Guidelines for the Management of Patients with Valvular Heart Disease: a report of the American College of Cardiology/American Heart Association Task Force on Practice Guidelines (Writing Committee to Develop Guidelines for the Management of Patients with Valvular Heart Disease). *Circulation*. 2006;114:e84–e231.

Garcia MJ, Ares MA, Asher C, et al. An index of early left ventricular filling that combined with pulsed Doppler peak E velocity may estimate capillary wedge pressure. *J Am Coll Cardiol*. 1997;29: 448–454.

Hatle L, Angelsen B, Tromsdal A. Noninvasive assessment of atrioventricular pressure half-time by Doppler ultrasound. *Circulation*. 1979;60:1096–1104.

Hatle LK, Appleton CP, Popp RL. Differentiation of constrictive pericarditis and restrictive cardiomyopathy by Doppler echocardiography *Circulation*. 1989;79:357–370.

Kircher BJ, Himelman RB, Schiller NB. Noninvasive estimation of right atrial pressure from the inspiratory collapse of the inferior vena cava. *Am J Cardiol*. 1990;66:493–496.

Lang RM, Bierig M, Devereux RB, et al. Chamber Quantification Writing Group; American Society of Echocardiography's Guidelines and Standards Committee; European Association of Echocardiography. Recommendations for chamber quantification: a report from the American Society of Echocardiography's Guidelines and Standards Committee and the Chamber Quantification Writing Group, developed in conjunction with the European Association of Echocardiography, a branch of the European Society of Cardiology. *J Am Soc Echocardiogr*. 2005;18: 1440–1463.

Libanoff AJ, Rodbard S. Atrioventricular pressure half-time. Measure of mitral valve orifice area. *Circulation*. 1968;38:144–150.

Nagueh SF, Appleton CP, Gillebert TC, et al. Recommendations for the evaluation of left ventricular diastolic function by echocardiography. *J Am Soc Echocardiogr*. 2009;22:107–133.

Nagueh SF, Middleton KJ, Kopelen HA, et al. Doppler tissue imaging: a noninvasive technique for evaluation of left ventricular relaxation and estimation of filling pressures. *J Am Coll Cardiol*. 1997;30:1527–1533.

Nakatani S, Masuyama T, Kodama K, et al. Value and limitations of Doppler echocardiography in the quantification of stenotic mitral valve area: comparison of the pressure half-time and the continuity equation methods. *Circulation*. 1988;77:78–85.

Pass RH, Hijazi Z, Hsu DT, et al. Multicenter USA Amplatzer patent ductus arteriosus occlusion device trial. *J Am Coll Cardiol*. 2004; 44:513–519.

Rakowski H, Appleton C, Chan KL, et al. Canadian consensus recommendations for the measurement and reporting of diastolic dysfunction by echocardiography: from the Investigators of Consensus on Diastolic Dysfunction by Echocardiography. *J Am Soc Echocardiogr*. 1996;9:736–760.

Reynolds HR, Tunick PA, Grossi EA, et al. Paradoxical septal motion after cardiac surgery: a review of 3,292 cases. *Clin Cardiol*. 2007; 30:621–623.

Rossvoll O, Hatle LK. Pulmonary venous flow velocities recorded by transthoracic Doppler ultrasound: relation to left ventricular diastolic pressures. *J Am Coll Cardiol*. 1993;21:1687–1696.

von Bibra H, Schober K, Jenni R, et al. Diagnosis of constrictive pericarditis by pulsed Doppler echocardiography of the hepatic vein. *Am J Cardiol*. 1989;63:483–488.

Xie GY, Berk MR, Smith MD, et al. Prognostic value of Doppler transmitral flow patterns in patients with congestive heart failure. *J Am Coll Cardiol*. 1994;24:132–139.

CHAPTER 8

Tissue Doppler and Strain

Steve L. Liao and Mario J. Garcia

1. Compared with standard Doppler, tissue Doppler settings make use of:
   A. The lesser reflectivity of tissue.
   B. The faster motion of tissue.
   C. Filters to exclude highly reflective tissue.
   D. Filters to exclude higher velocities.

2. Strain rate for tissue Doppler is defined as:
   A. Measured tissue velocity × time.
   B. Absolute difference in velocities.
   C. The change in velocity between two points divided by the end distance.
   D. The change in distance between two points divided by the initial distance.

3. Which is correct regarding Doppler strain?
   A. Doppler-derived strain may be obtained in any direction from a single view.
   B. Doppler-derived strain is more dependent on translational motion than tissue velocity imaging.
   C. Doppler-derived systolic strain rate correlates with indices of contractility.
   D. Doppler-derived strain has lower spatial and temporal resolution than magnetic resonance imaging strain.

4. Which is the best acoustic window to obtain the Doppler-derived radial strain of the anterior wall?
   A. Parasternal long axis.
   B. Parasternal short axis.
   C. Apical four chamber.
   D. Apical two chamber.
   E. Subcostal.

5. Which of the following hemodynamic parameters best correlates with a combination of mitral E-wave velocity and early diastolic longitudinal velocities of the myocardium (e′)?
   A. Superior vena cava pressure.
   B. Right atrial pressure.
   C. Right ventricular systolic pressure.
   D. Mean left atrial pressure.

6. Compared with Doppler-derived strain, speckle-tracking strain:
   A. Provides no discernible advantage.
   B. Can be performed independent of grayscale distribution.
   C. Is based on the Doppler shift of reflected sound waves.
   D. Does not rely on a particular angle of imaging with respect to tissue motion.

7. Which of the following radial strain rates obtained at the mid-inferior wall during systole of a patient with ischemic cardiomyopathy is consistent with dyskinesis?
   A. 0.
   B. 1.
   C. −1.
   D. 10.

8. In left ventricular (LV) torsion:
   A. During systole, the basal segments of the LV myocardium rotate counterclockwise.
   B. During systole, the apical segments rotate counterclockwise.
   C. During diastole, the basal segments of the LV myocardium rotate counterclockwise.
   D. Basal twisting is the main component of LV systolic torsion.

9. Which of the following is a true statement about Doppler tissue imaging (DTI)?
   A. It is more preload dependent than traditional Doppler imaging.
   B. A normal velocity and pattern of mitral annular velocities does not always indicate normal diastolic function.
   C. It is unable to discriminate passive motion from active motion.
   D. M-mode color DTI has lower spatial resolution than pulsed DTI.

10. Which of the following instrumental setting changes will not result in improved temporal resolution for strain imaging?
    A. Altering the sector width of interrogation.
    B. Selecting a point of interest at a closer image depth.
    C. Selecting a point of interest that typically suffers from echo dropout.
    D. Altering the harmonics setting.

11. In asymmetric septal hypertrophic cardiomyopathy, tissue Doppler e′:
    A. Is abnormal in the lateral wall.
    B. Is normal in the septum.
    C. Has an inverse relationship with septal thickness.
    D. Has a direct relationship with septal thickness.

12. In diabetic patients, which of the following statements is correct?
    A. HgbA1C correlates with E/e′.
    B. Diabetic patients have a higher Doppler E′.
    C. Asymptomatic diabetic patients do not demonstrate an abnormal E/e′.
    D. The mechanism for any diastolic dysfunction is thought to be related to concomitant renal dysfunction.

13. In which of the following conditions has e′ been shown to improve after treatment?
    A. Cardiac amyloidosis.
    B. Hypertrophic cardiomyopathy.
    C. Dyskinesis in ischemic heart disease.
    D. Aortic stenosis.

14. Which of the following tissue Doppler indices has been shown to carry the most prognostic value after myocardial infarction (MI)?
    A. E.
    B. e′.
    C. E/e′.
    D. S.

15. Which of the following parameters is not directly related to active LV relaxation?
    A. Isovolumic relaxation time.
    B. e′ velocity.
    C. A velocity.
    D. LV torsion.

16. Strain measurements obtained from color tissue Doppler:
    A. Are not affected by the angle of interrogation.
    B. May vary from one heart beat to another.
    C. Achieve higher temporal resolution when using a wider color sector angle.
    D. Achieve higher temporal resolution when extending the depth of the sampling region.
    E. Cannot be obtained in patients with atrial fibrillation.

17. Which of the following cardiac conditions is associated with a normal or high e′?
    A. Friedreich's ataxia.
    B. Fabry's disease.
    C. Hypertrophic cardiomyopathy.
    D. Cardiac amyloidosis.
    E. Myocardial hypertrophy in athletic hearts.

18. In a patient with a localized basal lateral infarct with evidence of akinesis by two-dimensional Doppler imaging, the expected longitudinal tissue Doppler velocities (m/sec) and strain rate (1/sec) would be:
    A. Tissue Doppler velocity = 0.2, strain rate = 0.
    B. Tissue Doppler velocity = 0, strain rate = 0.2.
    C. Tissue Doppler velocity = 0.2, strain rate = −0.5.
    D. Tissue Doppler velocity = 0, strain rate = 0.

19. The radial strain map in Figure 8-1 obtained from a patient with chest pain demonstrates:

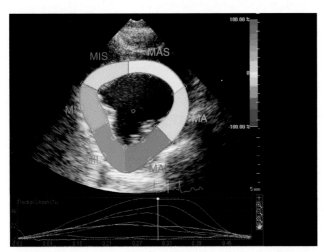

(MAL = mid anterolateral, MA = mid anterior, MAS = mid anteroseptal, MIS = mid iferoseptal, MI = mid inferior, MIL = mid inferolateral)

Fig. 8-1

A. Normal LV function.
B. Segmental dyskinesis.
C. Anterolateral hypokinesis.
D. Anteroseptal akinesis.

20. The strain rate pattern in Figure 8-2 is consistent with:

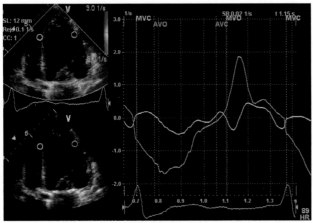

Fig. 8-2

A. Anteroseptal infarct.
B. Anterolateral infarct.
C. Extensive apical infarct.
D. Normal LV function.

21. A 70-year-old woman with ischemic heart disease and chronic obstructive pulmonary disease (COPD) presents for evaluation of dyspnea. What would you recommend on the basis of the echo Doppler findings in Figure 8-3?

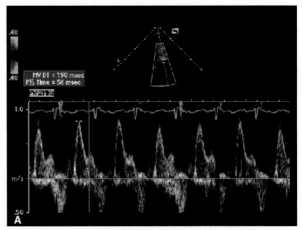

Fig. 8-3A

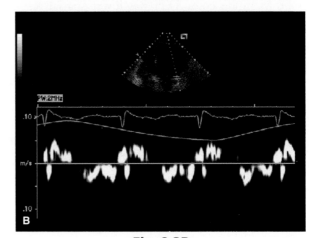

Fig. 8-3B

A. Evaluation for pulmonary embolism.
B. Intravenous diuresis and evaluation for ischemia.
C. Initiation of therapy for COPD exacerbation.
D. Right heart catheterization.

22. Two days after successful medical treatment in the previous case, symptoms of dyspnea have resolved. An echocardiogram is repeated, and the Doppler images are shown in Figure 8-4.

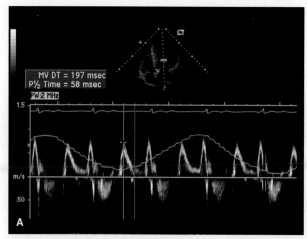

Fig. 8-4A

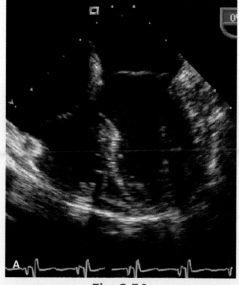

Fig. 8-5A

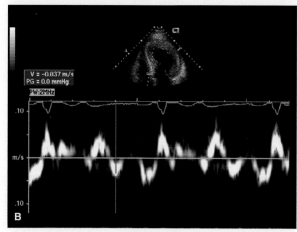

Fig. 8-4B

What can you conclude?

A. Patient requires more aggressive diuresis.

B. Patient has abnormal diastolic function.

C. Patient has a restrictive filling pattern.

D. Patient requires Doppler pulsed wave interrogation of her pulmonary veins to assess diastolic function.

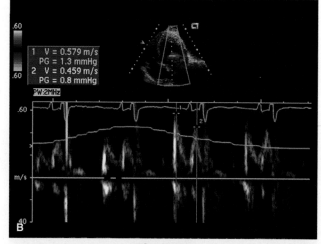

Fig. 8-5B

23. A 46-year-old woman with previous history of breast cancer treated with mastectomy, chemotherapy, and radiation therapy presents for evaluation of symptoms of fatigue. On examination she has a heart rate (HR) of 100 bpm, BP of 85/60 mm Hg, elevated jugular venous pressure (JVP), decreased breath sounds at the lung bases, ascites, and 3+ edema. Transesophageal and transthoracic echo Doppler images are shown in Figure 8-5. The most likely diagnosis is:

A. Hypertrophic cardiomyopathy.

B. Constrictive pericarditis.

C. Cardiac amyloidosis.

D. Restrictive cardiomyopathy postradiation.

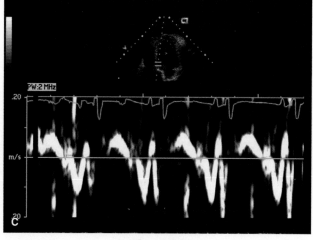

Fig. 8-5C

24. A 68-year-old woman presents for evaluation of dyspnea on exertion. Tissue Doppler images are shown in Figure 8-6.

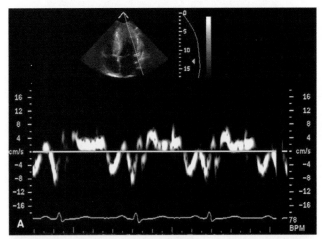

Fig. 8-6A

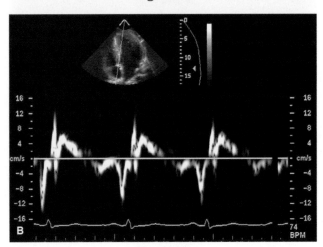

Fig. 8-6B

The most likely diagnosis is:
A. Asymmetric septal hypertrophic cardiomyopathy.
B. Anterolateral infarction.
C. Cardiac amyloidosis.
D. Constrictive pericarditis.

25. The image in Figure 8-7 was obtained from a 70-year-old patient presenting with chest pain. The longitudinal strain pattern suggests:
A. Anterior dyskinesis.
B. Apical dyskinesis.
C. Inferior dyskinesis.
D. Posterior dyskinesis.

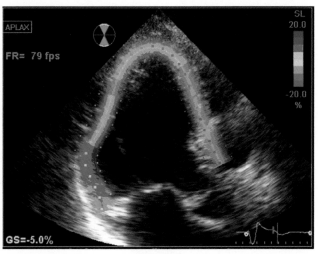

Fig. 8-7

26. A 64-year-old diabetic woman is referred for evaluation of heart failure symptoms. The two-dimensional (Fig. 8-8A), color tissue Doppler (Fig. 8-8B) images and strain (Fig. 8-8C) data obtained from the apical four-chamber view are consistent with:

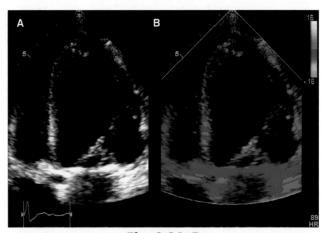

Fig. 8-8A–B

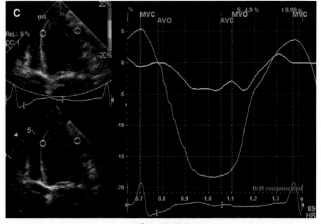

Fig. 8-8C

A. Dilated cardiomyopathy.

B. Ischemic heart disease.

C. Restrictive cardiomyopathy.

D. Hypertrophic cardiomyopathy.

27. A 35-year-old man is evaluated for palpitations. His BP is 120/70 mm Hg and his HR is 60 bpm. The findings from his physical examination are normal. An electrocardiogram shows increased voltage and diffused T-wave inversions. A transthoracic echocardiogram is performed. Two-dimensional (Fig. 8-9A), color Doppler (Fig. 8-9B) images and strain rate (Fig. 8-9C) measurements are obtained from the apical two-chamber view.

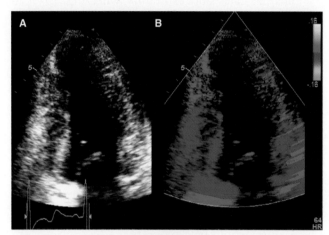

Fig. 8-9A–B

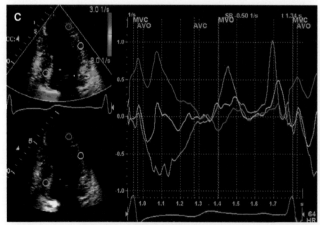

Fig. 8-9C

The most likely diagnosis is:

A. Asymmetric septal hypertrophic cardiomyopathy.

B. Apical hypertrophic cardiomyopathy.

C. LV dyssynchrony.

D. Normal structural heart.

28. A 72-year-old man is admitted to the hospital with decompensated heart failure. His BP is 100/70 mm Hg, and HR is 86 bpm. On examination, he has jugular venous distension, diffuse inspiratory rales, and 3+ pitting edema. He is taking carvedilol 25 mg twice daily, lisinopril 20 mg daily, furosemide 80 mg daily, and spironolactone 12.5 mg daily. Based on the two-dimensional (Fig. 8-10A) and color M-mode tissue Doppler (Fig. 8-10B) parasternal images, the most likely cause of heart failure is:

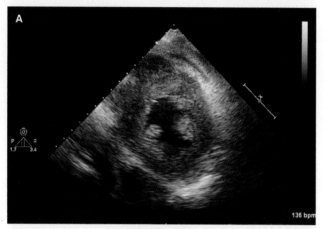

Fig. 8-10A

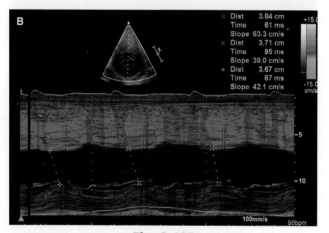

Fig. 8-10B

A. Atrial flutter.

B. Inferolateral MI.

C. Restrictive cardiomyopathy.

D. LV dyssynchrony.

29. A 62-year-old man with H/O rheumatic heart disease and previous mitral valve repair undergoes echocardiographic examination for evaluation of a heart murmur. The two-dimensional (Fig. 8-11A)

and color M-mode tissue Doppler (Fig. 8-11B) parasternal images are consistent with:

A. Anteroseptal MI.
B. Inferolateral MI.
C. LV dyssynchrony.
D. Normal postoperative findings.

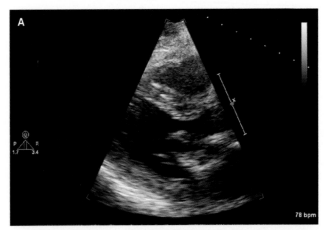

Fig. 8-11A

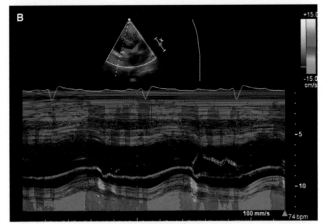

Fig. 8-11B

30. A 78-year-old woman with H/O diabetes, chronic renal insufficiency, sick sinus rhythm, congestive heart failure, and COPD presents to the emergency department with worsening symptoms of dyspnea. On her physical examination, BP is 160/90 mm Hg, HR is 60 bpm, and respiratory rate (RR) is 28. On auscultation, a II/VI ejection systolic murmur (ESM) is detected at the left upper sternal border (LUSB). Breath sounds are muffled, with both bibasilar rales and expiratory wheezing. Oxygen saturation is 90%. Initial blood work demonstrates hemoglobin count = 10 mg/dl, BUN = 50 mg/dl, and serum creatinine level = 2.0 mg/dl. An echocardiogram is performed immediately at the bedside while the patient has labored breathing. Apical four-chamber images obtained at end-diastole (Fig. 8-12A) and end-systole (Fig. 8-12B) as well as pulsed Doppler LV filling (Fig. 8-12C) and basal septal tissue Doppler (Fig. 8-12D) images are shown.

In addition to oxygen, you should initially recommend:

A. Intravenous furosemide.
B. Intravenous beta-blockers.
C. Inhaled bronchodilators.
D. Blood transfusion.

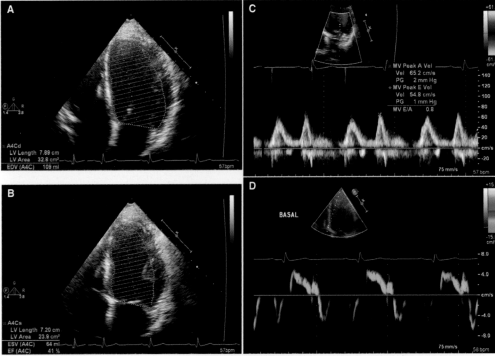

Fig. 8-12A–D

ANSWERS

1. ANSWER: D. Standard Doppler measures blood flow velocities on the basis of the Doppler effect. The change in frequency between transmitted sound and reflected sound is termed the "Doppler shift" and is used to calculate the velocity of the moving blood. Blood is a relatively weak reflector of sound waves and moves at a relatively high velocity; therefore, in standard Doppler, filters are used to exclude highly reflective and low-velocity objects, like myocardium so that the range of velocities to be measured is maximized. Conversely, since tissue moves at a slower velocity but has a higher reflectivity, DTI employs filters, which exclude low-intensity reflectors and higher velocities.

2. ANSWER: C. Based upon the information obtained from DTI about myocardial velocities, other variables related to myocardial motion can be determined. For example, the distance traveled by a measured point in the myocardium can be determined (velocity × time); and if two points are measured simultaneously, the velocity gradients between these two points can be determined. The change in distance of two points in the myocardium divided by the initial length or end diastolic length (end diastolic length—end systolic length/end diastolic length) is also known as myocardial *strain*. The *strain rate* (SR) is the first derivative of strain and is defined as the change in velocity between two points divided by the distance between the two points at the end of systole (L). SR $= (V_1 - V_2)/L$.

3. ANSWER: C. The standard Doppler equation is expressed as: $\Delta f = (2\,f_0 \times v \times \cos\theta)/c$ where Δf is the frequency shift, fo the transmitted frequency, c the speed of sound in blood, and θ the angle of the beam in relation to direction of blood flow. If $\theta = 0$ (parallel to direction of movement), then the cosine of 0 is 1. As the angle or θ increases, the cosine becomes progressively less than 1 resulting in an underestimation of Doppler shift and therefore peak velocity. Tissue Doppler is also dependent on θ when velocities are measured and is limited to interrogating segments aligned in parallel with the Doppler angle of incidence. Tissue velocity imaging is unable to discriminate passive motion from active deformation; however, strain is a measure of active tissue motion. Because of this ability to measure active tissue motion, there is a close correlation between strain rate and indices of LV contractility.

4. ANSWER: B. The spiral architecture of the myocardial fiber bundles determines strain deformation in multiple directions. Also, it is important to recall that the angle of incidence of the Doppler beam on the area of interest contributes to an accurate estimation of velocity by the Doppler equation:

$$\Delta f = (2\,f_0 \times v \times \cos\theta)/c.$$

Taking both the spiral architecture and the angle of incidence into account, changes in LV geometry during systole relate primarily to radial (short-axis), longitudinal (long-axis), and meridional (LV-torsion) strain. Therefore, radial strain (εr) of the anterior wall is best measured from the parasternal short-axis view (Fig. 8-13).

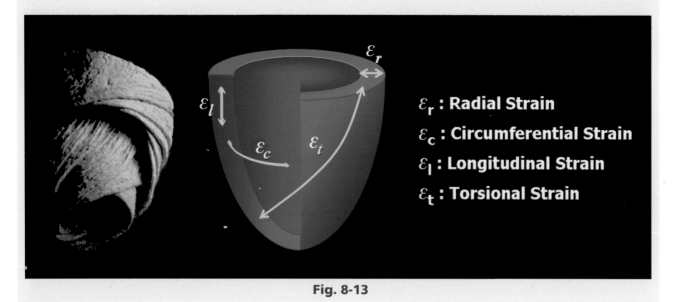

ε_r : **Radial Strain**

ε_c : **Circumferential Strain**

ε_l : **Longitudinal Strain**

ε_t : **Torsional Strain**

Fig. 8-13

5. ANSWER: D. The early diastolic velocity of the longitudinal motion of the myocardium (e') reflects the rate of myocardial relaxation. Decreased e' is one of the earliest signs of diastolic dysfunction and is present in all stages of diastolic dysfunction. Because e' velocity is reduced and mitral E velocity increase with higher filling pressures, the ratio between E and e' correlates well with LV filling pressures. This combination of early mitral E velocity and early diastolic longitudinal velocities of the myocardium has a linear relationship to the pulmonary capillary wedge pressure or mean left atrial pressure. This relationship persists even in patients with tachycardia as well as atrial fibrillation. There is debate to whether this relationship holds in the acutely decompensated patient with congestive heart failure.

6. ANSWER: D. One of the special characteristics of static B-scan ultrasound imaging is an appearance of speckle patterns within the tissue, which are the result of constructive and destructive interference of ultrasound back-scattered from structures smaller than a wavelength of ultrasound. This speckle pattern is unique for each myocardial region and is relatively stable throughout the cardiac cycle. Myocardial motion can be analyzed by tracking the movement of these speckles by filtering out random speckles and then performing an autocorrelation to estimate the motion of stable structures. Speckle-tracking technology has the advantage of measuring tissue velocities and deformation in an angle-independent fashion. It relies on a consistent and distinct grayscale pattern. This information is fed through a pattern recognition algorithm to tract the displacement of the speckles in both dimensions of the two-dimensional image. Because this analysis is not based on the Doppler shift of reflected sound waves, it is not angle dependent and can be performed on regular two-dimensional images.

7. ANSWER: C. Strain rate (ε) imaging simultaneously measures the velocities in two adjacent points as well as the relative distance between these two points. Expressed as: $\varepsilon = (V_1 - V_2)/L$. Positive radial strain rate represents active contraction. Negative values for radial strain represent either relaxation (if measured during diastole) or dyskinesis (if measured during systole).

8. ANSWER: A. The LV myocardium has a spiral architecture with myocardial fibers that vary in orientation depending on where in the myocardium they are located. Fiber direction is predominantly longitudinal in the endocardial region, transitioning into a circumferential direction in the mid wall and becoming longitudinal again over the epicardial surface. In addition to radial and longitudinal deformation, there is torsional deformation of the LV during the cardiac cycle due to the helical orientation of the myocardial fibers. During systole, the basal segments of the LV myocardium rotate or twist in counterclockwise direction, whereas the apical segments twist in clockwise direction. During diastole, untwisting occurs in the opposite direction. Systolic torsion represents the net effect of basal and apical twist. Apical twisting is the main component of global LV systolic torsion, and in the next diastole, the apical untwisting also plays the dominant role, whereas basal rotation is of less importance.

9. ANSWER: C. Standard Doppler measurement of mitral inflow velocities can be used to assess diastolic function by measuring the early rapid filling wave (E) and the late filling wave due to atrial contraction (A). The velocities and ratios of E/A are used to determine diastolic function, but as they are reflective of the pressure gradient between the left atrium and the left ventricle, they are directly related to preload and inversely related to ventricular relaxation. Doppler tissue myocardial diastolic velocities are less load dependent. In adults, an early diastolic longitudinal (e') velocity of >0.10 m/sec is associated with normal LV diastolic function. DTI measures only vector motion that is parallel to the ultrasound beam and is not able to differentiate between active motion (like myocardial contraction) and passive motion (like tethering). M-mode color DTI is acquired by color-coding images of tissue motion during an M-mode image acquisition. Different colors specify direction of motion and allow images to have both high temporal and spatial resolution.

10. ANSWER: C. Calculations of strain and strain rate from Doppler tissue data have several areas of possible error. Areas of echo dropout will be encoded slower than actual velocities. Deviation from the intended angle of interrogation alters the type of strain being measured. Areas of interest closer to the pulse source will have higher fidelity measurements, as there is less echo dropout present.

11. ANSWER: C. Tissue Doppler can also identify abnormal regional strain, predominantly in areas of localized hypertrophy. In fact, it appears that the greater the extent of segmental wall thickness, the greater is the reduction in myocardial strain. These abnormalities can often be found in asymptomatic carriers of hypertrophic cardiomyopathy genetic mutations, even in the absence of phenotypic expression. Pulsed Doppler LV filling usually shows impaired relaxation or pseudonormal patterns and rarely the restrictive patterns because of the markedly increased wall thickness and impaired relaxation.

12. ANSWER: A. Glycemic control in diabetic patients has been associated with microvascular complications. Microvascular disease may lead to ischemia and subsequent impaired LV relaxation and increased myocardial stiffness. Advance glycation end products have been associated with microvascular complications of type 1 diabetes mellitus and may be a pathophysiologic mechanism for diastolic dysfunction in these patients. Type I diabetic patients have worse diastolic function with lower tissue Doppler e'. Furthermore, HgbA1C was correlated with E/e'. These results demonstrate that asymptomatic diastolic dysfunction is common in patients with type I diabetes mellitus and that its severity is correlated with glycemic control. Furthermore, data suggest that asymptomatic diabetic patients have increased LV filling pressure as measured by E/e', and by a larger left atrial size.

13. ANSWER: D. In aortic stenosis, global LV dysfunction is common secondary to the increased afterload. This LV dysfunction may not be discernible based on standard two-dimensional echocardiography alone. Because the sensitivity of tissue Doppler imaging is superior, subclinical LV dysfunction has been detected by tissue Doppler imaging in patients with aortic stenosis despite good ejection fraction. In patients with aortic stenosis, the degree of abnormality in regional deformation correlates with aortic valve area. Once the aortic valve is replaced, e' can normalize.

14. ANSWER: C. After an MI, E/e' has been shown to be associated with an increased risk of death or need for heart transplant. Patients with an E/e' ratio of >17 had a mortality rate of approximately 40% at 36 months compared with 5% in those with an E/e' ratio of <17. In a study that included 250 nonselected patients who had an echocardiogram 1.6 days after an MI followed up for a median of 13 months, the most powerful predictor of survival was an E/e' ratio of >15. E/e' was a stronger predictor than other Doppler echocardiographic indices including the LV filling pulsed Doppler deceleration time. E/e' has also correlated with increased LV end-diastolic volume post-MI and has been attributed to a relationship to LV remodeling and progressive LV dilation.

15. ANSWER: C. Several studies have shown an inverse relationship between e' and LV relaxation in both patients with normal and elevated preload. Clinical studies suggest that e' is a better discriminator between diastolic dysfunction and normal patients, compared to any other single or combined index of transmitral filling and pulmonary venous Doppler flows. LV torsion and untwisting also correlate well with the relaxation time constant. Isovolumic relaxation time represents the earliest phase of diastole. It is defined as the time from aortic valve closure to mitral valve opening.

16. ANSWER: B. DTI differs from standard Doppler by eliminating the high-pass filter and using low-gain amplification to display the velocities of the myocardium. Tissue Doppler-derived strain is limited to interrogating segments aligned in parallel with the Doppler angle of incidence. Data should be recorded at the highest possible frame rate to maximize temporal resolution. This is accomplished by reducing sector size and depth. Ideally three consecutive heartbeats should be recorded in each view, to account for beat-to-beat variability. Strain measurements may be obtained in patients with atrial fibrillation.

17. ANSWER: E. Tissue Doppler velocities may help to differentiate myocardial hypertrophy seen in athletes from hypertrophic cardiomyopathy, where these velocities are abnormally decreased. Similar findings have been reported in Fabry's disease, a cardiomyopathy secondary to α-galactosidase A deficiency. Mutation-positive Fabry's patients have significant reduction of e' and higher E/e' compared with normal control subjects, even before the development of LV hypertrophy. Tissue Doppler has been used to study myocardial performance in patients with Friedreich's ataxia. Asymptomatic patients who are homozygous for the GAA expansion in the Friedreich's ataxia gene have reduced myocardial velocity gradients during systole and in early diastole. Patients with a restrictive cardiomyopathy from an infiltrative disease process like cardiac amyloidosis will have impaired relaxation and therefore reduced e' velocities.

18. ANSWER: A. Unlike tissue Doppler, which records myocardial motion and not necessarily contraction, strain rate measures the instantaneous velocities between two points within the myocardium. A strain rate of zero indicates akinesis. A strain rate of >0 indicates expansion, and a strain rate of <0 indicates compression. Velocities may be recorded in akinetic segments that are tethered by adjacent moving segments, in this example, from the apical and mid-lateral wall.

19. ANSWER: D. As the ventricle contracts, muscle fibers shorten in the longitudinal and circumferential directions and thicken or lengthen in the radial direction. Strain represents the change in segment length throughout a cardiac cycle. Strain rate or strain velocity is the local rate of myocardial deformation and can be derived from DTI velocities. DTI-derived strain rate is a strong index of LV contractility. In Figure 8-1, a parasternal short-axis image of the mid left ventricle is shown. The myocardium has been color coded by segment and by its percent strain value with a scale of 100% (red) and −100% (blue). The time plot at the bottom of the imaging graphs the percent radial strain of each color-coded segment. The color of the plot corresponds to the outlined color of the segment selected. Figure 8-1 shows that the best motion is seen in the mid-anterolateral wall, which has the darkest red coloring and is also plotted on the graph as the red line with a marked positive percent strain during systole. The mid-anteroseptal wall, colored white and outlined in orange, shows akinesis based upon the white color coding and the flat plot of the orange curve. Radial strain can provide quantitative data to assist in the interpretation of segmental wall motion and can be of particular use in the interpretation of stress echocardiograms.

20. *ANSWER: A.* Figure 8-2 shows strain rate imaging with regions of interest selected in the septum (yellow circle and corresponding plot) and lateral wall (blue circle and corresponding plot) in the apical four-chamber views. MVC = mitral valve closure, AVO = aortic valve opening, AVC = aortic valve closure, MVO = mitral valve opening. A strain rate of zero indicates akinesis. A strain rate of >0 indicates expansion, and a strain rate of <0 indicates compression. The strain rate of the selected area of the septum (yellow) shows that it maintains a strain rate of approximately zero throughout systole and diastole. This finding is consistent with akinesis and scar formation. The strain rate of the selected area of the lateral wall (blue), however, demonstrates a negative strain rate in systole (from MVC to AVC) signifying appropriate myocardial compression and a positive strain rate in diastole (from AVC to MVC) signifying appropriate myocardial expansion.

21. *ANSWER: B.* The common clinical presentation of dyspnea in an elderly patient with a history of heart disease with concurrent pulmonary pathology is a diagnostic dilemma that can be greatly clarified with echo Doppler tissue use. Specifically, Doppler and DTI can provide information regarding LV preload and relaxation. This information, in conjunction with standard information about biventricular size and function as well as assessment of right ventricular systolic pressure can provide a wealth of actionable information. Figure 8-3A shows an elevated E wave from standard Doppler interrogation of mitral inflow. Figure 8-3B shows decreased Doppler tissue velocities obtained from the lateral mitral annulus. The E/e' ratio in this example is 18. E/e' ratios of >15 have been correlated to pulmonary capillary pressures greater than 18–20 mm Hg. An elevated E/e' ratio has also been related to poor prognosis in both ischemic and nonischemic LV dysfunction.

22. *ANSWER: B.* Compared with the prior images, the mitral inflow E wave of the mitral inflow shows a markedly reduced velocity in early diastole after the patient was successfully treated with intravenous diuretics. This finding in combination with symptomatic improvement indicates that her LV end-diastolic pressure or preload has been reduced. This is further confirmed by the E/e' ratio. Despite normal preload conditions after diuresis, both the early to late diastolic filling waves in the standard Doppler as well as the tissue Doppler findings suggest that the patient has underlying diastolic dysfunction. As the deceleration time is >160 milliseconds, this pattern is not consistent with a restrictive filling pattern. Although pulmonary venous filling patterns may give additional information about LV filling patterns, the current information about mitral flow velocity and tissue Doppler allows for the diagnosis of diastolic function.

23. *ANSWER: B.* Diastolic dysfunction in constrictive pericarditis results from increased pericardial constraint on the LV that is related to the thickness and rigidity of the pericardium. Patients present with signs and symptoms of right-sided heart failure, which are similar to those found in restrictive cardiomyopathy. Two-dimensional echocardiography may not demonstrate increased pericardial thickness and the typical interventricular septal bounce. Right and left ventricular Doppler filling patterns may demonstrate respiratory variability. However, these findings are not always present and are not specific. Acute respiratory illnesses can increase intrathoracic pressure swings, and the respiratory flow variability also increases. Excessive preload may attenuate the effect of intrathoracic pressure swings and decrease respiratory variability, whereas low preload can decrease the constraining effect of the pericardium also masking the characteristic Doppler signs of constriction. Tissue Doppler myocardial velocities are useful in differentiating restrictive cardiomyopathy from constrictive pericarditis. In restrictive cardiomyopathy patients, both relaxation and stiffness are abnormal. On the other hand, relaxation is preserved in pure constrictive pericarditis, in the absence of other myocardial disease. Patients with constrictive pericarditis and normal systolic function have normal or elevated e' velocities (>8 cm/sec), reflecting their preserved ventricular relaxation. In this example, the mitral inflow demonstrates some respiratory variation and its morphology is suggestive of a restrictive filling pattern; however, Doppler tissue at the mitral annulus demonstrates preservation of relaxation making a cardiomyopathy such as cardiac amyloidosis and hypertrophic cardiomyopathy unlikely. The E/e' ratio is approximately 4, which does not correspond to an elevated left ventricular end-diastolic pressure.

24. *ANSWER: A.* Figure 8-6 shows tissue Doppler in the lateral wall and in the septal wall. The significant difference between the A and B can be seen in the early diastolic velocity. The most common form of hypertrophic cardiomyopathy is characterized by a prominent increase in global or segmental LV wall thickness and histologically by myocardial fiber disarray. Diastolic function is characterized by increased LV chamber stiffness and decreased relaxation of variable severity due to the asynchronous deactivation of the muscle fibers. This asynchronous deactivation is manifested in Doppler tissue as a decreased velocity seen in hypertrophic segments (septum in this example) in early diastole when compared with segments that do not demonstrate hypertrophy (lateral wall in this example).

25. ANSWER: D. This apical three-chamber view of the left ventricle is analyzed using a two-dimensional speckle-tracking algorithm. As reviewed in question number 8, speckle-tracking technology has the advantage of measuring tissue velocities and deformation in an angle-independent fashion, which enables it to track the movement of the speckle in both dimensions of the two-dimensional image. Figure 8-7 clearly shows that the posterior wall of the left ventricle has been colored in blue, denoting a positive longitudinal strain rate in systole, which indicates an inappropriate expansion during this phase of the cardiac cycle. The rest of the ventricle is colored in shades of red, denoting a negative strain rate in systole, which indicates an appropriate longitudinal compression.

26. ANSWER: B. The two-dimensional image in Figure 8-8 demonstrates a dilated LV cavity, consistent with either dilated or ischemic cardiomyopathy. The tissue Doppler image shows a different color velocity pattern in the septum and the lateral wall, and strain imaging shows reduced deformation in the apical septum (yellow curve) compared with the apical lateral wall (red curve); these findings have been consistent with a septal MI.

27. ANSWER: B. The strain rate images in Figure 8-9 demonstrate anteroapical dyskinesis (red curve), a pattern compatible with apical MI, a localized infiltrative disorder, or apical hypertrophic cardiomyopathy.

28. ANSWER: C. The two-dimensional short-axis images in Figure 8-10 demonstrate increased LV wall thickness with normal LV cavity size. The color M-mode tissue Doppler indicates a sinus rhythm pattern with both reduced septal and inferolateral velocities, findings consistent with a restrictive cardiomyopathy. LV dyssynchrony is a recognized cause of heart failure only in the setting of LV dilatation and reduced LV ejection fraction.

29. ANSWER: D. The color M-mode tissue Doppler in Figure 8-11 indicates paradoxical anterior systolic motion of the interventricular septum, a common finding after pericardiotomy.

30. ANSWER: C. In this patient, the E/e' ratio is 8, the E/A ratio is 0.9, and the E deceleration time is normal. All findings are consistent with normal LV filling pressures. Therefore, the most likely cause of the patient's symptoms is decompensated COPD.

SUGGESTED READINGS

Firstenberg MS, Greenberg NL, Main ML, et al. Determinants of diastolic myocardial tissue Doppler velocities: influences of relaxation and preload. *J Appl Physiol.* 2001;90:299–307.

Garcia MJ, Rodriguez L, Ares MA, et al. Differentiation of constrictive pericarditis from restrictive cardiomyopathy: assessment of left ventricular diastolic velocities in the longitudinal axis by tissue Doppler imaging. *J Am Coll Cardiol.* 1996;27:108–114.

Gilman G, Khandheria BK, Hagen ME, et al. Strain rate and strain: a step-by-step approach to image and data acquisition. *J Am Soc Echocardiogr.* 2004;17:1011–1020.

Greenberg NL, Firstenberg MS, Castro PL, et al. Doppler-derived myocardial systolic strain rate is a strong index of left ventricular contractility. *Circulation.* 2002;105:99–105.

Helle-Valle T, Crosby J, Edvardsen T, et al. New noninvasive method for assessment of left ventricular rotation: speckle tracking echocardiography. *Circulation.* 2005;112:3149–3156.

Ho CY, Sweitzer NK, McDonough B, et al. Assessment of diastolic function with Doppler tissue imaging to predict genotype in preclinical hypertrophic cardiomyopathy. *Circulation.* 2002; 105:2992–2997.

Nagueh SF, Middleton KJ, Kopelen HA, et al. Quinones MA. Doppler tissue imaging: a noninvasive technique for evaluation of left ventricular relaxation and estimation of filling pressures. *J Am Coll Cardiol.* 1997;30:1527–1533.

Ogawa K, Hozumi T, Sugioka K, et al. Usefulness of automated quantitation of regional left ventricular wall motion by a novel method of two-dimensional echocardiographic tracking. *Am J Cardiol.* 2006;98:1531–1537.

Oh JK, Hatle LK, Seward JB, et al. Diagnostic role of Doppler echocardiography in constrictive pericarditis. *J Am Coll Cardiol.* 1994;23:154.

Pieroni M, Chimenti C, Ricci R, et al. Early detection of Fabry cardiomyopathy by tissue Doppler imaging. *Circulation.* 2003;107: 1978–1984.

Rajogopalan N, Garcia MJ, Rodriguez L, et al. Comparison of new Doppler echocardiographic methods to differentiate constrictive pericardial heart disease and restrictive cardiomyopathy. *Am J Cardiol.* 2001;87:86–94.

Yang H, Sun JP, Lever HM, et al. Use of strain imaging in detecting segmental dysfunction in patients with hypertrophic cardiomyopathy. *J Am Soc Echocardiogr.* 2003;16:233–223.

Yu CM, Sanderson JE, Marwick TH, et al. Tissue Doppler imaging a new prognosticator for cardiovascular diseases. *J Am Coll Cardiol.* 2007;49:1903–1914.

Contrast-Enhanced Ultrasound Imaging

CHAPTER 9

Roxy Senior and Steven B. Feinstein

1. The first published work in the field of ultrasound contrast occurred in 1968 written by authors Gramiak and Shah. What was the initial use of ultrasound contrast agents in clinical cardiology?
   A. Myocardial perfusion.
   B. Doppler enhancement.
   C. Cardiac chamber definition.

2. Today, when the cardiac chambers are not adequately visualized, in both office- and hospital-based practices, cardiologists should establish policies and procedures for the appropriate use of FDA-approved ultrasound contrast agents. In the United States these agents include the following:
   A. Sonicated dextrose and sonicated sorbitol.
   B. Agitated saline and indocyanine green.
   C. PESDA and Berlex scan.
   D. Optison and Definity.

3. The first generation of ultrasound contrast agents exhibited limited in vivo persistence due primarily to the following instrumentation issue:
   A. Implementation of high mechanical indices (>1.0 MI).
   B. Preference of harmonic imaging software versus fundamental software.
   C. Presence of high molecular weight, relatively nondiffusible gases (perflutren).
   D. Power Doppler applications for perfusion imaging.

4. Today, what is the current FDA-approved application for the use of ultrasound contrast agents?
   A. Doppler signal enhancement.
   B. Left ventricular opacification (LVO).
   C. Therapeutic applications.
   D. Myocardial perfusion.

5. The American Society of Echocardiography (ASE) issued a report in 2008 on the current and future applications of contrast ultrasound applications. The guidelines focused on several applications of ultrasound contrast agents which included the following:
   A. Contrast-enhanced ultrasound imaging (CEUS) is indicated for use in difficult-to-image patients for LVO resulting in a reliable estimation of ejection fraction and regional wall motion abnormalities.
   B. CEUS is indicated for use with harmonic software resulting in quantification of myocardial perfusion.
   C. CEUS is indicated and should be used to triage patients on the basis of image quality for stress echocardiography or nuclear testing.
   D. CEUS is indicated as the first-line assessment when performing noninvasive imaging of the carotid arteries.

6. In 2009, the European Association of Echocardiography (EAE) published evidence-based recommendations for ultrasound contrast agents. The EAE document recommended to:
   A. Expand clinical use to include vascular indications and drug delivery applications.
   B. Limit the clinical uses of ultrasound contrast agents due to safety concerns.
   C. Deny the relevance and clinical uses of ultrasound on the basis of the lack of clinical efficacy.
   D. Confirm and sustain the ASE reports of 2008.

7. What are the current indications/criteria for the use of ultrasound contrast agents in clinical practice?
   A. Doppler signal is inadequate for the quantification of pressures (tricuspid, aortic).
   B. Detection of left ventricular (LV) pseudoaneurysms.
   C. Failure to visualize more than two LV endocardial regions.
   D. Detection of the no-reflow phenomena in post-myocardial infarction patients.

8. Based on expert opinions, approximately what percentage of transthoracic echocardiograms are considered technically inadequate on the basis of the ASE criteria?
   A. <5%.
   B. 10%–30%.
   C. 30%–50%.
   D. >75%.

9. In October of 2007, the FDA issued new product labeling changes for perflutren-containing ultrasound contrast agents. In May of 2008, the FDA reversed its decision and moved the new contraindications to the warning section. Therefore, as of May 2008, the new language in the product insert includes which of the following?
   A. Perflutren-based ultrasound agents are contraindicated in all cardiac patients.
   B. Ultrasound contrast agents require a consent form for each use.
   C. The use of ultrasound contrast agents should be considered experimental.
   D. Patients with pulmonary hypertension or unstable cardiopulmonary conditions require monitoring for 30 minutes post-injection.

10. In response to the decision of the FDA to institute labeling changes and the subsequent reversal and modifications implemented, an independent, grassroots organization along with the respective professional organizations (ASE and EAE) issued statements supporting the appropriate, safe use of ultrasound contrast agents. Subsequently, numerous editorials and peer-reviewed publications described the following:
    A. Ultrasound contrast agents should not be used in clinical medicine.
    B. The safety of using ultrasound contrast agents has been shown to be superior to that of noninvasive imaging agents and procedures.
    C. There remains a lack of peer-reviewed publications to understand the safety issues.
    D. Contrast ultrasound agent usage exceeds the risk of performing similar noninvasive imaging tests (transesophageal echocardiography [TEE], nuclear imaging, and computed tomography [CT]).

11. The safety issues regarding the clinical use of ultrasound contrast agents may be summarized as the following:
    A. Over the course of the last 2 years, the FDA identified a "safety" signal and therefore has subsequently restricted the use of ultrasound contrast agents for all clinical indications awaiting results of future clinical trails. Therefore, all ultrasound contrast agents remain under FDA review and should not be used clinically.
    B. Based on recent peer reviewed publications in which more than 228,611 patients received ultrasound contrast agents, the observed risk to patients is notably less than that of other comparable imaging agents and/or noninvasive tests. Therefore, ultrasound contrast agents should be used for appropriate indications.
    C. The clinical need to identify the LV endocardial surfaces has been eliminated through the use of three-dimensional and harmonic imaging systems.
    D. TEE, contrast-enhanced CT, X-ray, and nuclear imaging modalities all provide similar clinical information, whereas imposing less risk to the patient than the appropriate use of a contrast-enhanced ultrasound examination.

12. In 2009, the EAE published evidence-based recommendations regarding the clinical use of contrast echocardiography. The consensus document postulated the following:
    A. Contrast ultrasound may be used for additional clinical applications including myocardial perfusion imaging, viability, and detection of coronary flow in cardiac patients.
    B. Ultrasound contrast agents should not be widely used because of safety, concerns.
    C. Ultrasound contrast agents, when used for myocardial perfusion imaging, were inferior to the results obtained with nuclear imaging studies.
    D. The EAE consensus document did not propose additional uses on the basis of peer reviewed publications and suggested using other noninvasive imaging systems.

13. Contrast ultrasound has been used in carotid (vascular) applications. These agents are particularly useful due to the following:
    A. In the United States, vascular indications have received a CPT code, and accordingly, CMS provides reimbursement for "off-label" contrast-enhanced vascular applications.
    B. Ultrasound contrast agents have not been deemed useful because the agents obscure the measurement of the near and far wall intima-media-thickness (IMT) and consequently, do not adequately enhance the carotid artery lumen.
    C. When performing enhancement of the carotid IMT (c-IMT) measurement, in luminal morphology identification (ulcers/plaques), and the detection of intraplaque angiogenesis is possible
    D. The documented European experience with contrast-enhanced vascular imaging failed to provide evidence of clinical benefit.

14. Therapeutic uses of contrast ultrasound remain as a new application of ultrasound contrast agents and as such, represent a departure from diagnostic applications. In which of the following clinical applications, have there been clinical trials utilizing ultrasound-mediated therapy?
    A. Thrombolysis (deep vein thrombosis therapy).
    B. Cardiac stem cell transduction.
    C. Electrolysis for VEGF therapy.
    D. Nonviral, gene transduction for Parkinson disease.

15. Use of contrast agent in stress echocardiography:
    A. Is contraindicated.
    B. Requires prolonged monitoring.
    C. Results in an interaction of contrast agents and pharmacological stress agents.
    D. Requires no extra precautions beyond routine monitoring for stress echo.

16. This baseline apical four-chamber view of the left ventricle was obtained from examination of a patient (Fig. 9-1).

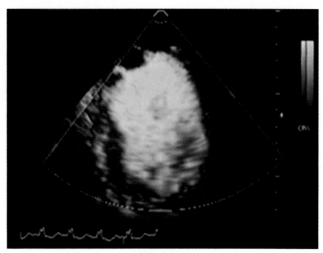

Fig. 9-1

The patient was referred for a dobutamine stress echo (DSE) and this image was obtained after injecting a contrast ultrasound agent to enhance the LV endocardial surfaces. Of note, these masses were not observed prior to the use of ultrasound contrast. What should one do next?
A. Continue the DSE, and alert the referring physician of the final results.
B. Call the referring physician and suggest a cardiac catheterization if the DSE result is positive for inducible ischemia.
C. Stop the DSE examination, call the referring physician, and initiate full anticoagulation, if there are no contraindications.
D. Pursue a malignancy work up following the completion of the DSE.

17. Figure 9-2 was obtained during an outpatient echocardiographic examination.

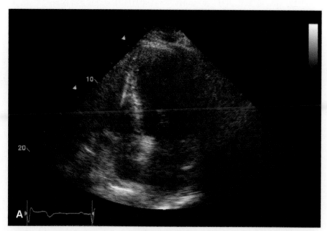

Fig. 9-2A

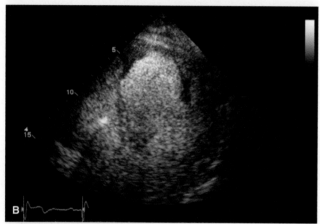

Fig. 9-2B

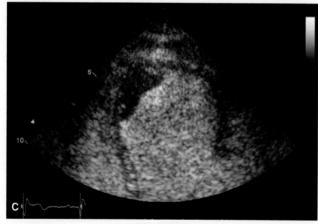

Fig. 9-2C

At the time of the study, scant past history was available. Because of the difficulty in obtaining a quality image of the ventricle, the patient received an ultrasound contrast agent. Figure 9-2A revealed a technically limited study. Figures 9-2B and C

were viewed following the intravenous injection of a contrast agent. What should one consider as the next step?

A. Call the referring physician and suggest a contrast-enhanced magnetic resonance imaging (MRI) or CT examination to confirm the images.

B. Perform a TEE to confirm the images.

C. Proceed with the study and suggest serial follow-up in 3 months.

D. Call the referring physician, suggest full anticoagulation, and schedule serial two-dimensional (2D) echocardiograms to assess therapeutic efficacy.

18. This patient was referred for an echocardiogram because of the symptoms of shortness of breath (Fig. 9-3).

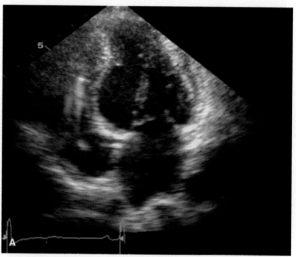

Fig. 9-3A

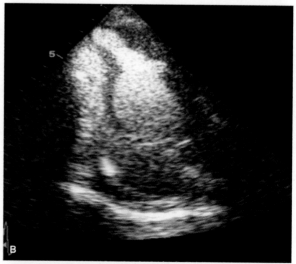

Fig. 9-3B

The initial image revealed an unusual apex. Because of the difficulty in identifying the true endocardial surfaces, an ultrasound contrast agent was indicated. Which of the following statements is correct?

A. The initial images were adequate to make the diagnosis.

B. The contrast-enhanced ultrasound images were diagnostic.

C. A TEE is needed to confirm the images.

D. A contrast-enhanced MRI or CT scan is indicated.

19. This outpatient examination revealed a strand-like mass in the apical region. In real-time, the linear object appeared to be quite mobile. To better define the apex, ultrasound contrast was used (Fig. 9-4).

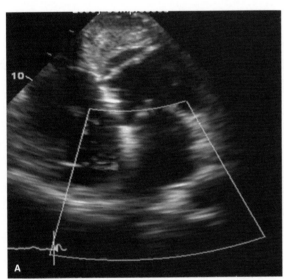

Fig. 9-4A

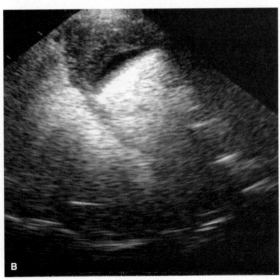

Fig. 9-4B

The likely diagnosis and/or procedures recommended include the following:

A. There is a false tendon at the apex.

B. A TEE or a contrast-enhanced MRI or CT scan is indicated to visualize the apex.

C. A new, soft thrombus is on the surface of an established apical thrombus.

D. The images represent an imaging artifact due to a technically difficult examination.

20. The series of images in Figure 9-5 was obtained from a patient who had a prior history of coronary artery disease and myocardial infarction. The contrast-enhanced images revealed an abnormality. What is the diagnosis/recommendation?

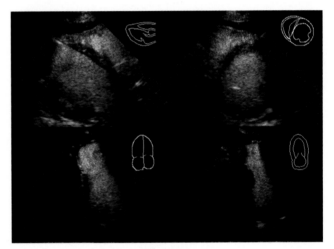

Fig. 9-5

A. Apical aneurysm.

B. Apical thrombus

C. Normal examination.

D. A TEE or contrast-enhanced MRI or CT scan should be obtained.

21. Figure 9-6 was obtained by the intravenous injection of an ultrasound contrast agent for luminal enhancement of a patient's carotid artery.

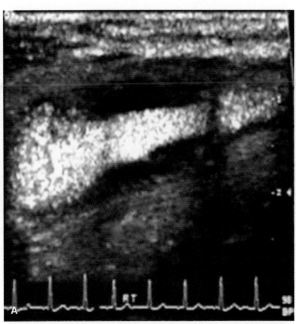

Fig. 9-6A

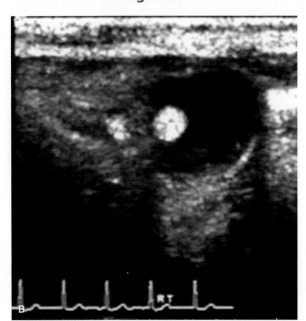

Fig. 9-6B

The use of contrast revealed the following observation:
A. The contrast agent produced shadowing of the far wall and no diagnostic information was obtained.
B. Unenhanced ultrasound images provide similar information and the added value of contrast is marginal.
C. The carotid artery revealed a significant, eccentric plaque in the common carotid artery.

22. The use of ultrasound contrast agents has been shown to be valuable for identifying the carotid artery luminal surfaces including plaques, ulcers, enhancement of c-IMT, and adventitial and plaque vasa vasorum.

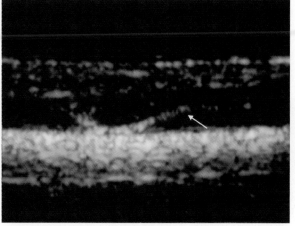

Fig. 9-10

Figure 9-10 illustrates the presence of the following (the structure indicated by the arrow):
A. Vasa vasorum within the arterial wall.
B. Carotid plaques.
C. Thickened IMT.
D. Imaging artifacts.

23. In this patient presented with heart failure, contrast was injected intravenously (four-chamber view is shown in Fig. 9-11).

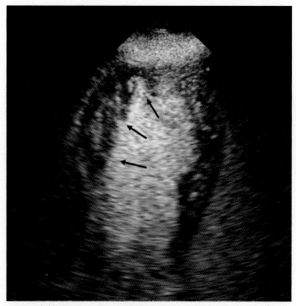

Fig. 9-11

What is the diagnosis?
A. Ischemic cardiomyopathy.
B. Apical hypertrophic cardiomyopathy.
C. Dilated cardiomyopathy.
D. Noncompaction cardiomyopathy.

24. Ultrasound contrast agents are used in vascular imaging for the detection of premature cardiovascular disease. What does the region highlighted by the arrow in Figure 9-12 show?

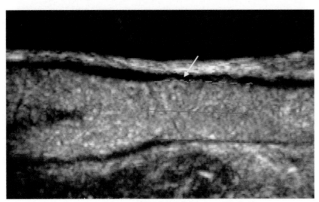

Fig. 9-12

A. Contrast ultrasound artifact (suggest contrast-enhanced MRI or CT image of the carotid artery).
B. Carotid ulceration highlighted by contrast ultrasound.
C. Carotid tumor with associated perfusion imaging.
D. Computed-aided, contrast-enhanced c-IMT measurements.

25. Contrast ultrasound can be used to highlight the carotid artery luminal surfaces (Fig. 9-13). After the use of intravenous ultrasound contrast, it is possible to identify the following as seen in this image.

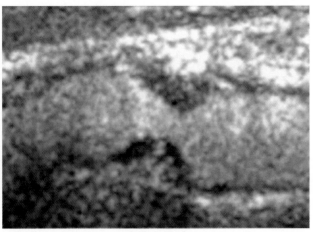

Fig. 9-13

A. Artifact of imaging.
B. Neurogenic carotid body tumor.
C. Dissection of the carotid artery.
D. Carotid artery stenosis.

CASE 1:

A 60-year-old woman is in the surgical intensive care unit (SICU). The cardiology consultation service was asked to see the patient for management of the deteriorating hemodynamic status. When initially seen in the SICU, the patient's vital signs revealed a tachycardic heart rate and systemic hypotension requiring aggressive medical treatment that included sympathomimetic therapies. The patient's cardiac output was reduced and the urine output was diminished; all consistent with diminished perfusion pressure.

As part of the cardiology consultation, a bedside 2D echocardiography was performed to assess the LV filling status and overall performance. The initial images were difficult to interpret and the overall LV systolic function was estimated at 10%–15% (see Video 9-1).

26. What should be done following the unenhanced echocardiogram?
A. TEE to assess LV function.
B. Contrast enhanced MRI to assess LV function.
C. Multigated acquisition scan to assess ejection fraction.
D. Contrast ultrasound injection to visualize the endocardial surfaces and assess the ejection fraction.

27. After the injection of an ultrasound contrast agent, the following assessment was made:
A. Hyperdynamic function >75% LVEF.
B. <15% LVEF.
C. Obtain contrast-enhanced MRI or CT scan.
D. Obtain TEE.

CASE 2:

An elderly woman was seen in the emergency department (ED) for nonspecific chest pain. Her presenting 12-lead ECG did reveal nonspecific ST segment changes and no evidence for acute changes consistent with the diagnosis of an acute myocardial infarction (AMI). The nonspecific clinical presentation and lack of ECG evidence for an AMI complicated the ensuing therapeutic decisions for the physicians.

A cardiology consultation was initiated; and following an initial history and physical examination, a 2D echocardiogram was ordered to identify regional wall motion abnormalities. The initial study revealed a relatively normal left ventricle without clear evidence for regional wall motion abnormalities (see Video 9-2).

28. Following the intravenous injection of an ultrasound contrast injection and based on the identification of the endocardial surfaces of the left ventricle, the following therapeutic approach was taken:
    A. Transfer to the cardiac catheterization laboratory for percutaneous intervention (PCI).
    B. Observe in the ED and monitor.
    C. The patient was discharged after monitoring in the ED.
    D. Conservative therapy that included oxygen, rest, and monitoring.

CASE 3:

A patient was scheduled for a pharmacologic echo stress examination. Prior to initiating the dobutamine agent, a baseline image of the heart was obtained with and without ultrasound contrast agents. As noted from the examination, the apical region of the left ventricle was dyskinetic, consistent with a prior myocardial infarction (see Video 9-3).

29. Based on the baseline, unenhanced images of the left ventricle, what clinical approach should be followed:
    A. Proceed with the study despite the lack of clear endocardial definition of the apex.
    B. Stop the test, and proceed with a nuclear imaging test (single photon emission computed tomography [SPECT]).
    C. Proceed but consider the test to be technically difficult and will likely require an additional imaging test (contrast-enhanced MRI or CT scan).
    D. Inject an ultrasound contrast agent to allow visualization of the LV endocardial surfaces.

30. After the injection of an ultrasound contrast agent, the following clinical decisions were made:
    A. Stop the test, consider beginning full anticoagulation.
    B. Proceed with low-dose infusions of dobutamine.
    C. Consider performing a contrast-enhanced MRI or CT scan.
    D. Convert the dobutamine study to a SPECT study.

CASE 4:

A 56-year-old male patient presents with atypical chest pain. He is hypertensive and hyperlipidemic on medication. The patient underwent rest and dipyridamole stress echo. Both rest and stress wall motions were normal (see Video 9-4).

31. What abnormalities are seen?
    A. Perfusion defect at rest.
    B. Transmural perfusion defect at stress.
    C. Subendocardial perfusion at stress.
    D. LV cavity dilatation at stress.

32. The abnormalities suggest:
    A. LAD disease.
    B. Right coronary artery disease.
    C. LCX.
    D. Multivessel disease.

CASE 5:

A 45-year-old woman with no other coronary risk factors presented with acute onset of chest pain. ECG showed significant ST depression in V_1–V_4. Troponin level was mildly raised at 12 hours. Real-time myocardial contrast echo was performed at rest and at 24 hours (see Video 9-5).

33. What is the likely diagnosis?
    A. Acute anteroseptal myocardial infarction.
    B. Noncardiac chest pain.
    C. Acute myocarditis.
    D. Takotsubo cardiomyopathy.

34. What is the prognosis?
    A. Excellent.
    B. Poor.
    C. Poor with improvement at 3 months.
    D. Unable to determine.

CASE 6:

A 62-year-old man with coronary risk factors presented with acute anteroseptal MI. The patient underwent primary PCI. Myocardial contrast echocardiography (MCE) was performed 48 hours after PCI. Apical four-chamber view is shown in Video 9-6.

35. What are the abnormalities seen?
    A. Normal perfusion.
    B. Mild apical-septal perfusion defect.
    C. Severe apical-septal perfusion defect.
    D. Severe lateral perfusion defect.

36. What is the probability that dyssynergic anteroseptal segments are unlikely to recover function?
A. High.
B. Low.
C. Intermediate.
D. Good initially with poor long-term outcome.

ANSWERS

1. ANSWER: C. The origins of Contrast-enhanced ultrasound imaging (CEUS) date to the earliest observations of Claude Joyner and publications of Gramiak and Shah in 1968. These authors used agitated solutions of saline and indocyanine green to identify the anatomic structures of the aortic root with M-mode ultrasound. Subsequent interest in the development of ultrasound contrast agents and clinical applications continues today, more than 40 years later.

In the early developmental phase of CEUS, nearly all diagnostic imaging modalities utilized blood pool, enhancement agents to define anatomic or physiologic structures including tissue perfusion. Today, due primarily to the unique physical parameters of the microbubbles, serve as true, intravascular indicators, capable of providing unparalleled access to the inherent spatial and temporal heterogeneity of tissue perfusion. Importantly, the microbubbles serve a dual role, they are promoted as a diagnostic enhancement agent but also serve as therapeutic delivery agents, which when fully realized have the potential to dramatically alter treatment of numerous diseases.

2. ANSWER: D. The two currently approved ultrasound contrast agents available in the United States are Optison and Definity. Levovist, SonoVue, and Sonazoid are approved for clinical use in Europe, Japan, and several other continents/countries.

3. ANSWER: A. Although unknown to clinicians at the time, the use of high mechanical indices (>1.0 MI) while useful in providing a higher signal to noise ratio for fundamental imaging and enhancing the 2D images, actually promoted ultrasound contrast agent destruction; hence, the observed reduced in vivo persistence of the first-generation agents. Today, implementation of sophisticated harmonic imaging systems and use of low mechanical indices prolongs persistence, leading to enhancement of the signal-to-noise ratio, and provides useful clinical information. The implementation of relatively persistent gases and the development of harmonic imaging systems significantly prolonged the efficacy of the second-generation agents.

The development of "second"-generation agents coupled with the harmonic imaging system satisfied the efficacy requirements for widespread clinical utility. These agents generally utilized high molecular weight, low soluble gases that promoted in vivo persistence. The second-generation ultrasound agents, coupled with harmonic imaging systems, appeared to fulfill the required clinical expectations for safe, efficient, and economical noninvasive imaging of the left-sided cardiac chambers (i.e., LVO and myocardial perfusion).

TABLE 9.1 Ultrasound Contrast Agents (Present and Past Agents)

Manufacturer	Name	Type	Development Stage
Acusphere		Polymer/perfluorocarbon	Clinical development
Alliance/Schering	Imavist	Encapsulated perfluorocarbon	Clinical development
Andaris	Quantison	Albumin/low-solubility gas	Clinical development
Bracco	SonoVue	Lipid/sulfur hexafluoride	Approved for clinical use
Byk-Gulden	BY963	Lipid/air (BY963)	Clinical development
Cavcon	Filmix	Lipid/air	Preclinical development
Lantheus Medical Imaging	Definity	Pentane/Octafluoropropane	Approved for clinical use
GE Healthcare	Optison	Sonicated albumin/octafluoropropane	Approved for clinical use
GE Healthcare	Sonazoid	Lipid/perfluorocarbon	Approved for clinical use
Point Biomedical	Bisphere	Perfluorocarbon/polymer bilayer	Clinical development
Porter MD/University of Nebraska	PESDA	Sonicated albumin/perfluoropropane	Not commercially available
Schering	Echovist		Approved for clinical use
Schering	Levovist	Lipid/air	Approved for clinical use
Schering	Sonavist	Polymer/air	Clinical development
Sonus	Echogen	Surfactant/perfluorocarbon	Withdrawn from development

The "third" generation of contrast agents may be considered as "designer" contrast agents. This latest group often involves the application of specific labeling chemistries to perform quantitative physiologic localization of inflammation and related disease states.

Ultimately, what could be considered the "fourth-generation" (therapeutic) contrast agents include systems that serve as therapeutic applications (site-specific drug/gene delivery systems).

4. *ANSWER: B.* In the United States today, there are two FDA-approved ultrasound contrast agents: Optison (GE Medical Diagnostics, Princeton, NJ) and Definity (Lantheus Medical Imaging, Billerica, MA). Several additional agents approved for clinical use in the world include Sonazoid, SonoVue, and Levovist (see Table 9-1). Ultrasound contrast agents are indicated for use in patients with suboptimal echocardiograms and to improve the delineation of the LV endocardial borders. The ASE in 2000 and 2008 and the EAE 2009 issued position papers focused on the indications for usage of ultrasound contrast agents in the clinics.

Left ventricular endocardial border detection

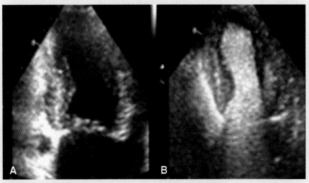

Fig. 9-14A   **Fig. 9-14B**

The still frame images in Figure 9-14 represent the apical four-chamber view obtained from a 2D echocardiogram. Figure 9-14A is that of an unenhanced image. The endocardial surfaces of the apical and lateral wall regions are difficult to visualize. Following the intravenous injection of an ultrasound contrast agent, the LV endocardial surfaces are fully visualized as shown in Figure 9-14B.

5. *ANSWER: A.* Based on the ASE Consensus Statement on the Clinical Applications of Ultrasonic Contrast Agents in Echocardiography (abstracted from the ASE document), the following criteria are listed for use:

- Difficult-to-image patients presenting for rest echocardiography with reduced image quality
  - Enable improved endocardial visualization and assessment of left ventricular (LV) structure and function when ≥2 contiguous segments are not seen on non-contrast images

- Reduce variability and increase accuracy in LV volume and LV ejection fraction (LVEF) measurements by 2-dimensional (2D) echocardiography
  - Increase the confidence of the interpreting physician in LV functional, structure, and volume assessments
- All patients presenting for rest echocardiographic assessment of LV systolic function (not solely difficult-to-image patients)
  - Reduce variability in LV volume measurements through 2D echocardiography
  - Increase the confidence of the interpreting physician in LV volume measurement
- Difficult-to-image patients presenting for stress echocardiography with reduced image quality
  - Obtain diagnostic assessment of segmental wall motion and thickening at rest and stress
  - Increase the proportion of diagnostic studies
  - Increase reader confidence in interpretation
- Confirm or exclude the echocardiographic diagnosis of the following LV structural abnormalities, when nonenhanced images are suboptimal for definitive diagnosis
  - Apical variant of hypertrophic cardiomyopathy
  - Ventricular noncompaction
  - Apical thrombus
  - Complications of myocardial infarction, such as LV aneurysm, pseudoaneurysm, and myocardial rupture
- Assist in the detection and correct classification of intracardiac masses, including tumors and thrombi
- For echocardiographic imaging in the ICU when standard imaging does not provide adequate cardiac structural definition.
  - For accurate assessment of LV volumes and EF
  - For exclusion of complications of myocardial infarction; i.e., LV aneurysm, pseudoaneurysm and myocardial rupture.
- Enhance Doppler signals when a clearly defined spectral pattern is not visible and is necessary to the evaluation of diastolic and/or valvular function

6. *ANSWER: D.* Contrast echocardiography: evidence-based recommendations published by EAE (abstracted from the EAE 2009): Indications for resting left ventricular opacification contrast echo in patients with suboptimal images

(1) Enable improved endocardial visualization and assessment of LV structure and function when two or more contiguous segments are NOT seen on non-contrast images.
(2) Allow accurate and repeatable measurements of LV volumes, and ejection fraction by 2D echo.
(3) Increase confidence of the interpreting physician in the LV function, structure and volume assessments
(4) Confirm or exclude the echocardiographic diagnosis of the following LV structural abnormalities, when non-enhanced images are suboptimal for definitive diagnosis:

  - Apical hypertrophic cardiomyopathy
  - Ventricular non-compaction

- Apical thrombus
- Ventricular pseudoaneurysm

Indications for use of contrast in stress echocardiography
    When two or more endocardial border contiguous segments of LV are not well visualized in order to:

- Obtain diagnostic assessment of segmental wall motion and thickening at rest and stress
- Increase the proportion of diagnostic studies
- Increase reader confidence in interpretation

7. ANSWER: C. Based upon established guidelines, ultrasound contrast agents are indicated for use when two or more LV endocardial surfaces cannot be visualized in any image plane (see Figure 9-14).

8. ANSWER: B. Today, with advanced ultrasound imaging systems including harmonic software modifications, experts agree that approximately 10%–30% of all transthoracic echo images are considered technically difficult or uninterruptible. Based on published ASE guidelines, the echo study is classified as technically difficult if two or more endocardial regions are not visualized.

Importantly, in 2009, Kurt et al. performed a large cohort, prospective study, which was designed to assess the efficacy of the routine use of ultrasound contrast for LV chambers enhancement. The authors concluded that the use of ultrasound contrast agents significantly and positively impacted diagnostic accuracy and resource utilization, ultimately benefiting patient management. In their study, ultrasound contrast agents were indicated in 14.5% of the cohort (total population = 4,362; 632 patients received ultrasound contrast). The impact of contrast usage resulted in a change in therapy, additional procedures, or both in 35.6%. Clearly, the highest benefit of the use of ultrasound contrast agents accrued to patients hospitalized in the SICU. In this critically ill population, the authors noted a change in therapy or procedures in 62.7% of the subjects. In addition, the authors commented on a reduction in subsequent testing, which included exposure to ionizing radiation and invasive imaging.

9. ANSWER: D. The two current ultrasound contrast agents that have been approved by the United States FDA include (1) Optison, approved in 1997 and (2) Definity in 2001. Following a series of self-reported adverse events over the last several years, the FDA officials responded in October 2007 issuing a "Black box" warning on both perflutren ultrasound contrast agents. This warning included language describing the risk of "serious cardiopulmonary reactions" within 30 minutes of administration of these agents. Several new contraindications were added to the package label including the following:

    (1) worsening or clinically unstable heart failure; (2) AMI or acute coronary syndrome; (3) serious ventricu-

lar arrhythmia or high risk for arrhythmias due to QT prolongation; (4) respiratory failure; and (5) severe emphysema, pulmonary emboli, or other conditions that cause pulmonary hypertension. In lieu of these new contraindications, a 30-minute monitoring period was mandated for all patients who received these agents.

Subsequent to the FDA's revised warnings, an international grassroots organization of physicians, sonographers, nurses, and interested parties appealed to the FDA to reconsider the new restrictions placed on the ultrasound contrast agents. Subsequently, recognized professional organizations (EAE and ASE) voiced strong concern over the new labeling limitations placed on the ultrasound contrast agents.

In May of 2008, the FDA officials revised the October 2007 "Contraindications" and subsequently changed the language to a warning. The 30-minute monitoring period following contrast administration continued to apply to those patients with pulmonary hypertension or who were deemed critically ill.

10. ANSWER: B. In direct response to the FDA labeling changes of ultrasound contrast agents, clinicians responded with peer-reviewed publications, which revealed the relative safety of using ultrasound contrast agents. As of May 2009, more than 228,611 patient experiences have been summarized in the literature. Further, the clinical community, grassroots organizations, and professional societies continue to provide leadership in producing scientific/clinical data highlighting the important clinical utility and safety of ultrasound contrast agents.

A summary of the clinical safety publications are as follows:

- Erb JM, Shanewise JS. Intraoperative contrast echocardiography with intravenous Optison does not cause hemodynamic changes during cardiac surgery. *J Am Soc Echocardiogr.* 2001;14:595–600.
- Herzog CA. Incidence of adverse event associated with use of perflutren containing contrast agents for echocardiography. *JAMA.* 2008;299:2023–2025. Hennepin County MC Registry.
- Kusnetzky LL, Khalid A, Khumri TM, Moe TG, Jones PG, Main ML. Acute mortality in hospitalized patients undergoing echocardiography with and without an ultrasound contrast agent: results in 18,671 consecutive studies. *J Am Coll Cardiol.* 2008;51:1704–1706.
- Main ML, Ryan AC, Davis TE, Albano MP, Kusnetzky LL, Hibberd M. Acute mortality in hospitalized patients undergoing echocardiography with and without an ultrasound contrast agent (multi-center registry results in 4,300,966 consecutive patients). *Am J Cardiol.* 2008;102:1742–1746.
- Wei K, Mulvagh SL, Carson L, et al. The safety of Definity and Optison for ultrasound image enhancement: a retrospective analysis of 78,383 administered contrast doses. *J Am Soc Echocardiogr.* 2008;21:1202–1206.

- Dolan MS, Gala SS, Dodla S, et al. Safety and efficacy of commercially available ultrasound contrast agents for rest and stress echocardiography a multicenter experience. *J Am Coll Cardiol.* 2009;53:32–38.
- Gabriel RS, Smyth YM, Menon V, et al. Safety of ultrasound contrast agents in stress echocardiography. *Am J Cardiol.* 2008;102:1269–1272.
- Main ML, Exuzides A, Colby C, et al. Abstract presented March 2009, American College of Cardiology Safety Studies OptisonTM does not increase mortality in critically ill patients: a retrospective matched case-control. *J Am Coll Cardiol.* 2009.
- Anantharam B, Chahal N, Chelliah R, Ramzy I, Gani F, Senior R. Safety of contrast in stress echocardiography in stable patients and in patients with suspected acute coronary syndrome but negative 12 hours troponin. *Am J Cardiol.* 2009;104:14–18.

11. ANSWER: B. Ultrasound contrast agent safety status (2009):

- The October 2007 FDA product label changes were substantially revised in May 2008.
- Multiple, clinical safety studies reported in 2008–2009 consistently revealed the fact that there existed no identifiable "safety signal" in more than 228,611 patients.
- Further reversal of the October 2007 product label changes awaits completion of the FDA mandated risk management plans.

12. ANSWER: A. In 2009, the EAE published a position paper on the clinical use of contrast echocardiography for the assessment of myocardial perfusion. The paper postulated that on the basis of present evidence, Myocardial Contrast Echocardiography (MCE) may now be used clinically both at rest and during stress for the detection of coronary artery disease, acute coronary syndrome, and myocardial viability. Coronary flow reserve may also be performed using quantitative MCE.

13. ANSWER: C. The vascular applications of ultrasound contrast agents are legion. Similar to the current clinical indications for echocardiography applications, ultrasound contrast agents provide enhanced images of the large vessels, and specifically, the aorta, carotid arteries, and peripheral venous systems. Recent reports have documented the added value of ultrasound contrast agents in providing a valuable alternative to more invasive imaging technologies. The clinical applications for vascular applications are not yet approved in the United States; however, these applications are approved in Europe.

Subsequently, investigators identified the presence of angiogenesis within the human carotid plaque. The published literature now reflects and international appreciation of the use of ultrasound contrast agents for detection and quantification of the vasa vasorum (angiogenic) vessels associated with atherosclerosis. It is now recognized that the initial vessel wall inflammation identified in such diverse disease states as diabetes, atherosclerosis, cancer, and inflammatory states have as a unifying requirement, a blood supply.

14. ANSWER: A. A clinical trial was initiated using ultrasound contrast agents for the dissolution of venous thrombi. The results are yet to be published. The therapeutic application of ultrasound contrast agents provides a distinct demarcation between diagnostic imaging and medical therapeutics. The key to this therapeutic application lies in the fact that the microbubble shell integrity can be externally altered via externally applied acoustic pressure leading to enhanced disruption of thrombi, and intriguingly enough, provides a mechanism to produce site-specific drug and gene delivery systems; providing access to a nonviral delivery system. Leading scientists have successfully demonstrated nonviral transduction through sonoporation in a variety of preclinical scenarios. Clearly, the exciting scientific developments are beyond the scope of this brief mention but command attention for the future applications of ultrasound contrast agents.

15. ANSWER: D. Several large studies clearly established the safety of contrast agents in stress echocardiography. In fact, contrast agents are used more in high-risk stress echo patients. In a recent study, it was shown that despite the use of contrast agents in higher risk patients compared with noncontrast stress echo studies, there was no difference in the side-effect profile.

16. ANSWER: C. Following the intravenous injection of an ultrasound contrast agent, this baseline apical four-chamber image revealed several masses in the apical region in a patient who had suffered a prior myocardial infarction. When seen in real-time, the dyskinetic apical segments likely served as a source for reduced blood flow, which may have lead to the formation of a mural thrombi. When confronted with these findings, it is reasonable to stop the DSE, call the referring physician, and begin full anticoagulation. If one chooses to continue the DSE, there may be an ill-defined risk of dislodging the mobile thrombi.

17. ANSWER: D. Note the presence of a large mass in the apical region of the left ventricle. Based on this finding, the patient may require full anticoagulation and subsequent follow up with contrast-enhanced echocardiograms. Generally, when LV masses are identified, it is prudent to ascertain the clinical history. The presence of a significant regional wall motion abnormality coupled with a history of a prior myocardial infarction, is consistent with the finding of apical thrombi. Although additional testing could be performed, the contrast-enhanced 2D echocardiogram provided a safe and cost-effective method for diagnosing this mass.

18. ANSWER: B. The appropriate and judicious use of ultrasound contrast in this case confirmed the diagnosis of an apical hypertrophy ("spade heart"). Although additional imaging modalities may be used to corroborate the findings, the use of a contrast-enhanced ultrasound examination provides a rapid, economical, and low-risk procedure. A TEE and/or a contrast-enhanced CT scan provide alternatives; however, the contrast-enhanced transthoracic echocardiogram provided diagnostic information without incurring additional risk of ionizing radiation exposure to the patient.

19. ANSWER: C. The images-reveal a mobile thrombus attached to the surface of a previous apical thrombus. When these baseline images were viewed without the use of an ultrasound contrast agent, it appeared that the band-like structure was a false tendon. However, following the use of an ultrasound contrast agent, it became obvious that the band was the "leading edge" of a newly developed apical thrombus.

20. ANSWER: A. The presence of an apical aneurysm was clearly demonstrated following the clinically indicated use of ultrasound contrast agents. When viewed in multiple planes and in real-time, the region of interest (apex) revealed a dyskinetic segment with outward motion and systolic expansion. These findings are consistent with the diagnosis of an apical aneurysm.

21. ANSWER: C. The contrast-enhanced carotid artery revealed a significant eccentric, carotid artery atherosclerotic plaque. The ultrasound contrast agent (white) appears to fully opacify the carotid artery lumen, and the unenhanced (black) regions represent the vessel wall and accompanying plaque.

22. ANSWER: A. The contrast-enhanced vascular image revealed vessel wall angiogenesis (vasa vasorum). The lumen is enhanced (white) following the intravenous injection of an ultrasound contrast agent. The extra-luminal structures represent the vasa vasorum. These images represent a physiologic response to vessel wall inflammation through the induction of angiogenesis (vasa vasorum). The vessel wall hypoxia (ischemia) likely triggered subsequent signaling of VEGF proteins and the growth of the vasa vasorum.

23. ANSWER: D. The contrast-enhanced image shows contrast microbubbles traversing the myocardial structure and delineating trabeculation in the inner third of the myocardium. This is characteristic of a non-compacted myocardium. Noncompaction is a congenital disorder of persistence of fetal spongiform myocardium. Normally this differentiates into normal myocytes. The persistence of the spongiform structure weakens the myocardium resulting in dysfunction.

24. ANSWER: D. The contrast-enhanced carotid image associated with the green computer line outlines the near wall c-IMT. Today, there are numerous commercially available, computer-aided algorithms for c-IMT detection. Although the near-wall c-IMT can be difficult to visualize, the use of ultrasound contrast agents provides an opportunity to fully analyze the entire carotid vascular system.

25. ANSWER: D. The use of ultrasound contrast agents revealed severe carotid stenosis due to the presence of atherosclerosis. The use of contrast ultrasound also provides a clearer definition of the luminal characteristics of the carotid artery and related atherosclerotic plaques. Of note, intraplaque angiogenesis (vasa vasorum) was identified following the intravenous use of ultrasound contrast agents.

26. ANSWER: D. The use of ultrasound contrast was clinically indicated for the detection of the LV endocardial surfaces to assist in the assessment of the ejection fraction.

27. ANSWER: A. The ejection fraction following the use of intravenous contrast was estimated at >75%. Minutes later, following the intravenous use of ultrasound contrast, it was clearly recognized that the LV chamber size was small and the overall systolic function was hyperdynamic. Thus, the use of diuretics and sympathomimetic therapy was not indicated for medical management. Following the CEUS, the therapy for the patient was changed to include intravenous fluids and beta-blocker therapy.

KEY POINT:
■ For accurate assessment of LVEF and LV volumes, contrast should be administered.

28. ANSWER: A. Following the clinical use of ultrasound contrast, the anterior apical region of the left ventricle was noted to be akinetic; suggestive of an acute coronary occlusion and myocardial infarction. Subsequently, the patient was taken to the cardiac catheterization laboratory for an urgent percutaneous coronary intervention.

KEY POINT:
■ Use contrast to enhance apical structure and function assessment.

29. ANSWER: D. Injection of an ultrasound contrast agent was indicated because of the lack of clear endocardial definition.

30. ANSWER: A. Following the intravenous injection of ultrasound contrast, the apex region revealed large, mobile masses, consistent with the presence of intracavitary thrombi.

KEY POINT:
■ This case demonstrated the use of ultrasound contrast for the detection of intracavitary masses (i.e., thrombi).

31. ANSWER: C. This is a typical subendocardial perfusion defect. Wall motion abnormalities are less common after a vasodilator stress as oxygen demand is only mildly increased. However, capillary derecruitment occurs early in the ischemic cascade.

32. ANSWER: C. The defect is in the lateral wall only and suggests left circumflex coronary artery disease.

KEY POINT:

■ Perfusion defect exceeds wall motion abnormalities during vasodilator stress.

33. ANSWER: D. The left ventricle demonstrated akinetic apex and septum with normal perfusion. Absence of a perfusion defect suggests minimal necrosis. The combination of presentation characteristics, that is, female, with no significant risk factors and large wall motion abnormality with mild rise in cardiac enzyme and normal perfusion suggests Takotsubo cardiomyopathy.

34. ANSWER: A. These patients are likely to have normal coronaries. The normal perfusion suggests minimal necrosis and hence recovery of LV function is complete.

KEY POINT:

■ It is important to assess both perfusion and function after an acute coronary event.

35. ANSWER: C. Very patchy perfusion is noted in the septum and apex. For the assessment of perfusion after AMI, intravenous contrast is administered. After attainment of a steady state in the myocardium, destruction and replenishment contrast imaging is performed. Imaging is continued for 15 seconds after destruction phase to assess collateral circulation. Marked perfusion defect at 15 seconds indicates very poor collateral and antegrade flow, which suggests myocardial necrosis.

36. ANSWER: A. Transmural perfusion defect suggests transmural infarction. Hence, recovery of function is expected to be limited.

KEY POINT:

■ Following AMI, assessment of perfusion and function at rest can accurately predict outcome.

SUGGESTED READINGS

Anantharam B, Chahal N, Chelliah R, et al. Safety of contrast in stress echocardiography in stable patients and in patients with suspected acute coronary syndrome but negative 12-hour troponin. *Am J Cardiol*. 2009;104:14–18.

Bommer WJ, Shah PM, Allen H, et al. The safety of contrast echocardiography: report of the Committee on Contrast Echocardiography for the American Society of Echocardiography. *J Am Coll Cardiol*. 1984;3:6–13.

Coli S, Magnoni M, Sangiorgi G, et al. Contrast-enhanced ultrasound imaging of intraplaque neovascularization in carotid arteries: correlation with histology and plaque echogenicity. *J Am Coll Cardiol*. 2008;52:223–230.

Feinstein SB. Contrast ultrasound imaging of the carotid artery vasa vasorum and atherosclerotic plaque neovascularization. *J Am Coll Cardiol*. 2006;48:236–243.

Feinstein SB. The powerful microbubble: from bench to bedside, from intravascular indicator to therapeutic delivery system, and beyond. *Am J Physiol Heart Circ Physiol*. 2004;287:H450–H457.

Feinstein SB, Ten Cate FJ, Zwehl W, et al. Two-dimensional contrast echocardiography. I. In vitro development and quantitative analysis of echo contrast agents. *J Am Coll Cardiol*. 1984;3:14–20.

Gramiak R, Shah PM. Echocardiography of the aortic root. *Invest Radiol*. 1968;3:356–366.

Kaul S, Pandian NG, Okada RD, et al. Contrast echocardiography in acute myocardial ischemia: I. In vivo determination of total left ventricular "area at risk". *J Am Coll Cardiol*. 1984;4: 1272–1282.

Kremkau FW, Gramiak R, Carstensen EL, et al. Ultrasonic detection of cavitation at catheter tips. *Am J Roentgenol Radium Ther Nucl Med*. 1970;110:177–183.

Kurt M, Shaikh KA, Peterson L, et al. Impact of contrast echocardiography on evaluation of ventricular function and clinical management in a large prospective cohort. *J Am Coll Cardiol*. 2009;53:802–810.

Kusnetzky LL, Khalid A, Khumri TM, et al. Acute mortality in hospitalized patients undergoing echocardiography with and without an ultrasound contrast agent: results in 18,671 consecutive studies. *J Am Coll Cardiol*. 2008;51:1704–1706.

Main ML, Exuzides A, Colby C, et al. Safety Studies OptisonTM does not increase mortality in critically ill patients: a retrospective matched case-control. *J Am Coll Cardiol*. 2009.

Main ML, Ryan AC, Davis TE, et al. Acute mortality in hospitalized patients undergoing echocardiography with and without an ultrasound contrast agent (multicenter registry results in 4,300,966 consecutive patients). *Am J Cardiol*. 2008;102: 1742–1746.

Mulvagh SL, DeMaria AN, Feinstein SB, et al. Contrast echocardiography: current and future applications. *J Am Soc Echocardiogr*. 2000;13:331–342.

Mulvagh SL, Rakowski H, Vannan MA, et al. American Society of Echocardiography Consensus Statement on the Clinical Applications of Ultrasonic Contrast Agents in Echocardiography. *J Am Soc Echocardiogr*. 2008;21:1179–1201; quiz 1281.

Powsner SM, Keller MW, Saniie J, et al. Quantitation of echocontrast effects. *Am J Physiol Imaging*. 1986;1:124–128.

Senior R, Becher H, Monaghan M, et al. Contrast echocardiography: evidence-based recommendations by European Association of Echocardiography. *Eur J Echocardiogr*. 2009;10:194–212.

Senior R, Monaghan M, Main ML, et al; RAMP-1 and RAMP-2 Investigators. Detection of coronary artery disease with perfusion stress echocardiography using a novel ultrasound imaging agent: two phase 3 international trials in comparison with radionuclide perfusion imaging. *Eur J Echocardiogr*. 2009;10:26–35.

Shohet RV, Chen S, Zhou YT, et al. Echocardiographic destruction of albumin microbubbles directs gene delivery to the myocardium. *Circulation*. 2000;101:2554–2556.

Unger EC, Hersh E, Vannan M, et al. Local drug and gene delivery through microbubbles. *Prog Cardiovasc Dis*. 2001;44:45–54.

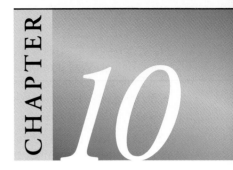
Systolic Function Assessment

Thomas H. Marwick

1. The change in left ventricular (LV) function attributable to cell therapy is sought in a postinfarct patient. Which of the following echocardiographic measures is the most feasible and closest analog of systolic elastance as a marker of myocardial contractility?
   A. Ejection fraction (EF).
   B. Systolic strain rate.
   C. Myocardial performance ("Tei") index.
   D. Systolic strain.
   E. dP/dt measured from the mitral regurgitant jet.

2. A patient after inferior infarction is thought on clinical grounds to have right ventricular (RV) infarction. Which parameters give a reliable assessment of RV function?
   A. 2D RV EF.
   B. Myocardial performance (Tei) index.
   C. Tricuspid annular plane displacement (TAPSE).
   D. RV S'.
   E. None of the above are reliable.

3. The development of end-systolic cavity obliteration during stress echocardiography reduces the development of ischemia, likely because of reduced wall stress. Wall stress is:
   A. Proportionate to transmural pressure and chamber size.
   B. Inversely proportionate to transmural pressure and chamber size.
   C. Proportionate to wall thickness.
   D. The same as systolic strain.
   E. Readily measured on a regional basis.

4. Visual assessment of EF is sometimes required (e.g., in an emergency). What are the potential limitations of visual EF?
   A. Inability to interrogate multiple imaging planes simultaneously.
   B. Image quality.
   C. Extremes of heart rate.
   D. Experience of the reviewer.
   E. All of the above.

5. A patient presenting with chest pain undergoes an echocardiogram during pain. The presence of segmental wall motion abnormality is:
   A. A marker of abnormal myocardium.
   B. Indicative of a high likelihood of myocardial ischemia.
   C. Identified with thickening of <50% or excursion <5 mm.
   D. Uninterpretable in the setting of left bundle branch block (LBBB).
   E. Useful in a diagnostic sense but not prognostically.

6. After implantation of a biventricular pacing device, a 55-year-old patient with dilated cardiomyopathy continues to complain of functional class III symptoms and there is no reduction of LV volumes. What factors are important in considering device optimization?
   A. There is no evidence to support its use.
   B. The role of mechanical dyssynchrony is in question since publication of the PROSPECT results.

C. The iterative technique for aortic valve (AV) optimization is based on observation of the LV filling curve at various pacing settings.

D. Site of previous infarction.

E. Site of the LV lead.

7. Following anterior myocardial infarction (MI), a 70-year-old man has an EF of 40% with an end-systolic volume (ESV) of 95 ml (50 ml/m^2). In what range is his 5-year mortality?

A. 10%.

B. 15%.

C. 20%.

D. 30%.

E. 50%.

8. In the course of auditing the activity of your echocardiography laboratory, you find that 18% of studies have had a previous echocardiogram. On investigating the matter further, you find that the majority are for inpatients with worsening heart failure (HF). Which of the following are true regarding repeat echocardiograms?

A. Repeat echo is a class I indication from the ACC/AHA guidelines.

B. 95% confidence intervals for EF are ±11%.

C. 95% confidence intervals for LV mass (LVM) are ±60 g.

D. All of the above.

E. None of the above.

9. LV strain has been proposed as a simple quantitative tool for assessing LV function. Which of the following is associated with reduced strain, irrespective of myocardial status?

A. Decreased afterload.

B. Decreased preload.

C. Decreased heart rate.

D. All of the above.

E. None of the above.

10. Measurement of midwall shortening provides information that is inconsistent with endocardial shortening in:

A. Normal hearts.

B. Dilated cardiomyopathy.

C. Concentric remodeling.

D. Eccentric LV hypertrophy (LVH).

E. Concentric LVH.

11. Accurate measures of LV volumes are needed in the course of follow-up of patients with asymptomatic mitral regurgitation (MR). Which is the most accurate option?

A. 2D echocardiogram.

B. 2D echocardiogram with contrast.

C. 3D echocardiogram.

D. 3D echocardiogram with contrast.

E. Transesophageal echocardiogram.

12. Given its high workload and distance from nutrient supply, the subendocardium is an important site of pathology. Which techniques could be used to assess subendocardial function?

A. Longitudinal, circumferential, and transverse strain.

B. Integrated backscatter.

C. Myocardial contrast echocardiography with high MI.

D. None of the above.

E. All of the above.

13. Which of the statements regarding the application of new technologies is true?

A. Systolic velocity is a useful marker of regional systolic function.

B. 3D measurements will be useful for the assessment of diastolic function.

C. Deformation analysis is useful for the assessment of myocardial viability.

D. None of the above.

E. All of the above.

14. Which of the following statements is true regarding the application of new technologies to the different stages of HF?

A. Myocardial deformation is of value in the detection of stage B HF.

B. 3D measurements are of most value in stages C and D.

C. Tissue velocity is of use in all stages.

D. None of the above.

E. All of the above.

15. A patient with hypertension has septal and posterior wall thickness of 12 and 13 mm, respectively, with an end-diastolic dimension of 52 mm. How would you characterize these LV dimensions?
A. Normal LV geometry.
B. Concentric remodeling.
C. Concentric hypertrophy.
D. Eccentric hypertrophy.
E. None of the above.

16. A 48-year-old woman presents to the hospital with chest pain following a motor vehicle accident. She has anterior ST segment elevation and an echocardiogram is performed because of pulmonary congestion. Color Doppler of the LV outflow tract shows aliasing. Echocardiographic images in the apical four- and two-chamber views are provided in Figure 10-1 and Videos 10-1A, B, and C.
The likely diagnosis is:
A. Hypertrophic cardiomyopathy (HCM).
B. Large anteroseptal MI.
C. Stress (Takotsubo) cardiomyopathy.
D. Multivessel ischemia.
E. Cardiac contusion.

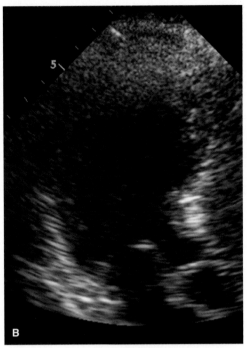

Fig. 10-1B

17. A systolic murmur is heard in a 67-year-old man, 3 days following MI. The echocardiogram in Figure 10-2 and Videos 10-2A and B show:
A. Papillary muscle rupture.
B. Postinfarct ventricular septal defect (VSD).
C. Congenital (perimembranous) VSD.
D. Congenital (muscular) VSD.
E. Ischemic MR.

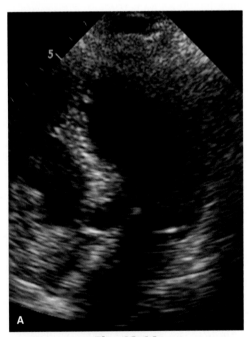

Fig. 10-1A

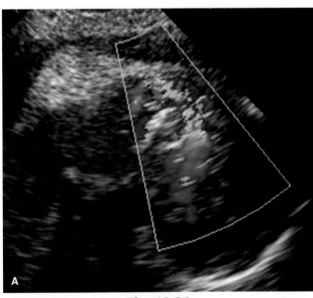

Fig. 10-2A

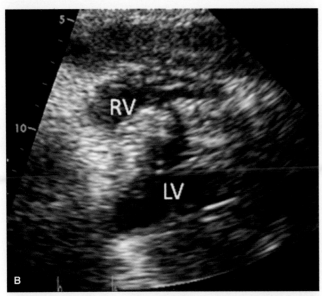

Fig. 10-2B

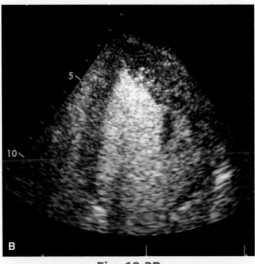

Fig. 10-3B

18. A 27-year-old man is found to have anterolateral T-wave inversions when an ECG is performed during a routine insurance physical examination. The echocardiogram with and without contrast in Figure 10-3 and Videos 10-3A, B, C and D shows:

A. Apical tumor (fibroma).

B. Apical muscular band.

C. Apical HCM (Yamaguchi variant).

D. Apical foreshortening.

E. Noncompaction cardiomyopathy.

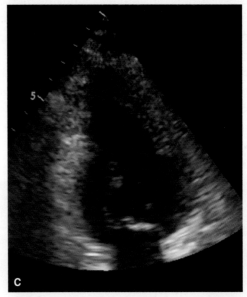

Fig. 10-3C

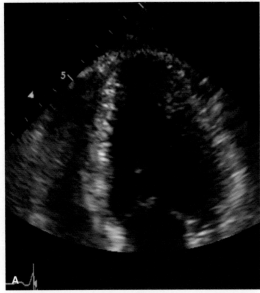

Fig. 10-3A

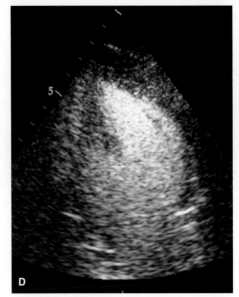

Fig. 10-3D

19. A 68-year-old woman presents with HF. There is no family history, she has previously been well and takes no medication. The ECG shows low voltage but is otherwise unremarkable. The echocardiogram in Videos 10-4A and B shows low tissue velocity (E' 4 cm/sec) with left atrial enlargement and a pseudonormal filling pattern.

   The likely diagnosis is:
   A. Fabry disease.
   B. Hypertensive heart disease.
   C. HCM.
   D. Amyloidosis.
   E. Sarcoidosis.

20. A 48-year-old man with renal impairment has presented late after an MI. There are no Q waves and preservation of R waves on the ECG but an apical wall motion abnormality. Coronary angiography has been withheld because of concerns regarding possible nephrotoxicity, so a myocardial contrast perfusion study is performed with a destruction-replenishment protocol (Fig. 10-4 and Videos 10-5A and B).

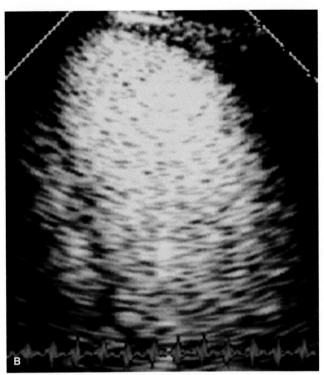

Fig. 10-4B

   The findings suggest:
   A. LCX scar.
   B. Medical management is appropriate.
   C. RCA scar.
   D. Stunned myocardium in the LAD territory.
   E. LAD scar.

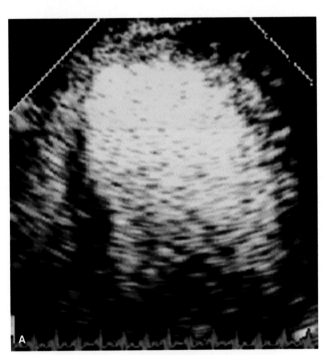

Fig. 10-4A

21. This 2D echocardiogram (apical four-chamber view in Video 10-6) was obtained following an out-of-hospital cardiac arrest in a 37-year-old man, who has continued to have episodes of ventricular tachycardia in the coronary care unit.

   The findings suggest:
   A. RV infarction.
   B. Pulmonary embolism (McConnell's sign).
   C. Arrhythmogenic RV dysplasia.
   D. Pulmonary hypertension and cor pulmonale.
   E. Cardiac rotation with off-axis imaging.

22. A 72-year-old patient becomes hypotensive following presentation with a myocardial infarction.

   The findings of this subcostal image in Video 10-7 suggest:
   A. RV infarction.
   B. Pulmonary embolism (McConnell's sign).
   C. Arrhythmogenic RV dysplasia.
   D. Pulmonary hypertension and cor pulmonale.
   E. Cardiac rotation with off-axis imaging.

23. A routine echocardiogram is performed 5 days following primary angioplasty to the left anterior descending coronary artery (Fig. 10-5 and Videos 10-8A–E).

The findings suggest:

A. Subacute rupture.
B. Apical muscle band.
C. Apical scar.
D. Apical thrombus.
E. Multivessel coronary artery disease.

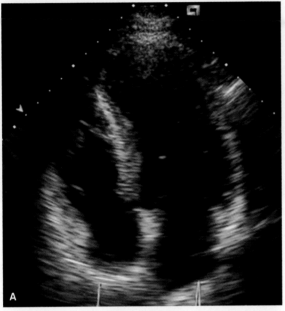

Fig. 10-5A

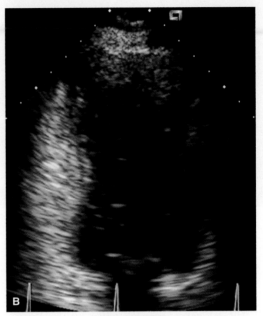

Fig. 10-5B

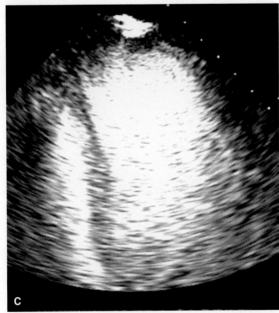

Fig. 10-5C

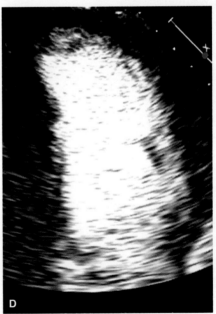

Fig. 10-5D

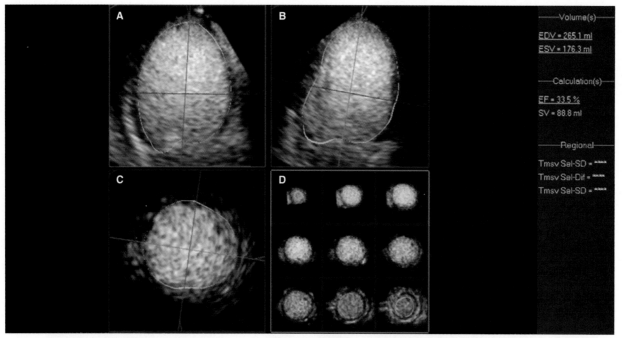

Volume(s)
EDV = 265.1 ml
ESV = 176.3 ml

Calculation(s)
EF = 33.5 %
SV = 88.8 ml

Regional
Tmsv Sel-SD = ^^^^
Tmsv Sel-Dif = ^^^^
Tmsv Sel-SD = ^^^^

Fig. 10-6A–D

24. A resting 3D echocardiogram was performed on a 62-year-old patient with type 2 diabetes who presented with dyspnea (Fig. 10-6 and Video 10-9).
    The findings suggest:
    A. Normal LV function.
    B. Diffuse LV dysfunction.
    C. Left anterior descending scar.
    D. Right coronary scar.
    E. Left circumflex scar.

25. **An** asymptomatic patient with normal LV function but severe MR has bileaflet prolapse. She is uncertain as to whether to proceed to mitral repair and undergoes an exercise echocardiogram.
    The apical four- and two-chamber views in Figure 10-7 and Video 10-10, before and after exercise findings, suggest:
    A. Normal LV response to stress.
    B. LAD scar.
    C. Loss of contractile reserve (CR).
    D. Right coronary scar.
    E. Left circumflex scar.

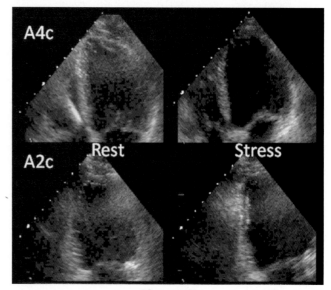

A4c
Rest
A2c
Stress

Fig. 10-7

CASE 1:

A 72-year-old woman undergoes an echocardiogram because of symptoms of HF (Fig. 10-8 and Video 10-11).

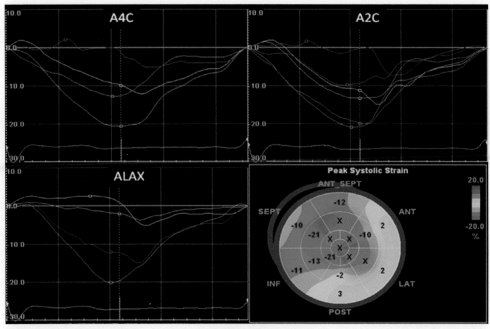

Fig. 10-8

26. The resting wall motion abnormalities suggest infarctions in:
    A. No discrete territory (nonischemic cardiomyopathy).
    B. Left anterior descending.
    C. Right coronary.
    D. Left circumflex.
    E. Multiple vessels.

27. The strain pattern in the posterior wall of Figure 10-9 suggests:
    A. No discrete abnormality.
    B. Loss of longitudinal function in the base but not the apex.
    C. Loss of longitudinal function in the apex but not the base.
    D. Loss of longitudinal function in both the apex and base.
    E. Loss of thickening in the whole posterior wall.

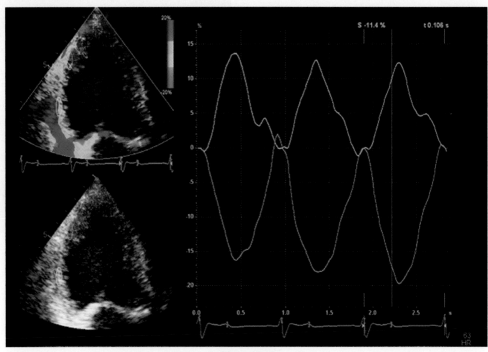

Fig. 10-9

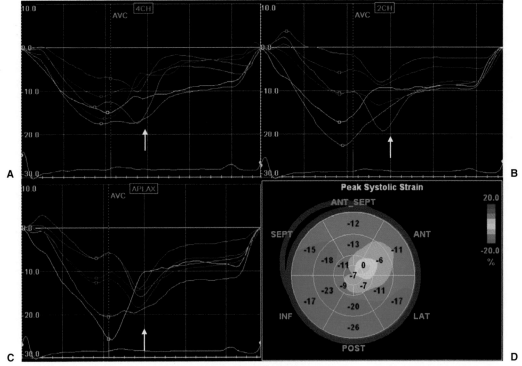

Fig. 10-10A–D

CASE 2:

A 63-year-old man undergoes an echocardiogram prior to a stress echocardiogram (Fig. 10-10 and Video 10-12). The biplane Simpson's EF was 37% (end-diastolic volume [EDV] 172, ESV 108).

28. In the presence of a mean global strain of -14% and segmental waveforms as shown:
    A. The findings are concordant in showing mildly reduced LV function.
    B. Show a discrepancy between radial and longitudinal function.
    C. Underestimate the severity of LV dysfunction.
    D. Show extensive late contraction (which may identify viability).
    E. The problem appears to be nonischemic.

29. The resting wall motion abnormalities in Video 10-13 suggest infarctions in:
    A. No discrete territory (nonischemic cardiomyopathy).
    B. Left anterior descending.
    C. Right coronary.
    D. Left circumflex.
    E. Multiple vessels.

CASE 3:

After an inferior MI, this 68-year-old woman developed HF and a new systolic murmur was noted.

30. The baseline echocardiogram in Figure 10-11 and Videos 10-14A–C demonstrates severe, posteriorly directed MR due to:

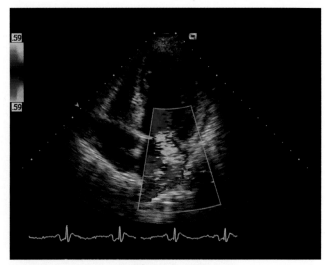

Fig. 10-11

    A. Papillary muscle rupture.
    B. Anterior prolapse.
    C. Severe LV dysfunction.
    D. Annular enlargement.
    E. Posterior leaflet restriction.

31. After 6 months, a follow-up echocardiogram is performed. What process do the findings in Figure 10-12A and B suggest?

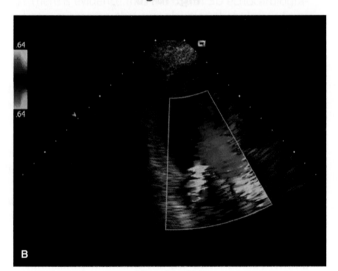

Fig. 10-12A

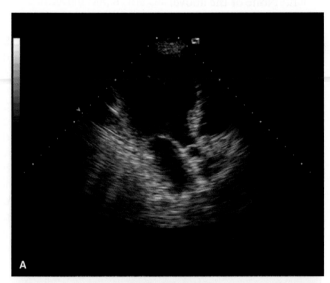

Fig. 10-12B

A. Scarring of the posterior wall.
B. Response to diuretics and vasodilators.
C. Mitral valve repair.
D. Percutaneous intervention and viable myocardium.
E. None of the above.

CASE 4:

A 61-year-old woman presents with fatigue and edema. The right heart border is prominent on CXR but PA pressure and pulmonary vascular resistance are normal. The echocardiogram is shown in Figure 10-13 and Videos 10-15A–C.

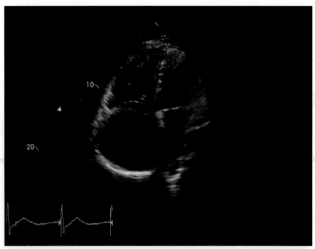

Fig. 10-13

32. The RV findings are consistent with:
A. RV infarction.
B. Pulmonary embolism (McConnell's sign).
C. Arrhythmogenic RV dysplasia.
D. Pulmonary hypertension and cor pulmonale.
E. Ebstein's anomaly.

33. The images in Figure 10-14 and Video 10-16 demonstrate a follow-up scan.

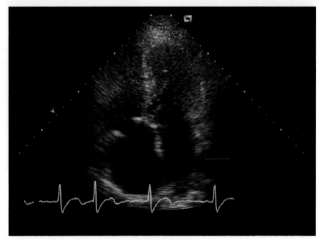

Fig. 10-14

What procedure has been undertaken?
A. Tricuspid valve replacement.
B. Heart transplant.
C. Tricuspid valve repair.
D. Heart-lung transplant.
E. None of the above.

SUGGESTED READINGS

Aikawa Y, Rohde L, Plehn J, et al. Regional wall stress predicts ventricular remodeling after anteroseptal myocardial infarction in the Healing and Early Afterload Reducing Trial (HEART): an echocardiography-based structural analysis. *Am Heart J.* 2001;141:234–242.

Armstrong WF, Pellikka PA, Ryan T, et al. Stress echocardiography: recommendations for performance and interpretation of stress echocardiography. Stress Echocardiography Task Force of the Nomenclature and Standards Committee of the American Society of Echocardiography. *J Am Soc Echocardiogr.* 1998;11:97–104.

Becker M, Hoffmann R, Kuhl HP, et al. Analysis of myocardial deformation based on ultrasonic pixel tracking to determine transmurality in chronic myocardial infarction. *Eur Heart J.* 2006;27:2560–2566.

Bonow RO, Carabello BA, Chatterjee K, et al. 2008 focused update incorporated into the ACC/AHA 2006 guidelines for the management of patients with valvular heart disease: a report of the American College of Cardiology/American Heart Association Task Force on practice guidelines (Committee on management of patients with valvular heart disease). *J Am Coll Cardiol.* 2008;52:e1–e142.

Greenberg NL, Firstenberg MS, Castro PL, et al. Doppler-derived myocardial systolic strain rate is a strong index of left ventricular contractility. *Circulation.* 2002;105:99–105.

Hayat SA, Senior R. Contrast echocardiography for the assessment of myocardial viability 4. *Curr Opin Cardiol.* 2006;21:473–478.

Horton KD, Meece RW, Hill JC. Assessment of the right ventricle by echocardiography: a primer for cardiac sonographers. *J Am Soc Echocardiogr.* 2009;22:776–792.

Hunt SA, Abraham WT, Chin MH, et al. ACC/AHA 2005 Guideline Update for the Diagnosis and Management of Chronic Heart Failure in the Adult: a report of the American College of Cardiology/American Heart Association Task Force on Practice Guidelines (Writing Committee to Update the 2001 Guidelines for the Evaluation and Management of Heart Failure): developed in collaboration with the American College of Chest Physicians and the International Society for Heart and Lung Transplantation: endorsed by the Heart Rhythm Society 5. *Circulation.* 2005;112:e154–e235.

Kozakova M, Palombo C, Distante A. Right ventricular infarction: the role of echocardiography. *Echocardiography.* 2001;18:701–707.

Lang RM, Bierig M, Devereux RB, et al. Recommendations for chamber quantification: a report from the American Society of Echocardiography's Guidelines and Standards Committee and the Chamber Quantification Writing Group, developed in conjunction with the European Association of Echocardiography, a branch of the European Society of Cardiology. *J Am Soc Echocardiogr.* 2005;18:1440–1463.

Lee R, Hanekom L, Marwick TH, et al. Prediction of subclinical left ventricular dysfunction with strain rate imaging in patients with asymptomatic severe mitral regurgitation. *Am J Cardiol.* 2004;94:1333–1337.

Otterstad JE, Froeland G, St John SM, et al. Accuracy and reproducibility of biplane two-dimensional echocardiographic measurements of left ventricular dimensions and function. *Eur Heart J.* 1997;18:507–513.

Prasad A, Lerman A, Rihal CS. Apical ballooning syndrome (Tako-Tsubo or stress cardiomyopathy): a mimic of acute myocardial infarction. *Am Heart J.* 2008;155:408–417.

Selvanayagam JB, Hawkins PN, Paul B, et al. Evaluation and management of the cardiac amyloidosis. *J Am Coll Cardiol.* 2007;50:2101–2110.

Stanton T, Hawkins NM, Hogg KJ, et al. How should we optimize cardiac resynchronization therapy? *Eur Heart J.* 2008;29:2458–2472.

Stanton T, Ingul CB, Hare JL, et al. Association of myocardial deformation with mortality independent of myocardial ischemia and left ventricular hypertrophy. *JACC Cardiovasc Imaging.* 2009;2:793–801.

Thanigaraj S, Schechtman KB, Perez JE. Improved echocardiographic delineation of left ventricular thrombus with the use of intravenous second-generation contrast image enhancement. *J Am Soc Echocardiogr.* 1999;12:1022–1026.

Voigt JU, Exner B, Schmiedehausen K, et al. Strain-rate imaging during dobutamine stress echocardiography provides objective evidence of inducible ischemia. *Circulation.* 2003;107:2120–2126.

White HD, Norris RM, Brown MA, et al. Left ventricular end-systolic volume as the major determinant of survival after recovery from myocardial infarction 16. *Circulation.* 1987;76:44–51.

Yoerger DM, Marcus F, Sherrill D, et al. Echocardiographic findings in patients meeting task force criteria for arrhythmogenic right ventricular dysplasia: new insights from the multidisciplinary study of right ventricular dysplasia. *J Am Coll Cardiol.* 2005;45:860–865.

Diastology

Andrew O. Zurick, David Verhaert, and Allan L. Klein

1. The best two-dimensional (2D) and Doppler echocardiographic finding to differentiate restrictive cardiomyopathy from constrictive pericarditis would be to evaluate:
   A. Mitral inflow pattern.
   B. Pulmonary venous flow pattern.
   C. Atrial size.
   D. Inferior vena cava dilatation.
   E. Early diastolic mitral annular velocity.

2. Echocardiography is performed on a 59-year-old male patient 3 months after having a large posterolateral wall infarction due to an acute stent thrombosis in his proximal circumflex coronary artery. Which of the following is associated with a better prognosis?
   A. Presence of moderate-to-severe mitral regurgitation (MR) (ERO = 0.3 cm²).
   B. Left ventricular ejection fraction of 33%.
   C. E/e′ = 21.
   D. Deceleration time of 123 ms.
   E. Lateral wall e′ of 7 cm/sec.

3. How will the pulmonary venous Doppler flow pattern immediately change in the case of left atrial stunning (e.g., after cardioversion for paroxysmal atrial fibrillation)? *S1: first velocity of systolic pulmonary venous flow; S2: second velocity of systolic pulmonary venous flow; D: diastolic velocity of pulmonary venous flow. AR: atrial reversal of pulmonary venous flow.*
   A. The systolic filling fraction (S1) will increase.
   B. The systolic filling fraction (S2) will increase.
   C. A decrease will be seen of the diastolic filling fraction (D).
   D. A decrease will be seen of the systolic filling fraction, particularly S1.
   E. An increase in the AR velocity.

4. Which of the following statements are true about the pulmonary venous flow pattern?
   A. Peak AR >35 cm/sec suggests elevated left ventricular (LV) filling pressures.
   B. The pulmonary S wave is related to LV relaxation.
   C. The S/D ratio provides an accurate estimation of LV filling pressures in patients with preserved and reduced systolic function.
   D. Pulmonary venous AR duration < mitral inflow A duration indicates an increased LV end-diastolic pressure.
   E. Pulmonary venous flow AR can be obtained in only 50% of patients.

5. In patients with atrial fibrillation, LV filling pressures could be best estimated using which of the following statements?
   A. E/e′ ≥11 correlates well with elevated pulmonary capillary wedge pressure (PCWP).
   B. Deceleration time in patients with a normal ejection fraction.
   C. Left atrial size. Higher left atrial size (>34 ml/m²) will reflect chronically elevated filling pressures.
   D. Peak velocity of the diastolic pulmonary venous flow, which will reflect atrial pressure in these patients.
   E. Impossible; there is no A wave and the variability in cycle length precludes any accurate estimation.

6. A 61-year-old male patient with a history of hypertension complains of exercise intolerance. His lung function tests are normal. His heart rate (HR) at rest is 60 bpm. He has a normal ejection fraction, mild LV hypertrophy, no valvular pathology. Doppler echocardiography data are included in Table 11-1.

TABLE 11-1

E-wave velocity	48 cm/sec
A-wave velocity	60 cm/sec
Deceleration time	300 msec
e' velocity	8 cm/sec
Tricuspid Regurgitation (TR) jet velocity	2.5 m/sec
E/e'	6

Based on this information:

A. The cause of his symptoms is unlikely cardiac. Refer him to internal medicine.

B. Consider a coronary angiography. Dyspnea is sometimes a symptom of underlying coronary artery disease.

C. We can conclude that the patient has elevated filling pressures and should be given a diuretic.

D. Consider a diastolic stress test.

E. BNP is 500 pg/ml.

7. The patient in Question 6 above undergoes stress testing with a supine bike protocol. Doppler echocardiography is performed 2 minutes after peak exercise (HR = 136 bpm, ~85% MPHR). Findings are included in Table 11-2:

TABLE 11-2

E-wave velocity	130 cm/sec
A-wave velocity	70 cm/sec
Deceleration time	160 msec
e' velocity	8 cm/sec
TR jet velocity	3.7 m/sec
E/e'	16

Which statement is true?

A. This patient has stage 1 diastolic dysfunction with exercise.

B. These findings raise concern for pulmonary embolism.

C. More information is needed to make any definite statement concerning the patient's diastolic function.

D. Normal values for this patient's age and gender given the fact that he just underwent stress testing and his HR is increased.

E. This patient has elevated LV filling pressures with exercise.

8. A dialysis patient undergoes cardiac catheterization. His ventricular angiogram shows normal systolic function. The pulmonary capillary wedge tracing shows significant v-waves. However, the ventriculogram and a carefully performed echocardiogram do not show significant MR. What is the most likely explanation?

A. MR can be very dynamic. In addition, there could be a very excentric jet.

B. Stage 3 diastolic dysfunction due to LV hypertrophy and volume overload.

C. Atrial rhythm disturbance.

D. Loss of left atrial reservoir function.

E. Congenital anomaly.

9. When performing pulsed wave Doppler imaging in the apical four-chamber view to acquire mitral annular velocities, which of the following is true?

A. The sample volume should be positioned at or 1 cm within the septal and lateral insertion sites of the mitral leaflets.

B. The sample volume should be small enough (usually 2–3 mm) to evaluate the longitudinal excursion of the mitral annulus in both systole and diastole.

C. In general, the velocity scale should be set at ~30 cm/s above and below the zero-velocity baseline.

D. Angulation up to 40 degree between the ultrasound beam and the plane of cardiac motion is acceptable.

E. Spectral recordings are ideally obtained during inspiration and measurements should reflect the average of three consecutive cardiac cycles.

10. Impaired elastic recoil is most consistent with which of the following?

A. Decrease in the isovolumic relaxation time (IVRT).

B. Decrease in left atrial pressure.

C. Impaired late diastolic filling.

D. Impaired active relaxation.

E. Decrease in the early diastolic intraventricular pressure gradient.

11. Which statement is false? First-degree AV block:
    A. May have the same effect on the mitral inflow pattern as sinus tachycardia.
    B. May lead to a pattern consistent with delayed relaxation even if there is no underlying diastolic dysfunction.
    C. May lead to diastolic MR in the presence of restrictive filling.
    D. May hamper evaluation of LV diastolic function when only pulsed Doppler interrogation of the mitral inflow is performed.
    E. Will decrease the LV diastolic filling period. Therefore, it may have an adverse effect on filling pressures and cardiac output in patients with severe systolic dysfunction.

12. Color Doppler M-mode (CMM) echocardiography provides information on flow propagation (Vp) which is unique in that it is relatively independent of which of the following?
    A. Cardiac output.
    B. LV compliance.
    C. Left atrial size.
    D. Loading conditions.
    E. HR.

13. What is the strongest determinant of mitral deceleration time?
    A. Left atrial mechanical function.
    B. LV operating stiffness.
    C. Left ventricular end-diastolic pressure (LVEDP).
    D. Ejection fraction.
    E. Left atrial reservoir function.

14. In patients with dilated cardiomyopathy, pulsed wave Doppler mitral flow velocity variables and filling patterns correlate with which of the following?
    A. Cardiac filling pressures and functional class, but not prognosis.
    B. Prognosis, but not filling pressures or functional class.
    C. Cardiac filling pressures, functional class, and prognosis, but less so than does LV ejection fraction.
    D. Cardiac filling pressures, functional class and prognosis better than does LV ejection fraction.
    E. Cardiac filling pressures, functional class, and prognosis, but to a lesser degree than in patients with LV ejection fraction >50%.

15. Which statement is most correct with respect to the application of the Valsalva maneuver in the assessment of diastolic function?
    A. The lack of reversibility in E/A ratio with Valsalva in patients with advanced diastolic dysfunction indicates irreversible restrictive physiology and implies a very poor prognosis.
    B. The Valsalva maneuver is a sensitive and specific way to differentiate normal from stage 1 diastolic function.
    C. The Valsalva maneuver should be used in every patient when assessing diastolic function.
    D. In cardiac patients, a decrease of ≥50% in E/A ratio is highly specific for increased LV filling pressures.

16. Figure 11-1 represents three different pulsed wave Doppler recordings of mitral inflow velocity in a 63-year-old male with a diagnosis of cardiac amyloidosis. The Doppler recordings were acquired at different stages in the progression of his disease. Atrial fibrillation is a common complication in these patients. At what stage in his disease would sudden onset of atrial fibrillation most likely cause a marked increase in symptoms in this patient?

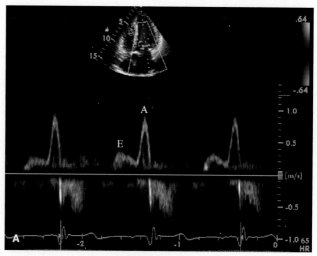

Fig. 11-1A

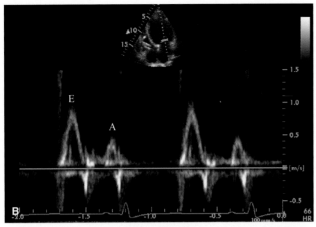

Fig. 11-1B

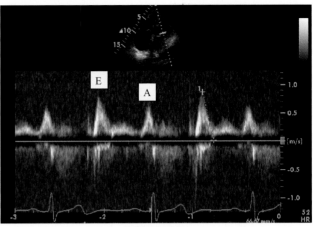

Fig. 11-2

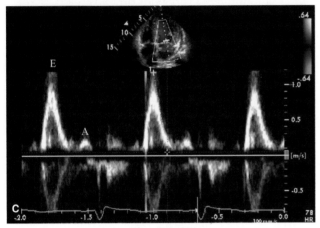

Fig. 11-1C

A. The transmitral gradient suddenly increases in mid-diastole because of a decrease in LV compliance.
B. This type of inflow pattern is sometimes seen in young individuals and can be explained by vigorous LV relaxation.
C. This finding represents a very early stage of diastolic dysfunction.
D. This patient has markedly delayed relaxation. Preload reduction will reveal stage 1 diastolic dysfunction.
E. The Doppler tracing is suggestive of atrial mechanical dysfunction, possibly due to a recent episode of atrial tachyarrhythmia.

A. Around the time of the Doppler recording represented in Figure 11-1A.
B. Around the time of the Doppler recording represented in Figure 11-1B.
C. Around the time of the Doppler recording represented in Figure 11-1C.
D. No matter how advanced the diastolic dysfunction, atrial fibrillation is always highly symptomatic in cardiac amyloidosis.
E. More information is needed to answer this question.

17. Based on Figure 11-2, what could you say about the underlying diastolic function in this patient?

18. A 53-year-old male with hypertension but no other cardiac events in the past complains of exercise intolerance. An echocardiogram shows a normal LV systolic function (ejection fraction = 60%), mild concentric LV hypertrophy and no valvular dysfunction. Based on the Doppler recording of his mitral inflow pattern in Figure 11-3, which additional echocardiographic parameter is most helpful in confirming whether his symptoms should be attributed to elevated filling pressure?

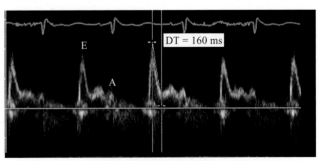

DT = Deceleration Time
Fig. 11-3

A. Left atrial volume index of 28 ml/m^2.

B. Tissue Doppler early diastolic velocity of the mitral annulus of 12 cm/s.

C. Tissue Doppler-derived early diastolic velocity of the mitral annulus of 6 cm/s.

D. Difference in duration of pulmonary venous flow AR and mitral inflow of 15 msec.

E. Transmitral flow propagation velocity assessed by color M-mode of 60 cm/s.

19. A patient with severe LV dysfunction due to long-standing untreated hypertension is referred for initiation of medical therapy. Based on the Doppler findings in Figure 11-4, one should be extra cautious when starting what medical therapy?

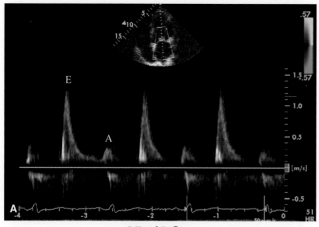

Mitral Inflow
Fig. 11-4A

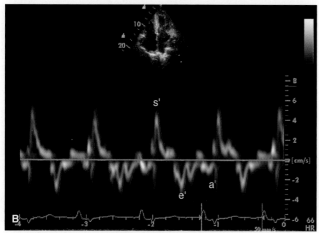

TDI Lateral Annulus
Fig. 11-4B

A. Diuretics.

B. Nitrates.

C. Angiotensin-converting enzyme (ACE) inhibitors.

D. Beta-blocking agents.

E. Hydralazine.

20. Figure 11-5 represents the transmitral flow propagation velocity (Vp) assessed by color M-mode (red line) in a patient with an acute myocardial infarction due to thrombotic occlusion of his mid-left anterior descending artery (LAD) 3 months ago. If it was possible to measure the intracavitary LV pressure with a high-fidelity pressure wire and compare measurements with values obtained prior to his infarction, what observation would be most likely?

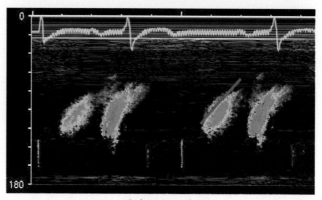

Color M-mode
Fig. 11-5

A. A decreased early diastolic pressure gradient between the tip of the mitral valve and the apex.

B. A higher absolute value for dP/dt.

C. A lower end-diastolic LV pressure.

D. A lower early diastolic pressure measured at the LV apex.

E. A lower late diastolic pressure measured at the LV apex.

21. A 61-year-old female with ischemic cardiomyopathy is referred for cardiac resynchronization therapy. Just before implantation of her biventricular device, she undergoes transthoracic echocardiography. Six months later, a new echocardiogram is obtained. Based on the LV Doppler filling pattern shown in Table 11-3 and Figure 11-6, which statement is correct?

TABLE 11-3	
Baseline	**6-Month Follow-Up**
E = 78 cm/s	E = 111 cm/s
A = 72 cm/s	A = 28 cm/s
E/A = 1.1	E/A = 3.6
DT = 180 ms	DT = 126 ms
Vp = 28 cm/s	Vp = 25 cm/s

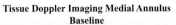

**Tissue Doppler Imaging Medial Annulus
Baseline**

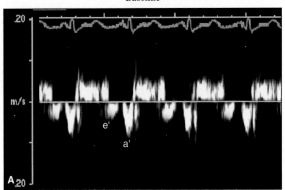

e' = 5 cm/s
Fig. 11-6A

6 Month Follow-up

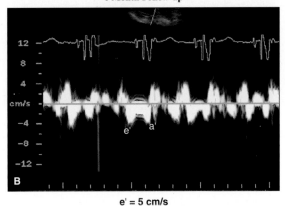

e' = 5 cm/s
Fig. 11-6B

A. LV relaxation has improved.
B. LV filling pressures are decreased.
C. Left atrial contractility has increased.
D. LV stiffness increased.
E. There is less dyssynchrony.

22. The Doppler findings in Figure 11-7 are most likely to be found in which clinical scenario?

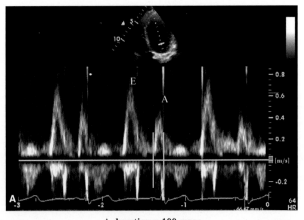

A duration = 100 msec
Mitral Inflow
Fig. 11-7A

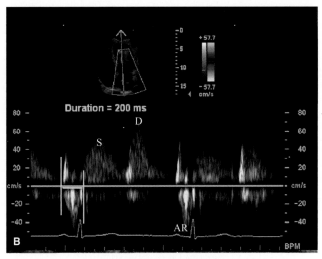

AR duration = 180 msec
Pulmonary Venous Flow
Fig. 11-7B

A. 35-year-old male athlete.
B. 50-year-old woman with 2+ MR.
C. 60-year-old man with advanced hypertensive heart disease.
D. 50-year-old man with recently diagnosed hypertrophic cardiomyopathy.
E. 50-year-old woman with constrictive pericarditis.

23. The mitral inflow pattern shown in Figure 11-8 is by itself suggestive of elevated filling pressures if:

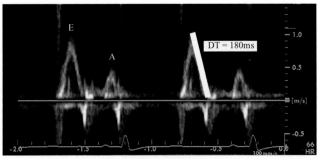

Fig. 11-8

A. The patient has an ejection fraction of 25%.
B. The patient has an ejection fraction of 60%.
C. The patient has a dilated left atrium and history of atrial fibrillation.

D. The patient has mitral valve prolapse and moderately severe MR.

E. The maximal jet velocity of the tricuspid regurgitant jet is 3.5 m/sec.

24. A 56-year-old patient was referred to you because of increasing shortness of breath. Pulsed-wave Doppler echocardiography in the hepatic veins reveals the tracing in Figure 11-9.

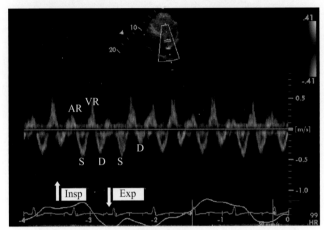

Fig. 11-9

What is the most appropriate statement?

A. There is evidence for an increased right ventricular end-diastolic pressure (RVEDP).

B. There must be severe tricuspid regurgitation.

C. This pattern can be seen in patients with constrictive pericarditis.

D. There is a right ventricular relaxation abnormality.

E. Chronic obstructive pulmonary disease can be the cause of this finding.

25. The mitral inflow filling pattern shown in Figure 11-10 should be considered abnormal for which of the following patients?

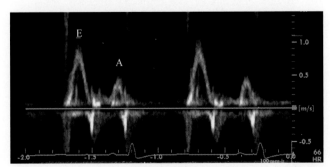

Fig. 11-10

A. A 41-year-old male with normal ejection fraction and an elective PCI of the RCA 2 years earlier.

B. A 46-year-old female with a bicuspid aortic valve and moderately severe aortic insufficiency.

C. A 28-year-old athlete complaining of atypical chest pain.

D. A 37-year-old obese female complaining of shortness of breath.

E. A 65-year-old male without medical history.

CASE 1:

A 48-year-old previously healthy male political lobbyist has recently started to notice increasing shortness of breath while walking up the US Capitol steps to lobby for health care reform over the past 4 weeks. He has no prior known history of cardiovascular disease or heart surgery.

Electrocardiogram (ECG) shows sinus tachycardia (108 bpm) without evidence of Q waves or ST segment alteration.

Physical examination is remarkable for blood pressure 90/50 mm Hg, HR 108 bpm, weight 87 kg. Cardiovascular examination demonstrates a laterally displaced LV apical impulse with an audible S3 on auscultation. Pulmonary examination is notable for faint crackles at bilateral bases. There is trace bipedal edema. Serum BNP is elevated at 1530 pg/ml (normal <100 pg/ml).

Transthoracic echocardiogram (parasternal long axis) movie images are shown in Video 11-1.

26. Baseline diastology assessment is shown in Figure 11-11. Based on the images, what can you conclude about LV compliance?

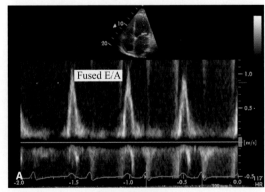

Mitral Inflow
Fig. 11-11A

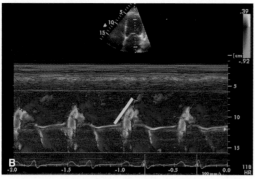

Vp = 20 cm/s

Color M-mode

Fig. 11-11B

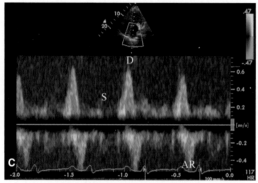

S = 20 cm/s, D = 60 cm/s, AR = 50 cm/s

Pulmonary Venous Flow

Fig. 11-11C

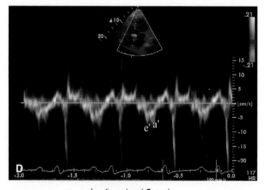

e' = 6 cm/s, a' 5 cm/s

TDI Medial Annulus

Fig. 11-11D

A. Increased.

B. Decreased.

C. Normal.

D. Cannot be assessed.

27. The gentleman is subsequently admitted to the hospital for evaluation of his newly documented dilated cardiomyopathy. Findings on a repeat echocardiogram 1 week later after intensive treat-

ment with IV diuretics, dobutamine, and nitroprusside are shown in Figure 11-12.

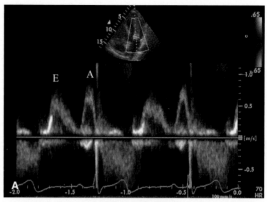

Mitral Inflow

Fig. 11-12A

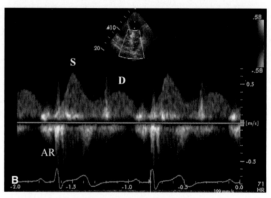

Pulmonary Venous Flow

Fig. 11-12B

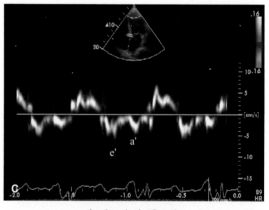

e' = 6 cm/s a' = 3 cm/s

TDI Medial Annulus

Fig. 11-12C

Which of the following statements is true?

A. Myocardial relaxation is now normal.

B. Myocardial compliance is now normal.

C. LV filling pressures are now normal.

D. Left atrial function has improved.

CASE 2:

A 48-year-old male commercial real estate developer presents to the hospital with increasing shortness of breath, abdominal swelling, and lower extremity edema developing over the past 6 months. For the last 2 years, he has been seen in clinic for evaluation of multiple episodes of syncope and atrial fibrillation has been documented on Holter monitoring.

ECG is notable for sinus tachycardia and low voltage. Physical examination is remarkable for blood pressure = 100/74 mm Hg, HR = 100 bpm, oral temperature = 37.9°C. Cardiovascular examination is notable for elevated neck veins at 8 cm, a normal S1 and S2 with a soft S4. In addition, he has a nondisplaced point of maximal impulse. Lungs are clear on auscultation. Abdomen does not demonstrate organomegaly. His extremities are cool, with mild pitting edema extending up to the mid tibia bilaterally.

Echocardiographic findings are shown in Figure 11-13 and in Video 11-2.

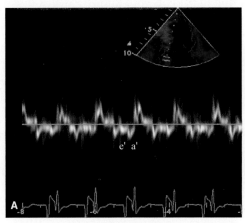

e' = 4 cm/s, a' = 4 cm/s

TDI Medial Annulus

Fig. 11-13A

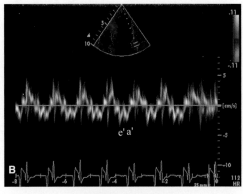

e' = 3.5 cm/s, a' = 3 cm/s

TDI Lateral Annulus

Fig. 11-13B

28. What finding in Video 11-2 could explain his symptoms?
    A. Pericardial effusion, suggesting imminent tamponade.
    B. Abnormal systolic function.
    C. Septal bounce, suggesting constrictive pericarditis.
    D. Restrictive cardiomyopathy.

29. Based on the Doppler information in Figure 11-14 and Table 11-4, which of the following statements is most consistent?

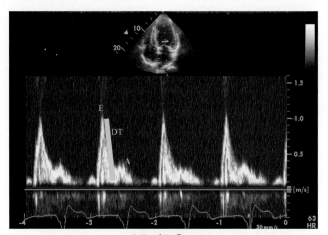

Mitral Inflow

Fig. 11-14

TABLE 11-4	
E-wave velocity	80 cm/sec
Deceleration time	106 msec
TDI medial annulus é velocity	4 cm/sec

A. The end-diastolic pressure–volume relationship in this patient is shifted downward and to the right.
B. These findings can be explained by a process of progressive myocardial stiffening.
C. Cardiac catheterization will likely reveal a difference of 10 mm Hg between PCWP and RVEDP.
D. It is imperative to maintain sinus rhythm in this patient to improve his symptoms.

CASE 3:

A 77-year-old woman with known coronary artery disease who is status post coronary artery bypass graft surgery in 2003 was scheduled for routine right rotator cuff surgery. However, due to marginal functional capacity, she undergoes a preoperative stress myocardial perfusion study that demonstrates a large area of septal ischemia. She is subsequently admitted for elective left heart catheterization and coronary angiography the following day. Overnight, she complains of somewhat atypical right-sided chest pain and is given sublingual nitroglycerin after which she rapidly becomes unresponsive.

Telemetry notes that she is now in junctional bradycardia (HR = 40 bpm) with markedly hypotension (BP = 75/43 mm Hg).

Subsequent coronary angiogram reveals patent bypass grafts with diffuse distal LAD disease after a left internal mammary artery (LIMA) anastomotic site, but deemed not suitable for revascularization.

Her transthoracic echocardiogram done 2 days prior to hospital admission is shown in Figure 11-15.

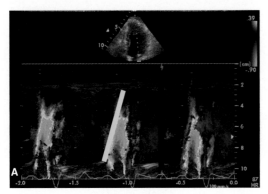

Color M-mode
Fig. 11-15A

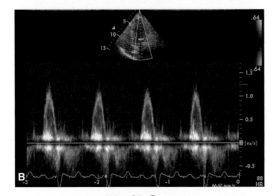

Mitral Inflow
Fig. 11-15B

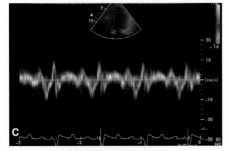

TDI Medial Annulus
Fig. 11-15C

30. What stage of diastolic dysfunction does this patient have?
   A. Stage 2 (pseudonormal).
   B. Stage 4 (irreversible–restrictive).
   C. Extreme stage 1 (impaired relaxation).
   D. Stage 3 (reversible–restrictive).

31. In patients with this stage of diastolic dysfunction, why are nitrates a therapy likely to cause hemodynamic abnormalities?
   A. These patients are extremely preload dependent, so venodilation associated with nitrate use can result in a leftward shift along the Frank–Starling curve resulting in decreased cardiac output.
   B. Reduction in afterload results in elevated LVEDP.
   C. Coronary vasodilation following nitrate administration leads to diffuse myocardial ischemia and subsequent decreased stroke volume.
   D. Nitrates, because they are endothelium-dependent mediated smooth muscle dilators, typically lead to more profound arterial hypotension in patients with known vascular disease.

CASE 4:

A 67-year-old male recently diagnosed with multiple myeloma has been complaining of worsening dyspnea with activity for approximately the last 6 weeks. In addition, he has been reporting intermittent episodes of chest discomfort that are not always associated with activity. His past medical history is otherwise only remarkable for hyperlipidemia and prior tobacco abuse, which he quit more than 10 years ago.

Physical examination is notable for a 2/6 systolic ejection murmur at the left lower sternal border. No S3 or S4 is audible. Neck veins are mildly elevated at 10 cm. There is mild lower extremity pitting edema that extends to the mid-tibias.

ECG is remarkable for relatively low voltage. In addition, there are Q waves present in the anteroseptal precordial leads.

An abdominal fat pad biopsy confirms the diagnosis of amyloidosis (type AL) with apple-green birefringence under a polarized light microscope after staining with Congo red.

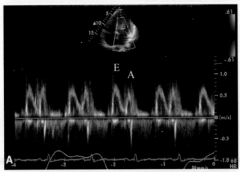

E wave velocity = 0.8 m/s, A wave velocity = 0.7 m/s

Mitral Inflow (supine)

Fig. 11-16A

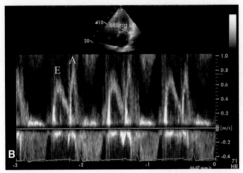

E wave velocity = 0.6 m/s, A wave velocity = 0.8 m/s

Mitral Inflow (sitting up)

Fig. 11-16B

32. Which of the findings listed below is considered a classical finding on transthoracic echocardiography in patients with amyloidosis?

A. Normal LV wall thickness.

B. Increased myocardial strain.

C. Short deceleration time associated with worsening prognosis.

D. Increased systolic and early diastolic velocities of the mitral annulus on tissue Doppler imaging.

E. Interventricular septal "bounce."

33. In patients with more advanced stages of amyloidosis, a combined relaxation abnormality and a mild increase in left atrial filling pressure will result in which of the following?

A. Grade 1 diastolic dysfunction (impaired relaxation).

B. Grade 2 diastolic dysfunction (pseudonormalized).

C. Decreasing pulmonary venous AR wave velocity.

D. Decreasing LVEDP.

CASE 5:

A 33-year-old Caucasian female, who is an avid runner, developed subacute onset of shortness of breath over a 2–3-month time period. She initially was evaluated at her local hospital and was demonstrated on transthoracic echocardiography to have a large circumferential pericardial effusion. When this failed to resolve with gentle diuresis, she subsequently underwent placement of a pericardial window. She was subsequently transferred to a tertiary care facility where her work-up for etiology of her pericardial effusion was unremarkable.

Her physical examination was only remarkable for a pericardial rub on auscultation without evidence of Kussmaul's sign.

Her initial cardiac magnetic resonance scan demonstrated diffuse enhancement of the pericardium on delayed imaging following gadolinium administration.

She was subsequently discharged home on scheduled nonsteroidal anti-inflammatory drugs (NSAIDs) and colchicine.

Her follow-up echocardiogram is shown in Figure 11-17.

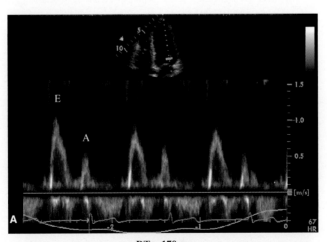

DT = 170 ms

Mitral Inflow

Fig. 11-17A

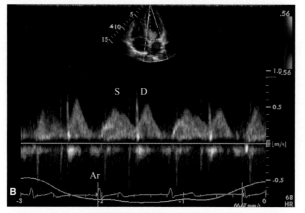

Pulmonary Venous Flow

Fig. 11-17B

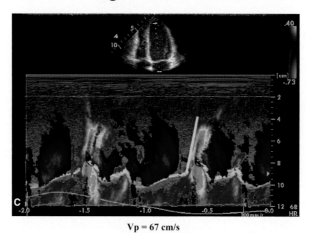

Vp = 67 cm/s

Color M-mode

Fig. 11-17C

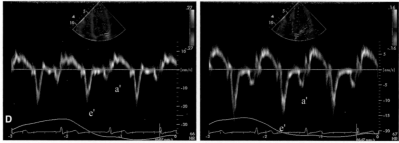

Lateral: e' = 19cm/s, a' = 7cm/s   Septal: e' = 15cm/s, a' = 6cm/s

TDI Lateral Annulus

Fig. 11-17D

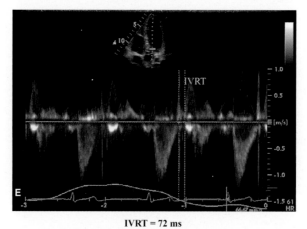

IVRT = 72 ms

Isovolumic relaxation time (IVRT)

Fig. 11-17E

34. Based on this woman's echocardiogram findings and following several months of therapy with NSAIDs, what can we say about her diastology?
   A. She appears to have normal diastolic function.
   B. She has stage 1a diastolic dysfunction.
   C. She has findings consistent with evolving constrictive pericarditis.
   D. We would expect to see a marked decrease in diastolic forward flow upon interrogation of the hepatic vein with increased diastolic reversals.
   E. She has markedly reduced LV compliance.

35. IVRT is the interval from aortic valve closure to mitral valve opening. It typically parallels the deceleration time. In our patient following therapy, the IVRT = 72 ms. What happens to IVRT with rapid relaxation or increased filling pressures or both?
   A. It shortens.
   B. It remains unchanged.
   C. It lengthens.

ANSWERS

1. ANSWER: E. Differentiating restrictive from constrictive pericarditis by echocardiography can be challenging. Mitral inflow, pulmonary venous flow, or tricuspid inflow does not always exhibit the typical respiratory changes displayed in textbook cases. The inferior vena cava is typically dilated in patients with constriction, but this can also be true in patients with advanced restrictive cardiomyopathy.

Atrial size will usually be increased in patients with restrictive cardiomyopathy but constrictive pericarditis will also eventually result in (particularly right-sided) dilatation. Apart from 2D features that give clues to the differentiation of diseases, tissue Doppler imaging (TDI) can provide important specific information. In patients with restrictive cardiomyopathy, myocardial relaxation (e') will be severely impaired; whereas patients with constriction usually have preserved annular vertical excursion. Radial left ventricular (LV) expansion is decreased in both groups: in restrictive cardiomyopathy because of the infiltrative disease process and in constrictive pericarditis because of the pericardial constraint. A septal e' velocity ≥7 cm/s has been shown to be highly accurate in differentiating patients with constrictive pericarditis from those with restrictive cardiomyopathy. Of note, the lateral annular e' velocity could be decreased if the constrictive

Restrictive cardiomyopathy

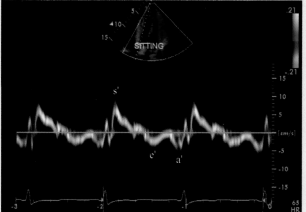

Fig. 11-18B

process involves the lateral mitral annulus. Figure 11-18 illustrates typical tissue Doppler tracings from a patient with constrictive pericarditis as opposed to a patient with restrictive cardiomyopathy.

2. ANSWER: E. Regional ischemic injury will decrease the longitudinal systolic and diastolic excursion of the affected wall. Therefore, a lower value of e' in the lateral wall of this patient is not an entirely unexpected finding (lateral e' should normally be ≥10 cm/sec). It is now recommended (and this is of particular importance in patients with regional wall motion abnormalities) to acquire and measure tissue Doppler signals at least at the septal and lateral sides of the mitral annulus and calculate their average to measure E/e'. The other possible answers each have been shown to carry important prognostic information in patients with a history (recent or not) of myocardial infarction.

3. ANSWER: D. There are two systolic velocities (S1 and S2), mostly noticeable when there is a prolonged PR interval since S1 is related to atrial relaxation. S2 should be used to compute the ratio of peak systolic to peak diastolic velocity. S1 velocity is primarily influenced by changes in left atrial pressure and left atrial relaxation or contraction, whereas S2 is related to stroke volume and pulse wave propagation in the pulmonary arterial tree. The diastolic velocity D is influenced by changes in

Constrictive Pericarditis

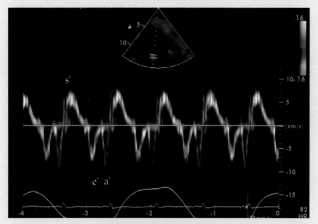

TDI Medial Annulus
Fig. 11-18A

LV filling and compliance and changes in parallel with mitral E velocity. Pulmonary venous atrial flow reversal (AR) velocity and duration are influenced by LV late diastolic pressures, atrial preload, and left atrial contractility. Atrial fibrillation or atrial stunning will result in a blunted S wave, mainly due to a loss of S1 with a decreased systolic fraction and absence of AR velocity (Fig. 11-19).

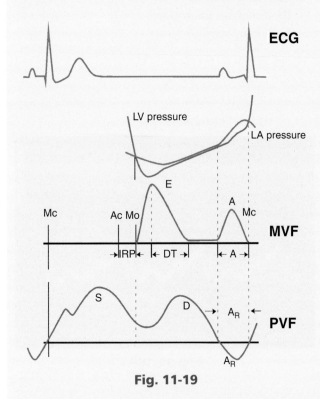

Fig. 11-19

4. ANSWER: A. AR may increase with age, but AR >35 cm/s is usually consistent with elevated LV filling pressures particularly at end diastole. The pulmonary D wave is related to LV relaxation. Young and healthy individuals can therefore exhibit large D waves indicating forceful elastic recoil of the LV rather than high left atrial pressure. The pulmonary S wave is related to LV contractility, atrial function, atrial pressure, and mitral regurgitation. Mitral and pulmonary vein inflow patterns are not very reliable for assessment of LV filling pressures in patients with an overall normal systolic function. ARdur–Adur >30 ms is, therefore, a more robust marker of elevated LV end-diastolic pressure (LVEDP) in this group of patients. Pulmonary venous atrial reversal can be obtained in more than 70% of patients. A commercially available contrast injection can help enhance the Doppler tracing.

5. ANSWER: A. Although sometimes challenging, an estimate of LV filling pressures can be obtained in patients with atrial fibrillation using the E/e' ratio. Different studies have shown good correlations in this population between filling pressures and the E/e' ratio (a ratio ≥11 predicting LVEDP ≥15 mm Hg), the mitral deceleration time (<150 ms in the presence of LV

systolic dysfunction) or the deceleration time (not the peak velocity) of the pulmonary venous diastolic velocity (≤220 ms associated with higher filling pressures).

6. ANSWER: D. This patient has evidence of stage 1 diastolic function with normal to low LV filling pressures at rest with a BNP of 100 pg/ml; however, it can be useful to evaluate LV filling pressure not only at rest but with exercise as well. The E/e' ratio will remain unchanged in subjects with normal myocardial relaxation because both E and e' velocities increase proportionally. However, in patients with impaired myocardial relaxation, the increase in e' with exercise is much less than that of mitral E velocity such that the E/e' ratio increases. Besides filling pressures, stress echocardiography also allows evaluation of systolic function in patients with coronary artery disease, of MR severity in patients with mitral valve disease, and of pulmonary artery pressures.

7. ANSWER: E. The stress test has provided evidence that the underlying relaxation abnormality can account for the patient's symptoms of dyspnea with exertion. With exercise, there is an increase in LV filling pressures (E/E' = 16). Many patients with diastolic dysfunction have exercise intolerance due to the rise in filling pressures needed to maintain adequate LV filling and stroke volume. Although the clinical implications of this finding have not yet been fully elucidated, one could consider starting therapy with a β-blocker, thereby preventing exercise-induced tachycardia and maximizing the diastolic filling period in these patients.

8. ANSWER: D. The presence of v-waves in absence of significant MR in this type of patient suggests severely decreased left atrial compliance. Classically, the left atrium has been ascribed to three different functions throughout the cardiac cycle: (1) reservoir function during ventricular systole and isovolumic relaxation (reflected by the pulmonary venous S wave); (2) conduit phase from the moment the mitral valve opens until onset of atrial contraction (reflected by the pulmonary venous D wave); and (3) contractile phase during atrial systole (reflected by the pulmonary venous AR wave and the mitral A wave).

9. ANSWER: A. The sample volume should be positioned at or 1 cm within the septal and lateral insertion sites of the mitral leaflets, and adjusted as necessary (usually 5–10 mm) to cover the longitudinal excursion of the mitral annulus in both systole and diastole. Attention should be directed to Doppler spectral gain settings because annular velocities have high signal amplitude. Most current ultrasound systems have tissue Doppler presets for the proper velocity scale and Doppler wall filter settings to display the annular velocities. In general, the velocity scale should be set at ~20 cm/s above and below the zero-velocity baseline, though lower settings may be needed when there is severe LV dysfunction, and annular velocities are markedly reduced (scale set to: 10–15 cm/s). Minimal angulation (<20°) should be present between the ultrasound beam and the plane of cardiac motion.

10. ANSWER: E. Elastic recoil does not directly affect active relaxation as suggested by answer D, but in combination with active relaxation, it is the driving force of early (and not late) diastolic filling. It acts by rapidly lowering the intraventricular pressure (thus creating a negative pressure gradient which results in diastolic "suction" of blood out of the left atrium). A decrease in recoil forces will increase the time needed to lower the ventricular pressure below the level of the left atrial pressure, resulting in an increase (not a decrease) of the isovolumic relaxation time (IVRT). Elastic recoil permits ventricular filling at low left atrial pressures. If elastic recoil is disturbed, ventricular filling can only be achieved by increasing the left atrial pressure.

11. ANSWER: B. First-degree AV block may lead to fusion of the E and A wave and therefore has a similar effect on mitral inflow as sinus tachycardia. A fused mitral inflow pattern can make an accurate interpretation of diastolic function impossible if no other information is available. In the presence of severely elevated LV filling pressures, first-degree AV block may lead to diastolic MR, as atrial contraction is not immediately followed by ventricular contraction, which is mandatory for complete mitral valve closure. Under these conditions, the atrioventricular pressure gradient may temporarily reverse during atrial relaxation, leading to diastolic MR. Fusion of E and A wave (leading to a decreased LV diastolic filling period) and diastolic MR may in turn have an adverse effect on cardiac output and filing pressures in patients with severe systolic dysfunction. Cardiac resynchronization therapy with restoration of optimal atrioventricular mechanical timing may improve LV filling in these patients. See Figure 11-20A and B for an illustration of the impact of PR prolongation on the mitral inflow pattern.

12. ANSWER: D. CMM echocardiography provides a spatiotemporal map of blood distribution (v(s,t)) within

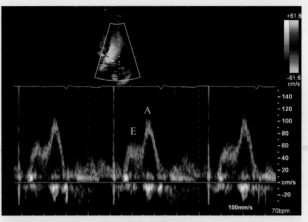

E-A fusion
Mitral Inflow
Fig. 11-20B

the heart with a typical temporal resolution of 5 ms, a spatial resolution of 300 microns and a velocity resolution of 3 cm/s. Assessment of diastolic flow propagation has offered novel information about LV filling dynamics. Vp is unique in that it appears to be relatively independent of loading conditions and therefore may overcome one of the main limitations of Doppler-based techniques. The earliest CMM velocities often occur during isovolumic relaxation. After the mitral valve opens, there is a rapid initial component (phase 1), often followed by a slower component (phase 2). Finally, the last component in late diastole is associated with atrial contraction. Please see Figure 11-21A and B for examples of CMM and determination of the Vp slope (white line).

First-Degree AV Block

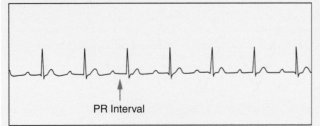

PR Interval

Fig. 11-20A

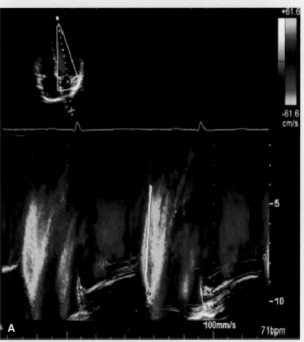

Color M-mode
Fig. 11-21A

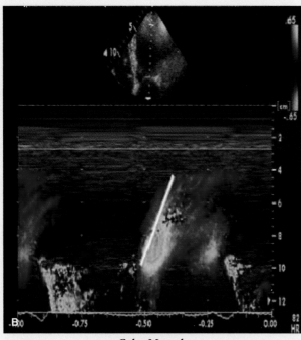

Color M-mode
Fig. 11-21B

13. ANSWER: B. E-wave deceleration time is mostly influenced by the operating stiffness of the LV. Changes in LV compliance (i.e., the relationship between LV pressure and volume) and also changes in ventricular relaxation or early (instead of late) diastolic ventricular pressures will affect the deceleration time. Left atrial mechanical function and ejection fraction are not or weakly and indirectly correlated with deceleration time (Fig. 11-22).

14. ANSWER: D. In patients with dilated cardiomyopathies, pulsed wave Doppler mitral flow velocity variables and filling patterns correlate better with cardiac filling pressures, functional class, and prognosis than with LV ejection fraction. Patients with impaired LV relaxation are the least symptomatic, while a short IVRT, short mitral deceleration time and increased E to A wave velocity ratio characterize advanced diastolic dysfunction, increased left atrial pressure and a worse functional class. A restrictive filling pattern is associated with a poor prognosis, especially if it persists after preload

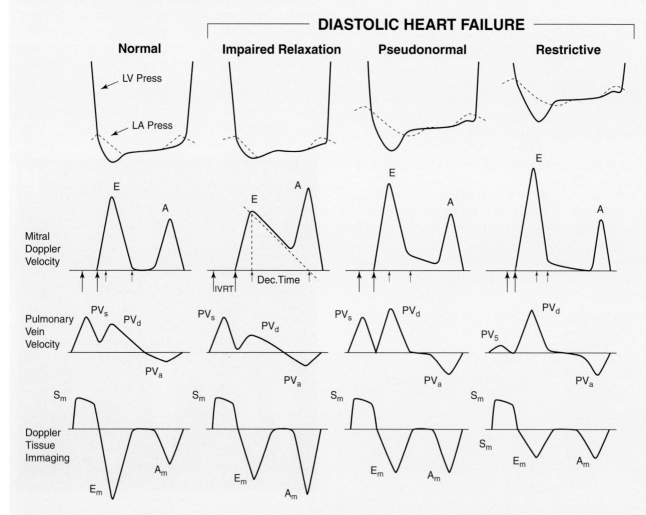

(From Zile MR, Brutsaert DL. New concepts in diastolic dysfunction and diastolic heart failure: part I. *Circulation.* 2002;105:1387–1393, with permission.)

Fig. 11-22

reduction. Likewise, a pseudonormal or restrictive filling pattern associated with acute myocardial infarction indicates an increased risk of heart failure, unfavorable LV remodeling, and increased CV mortality, irrespective of ejection fraction (Fig. 11-23).

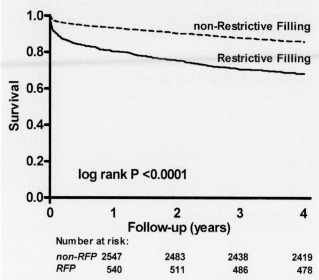

Event-Free Survival in Patients with Restrictive and Nonrestrictive Filling Patterns. (From Meta-Analysis Research Group in Echocardiography (MeRGE) AMI Collaborators. Independent prognostic importance of a restrictive left ventricular filling pattern after myocardial infarction: an individual patient meta-analysis: Meta-Analysis Research Group in Echocardiography Acute Myocardial Infarction. *Circulation*. 2008;117:2591–2598, with permission.)

Fig. 11-23

15. ANSWER: D. In cardiac patients, a decrease ≥50% in E/A ratio with application of the Valsalva maneuver is highly specific for increased LV filling pressure. However, a smaller magnitude of change does not always indicate normal diastolic function. One major limitation of the Valsalva maneuver is that not everyone is able to perform this maneuver adequately and it is not standardized. The Valsalva maneuver is performed by forceful expiration (about 40 mm Hg) against a closed nose and mouth. A decrease of 20 cm/s in mitral peak E velocity is usually considered an adequate effort in patients without restrictive filling. Lack of reversibility with Valsalva is imperfect as an indicator that the diastolic filling pattern is irreversible. In a busy clinical laboratory, the Valsalva maneuver can be reserved for patients in whom diastolic function assessment is not clear after mitral inflow and annulus velocity measurements. The Valsalva is obviously of little use in patients with stage 1 diastolic dysfunction but is useful to differentiate stage 2 diastolic function from normal (Fig. 11-24).

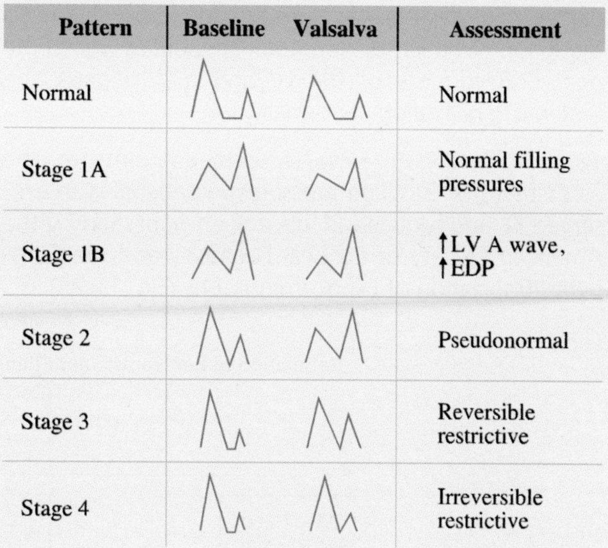

Pattern	Baseline	Valsalva	Assessment
Normal			Normal
Stage 1A			Normal filling pressures
Stage 1B			↑LV A wave, ↑EDP
Stage 2			Pseudonormal
Stage 3			Reversible restrictive
Stage 4			Irreversible restrictive

Fig. 11-24

16. ANSWER: A. According to the stage of the disease progress, a spectrum of filling abnormalities can be seen in cardiac amyloidosis that varies from delayed relaxation (Figure 11-1A) to pseudonormal (Figure 11-1B) to restrictive filling (Figure 11-1C). Panels B and C in Figure 11-1 represent these more advanced stages in the disease process where the operating stiffness of the LV becomes increasingly high due to a gradual loss in LV compliance. This is reflected in a short deceleration time (Figure 11-1C). In spite of the high left atrial pressure (suggested by a high E-wave velocity), atrial contraction itself hardly contributes to LV filling in the most advanced stages of diastolic dysfunction, as suggested by the diminutive A wave in restrictive filling. In contrast, although patients with delayed relaxation may be asymptomatic at rest or with mild exercise, their LV has become more dependent on atrial contraction (low E/A ratio). As such, these patients are most likely to feel a change in symptoms with sudden onset of atrial fibrillation due to loss of the atrial kick.

17. ANSWER: D. The Doppler tracing in Figure 11-2 shows transmitral flow during diastasis, often referred to as a mitral "L-wave." The result is a triphasic mitral inflow pattern that can be seen in patients with structural heart disease–particularly if the HR is relatively slow. It represents an advanced stage of diastolic dysfunction that is characterized by elevated filling pressures and loss of compliance (notice the high peak of early rapid filling and the short initial deceleration time) in combination with very delayed relaxation. The markedly prolonged relaxation, although not immediately obvious, results in a sudden decrease in LV diastolic pressure during mid-diastole, allowing further LV filling during mid-diastole. This explains the L-wave. Preload reduction will decrease left atrial pressure as well as the operating stiffness of the LV and may unmask the underlying relaxation abnormality.

18. ANSWER: C. New recommendations for the assessment of LV filling pressures in patients with preserved EF and reduced EF have been published by the American Society of Echocardiography and the European Association of Echocardiography (Fig. 11-25).

Elevated LV filling pressures in a patient with a normal EF can be confirmed with a decreased early diastolic velocity of the mitral annulus derived by tissue Doppler echocardiography (e′) <8 cm/s, reduced color M-mode slope of <40 cm/s, difference in duration of pulmonary venous AR and mitral inflow A wave duration of >30 msec, a change in mitral inflow E/A ratio of 0.5 with the Valsalva maneuver, or an increased left atrial volume index >34 ml/m^2.

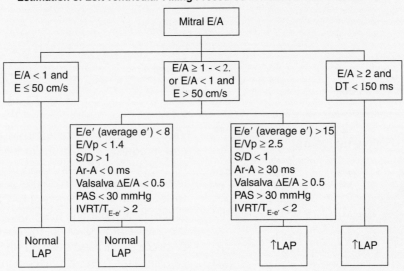

Estimation of Left Ventricular Filling Pressures in Patients with Reduced EF

Fig. 11-25A

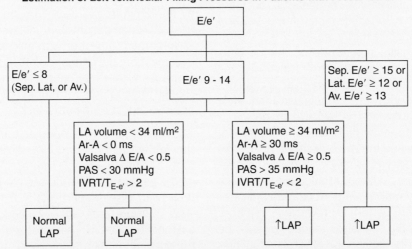

Estimation of Left Ventricular Filling Pressures in Patients with Preserved EF

(E) = Peak mitral flow velocity of the early filling wave. (A) = peak mitral flow velocity of the late filling wave due to atrial contraction. (Vp) = mitral inflow propagation velocity, IVRT = Isovolumic Relaxation Time, LAP = Left atrial pressure, PASS = Pulmonary artery systolic pressure. e′ = tissue Doppler early diastolic mitral annular velocity, (S) = pulmonary vein systolic flow velocity, (D) = pulmonary vein diastolic flow velocity, (Ar - A) = Time difference between pulmonary venous atrial reversal duration and peak mitral flow velocity of late filling duration, (DT) = deceleration time, LA = left atrium, (Av E/e′) = average E/e′ ratio.

Reprinted from Nagueh SF, Appleton CP, Gillebert TC, et al. Recommendations for the evaluation of left ventricular diastolic function by echocardiography. *JASE.* 2009;22:108–128, with permission from Elsevier.

Fig. 11-25B

As left atrial pressure increases, pulmonary vein flow velocity will show blunted systolic flow, and the presence or absence of this finding will therefore also point in the direction of elevated filling pressures. In addition, a prominent pulmonary venous flow AR (>35 cm/s) will also indicate high LVEDP.

Left atrial volume reflects the cumulative effect of filling pressures over time. A dilated left atrium (>34 ml/m²), without a clear history of atrial fibrillation or valvular dysfunction, is suggestive of chronically elevated filling pressures.

19. ANSWER: D. Although we have no information on the exact severity of his LV dysfunction nor his present hemodynamic state, Doppler findings show stage 3 or 4 diastolic dysfunction. Although these patients have a better long-term outcome if treated with beta blocking agents, the echocardiographic findings also indicate that the current operating stiffness of the heart is probably very high. The cardiac output in these patients can therefore be very dependent on HR, as it is almost impossible to increase cardiac output by an augmentation of their stroke volume which will increase their filling pressures even much more. Remember cardiac output = HR multiplied by stroke volume. Careful titration of the β-blocker therapy dose in these patients is therefore warranted.

20. ANSWER: A. Normal LV apical function is highly important in preserving the normal systolic twisting (torsion) and diastolic untwisting motion of the heart. A loss of apical untwisting (in this case due to ischemic injury) will likely have an adverse impact on the elastic recoil forces that generate LV suction, allowing LV filling during early diastole at low left atrial pressure. In normal conditions, a negative gradient from base to apex (with the lowest pressure in the apex) can be observed at early diastole, leading to an acceleration of blood toward the LV apex. In this patient, however, LV apical scar can disturb this mechanism, leading to a decrease and not an increase in the early diastolic pressure gradient (diastolic suction).

21. ANSWER: D. Note that color M-mode Vp and tissue Doppler E′ are essentially unchanged. A higher 6-month E/e′ ratio and E/Vp ratio both indicate increased LV filling pressures. A lower A-wave velocity indicates reduced left atrial contractility. The shorter deceleration time indicates increased LV operating stiffness. The association between tissue Doppler e′ and LV relaxation has been observed in both animal and human studies.

22. ANSWER: C. The Doppler findings demonstrate a large (>30 ms) difference between the duration of the mitral A-wave velocity and the duration of the late diastolic pulmonary venous flow reversal (AR), suggesting elevated end-diastolic LV filling pressures. This is usually seen in patients with stage 2 or stage 3 diastolic function. Of the four conditions stated earlier, the most likely is the 60-year-old man with advanced hypertensive heart disease. The other conditions including constrictive pericarditis would not cause stage 2 diastolic function.

23. ANSWER: A. The mitral inflow pattern can be used with relative accuracy to assess filling pressures in patients with depressed LV systolic function. In this population, changes in the inflow pattern will reflect changes in preload (e.g., due to volume overload or changes in medical therapy). Confusion between normal and pseudonormal filling should be absent as diastolic function is intrinsically disturbed in the presence of advanced systolic dysfunction.

In contrast, additional information is needed in the presence of preserved ejection fraction as this Doppler pattern could equally represent normal or pseudonormal filling. As mentioned earlier, the echocardiographer should assess tissue Doppler derived e′, Vp obtained by color M-mode Doppler, measure left atrial size, and finally evaluate the effect of Valsalva to detect an underlying relaxation abnormality in the case of pseudonormal filling. Left atrial dilatation can merely represent atrial remodeling independent of filling pressures in the setting of atrial fibrillation. Moderate and severe MR usually leads to an elevation of peak E velocity, representing the increased flow rate during diastole with a normal deceleration time. However, particularly with chronic MR, the left atrial will dilate and the increased left atrial compliance may be sufficient to maintain filling pressures at a normal level.

Finally, a high velocity tricuspid regurgitant jet may be suggestive of (but is not specific for) elevated left-sided filling pressures. Many other conditions may lead to pulmonary hypertension in the presence of normal diastolic function. (Refer to the answer to question 18; Nagueh et al.)

24. ANSWER: C. In normal patients, hepatic vein Doppler velocities reflect changes in pressure, volume, and compliance of the right atrium. Typically, hepatic vein Doppler velocities consist of four elements: (1) systolic forward flow (S), (2) diastolic forward flow (D), (3) systolic flow reversal (VR), and (4) atrial flow reversal (AR). In patients with normal hemodynamics, S is typically larger than D and there are no significant systolic or diastolic reversals. Typically, with myopathic conditions, flow reversals are accentuated with inspiration due to increased systemic venous return to the right heart. Diastolic flow reversal is seen most commonly in patients with pulmonary hypertension and constrictive pericarditis, and it is respiratory variation that helps to differentiate them from each other. In patients with constrictive pericarditis, there are increased right ventricular and right atrial pressures; and characteristically, these patients demonstrate augmentation of diastolic flow reversals with expiration. Patients with pulmonary hypertension typically do not have augmentation of diastolic flow reversals with respiration. In addition, constrictive pericarditis can be differentiated from restrictive cardiomyopathy with hepatic venous Doppler recordings. In patients with restrictive cardiomyopathy, inspiratory diastolic flow reversal is larger than expiratory. Alternatively, patients with severe tricuspid regurgitation, which by definition is occurring during systole, will typically demonstrate prominent systolic flow reversals (Fig. 11-26).

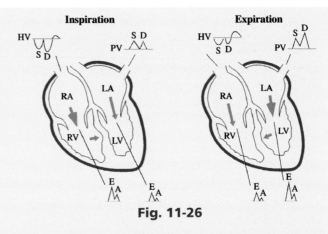

Fig. 11-26

25. ANSWER: E. Cutoff values for differentiating normal from abnormal cases should consider the age group from which the study sample is selected. In this case, E/A ratio is almost 2, which falls outside the range of normal values for patients older than 60 years.

26. ANSWER: B. In this case, there is clearly a reduced ejection fraction suggesting a nonischemic cardiomyopathy. There is a fused E and A wave, but the timing suggests an increased E wave with a shortened deceleration

TABLE 11-5   Stages of Diastolic Dysfunction

	Normal Young	Normal Adult	Stage 1, Delayed, Impaired, or Abnormal Relaxation	Stage II, Pseudonormal, Filling	Stage III, Restrictive, Filling	Stage IV, Irreversible Restrictive
E/A ratio	1–2	1–2	<1.0	1–1.5 (reverses with Valsalva maneuver)	>1.5	1.5–2.0 (Doppler values similar to stage III except no change with preload reduction maneuvers)
DT (msec)	<240	150–240	≥240	150–200	>150	<150
IVRT (msec)	70–90	70–90	>90	<90	<70	<70
PV S/D ratio	<1	≥1	≥1	<1	<1	<1
MVa/PVa duration	≥1	≥1	≥1 or <1	<1	<l	<1
PVs2/PVd ratio	≥1 or <1	≥1	≫1	<1	≪1	≪1
AR (cm/sec)	<35	<35	<35	≥35	≥35	≥35
CMM (cm/sec)	>55	>55	>45	<45	<45	<45
TDI (cm/sec)	>l0	>8	<8	<8	<8	<8
Anatomic abnormalities	None	None	Normal or mildly enlarged LA	Mild-to-moderate, LA enlargement. LVH, normal or abnormal EF	Severe LA enlargement, LV systolic dysfunction, MV or TV regurgitation	Severe LA enlargement, LV systolic dysfunction, MV or TV regurgitation with possible MV systolic regurgitation

AR, atrial reversal; CMM, color Doppler M-mode; DT, deceleration time; EF, ejection fraction; IVRT, isovolumic relaxation time; LA, left atrial; LV, left ventricle.

(From Bursi F, Weston SA, Redfiefd MM. Systolic and diastolic heart failure in the community. *JAMA.* 2006;296:2209–2216; Yamada H, et al. Prevalence of left ventricular diabolic dysfunction by Doppler echocardiography: Clinical application of the Canadian consensus guidelines. Adapted from *J Am Soc Echocardiogr.* 2002;15:1238–1244; Garcia MJ, et al. New Doppler echocardiographic applications for the study of diastolic function. *J Am Coll Cardiol.* 1998; 32:865–875.)

time. The blunted pulmonary vein systolic-to-diastolic flow with a large AR confirms that this indeed is an E wave with restrictive physiology and decreased LV compliance and elevated LV filling pressures. The decreased annular velocity and delayed Vp confirms impaired relaxation. The elevated E/e' of 17, and E/Vp of 5 also confirm elevated LV filling pressure. See Figure 11-27.

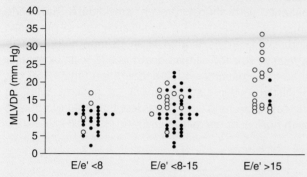

Mean left ventricular diastolic pressure (M-LVDP) versus groups defined by values of septal E/E'. ○ indicates patients with EF <50%; ● patients with EF >50%. (From Ommen SR, et al. Clinical utility of Doppler echocardiography and tissue Doppler imaging in the estimation of left ventricular filling pressures. *Circulation*. 2000;102:1788–1794, with permission.)

Fig. 11-27

27. ANSWER: C. E/e' is now <10, suggesting that LV filling pressures have been lowered.

This was subsequently confirmed by right heart catheterization (See Table 11-6):

TABLE 11-6

PASP	17 mm Hg
PADP	8 mm Hg
PCWP	8 mm Hg
CVP (mean)	0 mm Hg
CO (Fick)	4.7 L/min
CI (Fick)	2.1 L/min/m²

PASP, pulmonary artery systolic pressure; PADP, pulmonary artery diastolic pressure; PCWP, pulmonary capillary wedge pressure; CVP, central venous pressure; CO, cardiac output; CI, cardiac index.

The patient was subsequently discharged on a medical regimen of diuretics, ACE-inhibitors, spironolactone, and low-dose β-blockers. He continued to improve and at 6-month follow-up, echocardiogram showed mild improvement of systolic function with LVEF = 45%.

KEY POINTS:

■ In patients with decreased EF, mitral inflow and pulmonary vein flow can be used to assess LV filling pressures (see aforementioned ASE guideline recommendations).

■ If one wave is present in the mitral inflow, often the pulmonary vein flow will reveal which wave it is due the positive relationship of mitral E wave and pulmonary vein D wave (i.e., the larger the E wave, the larger the D wave).

■ Confirmatory variables will be elevated E/e' >15 and E/V$_P$ >2.

28. ANSWER: D. His symptoms can be explained by the constellation of preserved systolic function, normal ventricular size, and marked dilatation of both atria. These findings and a history of intermittent paroxysmal atrial fibrillation at an unusual young age suggest a form of restrictive cardiomyopathy.

29. ANSWER: B. Cardiac catheterization in this patient revealed normal coronary arteries but elevated filling pressures with a mean right atrial pressure of 20, pulmonary artery pressures of 57/25 mmHg, right ventricular pressures of 56/22 mmHg, PCWP 26 mm Hg, and a cardiac output of 4 L/min. An endomyocardial biopsy showed focal nonspecific interstitial fibrosis with no evidence of amyloidosis, hemochromatosis, or sarcoidosis. The patient eventually died 3 months later from progressive heart failure and ventricular arrhythmias

KEY POINTS:

■ An integrative Doppler assessment of diastolic function should be performed in every patient with unexplained shortness of breath. Advanced diastolic dysfunction and atrial dilatation in spite of normal LV size and function are the hallmarks of restrictive cardiomyopathy.

■ In idiopathic restrictive cardiomyopathy, the LV shows normal wall thickness with a preserved EF biatrial enlargement.

■ Restrictive physiology is noted by the shortened mitral E wave deceleration time and the E/A ratio is markedly increased (typically >2.0).

■ Restrictive cardiomyopathy is notable for restrictive (stage 3 or 4) diastolic filling with relatively normal systolic function.

■ Ventricular filling is notable for decreased compliance.

■ As left atrial pressure increases with disease progression, the mitral valve opens at a higher pressure, which results in a decrease in the IVRT. In addition, there is increased transmitral pressure gradient, increased E velocity on pulsed-wave Doppler, and decreased systolic pulmonary venous flow velocity.

30. ANSWER: C. This patient demonstrates a diastology picture consistent with extreme stage 1 diastolic dysfunction with a very large A wave. The mitral E velocity is severely decreased and the mitral A velocity is very prominently increased, producing an E/A ratio <1. The mitral flow propagation velocity is reduced (i.e., <50 cm/s). e' is also reduced (usually <7 cm/s at the septal annulus). However, it is unlikely that her filling pressures are increased because her E/e' ratio is ≤8. If her filling pressures were increased, we would more likely expect to see an E/e' ratio >15 and an E/A ratio <1 (stage 1a diastolic dysfunction).

31. ANSWER: A. In our patient with extreme stage 1 diastolic dysfunction, where the large majority of diastolic filling results from the atrial contraction, a reduction in preload via therapy with nitrates is likely to result in decreased venous return. This will decrease end-diastolic volume, thereby moving our patient to a leftward portion of the Frank–Starling curve (from point A to point B) and subsequently resulting in decreased stroke volume/cardiac output (Fig. 11-28). Reduction in afterload does not directly result in alteration in the LVEDP. Finally, nitrates are endothelium-INDEPENDENT vasodilators.

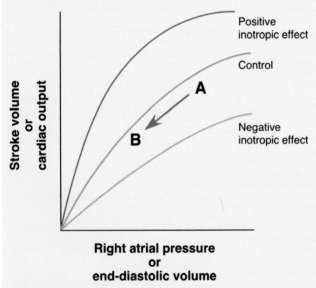

(Adapted from: http//totw.anaesthesiologists.org/2009/03/16/introduction-to-cardiovascular-physiology-125.)

Fig. 11-28

KEY POINTS:

- Decreased preload results in reduced end-diastolic volume; and in a patient with otherwise constant contractility, this will result in a reduced stroke volume/cardiac output.
- Nitrate use must be carefully considered in patients with known extreme stage 1 diastolic dysfunction.
- Stage 1 diastolic dysfunction is characterized by impaired myocardial relaxation.

- Typically, mitral E velocity is decreased with a deceleration time >200 ms, mitral A velocity is increased, E/A ratio is <1, and IVRT is increased.
- e' is usually <7 cm/s and mitral flow propagation velocity V_p on color M-mode is typically <50 cm/s.

32. ANSWER: C. Deceleration time ≤150 ms in patients with biopsy proven amyloidosis has been shown to correlate to a significantly worse prognosis and risk of cardiac death over an 18-month period with a relative risk for cardiac death nearly 5 times greater than those patients with a deceleration time >150 ms. Similarly, 1-year cardiac survival of patients with an increased E/A ratio (≥2.1) was less than that of patients with normal or decreased E/A ratio (<2.1) (Fig. 11-29).

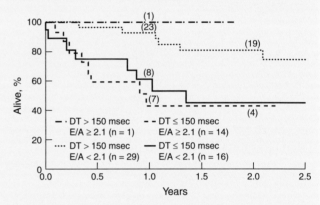

(From Klein AL, Hatle LK, Taliercio CP, et al. Prognostic significance of Doppler measures of diastolic function in cardiac amyloidosis: a Doppler echocardiography study. *Circulation.* 1991;83:808–816, with permission.)

Fig. 11-29

33. ANSWER: B. In most, if not all cardiac disease, as with cardiac amyloidosis, the initial diastolic dysfunction stage is impaired relaxation. With disease progression, continued impaired relaxation ultimately results in mild-to-moderate increases in left atrial pressure which can cause the mitral inflow velocity pattern to appear similar to normal filling ("pseudonormal") pattern. The E/A ratio is typically 1 to 1.5. The E-wave deceleration time is normal between 160 and 220 ms. The best way to identify a pseudonormal filling pattern is by demonstrating impaired myocardial relaxation by e' <7 cm/s and increased filling pressure by E/e' >15. In patients with known systolic dysfunction or abnormally increased wall thickness, a normal E/A ratio suggests that increased left atrial pressure is masking abnormal relaxation. By decreasing preload (i.e., via Valsalva maneuver), one may unmask the impaired LV relaxation by causing the E/A ratio to decrease by 0.5 or more and reversal of the E/A ratio. In addition, color M-mode of mitral inflow can determine rate of flow propagation in the LV; and with worsening diastolic function, myocardial relaxation is always impaired and flow propagation is slow even when left atrial pressure and mitral E velocity are increased.

KEY POINTS:

■ Deceleration time is an important prognostic factor in patients with cardiac amyloidosis.

■ Grade 2 diastolic dysfunction ("pseudonormal" pattern) represents a moderate stage of diastolic dysfunction, combining mildly-moderately elevated left atrial pressures and LV relaxation abnormality.

34. ANSWER: A. Normal diastole consists of four phases (see Figure 11-30) (1) Isovolumic relaxation (IVRT), (2) rapid early filling (corresponding to the E wave of the mitral and tricuspid inflow), (3) diastasis (which is largely affected by ventricular compliance), and (4) late filling from atrial contraction.

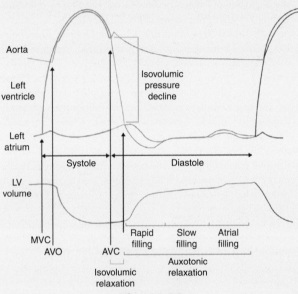

Fig. 11-30

Myocardial relaxation is an active energy-dependent process that requires removal of calcium from troponin C in the sarcoplasmic reticulum. Failure to re-uptake calcium can ultimately result in incomplete relaxation due to diastolic tension or stiffening. In addition, myocardial compliance is a passive property that influences all three filling phases of diastole and is capable of being affected by both intrinsic and extrinsic factors. The pulmonary veins, left atrium, and mitral valve are also all integral to diastole, as is HR.

The patient listed in the question has a normal E/A ratio >1. E-wave deceleration time (170 ms) is within the normal range (160–200 ms). Pulmonary venous flow velocities are normal (normal S wave = 0.6 m/s, normal D wave = 0.4 m/s). Color M-mode transmitral flow propagation velocity is within normal limits (normal flow propagation velocity is 50 cm/s or higher). Septal and lateral mitral annular velocities are also normal. IVRT is at the lower limits of normal (normal range 83 ±16 ms).

35. ANSWER: A. The IVRT is an important noninvasive index of LV diastolic function. IVRT is the interval from aortic valve closure to mitral valve opening and constitutes the first phase of diastole. As stated in the question, IVRT tends to parallel the mitral deceleration time. As such, IVRT shortens with rapid relaxation or increased filling pressures or both, whereas IVRT lengthens with abnormal relaxation. IVRT measurements are as follows: normal 70–90 ms, impaired relaxation >90 ms, pseudonormal <90 ms, restrictive <70 ms (Fig. 11-31).

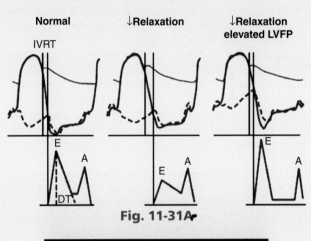

Fig. 11-31A

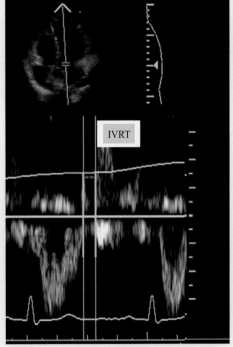

Fig. 11-31B

KEY POINTS:

▣ IVRT is the interval from aortic valve closure to mitral valve opening.

▣ IVRT shortens with rapid relaxation, increased filling pressures, or both.

▣ IVRT lengthens with abnormal relaxation.

▣ Diastole consists of four phases: (1) isovolumic relaxation (IVRT), (2) rapid early filling, (3) diastasis, and (4) late filling from atrial contraction.

▣ Various Doppler flow velocities provide assessment of diastolic function.

SUGGESTED READINGS

Abhayaratna WP, Seward JB, Appleton CP, et al. Left atrial size: physiologic determinants and clinical applications. *J Am Coll Cardiol.* 2006;47:2357–2363.

Appleton CP, Hatle LK, Popp RL. Relation of transmitral flow velocity patterns to left ventricular diastolic function: new insights from a combined hemodynamic and Doppler echocardiographic study. *J Am Coll Cardiol.* 1988;12:426–440.

Appleton CP, Jensen JL, Hatle LK, et al. Doppler evaluation of left and right ventricular diastolic function: a technical guide for obtaining optimal flow velocity recordings. *J Am Soc Echocardiogr.* 1997;10:271–292.

Greenberg NL, Vandervoort PM, Firstenberg MS, et al. Estimation of diastolic intraventricular pressure gradients by Doppler M-mode echocardiography. *Am J Physiol Heart Circ Physiol.* 2001;280:H2507–H2515.

Ha JW, Oh JK, Redfield MM, et al. Triphasic mitral inflow velocity with middiastolic filling: clinical implications and associated echocardiographic findings. *J Am Soc Echocardiogr.* 2004;17:428–431.

Hansen A, Haass M, Zugck C, et al. Prognostic value of Doppler echocardiographic mitral inflow patterns: implications for risk stratification in patients with chronic congestive heart failure. *J Am Coll Cardiol.* 2001;37:1049–1055.

Klein AL, Burstow DJ, Tajik AJ, et al. Effects of age on left ventricular dimensions and filling dynamics in 117 normal persons. *Mayo Clin Proc.* 1994;69:212–224.

Klein AL, Garcia MJ, editors. Diastology: clinical approach to diastolic heart failure. Philadelphia. Saunders Elsevier, 2008.

Nagueh SF, Appleton CP, Gillebert TC, et al. Recommendations for the evaluation of left ventricular diastolic function by echocardiography. *J Am Soc Echocardiogr.* 2009;22:107–133.

Nagueh SF, Lakkis NM, Middleton KJ, et al. Doppler estimation of left ventricular filling pressures in patients with hypertrophic cardiomyopathy. *Circulation.* 1999;99:254–261.

Nishimura RA, Appleton CP, Redfield MM, et al. Noninvasive Doppler echocardiographic evaluation of left ventricular filling pressures in patients with cardiomyopathies: a simultaneous Doppler echocardiographic and cardiac catheterization study. *J Am Coll Cardiol.* 1996;28:1226–1233.

Ommen SR, Nishimura RA, Appleton CP, et al. Clinical utility of Doppler echocardiography and tissue Doppler imaging in the estimation of left ventricular filling pressures: a comparative simultaneous Doppler-catheterization study. *Circulation.* 2000;102:1788–1794.

Rossvoll O, Hatle LK. Pulmonary venous flow velocities recorded by transthoracic Doppler ultrasound: relation to left ventricular diastolic pressures. *J Am Coll Cardiol.* 1993;21:1687–1696.

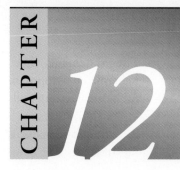

Stress Echocardiography

CHAPTER 12

Omar Wever-Pinzon and Farooq A. Chaudhry

1. The statement that best describes the ischemic cascade is:
   A. Wall motion abnormalities are preceded by electrocardiographic changes.
   B. Angina occurs prior to the development of wall motion abnormalities.
   C. Hemodynamic changes occur after electrocardiographic changes.
   D. Perfusion abnormalities precede the onset of wall motion abnormalities.
   E. Wall motion abnormalities precede diastolic dysfunction.

2. The statement that best describes the accuracy of stress echocardiography is:
   A. The sensitivity and specificity of exercise stress echocardiography to detect flow-limiting coronary artery stenosis is significantly lower compared to scintigraphic imaging.
   B. The specificity of stress echocardiography using vasodilators is lower than exercise and dobutamine stress echocardiography.
   C. During dobutamine stress echocardiography, the addition of atropine increases its specificity.
   D. The accuracy of stress echocardiography may be affected by the presence of significant aortic regurgitation.
   E. The accuracy of stress echocardiography to detect single-vessel disease is greater than its accuracy to detect multivessel disease.

3. Stress echocardiography and myocardial perfusion stress imaging are stress testing modalities based on different pathophysiologic concepts and techniques. The statement that best describes the relationship between both modalities is:
   A. The sensitivity of stress echocardiography to detect single-vessel coronary artery disease is lower compared to myocardial perfusion stress imaging.
   B. The specificity of stress echocardiography to detect flow-limiting stenosis is lower than myocardial perfusion stress imaging.
   C. Stress echocardiographic interpretation is less subjective than myocardial perfusion stress imaging.
   D. The cost of both modalities is comparable.

4. The following can decrease the specificity of stress echocardiography:
   A. Concomitant use of beta-blockers at the time of testing.
   B. Concentric left ventricular hypertrophy.
   C. Delay on image acquisition.
   D. Inadequate exercise with suboptimal peak heart rate.
   E. Hypertensive response.

5. The most appropriate indication to stop a dobutamine stress echocardiogram (echo) is:
   A. Chest pain.
   B. T-wave inversions.
   C. Bigeminy.
   D. New wall motion abnormality.
   E. Up-sloping ST-segment depressions.

6. The statement that best describes inducible ischemia on a dobutamine stress echo is:
   A. Normal resting wall motion that becomes hyperkinetic on stress.
   B. Akinetic segment that becomes dyskinetic on stress.
   C. Biphasic response.
   D. Hypokinetic segment that becomes hyperkinetic on stress.
   E. Monophasic response.

7. The sensitivity and specificity of stress echocardiography to detect ischemia is greatest in which coronary artery distribution?
   A. Left anterior descending artery.
   B. Left circumflex artery.
   C. Obtuse marginal branch.
   D. Right coronary artery.
   E. Septal perforators.

8. Which of the following statements about the prognostic value of stress echocardiography is correct?
   A. Left ventricular ejection fraction is not important if peak wall motion score index is increased.
   B. Development of wall motion abnormalities at lower heart rates does not have prognostic implications.
   C. Assessment of myocardial viability has no prognostic value.
   D. The event rate of a patient with intermediate pretest probability of coronary artery disease and a negative stress echo is < 1%/year.
   E. The event-free survival for diabetics and non-diabetics with a normal stress echo is similar.

9. The role of stress echocardiography in risk stratification of patients undergoing noncardiac surgery includes:
   A. Stress echo has a high positive predictive value.
   B. The territory of ischemia by stress echocardiography predicts the area of perioperative infarction.
   C. The negative predictive value of stress echocardiography is high.
   D. The perioperative event rate in patients undergoing exercise stress echocardiography is usually higher than those undergoing dobutamine stress echocardiography.
   E. The positive predictive value of stress echocardiography is better than stress myocardial perfusion imaging.

10. The use of contrast agents in stress echocardiography is best described by the following:
    A. Contrast increases intra- and interobserver variability of wall motion interpretation.
    B. The use of contrast in stress echocardiography is currently approved by the Food and Drug Administration.
    C. Dobutamine is the preferred method of stress for contrast myocardial perfusion imaging.
    D. The presence of a significant intracardiac shunt is an absolute contraindication for the use of echo contrast.
    E. Contrast should be used in all patients undergoing stress echocardiography.

11. Which of the following statements is correct about the basic concepts of myocardial viability assessment?
    A. Hibernating myocardium is a state of contraction-perfusion mismatch that can be seen after successful reperfusion therapy.
    B. A nontransmural infarction of 20% of myocardial thickness can impair wall thickening.
    C. Q waves in the ECG indicate absence of viable myocardium in the corresponding territory.
    D. In the presence of an open epicardial vessel, no reflow indicates consistent viable myocardium.
    E. Dobutamine stress echocardiography can differentiate viability in the endocardium versus epicardium.

12. The following statement about viability assessment by stress echocardiography is correct:
    A. The accuracy of exercise and dobutamine stress echocardiography is similar for the prediction of left ventricular function improvement, after revascularization in ischemic cardiomyopathy.
    B. The detection of inotropic contractile reserve relies on the intact metabolism within the myocytes to assess viability.
    C. In ischemic cardiomyopathy, biphasic response during dobutamine stress echocardiography is a better predictor of left ventricular function improvement than a monophasic response.
    D. The sensitivity of dobutamine stress echocardiography to detect viability is superior to that of Thallium redistribution studies.
    E. Dobutamine stress echocardiography can differentiate scar in the epicardium versus endocardium similar to magnetic resonance imaging.

13. The following portends a benign prognosis during stress echocardiography:
    A. Transient left ventricular cavity dilatation.
    B. Presence of wall motion abnormality at heart rates less than 100 bpm.
    C. Presence of wall motion abnormalities in both left and right ventricle.
    D. Drop in systolic blood pressure of 40 mm Hg during dobutamine stress echocardiography, without wall motion abnormalities.
    E. Peak wall motion score index >1.7.

14. Myocardial contrast echocardiography is a rapid and easy-to-perform technique for the assessment of myocardial perfusion. The statement that best describes the use of myocardial perfusion echocardiography on stress testing is:
    A. High-power imaging allows continuous imaging and wall motion analysis.
    B. The accuracy of nuclear scintigraphy and dobutamine stress echocardiography to detect flow-limiting coronary artery stenosis is superior to myocardial perfusion stress echocardiography.
    C. Attenuation artifacts do not affect myocardial perfusion stress echocardiography.
    D. The incidence of ventricular and supraventricular arrhythmias during dobutamine myocardial contrast stress echocardiography is lower than for dobutamine stress echocardiography.
    E. Myocardial perfusion during dobutamine stress imaging can detect subendocardial ischemia even when transmural wall thickening is normal.

15. Traditionally, the assessment of inducible ischemia by stress echocardiography has been based on the evaluation of systolic function post stress, either by subjective visual analysis or by quantitative techniques, such as tissue Doppler and strain. Recently, there is increasing interest in the assessment of diastolic echocardiographic parameters during stress echocardiography. The statement that best describes the application of diastology to stress echocardiography is:
    A. The passive nature of diastole makes its use in stress echocardiography a less sensitive technique than the assessment of systolic function.
    B. Relaxation abnormalities caused by inducible ischemia resolve earlier than systolic abnormalities.
    C. Unlike systolic function, the accuracy of diastolic function during stress echocardiography is not affected by the presence of cardiomyopathy or hypertensive heart disease.
    D. Regional diastolic abnormalities cannot be seen in the presence of a normal Early mitral valve inflow wave (E)/Early mitral annulus tissue Doppler wave (E′) ratio.
    E. Worsening left ventricular filling parameters during stress echocardiography correlate with lower exercise tolerance.

16. A 52-year-old female with a history of dyslipidemia and ex-smoker was referred for stress echo due to exertional dyspnea and a recent episode of syncope. She exercised for 6 minutes and had to stop due to shortness of breath. She reached 86% of her maximum predicted heart rate. What would be the cause of this patient's symptoms? See (Fig. 12-1 and Video 12-1A–C).

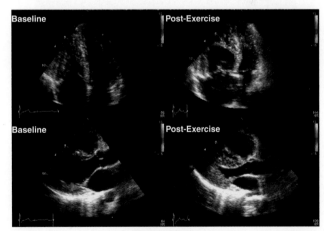

Fig. 12-1

    A. Severe proximal right coronary artery stenosis.
    B. Severe proximal left circumflex artery stenosis.
    C. Severe multivessel disease.
    D. Dynamic pulmonary hypertension.

17. A 50-year-old female with a history of dyslipidemia was referred for stress testing due to dyspnea on exertion. The resting echocardiogram showed left ventricular hypertrophy. She exercised for 4 minutes. Her heart rate and blood pressure changed from 69 bpm and 120/70 mm Hg to 111 bpm and 120/60 mm Hg, respectively, at peak exercise. A continuous-wave Doppler was done through the aortic valve post stress. Based on Figure 12-2, what would be the best next step in the management of this patient?

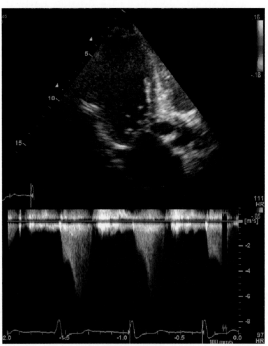

Fig. 12-2

A. Coronary angiography with revascularization.
B. Perform dobutamine stress echocardiography.
C. Perform pharmacologic nuclear stress imaging.
D. Medical therapy with beta blockers.
E. Valve replacement.

18. A 70-year-old male with a history of hypertension was admitted with chest pain and mild elevation of cardiac enzymes but no electrocardiographic changes. A dobutamine stress echo was performed. Based on Figure 12-3, which one is the most accurate statement? See also Video 12-2A–F.

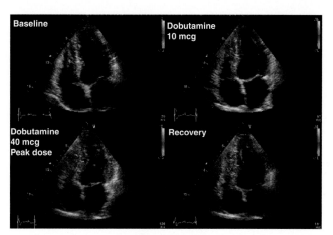

Fig. 12-3

A. Severe triple-vessel disease will be seen in coronary angiography.
B. Peak wall motion score index confers a bad prognosis.
C. Dobutamine stress echocardiography is consistent with ischemic response.
D. Dobutamine stress echocardiography shows a biphasic response.
E. Improvement in wall motion is likely.

19. A 58-year-old male with a history of hypertension and smoking presented with recurrent retrosternal chest pain for the last 3 weeks. Electrocardiogram and cardiac enzymes were normal. An exercise stress echo was performed. Which of the following statements best describes the findings on coronary angiography? (Video 12-3A–C and Fig. 12-4).
A. Left anterior descending artery stenosis of 70% without distal collateral circulation.
B. Left anterior descending artery stenosis of 70% with distal collateral circulation.
C. Right coronary artery stenosis of 70% without distal collateral circulation.
D. Left circumflex artery stenosis of 70% without distal collateral circulation.
E. Left circumflex artery stenosis of 70% with distal collateral circulation.

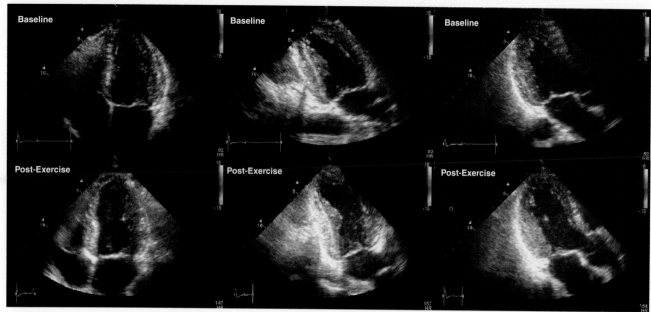

Fig. 12-4

20. A 71-year-old female with a history of diabetes and hypertension presented with dyspnea on exertion. A dobutamine stress echo was performed. Which of the following statements would best describe the findings on coronary angiography? (Video 12-4A–D and Fig. 12-5).

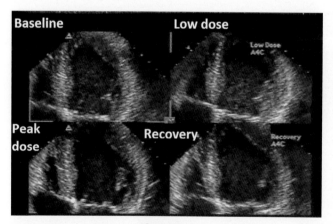

Fig. 12-5

A. Flow-limiting left anterior descending artery stenosis.
B. Flow-limiting left circumflex artery stenosis.
C. Flow-limiting right coronary artery stenosis.
D. Multivessel coronary artery stenosis.
E. Flow-limiting diagonal branch stenosis.

21. A 56-year-old asymptomatic male with a history of dyslipidemia and tobacco use was referred for a stress echo prior to elective cholecystectomy. The patient underwent dobutamine stress echo without chest pain or electrocardiographic changes. Based on the findings, which of the following is the most appropriate statement? (Video 12-5A–D and Fig. 12-6).

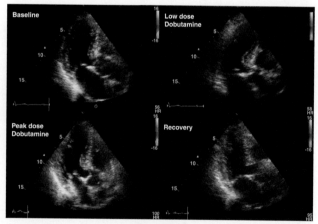

Fig. 12-6

A. This patient is at high risk for perioperative cardiac events.
B. This patient is at low risk for perioperative cardiac events.
C. Coronary angiogram and revascularization should be considered.
D. Myocardial perfusion imaging should be considered.
E. Computed tomography for calcium scoring should be considered.

22. A 55-year-old female with a previous history of hypertension and alcohol abuse presented with dyspnea, lower extremities edema, orthopnea, and paroxysmal nocturnal dyspnea. She was admitted and appropriate medical therapy was initiated. She was ruled out for acute coronary syndrome. A dobutamine stress echo was performed. Based on the findings in the dobutamine stress echo, which of the following statements is correct? (Fig. 12-7 and Video 12-6A–B).

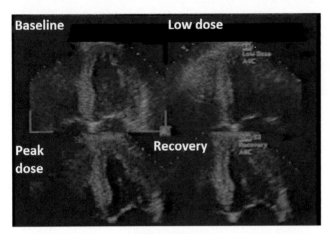

Fig. 12-7

A. A biphasic response is seen in this patient.
B. The probability of left ventricular functional recovery without revascularization is high.
C. The probability of left ventricular functional recovery with revascularization is high.
D. The probability of left ventricular functional recovery is low.
E. The peak wall motion score index in this patient predicts a high event rate.

23. A 56-year-old male complaining of dyspnea on exertion and only able to walk two blocks is referred for exercise stress echo. Based on the findings on the stress echo in Figure 12-8, what would be the next step in the management of this patient? (Video 12-7A [rest] and 12-7B [stress]).
A. Mitral valve repair.
B. Mitral valve replacement.
C. Monitor with serial echocardiography.
D. Work-up for pulmonary embolism.
E. Mitral valve repair after left ventricular function improves.

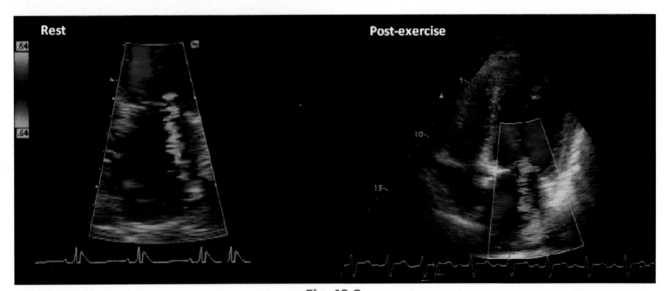

Fig. 12-8

24. A 79 year-old female was referred for a stress echo due to chest pain. She underwent dobutamine stress echo without chest pain or electrocardiographic changes. Which statement best describes the findings in Figure 12-9? (Video 12-8A–D).

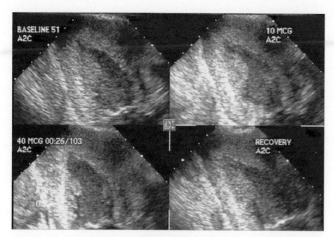

Fig. 12-9

A. No ischemia.
B. Anterior wall ischemia.
C. Lateral wall ischemia.
D. Apical ischemia.
E. Inferior and posterior wall ischemia.

25. A 72-year-old male was referred for an exercise stress echo due to chest pain. Which statement best describes the stress echo findings in Figure 12-10? See also Video 12-9A–C.
A. No ischemia.
B. Anterior wall ischemia.
C. Lateral wall ischemia.
D. Anteroseptal ischemia.
E. Inferior/posterior wall ischemia.

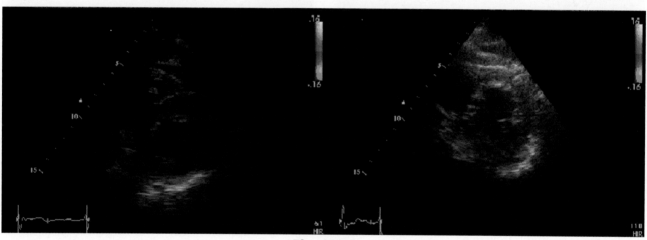

Fig. 12-10

CASE 1:

A 55-year-old man with a history of hypertension presented to the emergency department with left-sided chest discomfort lasting for 15 minutes. He started taking a diuretic and a calcium channel blocker 2 years ago. His BP was 155/90 mm Hg and the ECG revealed left ventricular hypertrophy without repolarization abnormalities. He was admitted and ruled out for myocardial infarction. A stress echocardiogram was ordered. He exercised on the treadmill for 6 minutes reaching a peak heart rate of 150 bpm and workload of 7 METS. The test was ended due to shortness of breath. His ECG at peak heart rate revealed 3 mm downsloping ST depressions in leads II, III, AVF, V5, and V6. He did not experience chest pain during the test. (Fig. 12-11 and Video 12-10A–C).

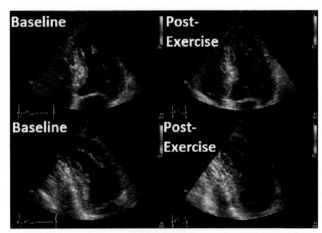

Fig. 12-11

26. Which of the following statements about the stress echo on this patient is correct?
    A. The ECG and echocardiographic findings are consistent with ischemia.
    B. The stress ECG is more specific for ischemia.
    C. The stress ECG changes make the results of this test equivocal.
    D. The ECG changes represent a false-positive result.
    E. The event rate in this patient approaches 5% per year.

27. Based on the stress echocardiographic findings, what would be the next step in the management of this patient?
    A. Discharge home.
    B. Refer the patient for coronary angiography.
    C. Order a dypiridamole nuclear stress test.
    D. Order a coronary CTA.
    E. Repeat the stress echo after optimal control of blood pressure.

CASE 2:

A 50-year-old man with a history of a previous myocardial infarction, diabetes, and dyslipidemia status post permanent pacemaker, presents to the emergency department complaining of shortness of breath and is found to be in pulmonary edema. He is admitted to the cardiac care unit. A transthoracic echocardiogram reveals moderate mitral regurgitation, dilated and severely hypokinetic left ventricle with an ejection fraction of 10%. A coronary angiogram reveals severe triple-vessel disease. A dobutamine stress echo is requested. (Fig. 12-12 and Video 12-11A–F).

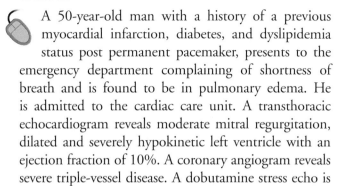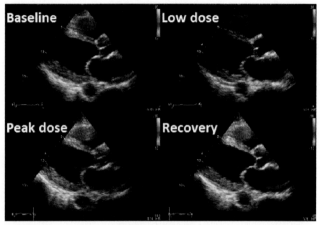

Fig. 12-12

28. Which of the following statements best describes the stress echo?
    A. Right ventricular ischemia.
    B. Septal wall ischemia.
    C. Marked viability in the inferior wall.
    D. Mild ischemia in the apex.
    E. Mild viability in the posterior wall.

29. Which of the following statements is correct?
    A. This patient will likely respond to beta-blocker therapy.
    B. The probability of left ventricular functional recovery in this patient is >80%.
    C. As the number of segments demonstrating inotropic contractile reserve in this patient is small, the probability of left ventricular function improvement is minimal.
    D. There is not enough information to predict the likelihood of cardiac events in this patient.
    E. This patient will likely respond to cardiac resynchronization therapy.

30. Based on the stress echocardiogram shown, what would be the most appropriate intervention?
   A. Coronary bypass graft surgery.
   B. Staged angioplasty.
   C. Coronary bypass graft surgery in addition to mitral valve repair.
   D. Referral for heart transplantation.
   E. Coronary bypass graft surgery with reduction left ventriculoplasty.

CASE 3:

A 69-year-old female with a history of diabetes, hypertension, end-stage renal disease, and previous MI presented to the emergency department with an episode of left-sided chest pain lasting 20 minutes. She was admitted and ruled out for acute myocardial infarction. A stress echo was requested. Her resting BP was 220/100 mm Hg. A dipyridamole stress echo was performed due to elevated blood pressure. The ECG did not show ischemic changes, but the patient experienced chest pressure. (Fig. 12-13 and Video 12-12A–F).

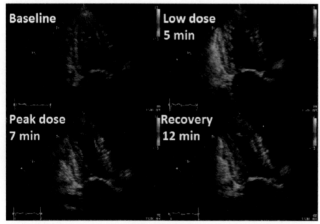

Fig. 12-13

31. Which of the following statements best describes the stress echo?
   A. Mild lateral wall ischemia.
   B. Moderate mid anteroseptal wall ischemia.
   C. Mild inferior wall ischemia.
   D. Mild right ventricular ischemia.
   E. There is no evidence of ischemia.

32. Which of the following statements is correct?
   A. The findings in this test are unreliable due to the low specificity of dipyridamole stress echocardiography.
   B. The sensitivity of dipyridamole stress echocardiography to detect ischemia is lower than for dobutamine stress echocardiography.

   C. The peak wall motion score index in this patient portends a low risk for cardiac events.
   D. The chest pain in this patient is most likely a side effect of dipyridamole.
   E. In women, dipyridamole stress echocardiography is preferred to dobutamine stress echocardiography as it is less likely to produce a left ventricular outflow tract gradient.

33. What would be the most likely finding on coronary angiogram?
   A. Severe flow-limiting mid left anterior descending artery stenosis.
   B. Severe flow-limiting mid left circumflex artery stenosis.
   C. Severe flow-limiting mid right coronary artery stenosis.
   D. Severe flow-limiting ramus intermedius artery stenosis.
   E. No flow-limiting coronary artery disease.

CASE 4:

A 63-year-old female with history of HIV, diabetes, dyslipidemia, and end-stage renal disease presented to the emergency department with retrosternal chest pressure. Her ECG did not reveal ischemic changes but her cardiac enzymes were mildly elevated. She was admitted for non-ST-segment elevation myocardial infarction. A dobutamine stress echo was performed using perflutren-based echo contrast. (Fig. 12-14 and Video 12-13A–E).

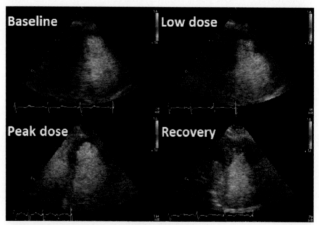

Fig. 12-14

34. Which of the following statements best describes the stress echo?
   A. Mild apical ischemia.
   B. Mild anterior wall ischemia.
   C. Mild lateral wall ischemia.
   D. Transient left ventricular cavity dilatation.
   E. Severe basal septum ischemia.

35. Which of the following statements is correct?
    A. High mechanical index during a contrast study can cause transient ischemic dilatation.
    B. The findings on the stress echo predict a cardiac event rate less than 1%/year.
    C. The severity of wall motion abnormality is not important if there is extensive ischemia.
    D. The peak wall motion score index in this patient is <1.7.
    E. A stress myocardial perfusion imaging study in this patient may be normal.

36. What findings would you expect on a coronary angiogram?
    A. Severe ramus intermedius artery flow-limiting stenosis.
    B. Severe left anterior descending artery flow-limiting stenosis.
    C. Severe triple-vessel disease.
    D. Severe right coronary artery + left circumflex artery flow-limiting stenosis.
    E. Good collateral circulation distal to the stenotic vessel.

CASE 5:

A 54-year-old male with a history of diabetes, dyslipidemia, and hypertension was referred by his primary care physician due to chest pressure after walking two blocks, which is relieved by rest. A dobutamine stress echo was performed due to low exercise tolerance. The ECG was nondiagnostic. The patient experienced chest pain during the test. (Fig. 12-15 and Video 12-14A–E).

37. Which of the following statements best describes the stress echo?
    A. Right ventricular hypokinesis.
    B. Mild hypokinesis of the anterior wall.
    C. Mild hypokinesis of the posterior wall.
    D. Mild hypokinesis of the apical septum.
    E. No evidence of new wall motion abnormalities.

38. Which of the following statements is correct?
    A. The exercise tolerance of this patient does not confer a higher risk for future cardiovascular events.
    B. The occurrence of chest pain, in light of the dobutamine stress echo findings does not suggest ischemia.
    C. The wall motion score index in this patient portends a favorable prognosis.
    D. The wall motion score index in this patient portends a poor prognosis.
    E. Right ventricular wall motion abnormalities do not confer additional prognostic information if the left ventricle is hyperkinetic.

39. What is the most probable finding on coronary angiography?
    A. Right coronary artery flow-limiting stenosis.
    B. Left anterior descending artery flow-limiting stenosis.
    C. Left circumflex artery flow-limiting stenosis.
    D. Triple-vessel coronary artery disease.
    E. No flow-limiting stenosis of the coronary arteries.

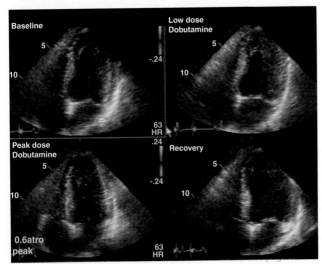

Fig. 12-15

ANSWERS

1. ANSWER: D. The use of stress echocardiography to diagnose flow-limiting coronary artery disease is based on a sequence of events known as the ischemic cascade, shown in Figure 12-16. The decrease in blood flow initially produces a perfusion abnormality, diastolic and systolic dysfunction, in that order, and then hemodynamic abnormalities occur. Electrocardiographic changes and symptoms occur late in the ischemic cascade, hence the lower sensitivity of these parameters to identify ischemia.

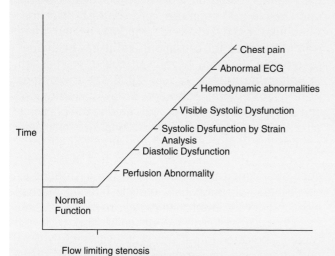

Fig. 12-16

2. ANSWER: D. The overall sensitivity and specificity of stress echocardiography is comparable to scintigraphic imaging. The sensitivity and specificity of stress echocardiography depends on multiple factors including significant coronary artery disease, pretest probability of coronary artery disease, mode of stress used, number of vessels involved, and medications used at the time of testing. The sensitivity of exercise stress echocardiography ranges from 80% to 88%, with specificities ranging from 82% to 90%. For dobutamine stress echocardiography, the sensitivity ranges from 68% to 95% with a specificity of 77% to 100%. The sensitivity of vasodilator-based stress echocardiography ranges from 40% to 91% but with a good specificity. Although the sensitivity of vasodilator stress echocardiography is lower than for exercise or dobutamine stress echocardiography, its specificity is good and comparable to both modalities. Atropine is frequently used during dobutamine stress echocardiography when the peak heart rate is suboptimal, to improve the sensitivity.

The sensitivity of stress echocardiography is proportionally related to the number of vessels involved, being the greatest for triple-vessel disease. Significant aortic regurgitation can produce regional wall motion abnormalities, thus reducing the specificity of stress echocardiography.

3. ANSWER: A. The sensitivity of stress myocardial perfusion imaging for single-vessel disease is better than stress echocardiography, while stress echocardiography has a greater specificity than stress myocardial perfusion imaging. Technically, stress echocardiography is a more challenging test compared to myocardial perfusion imaging, but has the advantage of being less costly and time-consuming for the patient, without the concern of radiation exposure. Interpretation of wall motion by stress echocardiography is subjective and requires some expertise.

4. ANSWER: E. It is important to recognize that not all wall motion abnormalities on stress are due to ischemia. Noncoronary causes of a false-positive study include the presence of a pacemaker, left bundle branch block, or prior cardiac surgery that can produce paradoxical septal motion. Hypertensive response, cardiomyopathy, dynamic right ventricular pressure overload, and aortic regurgitation can cause nonischemic wall motion abnormalities on stress. Inadequate workload with suboptimal peak heart rate, use of beta-blockers, delay on image acquisition, and concentric left ventricular hypertrophy decrease the sensitivity of the stress echo but not its specificity.

5. ANSWER: D. Symptoms not associated with objective evidence of ischemia (wall motion abnormalities) are not an indication to stop the test. Thus, chest pain or up-sloping ST-segment changes and T-wave inversions do not mandate termination of the test. Supraventricular or ventricular arrhythmias, such as atrial fibrillation or nonsustained ventricular tachycardia, are indications to stop the infusion of dobutamine, but not bigeminy.

6. ANSWER: C. The normal response of wall motion to stress is a hyperkinetic state with increase in myocardial thickening and endocardial excursion (greater than 5 mm). A normal or a hypokinetic segment that worsens on stress is considered abnormal and consistent with inducible ischemia. A hypokinetic segment that remains unchanged represents scar tissue. A hypokinetic segment that improves on stress represents viable myocardium (monophasic response). A hypokinetic segment that improves on low-dose dobutamine and deteriorates at peak dose represents viable myocardium and ischemia in this segment (biphasic response). Dyskinesis is the extreme degree of wall motion abnormality characterized by myocardial thinning and outward movement during systole.

7. ANSWER: A. The sensitivity of stress echocardiography to detect flow-limiting lesions depends not only on the degree of coronary stenosis, but also on the number of vessels involved or jeopardized myocardium. The sensitivity is superior for multivessel than for single-vessel disease. Likewise, the sensitivity to detect stenosis in the left anterior descending artery and right coronary artery territory is superior to the sensitivity for the left circumflex. The highest sensitivity is for left anterior descending artery stenosis.

8. ANSWER: D. Echocardiography is a complementary part of stress testing, and as such should be considered in conjunction with clinical and electrocardiographic variables for risk-stratifying patients. Stress echocardiography provides incremental value over clinical electrocardiography and resting echocardiographic parameters. The classification of stress echocardiography as normal and abnormal can effectively risk-stratify patients, but echocardiographic findings of ischemia, such as peak wall motion score index, are more important in the determination of risk. The event rate of a negative stress echo varies with the population studied, but overall in an intermediate risk population is <1%/year. The event rate and mortality are significantly increased (twofold), in diabetics versus nondiabetics with a negative stress echo (2.2% vs. 1%/ year). Left ventricular ejection fraction is a strong independent prognosticator. A wall motion abnormality at lower heart rates is consistent with multivessel disease and a worse prognosis. Viability has incremental prognostic value over clinical and resting echocardiographic variables.

9. ANSWER: C. The negative predictive value of a normal stress echo is very good (93%–100%). This high negative predictive value allows the identification of patients with a very low likelihood of experiencing perioperative events and thus can undergo noncardiac surgery without further testing. The positive predictive value of stress echocardiography (7%–33%) and myocardial perfusion imaging is low. Patients who can exercise generally have a better prognosis than those undergoing a dobutamine stress echo. The area of ischemia identified by stress echocardiography or myocardial perfusion imaging does not predict the perioperative region of infarction.

10. ANSWER: D. The use of echo contrast is currently approved by the Food and Drug Administration only for left ventricular opacification and endocardial border delineation. Echo contrast decreases intra- and interobserver variability in wall motion interpretation, thus increasing the accuracy of stress echocardiography. Myocardial perfusion imaging is another application of echo contrast in stress testing. Vasodilator agents are the preferred method of perfusion stress testing with echo contrast. The use of echo contrast agents has been shown to be a safe practice in multiple studies. In October 2007, the Food and Drug Administration issued new warnings and contraindications for the use of ultrasound contrast agents, based on reports of four deaths occurring within 30 minutes of contrast injection. Although these deaths were temporally related, there is little evidence for causation; and it has been suggested that they may have been due to progression of underlying disease. In July 2008, these warnings were relaxed by the Food and Drug Administration. The use of contrast is contraindicated in the presence of known right-to-left, bidirectional, or transient right-to-left cardiac shunts (other than patent foramen ovale). This is based on the fact that in the presence of a significant cardiac shunt the microbubbles can bypass the pulmonary particle filtering mechanism and directly enter the arterial circulation causing microvascular occlusion and ischemia. Also, their use is contraindicated in patients with hypersensitivity to perflutren; and hypersensitivity to blood products (Optison only). Additional monitoring of vital signs, oxygen saturation, and electrocardiography is recommended for 30 minutes after contrast administration, in patients with unstable cardiopulmonary conditions. Although the Food and Drug Administration has not approved the use of echo contrast agents for stress echocardiography, it is used in most laboratories and recommended by the American Society of Echocardiography.

11. ANSWER: B. Stunned myocardium is a state of contraction-perfusion mismatch that can be seen in the setting of acute myocardial infarction after successful reperfusion (Fig. 12-17). If recurrent chronic ischemia occurs, the dysfunctional but viable myocardium is called hibernating myocardium. Hibernating myocardium results from recurrent stunning of the myocardium. A nontransmural infarction of only 20% of the wall thickness can impair wall thickening. Up to 40% of regions showing Q waves in the electrocardiogram are viable. No reflow is consistent with capillary destruction, thus consistent with no viability. Dobutamine stress echocardiography cannot differentiate viability in the endocardium versus epicardium.

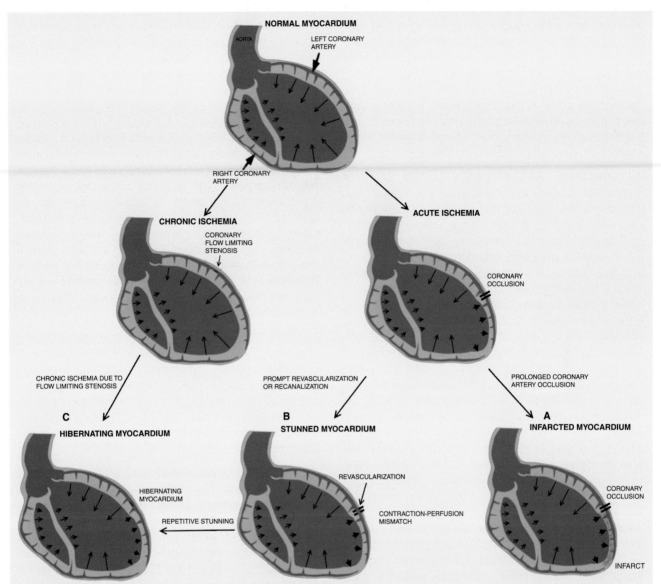

A normally perfused and functioning myocardium is depicted by normal coronary arteries and normal end-systolic and end-diastolic volumes. On the bottom, a complete left coronary artery occlusion has occurred in the setting of plaque rupture with acute thrombosis. If the lack of perfusion is prolonged enough, a myocardial infarction ensues, with loss of function, depicted here by regional increase in end-systolic volume (**A**). If reperfusion occurs, either due to recanalization or revascularization, the contractility initially abnormal due to ischemia may remain impaired in the acute and subacute stages, with subsequent improvement. This phenomenon is called stunning (**B**). Repetitive stunning leads to a state of chronic myocardial dysfunction called hibernation (**C**). On the top, a chronic flow-limiting coronary artery occlusion leads to downregulation of the regional wall motion abnormality, leading to hibernating myocardium (**C**).

Fig. 12-17

12. ANSWER: C. The predictive value of low-level exercise stress echocardiography for left ventricular function improvement is lower than dobutamine stress echocardiography. The use of dobutamine is based on the concept of inotropic contractile reserve in which a viable myocardium will improve its contractility, while nonviable myocardium will remain unchanged. Biphasic response has the highest predictive value of functional recovery. Sustained improvement or no change response can predict functional recovery, but with a lower positive predictive value than biphasic response. Dobutamine stress echocardiography unlike magnetic resonance cannot differentiate scar in the endocardium versus the epicardium.

13. ANSWER: D. Transient ischemic cavity dilatation of the left ventricle is defined as transient increase in the end-systolic dimensions from rest to peak stress. It is a marker of severe and extensive coronary artery disease and is associated with a high risk of cardiac events (19.7%/y event rate). Transient ischemic cavity dilatation occurs in patients with absent or limited collateral circulation. Peak left and right ventricular wall motion abnormalities, low ischemic threshold, and peak wall motion score index >1.7 are poor prognosticators associated with an increased cardiac event rate. Wall motion score index is derived from the cumulative sum score of all left ventricular wall segments, divided by the number of visualized segments. Hypotension occurring during exercise testing has been associated with an increased prevalence of multivessel coronary artery disease and a poor prognosis. Mild hypotension (a drop in systolic blood pressure < 50 mm Hg) occurs in 14%–38% of dobutamine stress echo. Unlike hypotension occurring with exercise stress echocardiography, mild hypotension during dobutamine infusion carries a good prognosis in the absence of new wall motion abnormalities.

14. *ANSWER: E.* The potential clinical utility of myocardial contrast echocardiography in conjunction with stress testing to diagnose hemodynamically significant coronary artery disease has been shown in numerous studies. The most commonly used stress agents for myocardial perfusion are adenosine, dipyridamole, and dobutamine. The accuracy of myocardial perfusion stress echocardiography to detect flow-limiting coronary artery stenosis is comparable to nuclear scintigraphy and dobutamine stress echocardiography, with a sensitivity of about 85% and a specificity of 74%. Myocardial perfusion stress echocardiography also provides prognostic information in patients with stable coronary artery disease. Patients with normal perfusion have a better prognosis than patients with normal wall motion. Xie et al., showed how in patients with significant left anterior descending artery disease, myocardial perfusion during dobutamine stress echocardiography was able to detect subendocardial ischemia even when transmural wall thickening appeared normal. Tsutsui et al. evaluated the safety of myocardial perfusion during dobutamine stress echocardiography in 1,486 patients and found no difference in adverse events, including cardiac arrhythmias, when compared to conventional dobutamine stress echocardiography. The image interpretation during myocardial perfusion stress echocardiography is affected by the lateral resolution of the ultrasound beam, which affects mainly the lateral wall; and also by attenuation, affecting the basal segments. Myocardial perfusion can be accomplished by using high-power (high mechanical index) or low-power (mechanical index < 0.2) modalities. Since high power destroys the microbubbles, high frame rates and continuous imaging cannot be performed without destroying most of the microbubbles, making impossible the simultaneous analysis of wall motion. On the other hand, low-power imaging causes minimal microbubble destruction, allowing continuous imaging and wall motion analysis.

15. *ANSWER: E.* Diastole is an active process. Myocardial contraction is initiated by cytosolic calcium binding troponin C, causing disinhibition of troponin I and actin–myosin cross-bridge formation. During relaxation, the interaction of adenosine triphosphate with myosin causing actin–myosin dissociation and the removal of cytosolic calcium by sarcoplasmic reticulum calcium adenosine triphosphatase, are energy-dependent

processes. As illustrated previously on the ischemic cascade, relaxation abnormalities occur earlier than systolic abnormalities making the assessment of stress-induced diastolic abnormalities a more sensitive technique than systolic abnormalities. Furthermore, diastolic abnormalities last longer than systolic abnormalities during ischemia. A recent study by Ishii et al. showed that at 10 minutes post exercise no systolic abnormalities were identified while delayed relaxation was seen in 85% of the territories supplied by stenotic coronary arteries. The accuracy of diastolic function assessment during stress echocardiography can be affected by conditions causing dyssynchrony, including cardiomyopathy and hypertensive heart disease. Regional diastolic abnormalities can be seen even if the global diastolic and systolic functions are normal. Patients whose left ventricle filling parameters worsen on stress have a lower exercise tolerance than those without diastolic abnormalities.

16. *ANSWER: D.* This case illustrates the hemodynamic pulmonary response to exercise in a patient with primary pulmonary hypertension who had only mild pulmonary hypertension at rest, with a pulmonary artery systolic pressure of 39 mm Hg that rose to 90 mm Hg during exercise. Post stress, there is right ventricular enlargement and hypokinesis due to a dynamic rise in right-side pressures.

17. *ANSWER: D.* An exercise stress echo is a useful tool to elicit a left ventricular outflow tract gradient in patients with latent hypertrophic cardiomyopathy. Patients without obstruction at rest or with provocation maneuvers may develop obstruction during exercise as evidenced in this patient, causing symptoms. The continuous-wave Doppler signal through the left ventricular outflow tract is a dagger-shaped, late peaking envelope characteristic of dynamic obstruction as opposed to aortic stenosis where the gradient usually peaks in early to midsystole.

18. *ANSWER: E.* Dobutamine stress echocardiography plays an important role in risk stratification of patients after myocardial infarction and for the assessment of myocardial viability. On baseline images, there is hypokinesis of the inferior, posterior, and lateral walls with marked inotropic contractile reserve at low-dose dobutamine stress echocardiography, without evidence of ischemia (monophasic response). The hypokinetic myocardium represents stunned myocardium without evidence of ischemia (biphasic response), indicating the absence of flow-limiting stenosis that may require revascularization. This phenomenon can be caused by spontaneous coronary recanalization. The presence of marked viability carries a good prognosis with a lower cardiac event rate, and predicts improvement in wall motion after restoration of coronary blood flow. The absence of ischemia confers a more favorable prognosis.

19. ANSWER: A. The echocardiographic images in Figure 12-4 show wall motion abnormalities at peak heart rate, in the mid to apical anterior and septal wall, as well as the apex. There is also evidence of transient ischemic cavity dilatation. This is typical of a left anterior descending artery flow-limiting stenosis. Transient ischemic cavity dilatation predicts severe and extensive coronary artery disease; and is most commonly seen in the absence of distal collateral circulation.

20. ANSWER: D. The echocardiographic images in Figure 12-5 show new wall motion abnormalities in the anterior, lateral, septal, inferior, and posterior walls, as well as evidence of transient ischemic cavity dilatation, consistent with extensive and severe ischemia. This distribution is consistent with multivessel disease.

21. ANSWER: B. The echocardiographic images in Figure 12-6 reveal mild apical ischemia. Note on the apical long-axis view, the difference in cavity size between the stages of low dose and peak dose of dobutamine, at the level of the apex. During the low-dose stage, there is a normal hypercontractile response with complete cavity obliteration; while during the peak dose, there is apical hypokinesis without complete cavity obliteration that indicates ischemia in this region. The absence of symptoms and mild degree of ischemia (<four segments) are factors that portend a low risk for perioperative cardiovascular events and further workup and delay in the surgical procedure is not warranted.

22. ANSWER: B. The dobutamine stress echo in this patient with severe left ventricular dysfunction was performed for diagnostic and prognostic purposes: It illustrates a case of nonischemic cardiomyopathy with marked inotropic contractile reserve. Gradual decrease in left ventricular cavity size can be appreciated from baseline to low and peak dose, consistent with a hypercontractile response. All left ventricular segments improve at low and peak dose, with normalization of the left ventricular ejection fraction at peak dose. Deterioration in wall motion contractility at peak dose is not seen, indicating the absence of ischemia (biphasic response). Inotropic contractile reserve, as determined by the change in wall motion score index from baseline to low or peak dose dobutamine, as well as the number of recruiting segments. It portends a favorable prognosis in this patient, with a high probability of left ventricular function recovery, good response to beta-blockers, cardiac resynchronization therapy, and a lower cardiac event rate.

23. ANSWER: A. This patient presents with symptoms not explained by the degree of mitral regurgitation seen on the resting echo. The exercise stress echo shows an increase in the severity of mitral regurgitation and a further increase in the pulmonary artery systolic pressure, both consistent with hemodynamically significant mitral regurgitation. Mitral valve repair is the treatment of choice due to the lower risk of thrombosis and endocarditis compared to a prosthetic valve.

24. ANSWER: E. The echocardiographic images in Figure 12-9 reveal new wall motion abnormalities consistent with ischemia in the inferior and posterior walls.

25. ANSWER: D. The echocardiographic images in Figure 12-10 reveal new wall motion abnormalities consistent with mild ischemia in the anteroseptum.

26. ANSWER: D; 27. ANSWER: A. The case illustrates a normal stress echo in a patient with left ventricular hypertrophy discordant with the stress ECG results. The specificity of the stress ECG can be affected by several factors including left ventricular hypertrophy which can cause nonischemic ST-segment depression, thus decreasing its specificity. The sensitivity and specificity of stress echocardiography are superior to that of ECG and given the normal results of the stress echocardiographic images, it can be assumed that the results of the ECG represent a false-positive one. The prognosis of an abnormal ECG in the face of a normal stress echo is good. There is no need for additional work-up.

KEY POINTS:
- Left ventricular hypertrophy can cause false-positive ECG changes.
- The sensitivity of stress echocardiography is superior to that of stress ECG.
- A normal stress echo, even in the presence of ECG changes, portends a good prognosis.

28. ANSWER: E; 29. ANSWER: C; 30. ANSWER: D. This case illustrates a patient with ischemic cardiomyopathy and severe left ventricular dysfunction with minimal inotropic contractile reserve and without evidence of inducible ischemia. The absence of inotropic contractile reserve, consistent with a scarred myocardium, portends a poor prognosis. Patients with significant viability demonstrate improved survival and improvement in left ventricular function after revascularization. A substudy of the β-blocker Evaluation of Survival Trial (BEST), where there was no clear survival benefit in patients with New York Heart Association functional class III and IV heart failure treated with bucindolol, examined whether myocardial contractile reserve as determined by dobutamine stress echocardiography could predict left ventricular function improvement after beta-blocker therapy. This study also showed a direct relationship between inotropic contractile reserve and left ventricular function improvement after beta-blocker therapy. The change in the wall motion score index was the most significant predictor of the change in left ventricular ejection fraction.

This patient is unlikely to benefit from revascularization or beta-blocker therapy. Likewise, it is unlikely that this patient with minimal inotropic contractile reserve will respond to cardiac resynchronization therapy.

KEY POINTS:

◼ Inotropic contractile reserve predicts left ventricular functional recovery after revascularization.

◼ Inotropic contractile reserve predicts response to beta-blocker therapy.

◼ Absence of inotropic contractile reserve portends a poor prognosis.

31. ANSWER: B; 32. ANSWER: B; 33. ANSWER: A.
This case illustrates a patient with moderate ischemia in the mid and apical septal and anterior walls, as well as the mid anteroseptum and apical inferior wall. Coronary angiography confirmed a severe mid left anterior descending artery stenosis. The sensitivity of dipyridamole stress echocardiography for single-vessel disease may be as low as 50%, but its specificity is excellent (88%–100%). The peak wall motion score index is about 1.7, which confers a high cardiovascular risk to this patient (>5%/year). Even though chest pain may represent a nonspecific symptom and a side effect of dipyridamole, the presence of new wall motion abnormalities indicates ischemia.

KEY POINTS:

◼ Dipyridamole stress has good specificity.

◼ Stress wall motion score index >1.7 confers a poor prognosis.

◼ Chest pain in conjunction with new wall motion abnormalities further supports ischemia.

34. ANSWER: D 35. ANSWER: E; 36. ANSWER: C.
This case illustrates a patient who underwent a dobutamine stress echo contrast study with the finding of ischemia involving multiple coronary artery territories and transient ischemic cavity dilatation, a marker of severe and extensive coronary artery disease. The peak wall motion score index as well as the evidence of transient ischemic dilatation put this patient in a high-risk group with an event rate as high as 19%. The severity and extent of wall motion abnormalities are independent and cumulative predictors of cardiac events. A coronary angiogram in this patient confirmed the presence of triple-vessel disease. The presence of collateral circulation distal to a flow-limiting lesion can affect the appearance of transient ischemic cavity dilatation on a stress echo. A myocardial perfusion imaging study may be normal in this patient due to balanced ischemia. While the myocardial perfusion study may not reveal segmental defects, transient ischemic dilatation may also be noted as a marker of multivessel disease.

Transient ischemic dilatation (terminology used in nuclear cardiology) and transient ischemic cavity dilatation (terminology used in echocardiography) denote severe and extensive coronary artery disease: They both a common pathophysiologic basis that includes a transient increase in the end-systolic dimensions from rest to peak stress, due to ischemic systolic dysfunction and is readily assessed by echocardiography. In addition, they both have diffuse subendocardial ischemia producing the appearance of a dilated cavity on perfusion images.

High mechanical index when used with echo contrast destroys more microbubbles, but does not cause transient ischemic cavity dilatation.

KEY POINTS:

◼ Transient ischemic cavity dilatation is a marker of severe and extensive coronary artery disease.

◼ Transient ischemic cavity dilatation portends a poor prognosis.

◼ Transient ischemic cavity dilatation appearance is affected by the presence of collateral circulation.

◼ Severe and extensive coronary artery disease is a cause of false-negative results on myocardial perfusion imaging studies.

37. ANSWER: A; 38. ANSWER: D; 39. ANSWER: D.
The dobutamine stress echo shows new wall motion abnormalities during the recovery stage. Note that the left ventricle at peak heart rate shows a normal hyperkinetic response, but during the recovery stage the left ventricle becomes diffusely and severely hypokinetic, with evidence of transient ischemic cavity dilatation. The right ventricle becomes diffusely hypokinetic in the recovery stage. Clinical variables, such as exercise capacity, chest pain on exertion, and comorbidities, put this patient into a high-risk category for cardiac events. The occurrence of chest pain in the setting of new wall motion abnormalities suggests ischemia. The wall motion score index in this patient confers a poor prognosis. The appearance of right ventricular wall motion abnormalities is an independent prognosticator for future cardiac events. This patient should undergo revascularization.

KEY POINTS:

◼ Wall motion abnormalities can present at any stage during the stress echo. Their appearance during the recovery stage also represents ischemia.

◼ Persistent wall motion abnormalities in recovery indicate severe flow-limiting stenosis.

◼ The appearance of right ventricular wall motion abnormalities is an independent predictor of future cardiac events.

◼ Transient ischemic cavity dilatation is a marker of severe and extensive coronary artery disease.

SUGGESTED READINGS

Afridi I, Kleiman NS, Raizner AE, et al. Dobutamine echocardiography in myocardial hibernation: optimal dose and accuracy in predicting recovery of ventricular function after coronary angioplasty. *Circulation.* 1995;91:663–670.

Allman KC, Shaw LJ, Hachamovitch R, et al. Myocardial viability testing and impact of revascularization on prognosis in patients with coronary artery disease and left ventricular dysfunction: a meta-analysis. *J Am Coll Cardiol.* 2002;39:1151–1158.

Armstrong WF, O'Donnell J, Ryan T, et al. Effect of prior myocardial infarction and extent and location of coronary disease on accuracy of exercise echocardiography. *J Am Coll Cardiol.* 1987;10:531–538.

Bangalore S, Yao SS, Chaudhry FA. Prediction of myocardial infarction versus cardiac death by stress echocardiography. *J Am Soc Echocardiogr.* 2009;22:261–267.

Bangalore S, Yao SS, Chaudhry FA. Role of right ventricular wall motion abnormalities in risk stratification and prognosis of patients referred for stress echocardiography. *J Am Coll Cardiol.* 2007;50:1981–1989.

Hoffer EP, Dewé W, Celentano C, et al. Low-level exercise echocardiography detects contractile reserve and predicts reversible dysfunction after acute myocardial infarction. *J Am Coll Cardiol.* 1999;34:989–999.

Mahenthiran J, Bangalore S, Yao SS, et al. Comparison of prognostic value of stress echocardiography versus stress electrocardiography in patients with suspected coronary artery disease. *Am J Cardiol.* 2005;96:628–634.

Marwick TH, Nemec JJ, Pashkow FJ, et al. Accuracy and limitations of exercise echocardiography in a routine clinical setting. *J Am Coll Cardiol.* 1992;19:74–81.

Mulvagh SL, Rakowski H, Vannan MA, et al. American Society of Echocardiography Consensus Statement on the Clinical Applications of Ultrasonic Contrast Agents in Echocardiography. *J Am Soc Echocardiogr.* 2008;21:1179–1201.

O'Keefe JH, Barnhart CS, Bateman TM. Comparison of stress echocardiography and stress myocardial perfusion scintigraphy for diagnosing coronary artery disease and assessing its severity. *Am J Cardiol.* 1995;75:25D–34D.

Poldermans D, Arnese M, Fioretti PM, et al. Improved cardiac risk stratification in major vascular surgery with dobutamine-atropine stress echocardiography. *J Am Coll Cardiol.* 1995;26:648–653.

Shah JS, Esteban MT, Thaman R, et al. Prevalence of exercise-induced left ventricular outflow tract obstruction in symptomatic patients with non-obstructive hypertrophic cardiomyopathy. *Heart.* 2008;94:1288–1294.

Wahi S, Marwick TH. Aortic regurgitation reduces the accuracy of exercise echocardiography for diagnosis of coronary artery disease. *J Am Soc Echocardiogr.* 1999;12:967–973.

Yao SS, Shah A, Bangalore S, et al. Transient ischemic left ventricular cavity dilation is a significant predictor of severe and extensive coronary artery disease and adverse outcome in patients undergoing stress echocardiography. *J Am Soc Echocardiogr.* 2007;20:352–358.

Yao SS, Qureshi E, Syed A, et al. Novel stress echocardiographic model incorporating the extent and severity of wall motion abnormality for risk stratification and prognosis. *Am J Cardiol.* 2004;94:715–719.

CHAPTER 13

Intraoperative Echocardiography

William J. Stewart

1. Air embolization to a coronary artery is associated with wall motion abnormalities in which coronary territory?
   A. Right coronary artery.
   B. Left anterior descending.
   C. Left circumflex.
   D. Global.
   E. No coronary territory.

2. In a patient who previously required dilation of an esophageal stricture, what should be done regarding intraoperative echocardiography?
   A. Passage of the transesophageal echo (TEE) probe can proceed as usual, because the stricture has been dilated.
   B. Use of a pediatric probe is the only way to do a TEE.
   C. The transesophageal probe should not be inserted. Epicardial echo is an alternative imaging modality.
   D. A standard TEE probe can be used, but it should not be passed beyond the gastroesophageal junction.
   E. Intraoperative echocardiography is not recommended.

3. In patients with aortic and mitral stenosis, the pre-pump TEE is less reliable than aortic and mitral valve continuous-wave Doppler gradients by preoperative transthoracic echo because:
   A. Mitral and aortic valve velocity cannot reliably be recorded by TEE.

B. Mitral valve velocity cannot reliably be recorded by TEE.
C. Aortic valve velocity cannot be reliably recorded by TEE.
D. Changes in loading conditions make recordings of the valvular velocities in the operating room unreliable.
E. Continuous-wave Doppler cannot be reliably recorded by TEE during electrocautery.

4. Intraoperative TEE during implantation of a left ventricular assist device (LVAD) is useful for:
   A. Exclusion of mitral regurgitation, which makes the LVAD ineffective.
   B. Deciding on location of the inflow cannula into the left ventricle.
   C. Exclusion of aortic regurgitation that causes a shunt to return back to the left ventricular (LV) cannula.
   D. Quantitation of tricuspid regurgitation (TR) that affects the amount of right atrial (RA) hypertension.
   E. Diagnosis of LV enlargement, which is necessary for allowing a large-enough outflow cannula size.

5. The midesophageal long-axis view subtends which walls of the left ventricle?
   A. Anterior and posterior.
   B. Lateral and anteroseptal.
   C. Inferior and anterior.
   D. Septal and inferior.
   E. Posterior and anteroseptal.

6. The midesophageal intercommissural view cuts through which portions of the mitral valve?

A. The middle scallop of the posterior leaflet and the medial portion of the anterior leaflet.

B. The middle scallop of the posterior leaflet and the lateral portion of the anterior leaflet.

C. The lateral portion of the anterior leaflet and the medial portion of the posterior leaflet.

D. The medial commissure and the lateral commissure.

E. The lateral commissure and the medial portion of the anterior leaflet.

7. When the left ventricle is underfilled, what happens to end-systolic volume (ESV) and ejection fraction (EF)?

A. Increased ESV, increased EF.

B. Decreased ESV, increased EF.

C. Increased ESV, decreased EF.

D. Decreased ESV, decreased EF.

E. No change in ESV, increased EF.

8. Immediately after implantation of a stented bioprosthesis, the most common transient abnormality is:

A. Small amounts of periprosthetic regurgitation.

B. Immobility of valve prosthetic leaflets.

C. Significant central prosthetic regurgitation.

D. LV outflow tract obstruction by prosthetic stents.

E. Dehiscence of the prosthesis.

9. If resistance is felt when trying to remove the TEE probe, the following measures should be taken:

A. Pull firmly with increasing pressure in a cranial direction.

B. Obtain gastroscopic assistance for removal.

C. Push the probe in further before attempting to remove it again.

D. Retroflex the probe tip and pull steadily and firmly.

E. Reopen the chest to remove suture material.

10. A 47-year-old woman in the intensive care unit, having just undergone aortic valve replacement (AVR) or mitral repair, develops decreased cardiac output, increased pulmonary artery wedge pressure, decreased oxygenation, and increased ventricular ectopy in the presence of hyperdynamic LV function. What can this be caused by?

A. Hypovolemia.

B. Massive myocardial infarction.

C. Systolic anterior motion of the mitral valve.

D. Protamine reaction.

E. Blood loss.

11. The physician taking care of a 66-year-old female patient did TEE imaging while the patient was still on cardiopulmonary bypass (CPB) and claimed that, as long as the aortic cross clamp was off, the assessment of LV EF would be the same as it would be in the postoperative period. Which statement is correct?

A. EF postoperatively will be higher than it looks while on CPB.

B. EF postoperatively will be lower than it looks while on CPB.

C. EF postoperatively may be higher or lower than it looks while on CPB.

12. A 66-year-old man has a history of infarction from distal left anterior descending coronary artery (LAD) occlusion with some apical hypokinetic segments. What is the most useful TEE imaging plane to see the LV apex?

A. Midesophageal long axis.

B. Transgastric short axis of the left ventricle.

C. Midesophageal four chamber.

D. Transgastric long axis of the left ventricle.

13. A 70-year-old man presents with chest and back pain and computerized tomographic imaging (CT) discovers a localized dissection of the ascending aorta. On arrival for the intraoperative TEE, you find aortic dilation but no dissection. What is the cause of the "blind spot" for TEE imaging?

A. The esophagus is between the aorta and the right mainstem bronchus.

B. The esophagus is between the aorta and the trachea.

C. The trachea is between the aorta and the esophagus.

D. The right mainstem bronchus is between the aorta and the esophagus.

14. Which imaging plane is most useful for determining whether posterior leaflet prolapse involves the medial, middle, or lateral scallop?
  A. The midesophageal long axis.
  B. The midesophageal two chamber.
  C. The midesophageal four chamber.
  D. The transgastric long axis.

15. Which is not a criterion for severe mitral regurgitation?
  A. A vena contracta of greater than or equal to 5 mm diameter.
  B. A regurgitant orifice area (ROA) of greater than or equal to 0.4 cm².
  C. Systolic reversal of pulmonary vein flow velocity.
  D. A density of the continuous-wave Doppler recording in systole equal to the antegrade signal.

A 62-year-old man develops new heart failure 8 weeks after AVR for endocarditis with aortic valve vegetations (Fig. 13-1).

16. What is the hemodynamic problem causing this patient's recurrent heart failure?
  A. Mitral regurgitation.
  B. Aortic regurgitation.
  C. Aortic prosthesis dehiscence.
  D. Aortic and mitral regurgitation.
  E. A coronary fistula to the LV outflow tract.

17. In the same patient, what is the mechanism of the valve process (Fig. 13-1)?
  A. Leaflet flail.
  B. Perforation of the leaflet.
  C. Disruption of sutures.
  D. Aortic dissection.
  E. LV dilation.

A 70-year-old woman with previous aortic and tricuspid valve replacements presents with leg edema and ascites, with clear lung fields. The frames in Figure 13-2 are recorded from a midesophageal transverse four-chamber view at a multiplane angle of 0 degrees, rotated to the right to view the right atrium and right ventricle.

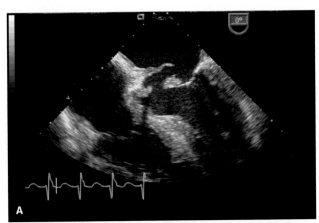

Fig. 13-1A

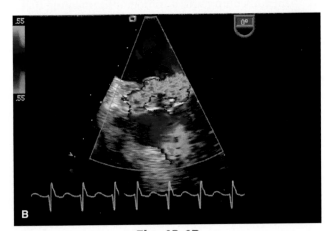

Fig. 13-1B

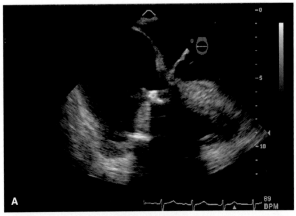

Fig. 13-2A

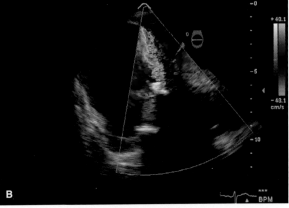

Fig. 13-2B

18. From where is the high velocity flow originating?
- A. Left ventricle.
- B. Aorta.
- C. Medial to the tricuspid prosthesis.
- D. Anterior to the tricuspid prosthesis.
- E. Right atrium.

19. What are the expected findings on abdominal examination?
- A. Normal liver and spleen.
- B. Hepatomegaly with nodularity.
- C. Hepatomegaly with pulsations.
- D. Small liver with splenomegaly.
- E. Normal liver with splenomegaly.

20. A patient undergoes aortic valve surgery and has the diastolic color image in Figure 13-3 recorded from the midesophageal long-axis view at 102 degrees, zoomed in to show the flow around the aortic valve. The two calipers marked (+) measure an aliasing radius of 0.63 cm.

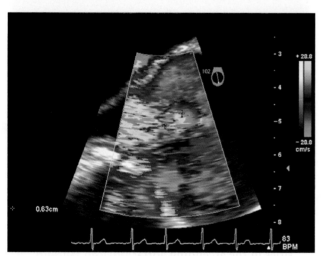

Fig. 13-3

Presuming the continuous-wave Doppler recording through this aortic regurgitation signal would have shown a maximum velocity of 4.0 m/sec, what is the maximum instantaneous ROA?
- A. 0.18 cm^2.
- B. 0.28 cm^2.
- C. 17.9 mm.
- D. 0.46 cm^2.

21. A 55-year-old woman was studied with a prepump TEE just prior to tricuspid and mitral valve surgery. Figure 13-4 was recorded from a long-axis view of the atrial septum after intravenous injection of agitated saline.

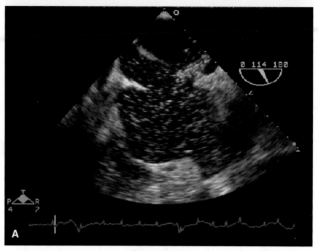

Fig. 13-4A

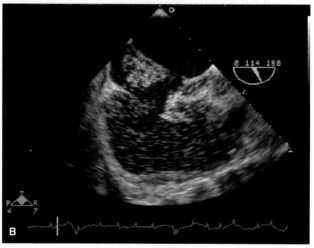

Fig. 13-4B

What can be said about the presence of shunting?
- A. There is a right-to-left shunt.
- B. There is a left-to-right shunt.
- C. There is no shunt.
- D. There is a bidirectional shunt.

CASE 2:

An 85-year-old woman, who is 5 feet 8 inches tall, and has controlled hypertension, began to have shortness of breath playing tennis with her 55-year-old friends. Evaluation found atrial fibrillation, pulmonary hypertension, trivial coronary narrowing, and mitral regurgitation.

33. Video 13-2A and B show her intraoperative transesophageal echocardiographic images in a transverse midesophageal view at 0 degree multiplane angle, before CPB (prepump). Video 13-2C shows her prepump intraoperative midesophageal imaging TEE images at a multiplane angle of 122 degrees. Video 13-2D shows her prepump midesophageal intraoperative images at a multiplane angle of 63 degrees. What is the primary mechanism of mitral regurgitation?
    A. Prolapse of the medial scallop of the mitral posterior leaflet.
    B. Flail of the middle scallop of the posterior leaflet.
    C. Restricted leaflet motion of the anterior leaflet.
    D. Flail of the A2 portion of the anterior leaflet.
    E. Bileaflet prolapse.

34. Video 13-2B shows a color Doppler image of the mitral regurgitation recorded in a transverse midesophageal imaging plane, from which the maximum aliasing radius was measured at 1.1 cm. The wall constraint was measured to be 90 degrees, meaning that exactly half of the hemispheric velocity isopleth converging into the regurgitant orifice was constrained by the adjacent ventricular wall. The maximum mitral regurgitation (MR) systolic velocity recorded by continuous-wave Doppler (not shown) was 5.5 m/sec.

    What is the regurgitant orifice area (ROA)
    A. 0.38 cm^2.
    B. 0.76 cm^2.
    C. 0.31 cm^2.
    D. 415 cm^2.
    E. 75.5 cm^2.

35. In addition to the mechanism of mitral regurgitation shown in this patient, the same jet direction might be caused by what type of MR (Video 13-2B)?
    A. Posterior leaflet restriction.
    B. Ischemic (functional MR).
    C. Anterior leaflet prolapse.
    D. Anterior leaflet flail.
    E. Posterior leaflet perforation.

36. Video 13-2E shows a transgastric short-axis view of the left ventricle. What is the approximate EF?
    A. 80%.
    B. 60%.
    C. 40%.
    D. 30%.
    E. 20%.

37. Videos 13-2E-G show the aortic valve. What would you conclude from these data?
    A. The aortic valve is normal.
    B. There is severe aortic stenosis and mild aortic regurgitation.
    C. There is mild aortic stenosis with mild to moderate aortic regurgitation.
    D. There is severe aortic stenosis and no aortic regurgitation.
    E. There is mild aortic stenosis and severe aortic regurgitation.

38. While the primary mission of the surgery is the mitral valve, what should be done to the aortic valve during the surgery?
    A. Nothing.
    B. Aortic bioprosthesis.
    C. Aortic homograft.
    D. Conduit replacement of the aorta with aortic valve resuspension.
    E. Mechanical aortic valve replacement.

39. Video 13-2H shows the proximal aortic arch. What is the abnormality shown?
    A. A large aortic atheroma.
    B. A large dissection flap.
    C. An intramural hematoma.
    D. A small dissection flap.
    E. A small aortic atheroma.

40. Video 13-2C and Figure 13-8 show the ascending aorta on the prepump intraoperative TEE. As indicated, the diameter of the tubular ascending aorta is 4.0 cm. What is the echo-free space posterior to the ascending aorta highlighted by the arrow Figure 13-8?
    A. A double lumen consistent with a small localized aortic dissection.
    B. A pericardial cyst.
    C. A reflection of pericardium with small amount of normal fluid.
    D. Part of the right upper pulmonary vein.
    E. The transverse portion of the hemiazygous vein.

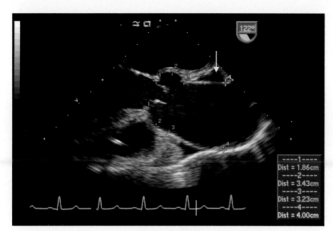

Fig. 13-8

41. What should be done surgically with the aorta and the surrounding area in this woman?

A. Nothing, the aorta is normal.

B. Nothing, the aorta is mildly dilated.

C. Ascending aortic replacement with a conduit.

D. Patch aortoplasty to reduce the wall stress and biopsy of the cyst.

E. Exploration of the area and excision of the cyst. Her mitral valve could not be repaired, due to extensive flail and friable leaflet tissue, so a bioprosthesis was implanted. The aortic valve and aorta were not touched surgically.

CASE 3:

A 37-year-old man has dyspnea and exertional presyncope. His TTE shows congenital aortic stenosis with a mean maximum gradient 52 mm Hg, mean gradient 28 mm Hg, and calculated valve area 0.77 cm². Angiography showed normal coronaries, although the aortic valve gradient was not re-evaluated at catheterization. As he undergoes TEE in the operating room, after the chest incision but before cannulation for CPB, the aortic valve gradient and short-axis planimetry suggest that the stenosis is not as bad as had been depicted on the preoperative studies. Video 13-3A shows a midesophageal long-axis view at 128 degrees, of the aortic valve, showing the doming in systole. Video 13-3B shows a similar view at 158 degrees with color Doppler, showing no significant aortic regurgitation. Figure 13-9A shows a continuous-wave Doppler recording through the aortic valve showing a mean gradient of only 14 mm Hg and a maximum gradient of 35 mm Hg. Figure 13-9B shows a short-axis view at 74

degrees with planimetry of the valve, calculating a valve area of 3.6 cm². Video 13-3C shows a short-axis view of the aortic valve at 49 degrees with the valve in motion. Figure 13-9C shows a short-axis view at 74 degrees with planimetry of the valve, calculating a valve area of 2.95 cm².

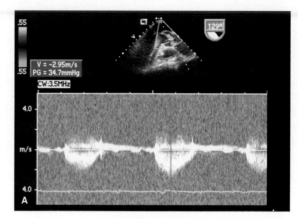

Fig. 13-9A

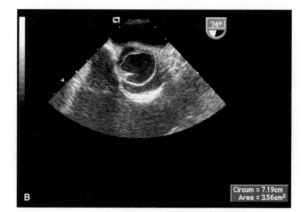

Fig. 13-9B

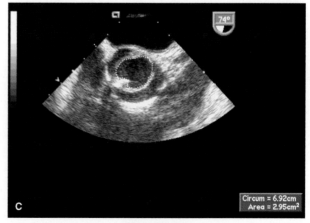

Fig. 13-9C

42. How severe is the aortic stenosis?
  A. Mild.
  B. Moderate.
  C. Moderately severe.
  D. Severe.

43. What should we do now?
  A. Close the chest and do no surgery.
  B. Replace the valve anyway.
  C. Do a valve sparing repair.
  D. Call in another cardiac surgeon.

ANSWERS

1. ANSWER: A. The right coronary artery is located anteriorly within the sinuses of Valsalva, which is the highest portion of the aorta (farthest off the ground) with the patient in the supine position for a midsternal thoracotomy. Therefore, air which enters the heart during open-heart surgery is pushed by pressure into this coronary preferentially. This occurs more commonly in mitral repair than other types of heart surgery, because of insufflation of the left ventricle (filling it with fluid under pressure) done to examine leaflet coaptation. Most cases of coronary air embolization can be treated conservatively. Sometimes, it is necessary to put the patient back on cardiopulmonary bypass (CPB), or to treat ventricular arrhythmias with medicines.

2. ANSWER: C. Epicardial echo is an alternative imaging modality. The need for intraoperative echo still exists for those who have a contraindication to blind transesophageal echo (TEE) passage, and these can readily be accomplished by epicardial echo. A standard transthoracic echo transducer is placed within a sterile sleeve with ultrasound gel inside the sleeve for elimination of air.

3. ANSWER: C. Continuous-wave Doppler recordings of mitral flow using TEE can accurately be recorded and relied upon for calculation of mitral gradients. Recording aortic valve gradients is less reliable. Sometimes, they can be recorded from the deep transgastric views, but the results are often underestimates of the true values. All gradients are affected by loading conditions, but such changes can be corrected for, by understanding hemodynamics, especially altered cardiac output and preload. Electrocautery does interfere with ultrasound recordings, but most transesophageal imaging can be obtained in between those interruptions.

4. ANSWER: C. Intraoperative TEE is an important monitoring tool in patients undergoing implantation of an left ventricular assist device (LVAD). The presence of aortic regurgitation makes an LVAD ineffective by creating a loop of ineffective flow. The presence of left ventricle (LV) enlargement and mitral regurgitation (MR) are irrelevant to the placement of the device. Placement of the inflow LVAD cannula into the left ventricle does not require TEE guidance. The presence and severity of tricuspid regurgitation (TR) are not important objectives of TEE imaging.

5. ANSWER: E. Like the apical transthoracic view of the same name, the midesophageal long-axis view usually cuts through the posterior and anteroseptal walls. This imaging plane is usually obtained at a multiplane angle of about 130 degrees (range 110–150 degrees).

6. ANSWER: D. The medial commissure and the lateral commissure. This view is usually obtained at a multiplane angle of about 60 degrees (range 35–75 degrees).

7. ANSWER: B. The hypovolemic patient usually has a small LV end-systolic size with increased ejection fraction (EF). The increased EF probably results from sympathetic stimulation, an attempt to maintain stroke volume despite the reduced end-diastolic volume. The small end-systolic LV size is probably the most reliable visual guide to the presence of underfilling.

8. ANSWER: A. It is common to see one or more small color jets of periprosthetic regurgitation early after cessation of CPB. When small, most of these resolve progressively after protamine administration, within a few hours.

9. ANSWER: C. A TEE probe may occasionally become looped, with its tip turned superiorly within the esophagus, up toward the patient's head. Traction of the probe to pull it out may cause the esophageal wall to tear. However, if the probe is advanced further, the loop comes out after it gains more room within the stomach, and the entire probe can then be extracted.

10. ANSWER: C. Hypovolemia, blood loss, and a protamine reaction would have lower wedge pressure. Massive myocardial infarction would not have hyperdynamic LV function. Systolic anterior motion (SAM) is a common (a few percent) complication of mitral valve repair, particularly when the LV cavity is small and hyperdynamic, catecholamine medications are being administered, and the posterior leaflet is redundant. Mitral SAM has also been reported after aortic valve replacement (AVR), probably because of the LV hypertrophy and the reduction in LV cavity size from relief of increased afterload. Initial treatment should consist of intravascular volume replacement, cessation of catecholamines (beta$_1$-agonists), appropriate diagnosis by TEE, and sometimes blood pressure support with phenylephrine.

11. ANSWER: C. Often the heart is underfilled on the pump, with lower cavity size in systole and diastole than in the ambulatory state, and therefore a higher EF.

However, on the pump, the patient may have metabolic abnormalities, or may have transient ischemia making the EF lower than it will be later when the patient has been weaned from CPB.

12. ANSWER: D. The transgastric short axis of the left ventricle does not cut through the apex. The midesophageal four-chamber view often foreshortens the left ventricle, and passes anterior and superior to the apex; what is seen is a pseudoapex which is really the anterior wall near but not at the apex. The midesophageal long axis view is not as likely to be foreshortened; but it is difficult to get a view of the true LV apex in many patients. Therefore, the transgastric long axis of the left ventricle is the preferred view.

13. ANSWER: C. The trachea is between the aorta and the esophagus. Because air provides a relatively poor propagation of ultrasound, the trachea does not transmit the reflecting images from the probe in the esophagus through the trachea to the mid ascending aorta.

14. ANSWER: B. Sometimes called the "intercommissural view," this plane is parallel to a line connecting the medial and lateral commissures of the mitral valve. Structural imaging or color flow information can be obtained using this view to make a determination of which portion of the anterior or posterior leaflet is abnormal. Arranged in the normal way with the inferior LV wall to the left of the screen, the medial scallop (P3) is located to the left on the upper portion of the screen, the middle scallop (P2) in the midupper part of the screen, and the lateral scallop (P1) to the upper right (Fig. 13-10).

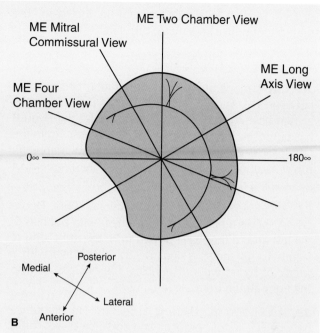

(Reprinted from Shanewise JS, Cheung AT, Aronson S, et al. Guidelines for performing a comprehensive intraoperative multiplane transesophageal echocardiographic examination recommendations of the American Society of Echocardiography Council on Intraoperative Echocardiography. *J Am Soc Echocardiogr.* 1999;12:884–900, with permission from Elsevier.)

Fig. 13-10B

15. ANSWER: A. The valid criterion for severe MR is a vena contracta of greater than or equal to 7 mm diameter. The other criteria listed are correct ones for the threshold of severe MR.

16. ANSWER: A; 17. ANSWER: B. The midesophageal transverse images in Figure 13-1 show that this patient has a perforation in the anterior mitral leaflet. This was likely caused by the jet of aortic regurgitation that was presumedly present prior to the AVR. Such a "jet lesion" causes endocardial abrasion of the LV surface of the base of the anterior mitral leaflet, allowing infection to set up locally, which may cause a perforation, leading to the MR, which is seen in the color flow image.

18. ANSWER: C. 19. ANSWER: C. The patient has a partially dehisced tricuspid prosthesis, with a periprosthetic leak of TR, located medial to the valve. For this reason, his exam would show pulsatile hepatomegaly. The key in this case is to understand the imaging plane, which is stated in the question given. Note that the right atrium is very large and that the interatrial septum bows toward the left atrium due to right atrial hypertension. The anterior mitral leaflet is shown in the image, while the aortic prosthesis is not shown.

20. ANSWER: A. The correct answer to the question is 0.18 cm². The formula is two times π, times the radius squared, times the aliasing velocity (Nyquist limit),

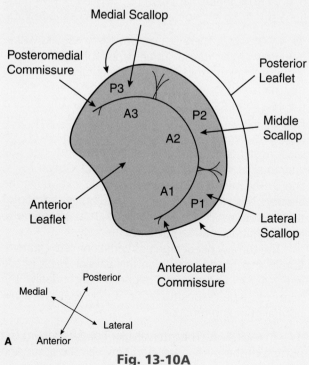

Fig. 13-10A

divided by the maximum velocity. In this case, the regurgitant orifice area (ROA) calculates to 0.18 cm^2

$$ROA = 2\pi r^2 v/V_{max}.$$

This is moderate aortic regurgitation because it is between 0.1 and 0.2 cm^2. Note that the size of the aliased flow convergence is larger because the Nyquist has purposely been decreased to 28.8 cm/sec (from the nominal 50–60 cm/sec level used for spatial mapping); this was done in order to make the measurement of the aliasing radius more feasible and accurate.

21. ANSWER: D. There is a bidirectional shunt. Figure 13-4A shows a positive contrast effect with bubbles in the left atrium that have passed from the right atrium. Figure 13-4B shows a negative contrast effect with a streak of blood without bubbles that has passed into the right atrium from the left atrium.

22. ANSWER: B. There is a 64 mm Hg difference between LV systolic pressure and aortic pressure. This is a patient with aortic valve stenosis in addition to MR. The deep transgastric views are the usual and best ones with which to record LV outflow velocities using TEE. Figure 13-5 shows that the cursor extends through the left ventricle to the LV outflow tract. In addition, the continuous-wave recording itself shows a key factor there is a blank period lasting about 80 milliseconds, during isovolumic relaxation. This blank period on the tracing starts immediately at the cessation of the AS signal, occurring at the time of aortic valve closure. It ends at the beginning of the mitral valve antegrade flow signal. The separation of these two events in time, separated by isovolumic relaxation, confirms the systolic jet to be AS, not MR or TR.

23. ANSWER: D; 24. ANSWER: C. This is a patient without fever or any signs of infection. He has a congenital bicuspid aortic valve of the horizontal type, with fusion of what would have been the right and left coronary cusps. In patients like this, the conjoined cusp has a longer length of its free edge, causing it to prolapse back into the outflow tract, causing aortic regurgitation. His right coronary artery is normal, and well-visualized on Figure 13-6.

25. ANSWER: C. Figure 13-7 shows artifacts from the electrocautery. Note that these artifacts extend across tissue planes, appearing as a stripe through the aorta and left ventricle. The discoloration of the external surface of the ascending aorta was not related to this image.

26. ANSWER: B. There is mild TR. This is based on spatial mapping alone. Not shown here is that the mitral repair looks OK, with only trivial MR. No vegetations were noted.

27. ANSWER: D. He has become volume depleted and hypotensive. All valve lesions are load-dependent, especially TR and MR with TR being the most load-dependent of all of them. Many ambulatory patients have excess sympathetic tone during heart failure with activation of the renin-angiotensin system and the sympathetic nervous system. This patient was hypertensive at the time of admission. In the next few days, he was probably diuresed and put on various vasodilators. In the operating room, he may have been volume depleted, at least, relative to his hemodynamics when he initially was admitted. Anesthesia lyses sympathetic tone, often resulting in a drop in systemic and pulmonary arteriolar resistance; therefore, some lesions decrease in severity. This accounts for the reduction in the severity of TR. The severity of the valve dysfunction seen under "street conditions" is more likely to be of use in deciding long-term plans like valve surgery.

28. ANSWER: A. There is functional TR from apical tethering of normal leaflets. When RV enlargement occurs from any cause, the normal tricuspid leaflets become apically tethered, a feature of "functional TR," similar to functional MR that occurs in ischemic heart disease or cardiomyopathy when the mitral valve is tethered apically by the LV enlargement.

29. ANSWER: C. There is an abscess of the atrial septum near the aortic prosthesis. It is obviously a pulsatile mass with continuous flow within a cystic area. The history of infection and a previous prosthetic valve helps here. From Video 13-1C, we cannot determine exactly what type of flow is present, where it came from, or where it is exiting. Video 13-1D suggests that the flow in the atrial septum comes from the left ventricle. Note that it is systolic, with expansion of the mass due to transmission of flow from ventricular pressure. There is no flow in the right atrium, so it is not an AV fistula or a Gerbode VSD.

30. ANSWER: B. There is a periprosthetic abscess within the intervalvular fibrosa. Three-dimensional echo allows postexamination exploration of different imaging planes than had been found during active imaging, especially in the operating room. The images show that the abscess extends almost 180 degrees around the prosthesis, and extends superiorly along the area of the sinuses of Valsalva posteriorly. This is why it extended up into the interatrial septum as shown previously in Videos 13-1C and D. The intervalvular fibrosa is indeed involved in the abscess. This structure is part of the fibrous skeleton of the heart, to which the aortic valve is attached anteriorly, and the mitral valve is attached posteriorly.

The surgery needed begins with complete exoneration of the infected tissue. In this patient, most of the intervalvular fibrosa was débrided. Secondarily, the heart must be reconstructed in a way that will allow normal pumping function.

31. ANSWER: A. The intervalvular fibrosa contains the portion of the cardiac skeleton between the aortic and mitral valves, and represents a portion of the annulus of both valves.

32. ANSWER: A. Actually, the homograft is less available, and more difficult to implant than a standard prosthesis, and the systolic gradient from a homograft is lower than a stented prosthetic valve of the same size. There is often trivial regurgitation of either a homograft or a stented bioprosthesis. There is an advantage of lower rates of persistent infection with a homograft. Videos 13-1I and J show the results of surgery on the postpump TEE, with no TR or AR, and only mild MR. Note that the normal homograft has a unique appearance, which is different than stented aortic prostheses. Note the double density at the walls of the homograft tissue. This results from its implantation as an "inclusion cylinder" which includes the walls of the aortic sinuses from the donor. The band of soft tissue between the double densities should be relatively uniform in thickness and free of any flow in that space demonstrable by color Doppler.

KEY POINTS:

■ This case shows severe perivalvular regurgitation and an abscess that started around the aortic prosthesis, in the intervalvular fibrosa, and extended up into the atrial septum. It was fixed by extensive debridement of infected tissue and placement of an aortic homograft, with its posterior tissue accessible for attaching the mitral valve, which itself was not infected.

■ Abscesses of the heart most commonly occur in the area of an infected prosthesis.

■ The patient also had severe functional TR at the time of admission; though it diminished to mild TR prior to the surgery, due to diuresis and lysis of sympathetic tone by the anesthesia, the risk of postoperative TR warranted tricuspid annuloplasty.

33. ANSWER: B. There is a flail of the middle scallop of the posterior leaflet. Both long-axis views show an untethered portion of the posterior leaflet reflecting chordal rupture. The anterior leaflet is normal. Video 13-2D is the intercommissural view. Though the left ventricle is forshortened, the image is aligned parallel to a line connecting the medial commissure and the lateral commissure. The medial commissure is on the left side of the image and the lateral commissure is on the right. The image shows that the middle scallop of the posterior leaflet is the primary abnormality. The magnitude (width) of the flail is very large, almost 2 cm in medial-lateral diameter.

34. ANSWER: A. The correct answer is 0.38 cm^2. The formula for ROA, prior to correcting for wall constraint, is:

$$ROA = 2\pi \underline{r}^2 v / V_{max}.$$

The term v is the aliasing velocity derived from the color bar scale setting shown on the image, which is 55 cm/sec in this case. The value for π is 3.14, a constant. V_{max} is 550 cm/sec; keeping all units in centimeters.

So: the <u>uncorrected</u> ROA = 2 × 3.14 × 1.1 × 1.1 × 55/550 which is equal to 0.76 cm^2. The way to correct for wall constraint is to divide the angle, in this case 90 degrees, by 180 degrees, implying that only 50 percent of the hemisphere has its surface area involved with flow at that velocity. So, the presence of an aliasing pattern with wall constraint leads us to multiply the uncorrected ROA by the observed angle divided by 180 degrees. In this case, the constraint angle of 90 degrees, derives a ratio of ½ (90/180). So the ROA is one-half of what it would have been if the flow convergence with the same radius had no wall constraint. Therefore, the calculated ROA is 0.38 cm^2. Severe MR is defined as an ROA > 0.40 cm^2.

35. ANSWER: E. The correct answer is posterior leaflet perforation. Posterior leaflet restriction, anterior leaflet flail, and an anterior leaflet prolapse would usually cause a posterior jet direction. In ischemic (functional) MR, the jet is most commonly central in direction, and sometimes posteriorly directed.

36. ANSWER: B. The correct answer is 60%. The EF on this patient appears normal, which is often quoted at 55–65%.

37. ANSWER: C. There is mild aortic stenosis with mild to moderate aortic regurgitation. Notice the anterior leaflet doming of the anterior portion of the valve in Video 13-2G, and the restriction of opening of the right coronary cusp in the short-axis view of Video 13-2F. Not shown here are the data from the preoperative transthoracic continuous-wave Doppler recording, which showed a maximum systolic velocity of 2.2 m/sec.

38. ANSWER: A. Most experts would not replace the aortic valve in this case. This threshold would usually be aortic regurgitation that is at least moderately severe (3+) or aortic stenosis that is at least moderate (valve area of less than about 1.3 cm^2). Remembering this patient's age of 85 years, the threshold for doing concomitant surgery on her aortic valve, "while we are there" for the primary mission of the mitral surgery, might be higher than in a younger patient.

39. ANSWER: E. The correct answer is "a small aortic atheroma." This aortic atheroma protrudes only 1–2 mm from the intimal surface which seems smooth and normal in all other areas than the one location. Atheromas that protrude into the lumen by 4 mm or more, and ones that show mobility, are considered severe, and are associated with a marked increase in perioperative mortality, mostly from atheroembolic events that shower cholesterol plaques to the liver, kidneys, brain, and skin.

The embolic risk of this mild atheroma is low, though risk of atheroemboli is increased by the patient's age.

40. *ANSWER: C;* **41.** *ANSWER: B.* The images show a reflection of the pericardium with a small amount of normal fluid. Although her aorta is abnormal with mild enlargement, most experts would not replace the aorta or even do an elliptical aortoplasty unless it was larger than this. The threshold for doing so might be lower as a concomitant procedure "while we are there," and it might be lower because she does have some effacement of the sinotubular junction. With her height of about 174 cm, the ratio of the cross-sectional area of her aorta to her height in meters would not be over 10, unless her aortic diameter was over 4.7 cm. Using this ratio to obtain a height-corrected threshold for surgery is a fairly aggressive criterion but it does improve on an arbitrary diameter of 5.0 cm that does not correct for body size.

KEY POINTS:

- Having identified P2 prolapse with MR quantitated to be moderately severe, with a ROA of 0.38 cm^2 and a normal left ventricular ejection fraction (LVEF), a mitral valve repair was anticipated. However, friable mitral valve tissue in this elderly lady led to implantation of a mitral prosthesis.

- AVR was not felt to be required in an elderly woman with nonsevere aortic regurgitation. The natural history of degenerative aortic regurgitation is to remain stable for many years and the additional risk of a two-valve surgery would significant.

42. *ANSWER: C;* **43.** *ANSWER: B.* In this case, the skin incision was closed and the patient was awakened with the news that his aortic stenosis was not as bad as originally thought. However, over the next few months, he became even more symptomatic, with exertional angina and dyspnea. Repeat transthoracic echo again showed aortic stenosis with peak/mean gradients of 65/38 mm Hg, and aortic valve area = 0.8 cm^2. The patient underwent successful AVR 8 months after the initial surgery that was abbreviated. His symptoms resolved after the valve replacement.

In this case, the aortic stenosis is best characterized by the transthoracic echocardiography. One could call it severe, on the basis of the valve area of 0.77 cm^2, or moderately severe, on the basis of the mean gradient derived by transthoracic echo of 28–38 mm Hg. The continuity equation for valve area calculation is well-validated and reliable, relying on recording the maximum velocity using the highest of multiple windows. The TEE-derived gradient recorded in the operating room was an underestimate of true valvular velocity; see figures. Short-axis planimetry of the valve area has also been validated in senile calcified valves, but is less reliable due to gain dependence. Particularly problematic in congenital noncalcified aortic stenosis, short-axis planimetry of valve area may overestimate valve area if the plane cuts through the "base of dome," as was done here.

KEY POINTS:

- Listen to the patient. Symptoms do not result from mild aortic stenosis.

- Gradients are not the whole story and maximum velocity recordings may underestimate the gradient if they are angulated.

- Short-axis planimetry may overestimate valve area if it cuts through the "base of the dome."

- TEE often underestimates aortic valve gradients.

- Talk to the clinician who knows the patient if any change occurs in operative plan.

SUGGESTED READINGS

Obarski TP, Loop FD, Cosgrove DM, et al. Frequency of acute myocardial infarction in valve repairs vs. valve replacement for pure mitral regurgitation. *Am J Cardiol.* 1990;65:887–890.

Pu M, Vandervoort PM, Griffin BP, et al. Quantification of mitral regurgitation by the proximal convergence method using transesophageal echocardiography clinical validation of a geometric correction for proximal flow constraint. *Circulation.* 1995;92: 2169–2177.

Shanewise JS, Cheung AT, Aronson S, et al. Guidelines for performing a comprehensive intraoperative multiplane transesophageal echocardiographic examination recommendations of the American Society of Echocardiography Council on Intraoperative Echocardiography. *J Am Soc Echocardiogr.* 1999;12: 884–900.

Stewart WJ, Currie PJ, Salcedo EE, et al. Evaluation of mitral leaflet motion by echocardiography and jet direction by Doppler color flow mapping to determine the mechanism of mitral regurgitaiton. *J Am Coll Cardiol.* 1992;20: 1353–1361.

Zoghbi WA, Enriquez-Sarano M, Foster E, et al. Recommendations for evaluation of the severity of native valvular regurgitation with two-dimensional and Doppler echocardiography. *J Am Soc Echocardiogr.* 2003;16:777–802.

Dyssynchrony Evaluation/AV Optimization

Victoria Delgado and Jeroen J. Bax

1. Which of the following statements about the echocardiographic assessment of cardiac dyssynchrony in patients with heart failure is correct?
   A. Atrioventricular (AV) dyssynchrony can be identified by a long left ventricular (LV) filling time (LVFT) (>40%).
   B. Interventricular dyssynchrony is defined by a prolonged delay between the right ventricular (RV) and LV ejections as assessed with pulsed-wave Doppler echocardiography (≥40 milliseconds).
   C. An early diastolic notching of the interventricular septum at M-mode LV parasternal long-axis recordings is observed in patients with left bundle branch block and indicates LV dyssynchrony.
   D. Intra-LV dyssynchrony is observed only in patients with left bundle branch block, whereas interventricular dyssynchrony is observed only in patients with right bundle branch bock.

2. AV dyssynchrony is characterized by prolonged AV conduction. Which of the following echocardiographic signs can be observed?
   A. LV diastolic filling is reduced because atrial contraction occurs against a closed mitral valve.
   B. The diastolic LVFT lengthens as indicated by a relative early E wave on transmitral Doppler recordings.
   C. A truncated A wave is observed on transmitral Doppler recordings.
   D. The diastolic LVFT shortens with fusion of E and A waves.

3. Which is the echocardiographic method used to measure interventricular dyssynchrony?
   A. M-mode echocardiography, measuring the time delay between peak systolic thickening of the interventricular septum and the RV free wall.
   B. Pulsed-wave Doppler echocardiography, measuring the time delay between the onset of LV ejection and RV ejection.
   C. Continuous-wave Doppler echocardiography, measuring the time difference between closure of tricuspid valve and mitral valve.
   D. Tissue Doppler imaging (TDI), measuring the time delay between peak systolic velocity of the interventricular septum and the LV lateral wall.

4. LV dyssynchrony can be measured with M-mode echocardiography obtaining the so-called septal-to-posterior wall motion delay (SPWMD) index. Which of the following statements about this method is correct?
   A. This index is derived by measuring the time delay between the peak inward motion of the interventricular septum and the LV posterior wall.
   B. This index is measured by applying anatomic M-mode to the LV apical four-chamber view.
   C. A cutoff value of ≥65 milliseconds predicts favorable response to cardiac resynchronization therapy (CRT).
   D. This method is highly feasible in patients with ischemic heart failure with prior myocardial infarction of the posterolateral wall.

5. TDI techniques have been extensively used to quantify LV dyssynchrony. Which of the following statements about these methodologies is correct?
    A. Pulsed-wave TDI permits simultaneous interrogation of two opposing LV walls online.
    B. TDI techniques permit the angle-independent assessment of LV myocardial velocities.
    C. TDI data should be acquired at a frame rate of <90 frames/sec.
    D. LV dyssynchrony can be measured by calculating the time delay between peak systolic velocities of two or four opposing walls.

6. Which of the following recommendations to measure LV dyssynchrony with color-coded TDI is correct?
    A. Color-coded TDI data acquisition should be performed at a low frame rate (<90 frames/sec).
    B. The timing of LV ejection should be determined from the beginning to the end of the pulsed-wave Doppler recordings of the transmitral flow.
    C. LV dyssynchrony is calculated as the difference in time to isovolumic contraction velocity from opposing walls.
    D. The components of the velocity curve should be identified and include the isovolumic contraction velocity, the systolic wave (S), the early diastolic wave (E), and the late diastolic wave (A).

7. Which of the following sentences about the measurement of LV dyssynchrony based on color-coded TDI is correct?
    A. An opposing wall delay of ≥65 milliseconds predicts favorable response to CRT and long-term outcome.
    B. The standard deviation of time to peak systolic velocities of 12 segments of the LV apical two- and four-chamber views (basal, mid, and apical segments) yields the most accurate measurement of LV dyssynchrony.
    C. A standard deviation of time to peak systolic velocities of 12 LV segments of ≥65 milliseconds predicts clinical improvement after CRT.

D. A septal-to-lateral wall delay of ≥31 milliseconds predicts LV reverse remodeling after CRT.

8. TDI-derived strain rate imaging has been demonstrated to identify LV dyssynchrony. Which of the following sentences is correct?
    A. TDI-derived strain rate imaging evaluates myocardial displacement.
    B. TDI-derived strain rate imaging enables the measurement of time from QRS onset to peak strain in all LV segments (basal, mid, and apical) since this technique is not influenced by the insonation angle of the ultrasound beam.
    C. In patients with ischemic heart failure, TDI-derived strain rate imaging permits detection of myocardial segments with active contraction and segments that are passively tethered (myocardial scar).
    D. Applied to LV short-axis images, a time delay of ≥33 milliseconds between peak systolic strain of the septal wall and the posterior wall predicts acute improvement in LV stroke volume after CRT.

9. Which of the following sentences about LV dyssynchrony assessment with two-dimensional (2D) speckle tracking echocardiography is true?
    A. The measurement of time to peak strain with 2D speckle tracking echocardiography is highly dependent on the angle of insonation of the ultrasound beam.
    B. Two-dimensional speckle tracking echocardiography permits the assessment of LV dyssynchrony in the radial, circumferential, and longitudinal directions.
    C. A peak radial strain-time delay between the (antero) septal and the (postero) lateral region of ≥31 milliseconds predicts LV reverse remodeling.
    D. Two-dimensional speckle tracking echocardiography does not distinguish between myocardial segments with active contraction and myocardial segments passively tethered.

10. Three-dimensional (3D) echocardiography enables LV dyssynchrony assessment. Which of the following statements is correct?
    A. Currently, the evaluation of LV dyssynchrony with 3D echocardiography techniques relies only on qualitative assessment of LV wall motion of 3D full volume data.
    B. With triplane tissue synchronization imaging (TSI), the standard deviation of time to minimum systolic volume of 16 segments (so-called systolic dyssynchrony index [SDI]) is calculated to quantify LV dyssynchrony.
    C. With real-time 3D echocardiography, the time to peak systolic velocity of 16 segments is displayed in a polar map and time delays between two or four opposing walls as well as the standard deviation of 16 segments can be calculated.
    D. The presence of substantial LV dyssynchrony defined by an SDI of ≥6.4% measured with real-time 3D echocardiography or ≥33 milliseconds measured with triplane TSI predicts response to CRT.

11. Which of the following statements about AV delay optimization is correct?
    A. The optimal AV delay is the shortest AV interval without truncation of A wave.
    B. An optimized AV synchrony is achieved by the shortest AV delay with fusion of the E and A waves.
    C. In the optimal AV delay, the end of the left atrial contraction should coincide with the onset of the diastolic mitral regurgitation spectral signal.
    D. The optimal AV delay is the longest AV delay that permits the longest LVFT regardless of whether A-wave truncation occurs.

12. Which of the following echocardiographic signs can be observed when a short AV delay is programmed?
    A. Diastolic mitral regurgitation.
    B. E and A wave fusion on transmitral pulsed-wave Doppler recordings.
    C. Reduced LVFT.
    D. Truncated A wave on transmitral pulsed-wave Doppler recordings.

13. Which of the following echocardiographic methods can be used to optimize the AV delay?
    A. Pulsed-wave TDI, placing the sample volumes at the septal and lateral mitral annulus.
    B. M-mode recordings of the mitral annulus.
    C. Color-coded TDI, placing the sample volumes at the lateral wall of the left atrium and the LV lateral wall.
    D. Pulsed-wave Doppler recordings of the transmitral blood flow.

14. Which of the following statements about echocardiographic AV delay optimization is true?
    A. The Ritter's method can always be performed regardless of the duration of the intrinsic PR interval.
    B. The iterative method involves programming a long AV delay and then shortening it by 20-millisecond increments until the A wave is truncated.
    C. The peak rate of rise of LV pressure during isovolumic contraction, the so-called dP/dt_{max}, is the most feasible method to optimize the AV delay.
    D. The shortest velocity-time integral of the flow across the LV outflow tract indicates the optimal AV delay.

15. Which of the following sentences about interventricular (VV) delay optimization is true?
    A. The measurement of velocity-time integral of the LV outflow tract on pulsed-wave Doppler recordings can be used to optimize VV delay.
    B. Color-coded TDI is the most used method to optimize VV delay, placing the sample volumes at the basal segments of the free right ventricular wall and the LV lateral wall.
    C. The VV delay optimization can be performed only by electrocardiographic methods.
    D. M-mode recording of the LV parasternal long-axis view, measuring the time delays between the peak inward motion of the septum and the posterior wall, is highly feasible in patients with ischemic heart failure.

16. Based on Figure 14-1, which of the following sentences on AV dyssynchrony is true?

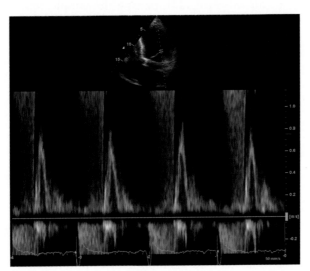

Fig. 14-1

A. The AV delay is optimal and maximizes diastolic LVFT by starting the LV contraction at the end of the A wave.

B. The AV delay is too short and the A wave is truncated.

C. The AV delay is too long and, consequently, the E and A waves are fused reducing the diastolic LVFT.

D. The AV delay cannot be assessed because the patient is in atrial fibrillation.

17. Figure 14-2 shows an example of LV dyssynchrony assessed with pulsed-wave TDI. Based on this example, which of the following statements is correct?

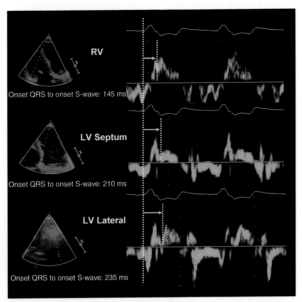

Fig. 14-2

A. Time from Q wave to onset of the first positive systolic velocity (isovolumic contraction) should be measured at the basal segments of the right ventricle, septum, and LV lateral wall.

B. There is substantial LV dyssynchrony indicated by the difference in systolic velocities of LV septal and lateral walls.

C. The measurement of the electromechanical delay in the septal wall is incorrect because the ultrasound beam is not aligned properly.

D. There is substantial interventricular dyssynchrony (RV free wall to LV lateral wall delay of 90 milliseconds) but not LV dyssynchrony with a time delay of 25 milliseconds between LV septal and lateral walls.

18. In Figure 14-3, LV dyssynchrony is evaluated with color-coded TDI. What conclusion can be drawn from this example?

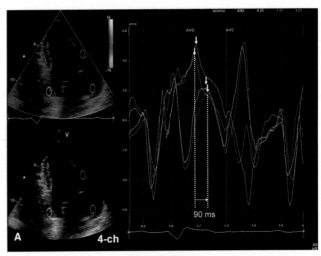

Fig. 14-3A

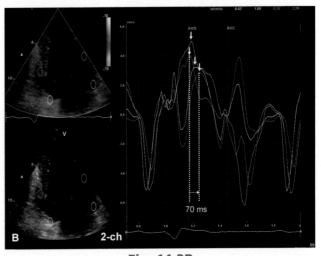

Fig. 14-3B

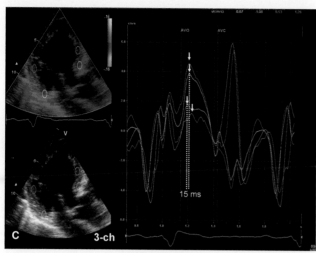

Fig. 14-3C

A. The likelihood of response to CRT is low.
B. The timing of LV ejection does not include the first positive peak velocity and, therefore, LV dyssynchrony cannot be evaluated.
C. There is substantial LV dyssynchrony with a maximum delay of 90 milliseconds between two opposing walls and, therefore, the likelihood of response to CRT is high.
D. The LV segments where the sample volumes are placed show very high systolic velocities indicating active contraction and, therefore, the likelihood of response to CRT is high.

19. Doppler-derived strain imaging has been proposed to measure LV dyssynchrony. What is incorrect about Figure 14-4?

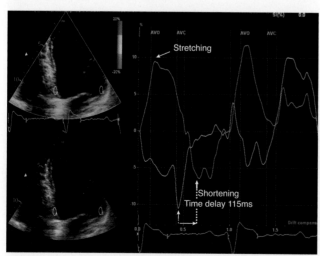

Fig. 14-4

A. There is substantial LV dyssynchrony with the lateral wall stretching while the septal wall shortens.
B. In this example, strain imaging is not the best method to assess LV dyssynchrony since the lateral wall seems to be tethered by the adjacent segments.
C. There is substantial LV dyssynchrony with a peak systolic strain-time delay of 115 milliseconds between the septal and the lateral walls.
D. Strain (rate) imaging enables the assessment of active myocardial contraction and reflects, therefore, myocardial viability.

20. LV dyssynchrony assessed with TDI-derived radial strain has been shown to be predictive of improvement in LV stroke volume after CRT. Which sentence about Figure 14-5 is correct?

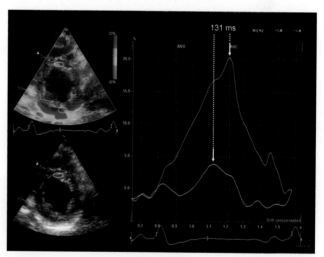

Fig. 14-5

A. The example shows circumferential strain-time curves and, therefore, LV dyssynchrony cannot be assessed.
B. Septal peak radial strain is earlier than the posterior peak radial strain indicating significant LV dyssynchrony.
C. The sample volumes are not correct and should be placed in the inferior and lateral walls.
D. Radial strain-time curves in this example are too noisy and, therefore, LV dyssynchrony assessment results are inaccurate.

21. Based on Figure 14-6, which of the following sentences about 2D speckle tracking is correct?

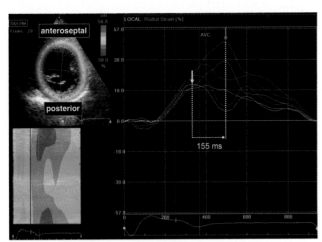

Fig. 14-6

A. LV dyssynchrony can only be assessed by measuring the time delay between peak radial strain of the anteroseptal segment and the posterior segment since those are the segments aligned along the ultrasound beam.

B. With this method, the latest activated segment can be identified and may be useful to indicate where the LV pacing lead should be placed.

C. There is no significant LV dyssynchrony since the time delay between peak radial strain of the anteroseptal and posterior segments is <130 milliseconds.

D. The low values of radial strain of the septal, anteroseptal, and anterior segments indicate that these segments are tethered by the adjacent segments and they do not show active contraction.

22. Triplane TSI permits to characterize LV mechanical activation. Based on Figure 14-7, which of the following statements is correct?

A. In patients with ischemic heart failure, triplane TSI is the best tool to distinguish those segments with active contraction from those that are passively tethered.

B. Activation time intervals from 16 LV segments (six basal, six mid, and four apical segments) are obtained simultaneously during the same heartbeat.

C. The site of maximal mechanical delay cannot be identified.

D. The TSI algorithm calculates time to peak myocardial systolic velocities in 12 LV segments and converts these time intervals into color codes.

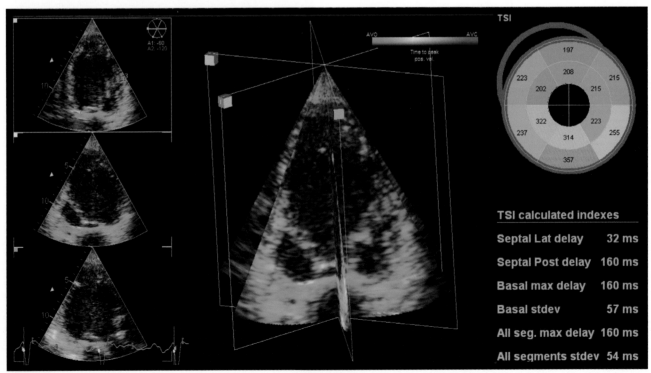

Fig. 14-7

23. Figure 14-8 illustrates the analysis of LV dyssynchrony with real-time 3D echocardiography. Which of the following sentences about this technique is correct?

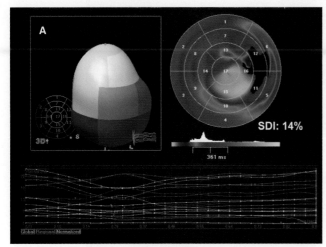

Fig. 14-8A

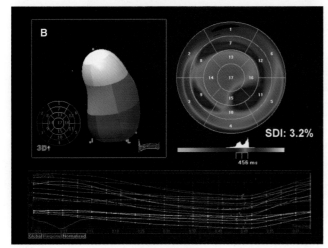

Fig. 14-8B

A. LV dyssynchrony is quantified by calculating the standard deviation of time to minimum systolic volume of 16 LV subvolumes, the so-called SDI.

B. The polar maps show the time to minimum systolic volume of the 16–17 LV subvolumes, but the latest activated region cannot be identified.

C. The time-volume curves indicate which segments show active contraction and which segments are tethered by the adjacent segments.

D. After 6-month follow-up (panel B), there is still substantial LV dyssynchrony.

24. The iterative method to optimize AV delay has been used in several single-center and randomized multicenter CRT studies. Based on the sequence shown in Figure 14-9, which of the following sentences is correct?

A. The sequence is incorrect since this method starts with the shortest AV delay and lengthens in 10-millisecond steps until the E and A waves are fused.

B. The optimal AV delay is 120 milliseconds.

C. The optimal AV delay is defined by the longest AV delay with truncation of the A wave.

D. This method cannot be applied if there is no mitral regurgitation signal.

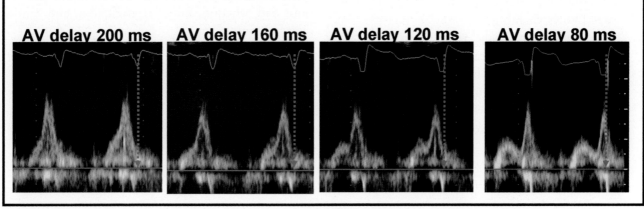

Fig. 14-9

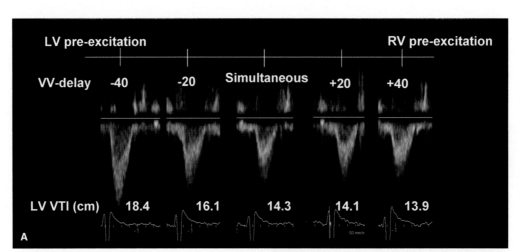

Fig. 14-10A

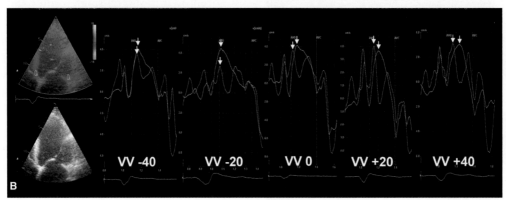

Fig. 14-10B

25. Optimization of VV delay can be performed with pulsed-wave Doppler recordings of the LV outflow tract, by measuring the cardiac output; and with TDI, by evaluating LV dyssynchrony. Based on Figure 14, which of the following statements is correct?

A. The VV delay that provides the highest cardiac output does not provide the smallest amount of LV dyssynchrony.

B. Prestimulation of the right ventricle usually provides the highest cardiac output.

C. In this example, the best VV delay should be set at −40 milliseconds (prestimulation of the LV) since it yields the highest cardiac output and the more LV synchronous contraction.

D. Once the optimal VV delay is programmed, it remains stable and no further adjustments are needed.

CASE 1:

A 56-year-old man with New York Heart Association heart failure functional class II was referred to the echocardiography laboratory to evaluate LV dimensions and function, mitral regurgitation, and cardiac dyssynchrony.

26. Based on Figure 14-11, what conclusions about cardiac dyssynchrony can be drawn?

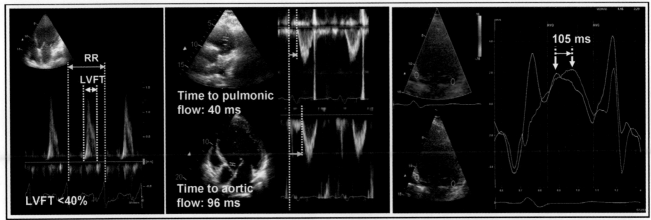

Fig. 14-11

A. The patient shows normal LV diastolic filling pattern and optimal AV synchrony.

B. There is a perfect interventricular synchrony with the onset of the RV ejection after the onset of the LV ejection.

C. Color-coded TDI image does not show LV dyssynchrony.

D. The patient shows a restrictive LV diastolic filling pattern with shortened diastolic LVFT (<40%) and significant interventricular and LV dyssynchrony.

27. On color Doppler images, the patient showed severe functional mitral regurgitation (Fig. 14-12A and Video 14-1A). Two-dimensional speckle tracking echocardiography was used to evaluate mechanical dyssynchrony between the LV segments underlying the papillary muscles (panel B) (Fig. 14-12B and Video 14-1B).

Which of the following statements regarding the assessment of mitral regurgitation in this patient is correct?

A. The ischemic etiology can be excluded because the most frequent cause of functional mitral regurgitation in patients with heart failure is isolated mitral annulus dilatation.

B. A significant reduction in mitral regurgitation can be observed by resynchronizing the LV segments underlying the papillary muscles.

C. Two-dimensional speckle tracking echocardiography cannot distinguish between segments with active contraction and segments that are tethered and, therefore, ischemic etiology cannot be excluded.

D. The evaluation of LV dyssynchrony should be performed at the level of the mitral valve (basal short-axis view).

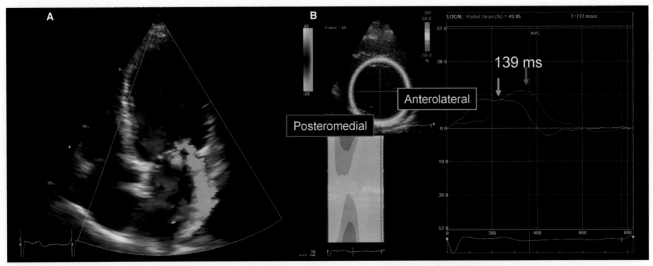

Fig. 14-12A   **Fig. 14-12B**

CASE 2:

An 87-year-old man was admitted at the emergency department because of heart failure symptoms 1 week after dual-chamber pacemaker implantation. Figure 14-13 shows the pulsed-wave Doppler recordings of the transmitral flow.

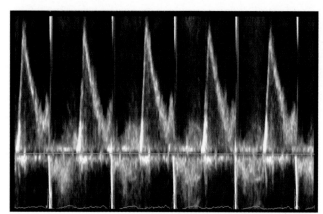

Fig. 14-13

28. Based on Figure 14-13, which of the following statements about the transmitral flow pattern is correct?
    A. The transmitral flow pattern demonstrates normal LV diastolic filling.
    B. The cardiac rhythm is atrial fibrillation and, therefore, only the E wave is observed.
    C. The AV delay is programmed too short and, therefore, the A wave is truncated.
    D. The AV delay is programmed too long and, consequently, the E and A waves are fused reducing the LVFT.

29. What would be the correct management of this patient?
    A. Turn off the pacemaker because it induces heart failure.
    B. A cardioversion is indicated because the patient is in atrial fibrillation.
    C. Program a longer AV delay to assure completion of the diastolic LV filling without truncation of the A wave.
    D. Program a shorter AV delay to lengthen the LVFT separating the E and A waves.

CASE 3:

A 67-year-old man with prior inferoposterior myocardial infarction was admitted to the coronary care unit because of acute pulmonary edema. After stabilization, a transthoracic echocardiogram was performed to evaluate LV volumes, ejection fraction, and LV dyssynchrony. When the sonographer applied M mode to quantify SPWMD, Figure 14-14 was observed:

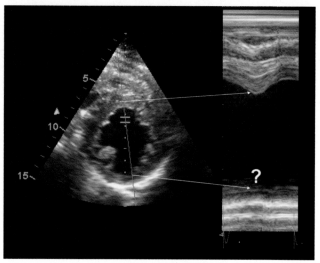

Fig. 14-14

30. Based on Figure 14-14, which of the following statements about LV dyssynchrony assessment with M mode is correct?
    A. In this case, the amount of LV dyssynchrony is extremely large because the posterior wall does not show peak inward motion.
    B. LV dyssynchrony cannot be assessed with this method because the posterior wall may not contract actively and, therefore, the peak inward motion cannot be defined.
    C. Myocardial velocities based on color-coded TDI may distinguish myocardial segments with active contraction and segments passively tethered and, therefore, may constitute a better tool to evaluate LV dyssynchrony.
    D. Two-dimensional speckle tracking echocardiography cannot evaluate LV dyssynchrony in this case due to the high angle-dependency of the technique.

31. A second, more experienced observer performed 2D speckle tracking analysis on short-axis images to evaluate LV activation mechanical pattern and obtained Figure 14-15:

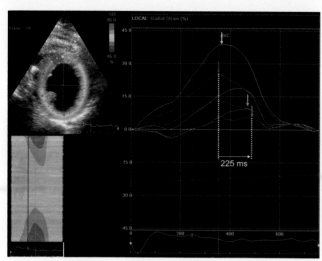

Fig. 14-15

Which of the following sentences about this case is correct?

A. There is substantial LV dyssynchrony as indicated by the radial strain-time curves with the earliest activated segments at the septal and anteroseptal walls and the latest activated segments at the lateral and posterior walls.

B. The likelihood of favorable response to CRT is high regardless of the location and extent of myocardial scar since there is substantial LV dyssynchrony.

C. The analysis is not properly performed because the region of interest is not narrow enough to evaluate the endocardium.

D. After CRT, a responder should demonstrate postsystolic thickening in the anteroseptal and the septal segments.

CASE 4:

A 54-year-old man with ischemic heart failure, LV ejection fraction of 28%, and left bundle branch block received CRT. At 6-month follow-up, the patient did not experience any clinical or echocardiographic improvement.

32. According to Figure 14-16, which of the following sentences is correct?

A. LV diastolic filling pattern is normal, as indicated by the transmitral pulsed-wave Doppler recordings, but there is substantial LV dyssynchrony indicated by the large septal-to-lateral wall delay on TDI data.

B. LV diastolic filling is compromised by a long AV delay with fusion of E and A waves.

C. LV diastolic filling is compromised by a short AV delay with truncation of A wave, and there is still substantial LV dyssynchrony with large septal-to-lateral wall delay on TDI recordings.

D. LV dyssynchrony is incorrectly measured with wrong alignment of the ultrasound beam, very small sample volumes, and very noisy time-velocity curves.

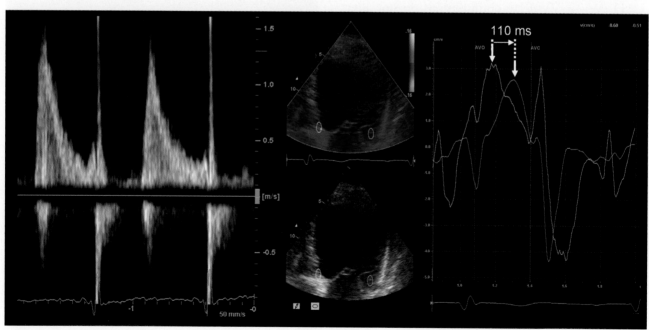

Fig. 14-16

33. On color-coded TDI tracings, substantial diastolic LV dyssynchrony could also be observed (Fig. 14-17). The time delay between septal and lateral early diastolic peak velocities (E) was 98 milliseconds. Which of the following statements about diastolic LV dyssynchrony is correct?

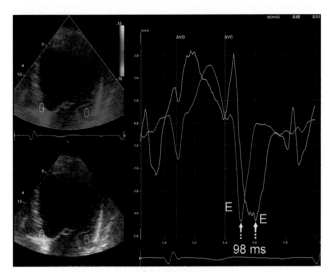

Fig. 14-17

A. Diastolic LV dyssynchrony is uncommon in patients with heart failure.
B. Diastolic LV dyssynchrony is strongly related to the QRS complex duration.
C. After CRT, persistent diastolic LV dyssynchrony may explain the lack of clinical improvement despite systolic LV resynchronization.
D. AV- or VV-delay optimizations do not affect diastolic LV dyssynchrony.

34. An AV-delay optimization was performed first (Fig. 14-18). Which of the following sentences about AV-delay optimization is correct?

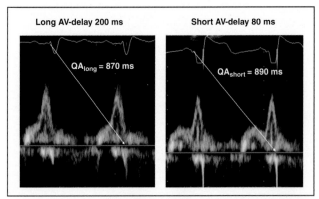

Fig. 14-18

A. AV-delay optimization by the Ritter's method requires continuous-wave Doppler recordings of the transmitral flow and the presence of mitral regurgitation to measure the dP/dt_{max}.
B. The Ritter's method is the most accurate method to optimize AV delay, and it is applicable in all patients regardless of the intrinsic AV conduction.
C. The iterative method starts from a long AV delay and shortens by 20-millisecond steps until the E and A waves are fused.
D. The Ritter's method calculates the optimal AV delay with the formula: AV short + ([AV long + QA long] − [AV short + QA short]). In this case, the optimal AV delay was 100 milliseconds.

35. After AV-delay optimization, the VV delay was optimized by measuring the velocity-time integral of the flow at the LV outflow tract (Fig. 14-19). Which of the following statements about VV-delay optimization is correct?

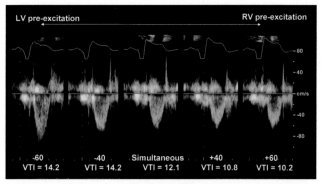

Fig. 14-19

A. Optimization of the VV delay in this case is not necessary since changes in AV delay may favorably affect interventricular and LV dyssynchrony.
B. Preexcitation of the left ventricle with a VV delay of −60 milliseconds provides the highest cardiac output.
C. Preexcitation of the right ventricle, regardless of the VV delay programmed, yields usually the highest cardiac output.
D. Changes in the angle of incidence between the outflow jet and the ultrasound beam do not affect the accuracy of the velocity-time integral measurement.

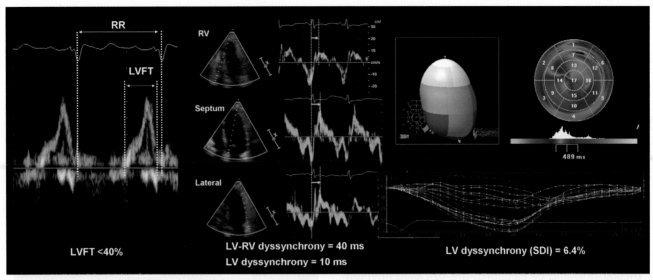

LVFT <40%

LV-RV dyssynchrony = 40 ms
LV dyssynchrony = 10 ms

LV dyssynchrony (SDI) = 6.4%

Fig. 14-20

CASE 5:

A CRT device was implanted in a 67-year-old woman with dilated cardiomyopathy, New York heart Association heart failure functional class III, LV ejection fraction of 30% (see Video 14-2), and QRS duration on surface electrocardiogram of 120 milliseconds. Figure 14-20 shows the key issues to evaluate cardiac dyssynchrony.

36. Based on Figure 14-20, which of the following sentences about cardiac dyssynchrony is correct?
    A. There is no AV, interventricular, or LV dyssynchrony.
    B. There is only AV dyssynchrony with a diastolic LVFT of <40%.
    C. There is substantial LV dyssynchrony as assessed with real-time 3D echocardiography with the inferoposterior segments as the most delayed activated segments.
    D. Pulsed-wave TDI does not indicate the presence of LV dyssynchrony because the ultrasound beam was not properly aligned.

37. At 6-month follow-up, the patient was in New York Heart Association functional class I and LV ejection fraction improved to 38%. Figure 14-21 illustrates the changes in cardiac dyssynchrony.

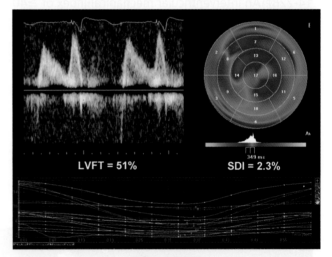

LVFT = 51%   SDI = 2.3%

Fig. 14-21

In this particular case, which of the following statements about response to CRT is correct?
A. The patient showed improved LV synchronicity with a reduction in SDI, but LV diastolic filling pattern was still impaired with restrictive filling pattern.
B. LV dyssynchrony did not improve.
C. The AV delay is too short and, therefore, the A wave is truncated.
D. The improvement in LV ejection fraction may be secondary to improved AV and LV synchrony.

5. ANSWER: D. LV dyssynchrony has been extensively studied with TDI. Among several TDI modalities, assessment of LV longitudinal velocities is the principal method used in clinical practice. Pulsed-wave TDI or color-coded TDI are the main approaches to evaluate LV longitudinal velocities. Pulsed-wave TDI permits interrogation of only one region at a time and precludes simultaneous comparison of two opposite regions. This technical issue may reduce the accuracy of LV dyssynchrony assessment. In contrast, color-coded TDI permits the assessment of LV longitudinal velocities in multiple regions simultaneously. Myocardial velocities are obtained by postprocessing color-coded TDI data, and, subsequently, LV dyssynchrony is evaluated by means of time delay to peak systolic velocity between two to four opposing regions or calculating the standard deviation of time to peak systolic velocity of 6–12 LV segments. As all Doppler-based techniques, TDI data analysis is highly dependent on the angle of insonation of the ultrasound beam, and, therefore, accurate LV dyssynchrony assessment requires proper alignment of ultrasound beam with the direction of the motion.

6. ANSWER: D. To assure proper analysis of LV dyssynchrony with TDI techniques, tissue Doppler data acquisition and postprocessing require the following actions:

- Acquire high frame rate color tissue Doppler (>90 frames/sec).
- Optimize gain and time gain control settings for clear myocardial definition.
- Position the LV cavity in the center of the sector and align with the Doppler ultrasound beam for optimal LV longitudinal motion assessment.
- Have patients hold breathing for 5 seconds while a three-to-five-beat digital acquisition is performed.
- Record standard apical two-, four-, and three-chamber views.
- Determine the LV ejection interval; from pulsed-wave Doppler recordings of the LV outflow tract, the aortic valve opening and closure timings can be defined.
- Place the regions of interest (5 × 10 mm to 7 × 15 mm size) at the basal and midventricular segments of opposing LV walls to obtain time-velocity tracings.
- Check physiologic signal quality identifying the components of the velocity curve: isovolumic contraction positive curve (<60 milliseconds from the Q wave), the systolic wave (S), and the early (E) and late (A) diastolic waves (Fig. 14-24).
- Adjust the regions of interest to obtain the most reproducible peak systolic velocity. Time from the onset of QRS to peak S wave should be measured for basal and midventricular segments of the three apical views (12 segments). Alternatively, the difference in time to peak S wave from opposing walls can define LV dyssynchrony.

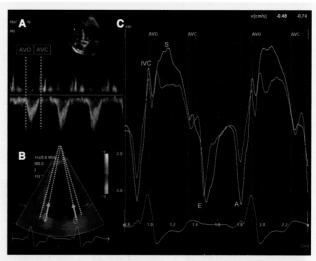

LV dyssynchrony assessment with color-coded TDI. First, LV ejection interval should be defined (panel **A**). TDI data acquisition requires proper alignment of the ultrasound beam along the LV motion direction (panel **B**). Postprocessing of TDI data provides velocity-time curves of two opposing LV walls. The components of the velocity-time curves should be identified (panel **C**): the isovolumic contraction (IVC) curve, systolic velocity (S), and early (E) and late (A) diastolic velocities. Finally, time delay between peak systolic velocities (S wave) can be measured to assess LV dyssynchrony.

Fig. 14-24A–C

7. ANSWER: A. Color-coded TDI is the technique most frequently used to evaluate LV dyssynchrony and to predict mid- and long-term prognosis after CRT. Several LV dyssynchrony parameters have been developed in the last decade. The measurement of time delay in peak systolic velocity between the basal septal and basal lateral segments of the apical four-chamber view is the simplest parameter to identify LV dyssynchrony. A cutoff value of ≥60 milliseconds predicts favorable echocardiographic response to CRT with a sensitivity and specificity of 76% and 78%, respectively. In addition, LV dyssynchrony can be defined by the time delay between 4 opposing walls (basal segments of the anterior, inferior, septal, and lateral walls). A cutoff value of ≥65 milliseconds predicts favorable clinical and echocardiographic response to CRT at midterm follow-up and improved long-term prognosis (Table 14-1). Finally, Yu et al. developed an LV dyssynchrony index that integrates information from the 3 apical views (two-, four-chamber and log-axis views). This index is derived by calculating the standard deviation of time to peak systolic velocity of 12 segments (basal and midventricular segments). A cutoff value of ≥31.4 milliseconds predicts favorable response to CRT with a sensitivity and specificity of 96% and 78%, respectively (Table 14-1).

8. ANSWER: C. Strain and strain rate imaging evaluate myocardial deformation and permit distinction of myocardial segments with active contraction from segments that are passively tethered (scar segments). From

TDI data, strain and strain rate-time curves can be obtained. As all Doppler techniques, TDI-derived strain and strain rate measurements are highly dependent on the angle insonation of the ultrasound beam. At the apical views of the left ventricle, only longitudinal strain or strain rate can be measured; whereas from the short-axis views, radial strain and strain rate can be measured at the (antero)septal and posterior walls and circumferential strain and strain rate can be measured at the inferior and lateral walls. Several studies have evaluated the role of strain and strain rate imaging to define LV dyssynchrony and to predict response to CRT. LV dyssynchrony can be evaluated either with longitudinal or radial strain and strain rate by measuring the time delay between the peak strain of two opposing walls. A time delay of ≥130 milliseconds between the (antero)septal and the posterior walls measured on radial strain-time curves has been predictive of acute improvement in stroke volume after CRT while longitudinal strain failed to predict LV reverse remodeling after CRT.

9. ANSWER: B. Two-dimensional (2D) speckle tracking echocardiography permits angle-independent myocardial strain and strain rate assessment in three orthogonal directions (radial, circumferential, and longitudinal) and in all LV segments. Strain analysis, based on this novel modality, also enables the differentiation of myocardial segments with active contraction from segments that are passively tethered by the adjacent segments. From radial strain-time curves, a time delay between peak strain of the anteroseptal and posterior walls of ≥130 milliseconds predicts LV reverse remodeling after CRT (Fig. 14-25). In addition, strain analysis based on 2D speckle tracking echocardiography permits the detection of the latest activated segment. This has important clinical implications since positioning the LV pacing lead at the latest activated site provides a high likelihood of favorable response to CRT and superior clinical outcome.

10. ANSWER: D. Three-dimensional (3D) echocardiography allows for the assessment of LV dyssynchrony in the entire left ventricle and in the same cardiac cycle. 3D echocardiography analysis of LV dyssynchrony can be performed by direct volumetric analysis (real-time 3D echocardiography) or by triplane TSI analysis. With real-time 3D echocardiography, an LV full volume is obtained and, subsequently, divided in 17 subvolumes. LV dyssynchrony is calculated as the standard deviation of time to minimum regional systolic volume for 16 segments, the so-called systolic dyssynchrony index (SDI). A cutoff value of ≥6.4% predicts LV reverse remodeling after CRT. Triplane TSI automatically calculates time to peak systolic velocity in basal and midventricular segments of the septal, lateral, inferior, anterior, posterior, and anteroseptal walls. This method selects a specific interval of the cardiac cycle to calculate time delays (only in the LV ejection interval) and excludes the early isovolumic contraction and the late postsystolic shortening. A color-coded overlay is added onto 2D images to visually identify the regional mechanical delay. The earliest activated areas are coded in shades of green, whereas the latest activated areas are coded in shades of red. Time to peak systolic velocities are displayed in a 12-segment polar map and LV dyssynchrony is defined by the septum and lateral walls and the standard deviation of 12 segments. A standard deviation of time to peak systolic velocity of 12 segments of ≥33 milliseconds has been shown to predict a favorable clinical and echocardiographic response to CRT at midterm follow-up.

11. ANSWER: A. The optimal AV delay is defined by the shortest AV interval achievable without compromising the left atrial contribution to LV filling. On pulsed-wave Doppler recordings of the transmitral flow, the end of the A wave should coincide with the onset of rise in LV pressure. The optimal AV delay settings provide a complete late-diastolic filling by atrial contraction and the maximum diastolic LVFT resulting in maximal LV stroke volume.

12. ANSWER: D. When the AV delay is programmed too short, LV contraction occurs earlier and MVC prematurely compromising the left atrial contribution to LV filling. On pulsed-wave Doppler recordings of transmitral flow, a truncation of the A wave is observed together with a relatively early E wave. As a consequence, LVFT lengthens with widely separated E and A waves (Fig. 14-26).

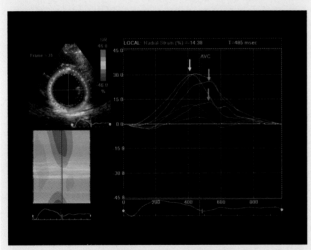

LV dyssynchrony assessed with 2D speckle tracking analysis. From the midventricular LV parasternal short-axis view, time-radial strain tracings of the 6 LV segments are obtained. A time delay of ≥130 milliseconds between peak radial strain of the anteroseptal (yellow arrow) and the posterior (purple arrow) segments define the presence of substantial LV dyssynchrony. In addition, the latest activated segments can be identified (purple and green arrows) indicating where the LV pacing lead should be preferably placed.

Fig. 14-25

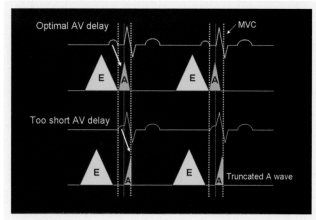

Too short AV delay compromises left atrial contribution to LV filling. Left atrial contraction is interrupted by an early LV contraction. On transmitral pulsed-wave Doppler recordings, A wave is truncated and LV filling time lengthens with widely separated E and A waves.

Fig. 14-26

13. ANSWER: D. The echocardiographic methods used to optimize the AV delay aim to improve either diastolic LVFT or hemodynamic markers of LV systolic function. Diastolic LVFT is usually evaluated using pulsed-wave Doppler recordings of the transmitral flow. LV hemodynamics are usually evaluated using the following: (1) continuous-wave or pulsed-wave Doppler recordings of the LV outflow tract, measuring the velocity-time integral of the flow and calculating the cardiac output or (2) continuous-wave Doppler recordings of the mitral regurgitation, measuring the peak rate of rise of LV pressure during isovolumic contraction (dP/dt_{max}).

14. ANSWER: B. Echocardiographic AV optimization techniques aiming to improve LV diastolic filling include the iterative method, the Ritter's method, the mitral inflow velocity-time integral method, and the simplified (Meluzin) mitral inflow method. Echocardiographic AV optimization methods aiming to improve LV hemodynamics include the assessment of aortic valve or LV outflow tract velocity-time integral, dP/dt_{max}, and myocardial performance index. Figure 14-27 summarizes and illustrates these methods.

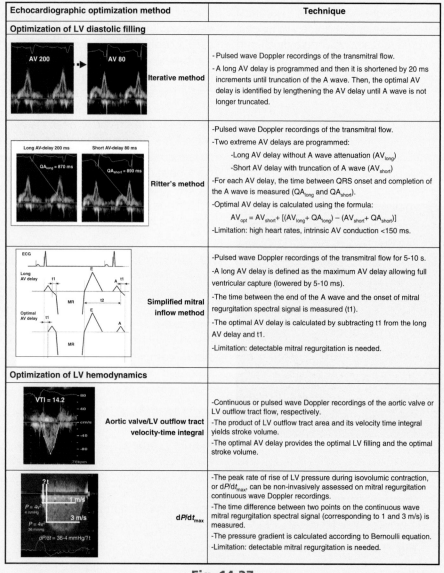

Echocardiographic optimization method		Technique
Optimization of LV diastolic filling		
	Iterative method	- Pulsed wave Doppler recordings of the transmitral flow. - A long AV delay is programmed and then it is shortened by 20 ms increments until truncation of the A wave. Then, the optimal AV delay is identified by lengthening the AV delay until A wave is not longer truncated.

	Ritter's method	-Pulsed wave Doppler recordings of the transmitral flow.
		-Two extreme AV delays are programmed:
		    -Long AV delay without A wave attenuation (AV_{long})
		    -Short AV delay with truncation of A wave (AV_{short})
		-For each AV delay, the time between QRS onset and completion of the A wave is measured (QA_{long} and QA_{short}).
		-Optimal AV delay is calculated using the formula:
		  $AV_{opt} = AV_{short} + [(AV_{long} + QA_{long}) - (AV_{short} + QA_{short})]$
		-Limitation: high heart rates, intrinsic AV conduction <150 ms.

	Simplified mitral inflow method	-Pulsed wave Doppler recordings of the transmitral flow for 5-10 s. -A long AV delay is defined as the maximum AV delay allowing full ventricular capture (lowered by 5-10 ms). -The time between the end of the A wave and the onset of mitral regurgitation spectral signal is measured (t1). -The optimal AV delay is calculated by subtracting t1 from the long AV delay and t1. -Limitation: detectable mitral regurgitation is needed.
Optimization of LV hemodynamics		
	Aortic valve/LV outflow tract velocity-time integral	-Continuous or pulsed wave Doppler recordings of the aortic valve or LV outflow tract flow, respectively. -The product of LV outflow tract area and its velocity time integral yields stroke volume. -The optimal AV delay provides the optimal LV filling and the optimal stroke volume.
	dP/dt_{max}	-The peak rate of rise of LV pressure during isovolumic contraction, or dP/dt_{max}, can be non-invasively assessed on mitral regurgitation continuous wave Doppler recordings. -The time difference between two points on the continuous wave mitral regurgitation spectral signal (corresponding to 1 and 3 m/s) is measured. -The pressure gradient is calculated according to Bernoulli equation. -Limitation: detectable mitral regurgitation is needed.

Fig. 14-27

15. ANSWER: A. The most common echocardiographic methods to optimize the VV delay include the measurement of velocity-time integral on pulsed-wave Doppler recordings of the LV outflow tract and the evaluation of LV dyssynchrony on color-coded TDI data by measuring septal-to-lateral peak systolic velocity time delay.

16. ANSWER: C. Prolonged AV conduction induces late ventricular contraction. Left atrial contraction occurs relatively early in diastole and, on pulsed-wave Doppler recordings of the transmitral flow, the E and A waves appear fused (superimposition of atrial contraction on the early diastolic LV filling phase). Subsequently, diastolic LVFT is reduced. In addition, after left atrial contraction, the mitral valve remains open and diastolic mitral regurgitation can be observed.

17. ANSWER: D. Interventricular and LV dyssynchrony can be assessed with pulsed-wave TDI. Interventricular dyssynchrony is measured as the peak systolic velocity time delay between the basal segment of RV free wall and the most delayed basal LV segment. LV dyssynchrony is calculated as the peak systolic velocity time delay between 2, 4, or 6 basal LV segments. The combination of both, interventricular and LV dyssynchrony, predicts favorable response to CRT with high sensitivity and specificity (Table 14-1). In this case, the sum of both delays results in 115 milliseconds and, therefore, the likelihood of favorable response to CRT is high.

18. ANSWER: C. Color-coded TDI is one of the most used echocardiographic techniques to evaluate LV dyssynchrony. The time delay between 2 (septal-to-lateral) or 4 opposing walls (anterior, inferior, septal, and lateral) as well as the standard deviation of time to peak systolic velocity of 12 segments define LV dyssynchrony and predict favorable response to CRT (Table 14-1). In this case, a septal-to-lateral wall delay of 120 milliseconds ($\geq$65 milliseconds) is highly predictive of LV reverse remodeling.

19. ANSWER: B. In this example, there is substantial LV dyssynchrony as assessed with TDI-derived longitudinal strain: the lateral wall stretches, whereas the septal wall shortens. Peak shortening of the lateral wall occurs after aortic valve closure. TDI-derived strain imaging is a valuable technique to evaluate patients with heart failure who are candidates for CRT since it provides information not only on LV dyssynchrony but also on myocardial active contraction. TDI-derived strain imaging permits differentiation of myocardial segments with active deformation or contraction (viable segments) from those segments with a substantial amount of scar tissue that are usually tethered by the adjacent segments. Previous studies have demonstrated the importance of assessing the extent and location of scar tissue before CRT implantation. Thus, when the LV pacing lead is placed at a region with transmural scar or when the LV content of scar tissue is excessive, the likelihood of favorable response to CRT reduces dramatically. In this example, the LV lateral wall shows active contraction, although more delayed as compared to the septal wall.

20. ANSWER: B. From midventricular short-axis images of the left ventricle, radial or circumferential strain can be assessed. Although TDI-derived strain is highly dependent on the ultrasound angle of incidence, radial strain can be assessed at the (antero)septal and posterior walls. With radial strain, myocardial thickening is evaluated and scored as positive values. Circumferential strain can be assessed only at the lateral and inferior(septum) walls and evaluates myocardial shortening along the curvature of the left ventricle. Circumferential shortening is scored as negative values. In this example, LV dyssynchrony is evaluated with TDI-derived radial strain and demonstrates the presence of substantial LV dyssynchrony with a peak radial strain-time delay between the septum and the posterior wall of $\geq$130 milliseconds.

21. ANSWER: B. Strain imaging based on speckle tracking echocardiography has emerged as a powerful technique to evaluate patients with heart failure who are candidates for CRT. This imaging technique enables angle-independent multidirectional LV strain and strain rate assessment. LV dyssynchrony can be assessed with radial strain speckle tracking analysis. In addition, the latest activated segment can be identified having important implications on CRT response. In patients with an LV pacing lead placed at the latest activated areas, a higher response rate to CRT and superior long-term outcome have been demonstrated. Finally, as all strain imaging techniques, viable LV segments, showing active contraction, may be identified and differentiated from those scar segments passively tethered.

22. ANSWER: D. The assessment of LV dyssynchrony can be performed with triplane TSI. First, the apical two-, four-, and three-chamber views of the left ventricle are simultaneously acquired rendering an LV 3D volume. Color-coded TSI is applied to the triplane view to assess myocardial longitudinal velocities. The time from onset of QRS complex to peak systolic velocity in every segment of the left ventricle is calculated automatically, and LV dyssynchrony is expressed as time delays between the septum and the lateral wall and the standard deviation of 12 segments. In addition, the TSI algorithm color codes the time delays ranging from the green (earliest activated) over yellow-orange to red (latest activated) within the systolic period. The electromechanical activation times are presented in a polar map allowing for the identification of the earliest and latest activated segments. Figure 14-7 illustrates an example of a patient with substantial LV dyssynchrony,

Coronary Artery Disease

Ronald Mastouri and Stephen G. Sawada

1. A false-positive stress-induced wall motion abnormality is most commonly seen in which of the following myocardial segments?
A. Basal inferior.
B. Apical septum.
C. Mid lateral.
D. Mid septum.

2. Which one of the following is not a high-risk feature on a dobutamine stress echo?
A. Stress-induced wall motion abnormalities in more than one coronary territory.
B. Dilation of the left ventricular (LV) cavity with stress.
C. Dobutamine-induced ventricular arrhythmias.
D. Decrease in global LV systolic function with stress.

3. A 40-year-old man is referred for two-dimensional echocardiography for evaluation of an incidentally found left bundle branch block (LBBB) on ECG. Global LV function is normal. Which of the following is true concerning wall motion abnormalities due exclusively to LBBB?
A. There is absent myocardial thickening.
B. Wall motion abnormalities are most prominent in the proximal and mid anterior septum.
C. Wall motion abnormalities frequently involve the apex and anterior wall.
D. Two-dimensional imaging provides the most accurate information for recognition of LBBB wall motion.

4. The false-negative rate for dobutamine stress echocardiography is higher for patients who have:
A. Multivessel coronary disease due to balanced ischemia.
B. Concentric LV remodeling.
C. Hypertensive blood pressure response to stress.
D. Eccentric LV hypertrophy.

5. A 65-year-old patient presented with an inferior ST elevation and right ventricular (RV) myocardial infarction. Angioplasty of a proximally occluded right coronary artery (RCA) was unsuccessful. The patient received generous intravenous fluid for hypotension, which eventually resolved. Later that night, the patient developed progressive shortness of breath and worsening hypoxia not responding to oxygen supplementation. Cardiovascular examination revealed a faint apical systolic murmur and marked jugular venous distention. A stat echocardiogram was ordered. Which of the following needs to be performed?
A. Color Doppler interrogation of the mitral valve.
B. Agitated saline contrast to rule out right-to-left shunt.
C. Color Doppler interrogation of the interventricular septum.
D. Color Doppler interrogation of the tricuspid valve.

6. Which of the following is true about a pseudo-aneurysm?
   A. It is most frequently located in the apex.
   B. It is characterized by a small neck communicating with the LV cavity.
   C. It has a lower risk of rupture compared with a true aneurysm.
   D. It has a thin wall of myocardium.

7. Commercially available echo contrast agents pass through the pulmonary circulation into the left atrium and left ventricle providing image enhancement of these structures. An accurate statement about the use of echo contrast agents is:
   A. They are approved for evaluation of myocardial perfusion in acute infarction and are useful in identifying no-reflow phenomenon.
   B. Contrast agents can be used in patients with intracardiac right-to-left shunts.
   C. Contrast agents persist longer in the circulation if low power, low mechanical index imaging techniques are used.
   D. They can be safely used in any patient with decompensated congestive heart failure.

8. Tissue Doppler imaging is a newer technology that enables quantitative assessment of longitudinal systolic function of segments of the right and left ventricle. A true statement regarding assessment of segmental myocardial velocity by tissue Doppler imaging using the apical views is:
   A. In normal individuals, basal LV lateral wall velocity typically exceeds basal RV free wall velocities.
   B. In normal individuals, LV apical segment velocities exceed LV basal segment velocities.
   C. LV twist or torsion can be assessed by tissue Doppler imaging using the apical views.
   D. In normal individuals, there is a base-to-apex gradient in velocities whereby apical segment velocities are significantly lower than basal segment velocities.

9. Resynchronization therapy has been shown to promote reverse remodeling and improve symptoms in patients with ischemic cardiomyopathy who have dyssynchrony and severely reduced global LV systolic function. Which of the following group of patients is likely to have the highest frequency of improvement from resynchronization therapy?
   A. Patients with ischemic myopathy with QRS duration of >130 milliseconds and dobutamine echo evidence of viability in both the septal and lateral walls.
   B. Patients with ischemic myopathy with QRS duration of <130 milliseconds and Ts-SD (standard deviation of time to peak ejection tissue Doppler velocity of 12 segments) of >32 milliseconds.
   C. Patients with ischemic myopathy with QRS duration of >130 milliseconds and nonviable inferolateral wall by dobutamine echo.
   D. Patients with ischemic myopathy with QRS duration of >130 milliseconds and M-mode septal to posterior wall delay <130 milliseconds.

10. After an acute interruption of coronary blood flow, which sign of ischemia will appear first?
    A. ECG changes.
    B. Wall motion abnormality by visual assessment.
    C. Angina.
    D. Diastolic dysfunction.

11. A 67-year-old patient presents with new-onset chest pain. A two-dimensional echocardiogram showed akinesis of the septum, anterior wall, and apical inferior segment. This distribution of wall motion abnormalities is most often the result of obstruction of:
    A. The RCA.
    B. The left anterior descending (LAD) and RCAs.
    C. The left circumflex (LCX) and LAD arteries.
    D. The LAD artery.

12. A 45-year-old man presents with worsening shortness of breath. A two-dimensional echocardiogram shows reduced LV systolic function with an ejection fraction of 35%. Which of the following echocardiographic parameters best differentiates ischemic from idiopathic dilated cardiomyopathy?
    A. Presence of regional wall motion abnormalities.
    B. LV generalized hypokinesis.
    C. Apical dilatation.
    D. Extensive transmural myocardial scar.

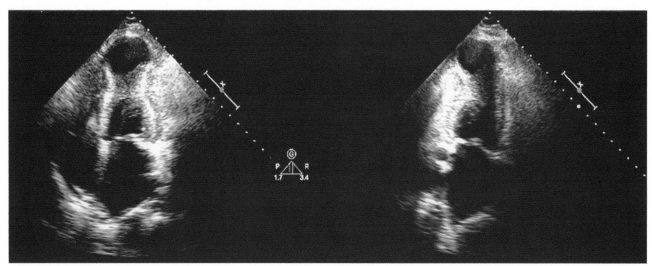

Fig. 15-1

13. A failure to decrease LV end-systolic volume during stress may be a normal finding in which one of the following stress echo modalities?
  A. Dobutamine stress echo.
  B. Treadmill stress echo.
  C. Bicycle stress echo.
  D. Vasodilator stress echo.

14. In patients who cannot perform exercise, various stress methods have been used in combination with echocardiography for the detection of coronary artery disease. Of the stress methods listed below, which is the least effective when employed in stress echocardiography?
  A. Dobutamine-atropine.
  B. High-dose dipyridamole.
  C. Adenosine.
  D. Transesophageal atrial pacing.

15. Which of the following is an appropriate indication for performing stress echocardiography?
  A. Asymptomatic patient <2 years postpercutaneous revascularization.
  B. Asymptomatic patient <1 year after normal noninvasive study scheduled to undergo high-risk nonemergent surgery.
  C. Asymptomatic patient with a low to moderate coronary artery disease risk by Framingham Score.
  D. New-onset atrial fibrillation in a patient with moderate to high coronary artery disease risk.

16. A 60-year-old woman suffered an anterior ST elevation myocardial infarction. She underwent

percutaneous revascularization of the LAD artery. The patient presents for follow-up 2 months later without symptoms. A late systolic frame of an apical four- and two-chamber view obtained at follow-up is shown in Figure 15-1. A 12-lead ECG showed ST elevation in the anterior leads. The most likely reason for this finding is:
  A. Recurrent infarction due to acute stent thrombosis.
  B. The ECG finding is consistent with the normal evolutionary changes of an anterior infarction.
  C. The ECG finding is due to an apical aneurysm.
  D. The ECG finding is due to Dressler's syndrome.

17. A 75-year-old patient with a transmural anterior myocardial infarction and ischemic heart disease is seen in clinic 3 weeks after his event. His current medical regimen includes aspirin, metoprolol, simvastatin, and lisinopril. A routine two-dimensional echocardiogram is performed (Fig. 15-2). What is the most appropriate next step?

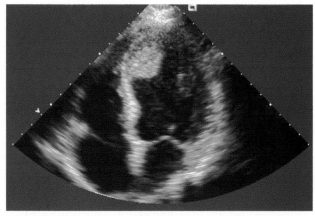

Fig. 15-2

A. Warfarin needs to be added to the medical regimen with a goal INR of 2–3 with a repeat echocardiogram in 3 months.
B. Clopidogrel needs to be started for at least 1 year.
C. Commercial contrast is needed for better assessment of the LV apex.
D. Continue current medical regimen.

18. An echocardiogram in a 60-year-old man is performed because of dyspnea. The two-dimensional image is an end-systolic frame. Pulsed-tissue Doppler recordings from the basal inferior (Fig. 15-3A) and basal anterior (Fig. 15-3B) walls. A true statement about the tissue Doppler recordings is:
A. Both the inferior and anterior wall signals are normal.
B. There is too much artifact to render an interpretation.
C. There is evidence for postsystolic shortening of the inferior wall.
D. There is prominent inferior and anterior wall dyssynchrony.

19. A 65-year-old man with no history of heart disease had a two-dimensional echocardiogram performed for palpitations. The finding of interest in the parasternal long- and short-axis end-diastolic image in Figure 15-4 is:

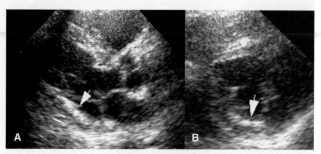

Fig. 15-4A-B

A. Mitral annular calcification.
B. Rheumatic mitral valve disease with subvalvular calcification.
C. Subendocardial scar due to prior silent myocardial injury.
D. Pericardial calcification.

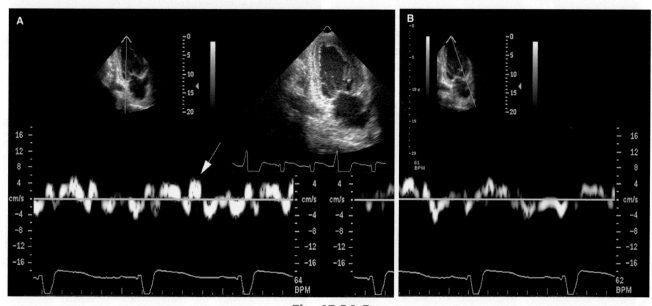

Fig. 15-3A-B

Septal wall motion is normal at rest and becomes hyperdynamic poststress suggesting no ischemia in the LAD circulation.

26. ANSWER: C. Mitral regurgitation (MR) due to papillary muscle migration or displacement is referred to as "functional MR." Progressive LV remodeling and dilatation lead to both apical and medial/lateral displacement of the papillary muscles from their usual position relative to the mitral annulus. This results in tethering (restriction) of the mitral leaflets with the characteristic appearance of tenting of the valve. The coaptation point is displaced into the ventricle. Often restriction of the mitral leaflets is asymmetric (as in this case) with the posterior leaflet more tethered. This result in an asymmetric mitral regurgitation jet directed toward the lateral wall of the left atrium.

27. ANSWER: C. Ischemic MR is traditionally a complex lesion to repair which has usually been attempted with an annuloplasty ring. The failure of true-sized annuloplasty rings has led to the use of down-sized rings, which in some cases of functional regurgitation provides adequate repair. However, in cases where there is significant leaflet tenting, the primary mechanism of MR is papillary muscle migration rather than annular dilatation. Annuloplasty alone is insufficient. A mitral annulus to coaptation point distance of >1 cm (in this case 1.5 cm) is associated with persistent MR and symptoms after annuloplasty. In some cases, such as this one with more restriction of posterior versus anterior leaflet motion, placement of a ring may further restrict posterior leaflet motion. Recently more complex techniques, involving resection of myocardium, repositioning of the papillary muscles, chordal cutting, etc., have been combined with annuloplasty to improve the results in tented valves.

KEY POINTS:

■ LV remodeling with apical and medial/lateral papillary muscle displacement can lead to marked leaflet tenting and MR.

■ Reduction annuloplasty has been the traditional therapeutic approach.

■ A more sophisticated surgical technique involving resection of myocardium, repositioning of the papillary muscles, chordal cutting, etc. may be needed in cases of severe mitral valve tenting or asymmetric tethering.

28. ANSWER: B. The dense continuous wave spectral display shown in this example and the elevated inflow velocity (1.5 m/sec) indicate severe MR. The peak velocity of the mitral regurgitant jet is 3.5 m/sec. The pressure difference between the left ventricle and left atrium in systole from the modified Bernoulli equation $(4V^2)$ is $4 \times (3.5)^2 = 50$ mm Hg. The estimated left atrial pressure is 90 mm Hg − 50 mm Hg = 40 mm Hg.

Although the mitral E velocity is elevated, the deceleration time is rapid indicating no significant mitral stenosis.

29. ANSWER: C. The leading slope of the mitral regurgitant jet is more gradual than usual. Left ventricle pressure (dP/dt) can be assessed from the slope of the mitral regurgitant jet. The time difference between the leading edge of the jet between 1 and 3 m/sec is determined. This time difference is divided into 32 mm Hg, which is the pressure difference between 1 and 3 m/sec. Normal dP/dt is >1000 mm Hg/sec, corresponding to a time difference of <0.03 seconds. In this case, the slope is so gradual that the time difference is >0.06 seconds, corresponding to a dP/dt of approximately 500 mm Hg/sec, which is markedly reduced. The LV outflow tract pulsed-wave Doppler velocity is significantly reduced. Forward stroke volume in this case was approximately 25 ml.

KEY POINTS:

■ Using the modified Bernoulli equation, left atrial pressure can be estimated using the MR peak velocity.

■ The slope of the mitral regurgitant jet can be used for the assessment of LV systolic function.

■ Forward stroke volume and cardiac output may be severely reduced in some cases of severe MR, and this can be recognized by the assessment of LVOT velocity and time-velocity integral.

30. ANSWER: A. The four view two-dimensional cine loop confirms the presence of extensive inferior and posterior wall motion abnormality. The short-axis view suggests a ventricular septal rupture, which is confirmed by color Doppler. Ventricular septal rupture occurs as a complication of infarction in about 0.2% of cases in fibrinolytic trials. Septal rupture is more common in elderly women presenting with their first myocardial infarction. The size of the rupture dictates the magnitude of the left-to-right shunt and the subsequent hemodynamic consequence. Anterior infarctions tend to cause apical interventricular septal rupture, whereas inferior infarctions are associated with perforations of the basal septum. The physical examination characteristically reveals a new harsh, loud holosystolic murmur that is best heard at the left sternal border.

31. ANSWER: D. Circulation should be supported at first with intra-aortic balloon counterpulsation and intravenous dobutamine or dopamine. Nitroprusside can be used if hypotension is not severe. The timing of surgical repair in patients with postinfarction ventricular septal rupture is controversial and the optimal approach varies with the clinical presentation. In patients with cardiogenic shock, death is inevitable in the absence of urgent surgical intervention. Stabilization is attempted, followed by coronary angiography to define the coronary anatomy and then surgical repair. Operative mortality is high in this setting, but late results in survivors are excellent. Delayed elective surgical repair is feasible in patients without shock, but the potential for unpredictable and rapid clinical deterioration is always possible.

KEY POINTS:

- Ventricular septal rupture is a rare complication of acute myocardial infarction.
- Diagnosis can be confirmed by color Doppler echocardiography.
- Treatment includes hemodynamic support along with early surgical consultation.

32. ANSWER: B. A freely mobile portion of the posteromedial papillary muscle is seen attached to the mitral chordae. A portion of the valve appears to prolapse. This is due to lack of traction on a portion of the mitral valve from chordal attachments from the free portion of the papillary muscle rather than chordal rupture or myxomatous disease. Papillary muscle rupture is a life-threatening complication of acute myocardial infarction. It usually occurs 2 to 7 days after the infarct and can follow both ST elevation and non-ST elevation myocardial infarction. Rupture of the posteromedial papillary muscle occurs 6–12 times more frequently than rupture of the anterolateral papillary muscle. This is related to the difference in blood supply. The posteromedial papillary muscle is supplied with blood from the posterior descending artery, whereas the anterolateral papillary muscle has a dual blood supply from the LAD and LCX arteries.

33. ANSWER: B. Prompt diagnosis and initiation of medical therapy and emergent surgery are all necessary for a favorable outcome. Medical therapy may include the use of nitrates, sodium nitroprusside, diuretics, dobutamine, and intra-aortic balloon pump counterpulsation if necessary. Despite high operative mortality (20%–25%), emergent surgical intervention remains the treatment of choice. If possible, mitral valve repair is preferable over replacement.

KEY POINTS:

- A ruptured papillary muscle head will be seen as a mobile structure attached to the chordal apparatus.
- Rupture of the posteromedial muscle occurs 6–12 times more frequently than rupture of the anterolateral papillary muscle due to differential blood supply.
- Emergent surgical intervention remains the treatment of choice.

34. ANSWER: B. In this case, there is progressive improvement of global systolic function and regional wall motion with increasing doses of dobutamine. The exception is function of the apical septum which exhibits initial improvement and then deterioration of function at peak dose (biphasic response). Testing for viability is usually reserved for patients with significant ischemic LV dysfunction who are potential candidates for revascularization in the hope that ventricular function and prognosis will improve with revascularization of viable myocardium. Low-dose dobutamine stress echocardiography is one of the established modalities used for viability assessment. The uncoupling of the inotropic and chronotropic effects of dobutamine at low doses ($\leq$10 μg/kg/min) permits improvement of contractile function in stunned or hibernating myocardium without major increases in heart rate and myocardial oxygen demand. Viable myocardium will show increased wall thickening or increased endocardial excursion.

35. ANSWER: C. Dobutamine echocardiography protocols that utilize both low and stress doses of dobutamine have been advocated for prediction of functional recovery. The biphasic response (improvement of contractility at low dose with subsequent deterioration at high dose) has the highest positive predictive value for functional recovery compared with other wall motion responses. However, in many studies utilizing only low-dose (up to 20 μg/kg/min) dobutamine infusion, the presence of contractile reserve with low-dose dobutamine has been shown to have good positive predictive value (mean value of 77%) for functional recovery without determination of the presence or absence of the biphasic response. In addition, a third or more of segments exhibiting a sustained response may have functional recovery. The patient underwent surgical revascularization. A two-dimensional echocardiogram done a few months later showed marked improvement of LV systolic function (Video 15-10). The estimated ejection fraction improved from 18% to 40%.

KEY POINTS:

- Dobutamine stress echocardiography is a well-established modality for the assessment of myocardial viability.
- A biphasic response, which is improvement of contractility at low dose with subsequent deterioration at high dose, has a high positive predictive value for functional recovery. However, some patients with sustained responses also have significant functional recovery. Demonstration of improvement of wall motion with low-dose dobutamine alone has good positive predictive value for functional recovery.

SUGGESTED READINGS

Bax JJ, Poldermans D, Elhendy A, et al. Sensitivity, specificity, and predictive accuracies of various noninvasive techniques for detecting hibernating myocardium. *Curr Probl Cardiol*. 2001; 26:147–186.

Bax JJ, Wijns W, Cornel JH, et al. Accuracy of currently available techniques of functional recovery after revascularization in patients with left ventricular dysfunction due to chronic artery disease: comparison of pooled data. *J Am Coll Cardiol*. 1997; 30:1451–1460.

Calafiore AM, Gallina S, Di Mauro M, et al. Mitral valve procedure in dilated cardiomyopathy: repair or replacement? *Ann Thorac Surg*. 2001;71:1146–1152.

Chung ES, Leon AR, Tavazzi L, et al. Results of the Predictors of Response to CRT (PROSPECT) trial. *Circulation*. 2008;117: 2608–2616.

Douglas, PS, Khandheria B, Stainback R, et al. ACCF/ASE/ACEP/AHA/ASNC/SCAI/SCCT/SCMR 2008 appropriateness criteria for stress echocardiography. *J Am Coll Cardiol*. 2008; 51:1127–1147.

Levine RA, Schwammenthal E. Ischemic mitral regurgitation on the threshold of a solution: from paradoxes to unifying concepts. *Circulation*. 2005;112:745–758.

Medina R, Panidis IP, Morganroth J, et al. The value of echocardiographic regional wall motion abnormalities in detecting coronary artery disease in patients with or without a dilated left ventricle. *Am Heart J*. 1985;109:799–803.

Mulvagh Sl, Rakowski SH, Vannan MA, et al. American Society of Echocardiography consensus statement on the clinical applications of ultrasound contrast agents in echocardiography. *J Am Soc Echocardiogr*. 2008;21:1180–1281.

Pellikka PA, Nagueh SF, Elhendy AA, et al. American Society of Echocardiography recommendations for performance, interpretation and application of stress echocardiography. *J Am Soc Echocardiogr*. 2007;20:1021–1034.

Santoro GM, Valenti R, Buonamici P, et al. Relation between ST-segment changes and myocardial perfusion evaluated by myocardial contrast echocardiography in patients with acute myocardial infarction treated by direct angioplasty. *Am J Cardiol*. 1998;82: 932–937.

Smart SC, Knickelbine T, Malik F, et al. Dobutamine-atropine stress echocardiography for the detection of coronary artery disease in patients with left ventricular hypertrophy: importance of chamber size and systolic wall stress. *Circulation*. 2000;101:258–263.

Sutter J, Poldermans D, Vourvouri E, et al. Long-term prognostic significance of complex ventricular arrhythmia induced during dobutamine stress echocardiography. *Am J Cardiol*. 2003;91: 242–244.

Yao SS, Shah A, Bangalore S, et al. Transient ischemic left ventricular cavity dilation is a significant predictor of severe and extensive coronary artery disease and adverse outcome in patients undergoing stress echocardiography. *J Am Soc Echocardiogr*. 2007;20: 352–358.

Yu CM, Fung WH, Lin H, et al. Predictors of left ventricular reverse remodeling after cardiac resynchronization therapy for heart failure secondary to idiopathic dilated or ischemic cardiomyopathy. *Am J Cardiol*. 2003;91:684–688.

CHAPTER 16

Pulmonic and Tricuspid Valvular Disease

Brian P. Griffin

1. In which of the following clinical scenarios is transesophageal echocardiography (TEE) usually indicated in addition to transthoracic echocardiography (TTE) in the diagnostic assessment?
   A. Pulmonary artery (PA) pressure in primary pulmonary hypertension.
   B. Inferior vena cava (IVC) thrombus.
   C. Suspected pacemaker endocarditis.
   D. Right ventricular (RV) function.

2. A patient is undergoing an examination of the heart following a heart transplant. Severe tricuspid regurgitation (TR) is present but no turbulence in the jet is appreciated. RV function is moderately reduced. The tricuspid regurgitant velocity is 1 m/sec. What other finding is most likely to be evident in this patient?
   A. McConnell's sign.
   B. Flail tricuspid valve leaflet.
   C. Tricuspid stenosis.
   D. Atrial septal defect (ASD).
   E. Severe pulmonary insufficiency.

3. In the patient in question 2, the estimated RV systolic pressure from the tricuspid regurgitant velocity is:
   A. Low (<30 mm Hg).
   B. Mildly increased (30–50 mm Hg).
   C. Moderately increased (51–70 mm Hg).
   D. High (>70 mm Hg).
   E. Cannot be accurately estimated by this technique.

4. A young man with mild pulmonary valve stenosis is seen. He has a peak gradient across the pulmonary valve of 20 mm Hg. His tricuspid regurgitant velocity is 3 m/sec and his right atrial size is normal. His IVC is not enlarged and decreases further on sniffing. Which of the following is true?
   A. His PA systolic pressure is normal.
   B. His PA systolic pressure is moderately elevated.
   C. His PA systolic pressure cannot be estimated when pulmonic stenosis is present.
   D. He has severe PA hypertension that will require treatment.
   E. None of the above.

5. The tricuspid valve consists of the following leaflets:
   A. Anterior, lateral, medial.
   B. Anterior, posterior, septal.
   C. Left, right, posterior.
   D. Moderator, anterior, posterior.
   E. Moderator, posterior, septal.

6. A Gerbode defect is:
   A. Atrialization of the right ventricle in Ebstein's anomaly.
   B. An unroofed coronary sinus with resultant bidirectional ASD at the level of the AV groove.
   C. A left-sided superior vena cava entering and enlarging the coronary sinus.
   D. A communication between the right atrium and left ventricle that may encompass the tricuspid valve leaflets.
   E. A sinus of Valsalva aneurysm that communicates with the right atrium.

7. A patient with prior rheumatic disease is seen. An echocardiogram is performed. Which of the following is true about the Doppler echocardiographic assessment of tricuspid stenosis in this condition?
   A. Doming and thickening of the valve in systole are seen.
   B. The mean pressure gradient is at least 10 mm Hg in severe stenosis.
   C. The valve area may be estimated by dividing 190 by the pressure halftime.
   D. Planimetry of the valve area is readily obtained.
   E. Tricuspid stenosis is clinically significant in 25% of patients with rheumatic mitral stenosis.

8. Severe TR is associated with all of the following except:
   A. Paradoxical motion of the interventricular septum.
   B. Regurgitant orifice area by proximal isovelocity surface area of 0.25 cm^2.
   C. Flow reversal in the hepatic veins in systole.
   D. A color flow jet area of >10 cm^2 in the right atrium.
   E. A vena contracta dimension of 0.8 cm.

9. The most common cause of significant TR is:
   A. Myxomatous change or prolapse.
   B. Rheumatic disease.
   C. Endocarditis.
   D. Secondary to pulmonary hypertension and/or RV dilatation.
   E. Trauma.

10. Which of the following is consistent with the diagnosis of severe pulmonic stenosis?
    A. Peak velocity of >4 m/sec across the valve.
    B. Normal RV systolic pressure.
    C. RV wall thickness of 0.3 cm.
    D. Normal size of the PA.

11. A 25-year-old asymptomatic man presents with a systolic murmur at the second right interspace. An echocardiogram is performed and he is found to have pulmonic stenosis. A peak pressure gradient is measured and is 20 mm Hg. Which of the following statements about his condition is most likely to be true?
    A. He is likely to require surgical or balloon valvuloplasty in the next decade.
    B. He should undergo yearly examination and echocardiography and a baseline transesophageal echocardiogram.
    C. Cardiac catheterization is indicated to more accurately determine his pulmonic pressure gradient.
    D. Systolic doming of the pulmonary valve is present.

12. Which of the following statements about pulmonary insufficiency is correct?
    A. Pulmonary insufficiency detected by Doppler of any degree is abnormal.
    B. Severe pulmonary insufficiency leads to a highly turbulent jet on color flow Doppler.
    C. Severe pulmonary insufficiency most commonly occurs in the setting of prior treatment of congenital heart disease.
    D. Pulmonary insufficiency may be used to measure the PA systolic pressure.

13. Which of the following is the most likely cause of a mobile tricuspid valve mass?
    A. Sarcoma.
    B. Fibroelastoma.
    C. Myxoma.
    D. Chiari network.
    E. Carcinoid syndrome.

14. Which of the following conditions may not cause hemodynamically significant lesions at both the tricuspid and pulmonary valve?
    A. Carcinoid syndrome.
    B. Staphylococcal infection.
    C. Rheumatic fever.
    D. Ebstein's anomaly.

15. Which of the following statements about infundibular pulmonic stenosis is correct?
   A. Infundibular pulmonic stenosis is always part of a congenital syndrome.
   B. Infundibular stenosis may cause a high-velocity jet that impinges on the pulmonary valve causing pulmonary insufficiency.
   C. The site of stenosis is usually discrete.
   D. Doppler estimation of the pressure gradient across the infundibular stenosis is inaccurate except when valvar stenosis coexists.
   E. Infundibular stenosis is most easily assessed from a parasternal short-axis imaging plane.

16. A young man presents with fatigue and a history of occasional near syncope with onset of a fast heart rhythm. Based on the apical four-chamber image in Figure 16-1, which is the least likely finding in this patient?

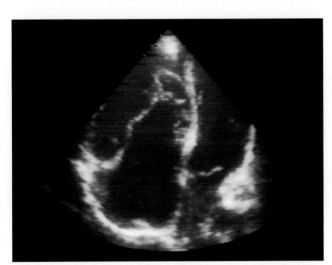

Fig. 16-1

   A. Wolff-Parkinson-White pattern on electrocardiogram.
   B. Intracardiac shunt.
   C. Parchment-like RV wall.
   D. Severe TR.
   E. Atrialization of a portion of the right ventricle.

17. You see a young man with prior open heart surgery for the first time. He is unaware of what surgery he had performed in the past. He has significant RV dilatation and some RV dysfunction. Based on the accompanying parasternal short-axis image of the pulmonary valve in Figure 16-2, which of the following statements is most likely to be correct?

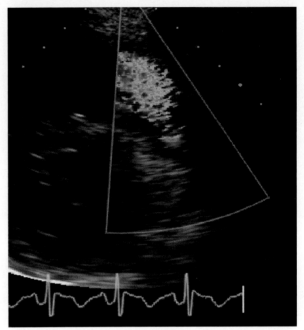

Fig. 16-2

   A. Mild pulmonary regurgitation is present. No further work-up is indicated.
   B. He likely has an ASD with RV overload and high flow through the pulmonary circuit.
   C. He has severe pulmonary regurgitation likely as a result of prior surgery on his pulmonary valve or RV outflow tract.
   D. This represents a patent ductus arteriosus and requires reoperation.
   E. If replacement of the pulmonic valve is required, a mechanical valve should be contemplated.

18. A 57-year-old man is undergoing mitral valve repair for severe mitral regurgitation from mitral valve prolapse. He has an intraoperative TEE before the surgical repair and you are asked to consult regarding the image of the TR and tricuspid valve in the midesophageal four-chamber view (Fig. 16-3). Which of the following is correct?

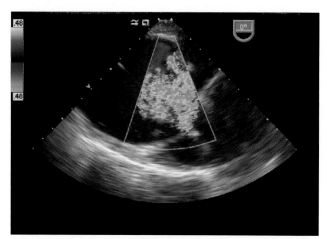

Fig. 16-3

A. The TR detected intraoperatively will likely overestimate that detected on routine ambulatory examination and should not be used in the decision making regarding concomitant tricuspid valve surgery.

B. Surgical intervention on the tricuspid valve is rarely required in this situation as it always improves after surgical correction of the mitral valve.

C. Surgical correction of the tricuspid valve should be considered as the regurgitation appears severe with a significant flow convergence area, and TR is more likely underestimated in the operative setting.

D. The most likely cause of severe TR in this situation is a flail tricuspid valve.

E. TR only occurs in this situation in the presence of severe pulmonary hypertension.

19. A 35-year-old woman has a history of recurrent fever of unknown origin and fleeting pleuritic chest pain. Multiple blood cultures have been negative, and a transthoracic echocardiogram of reasonable quality has been unremarkable. A chest X-ray has shown a small pleural effusion but an ultrasound has shown that this is too small to aspirate. She undergoes TEE. A representative image of the RV outflow tract is shown in Figure 16-4

and constitutes the only abnormality detected. Which of the following would be the most appropriate next step in managing this patient?

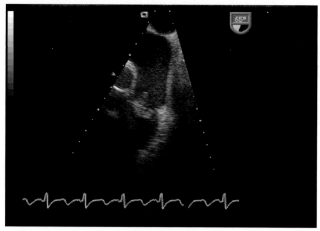

Fig. 16-4

A. Hypercoagulability work-up.

B. Venous duplex of lower limbs to exclude venous thrombosis.

C. CT scan with contrast of the chest to exclude pulmonary emboli.

D. Noncontrast chest CT.

E. Broad spectrum antibiotic treatment including antifungal coverage.

20. The hepatic vein pulsed Doppler profile shown in Figure 16-5 is most likely associated with which of the following clinical profiles?

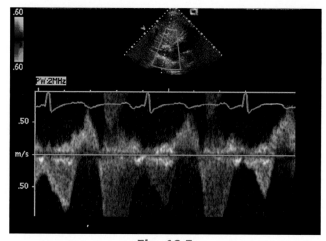

Fig. 16-5

A. Large "v" waves in the jugular venous profile.

B. Pulsus paradoxus.

C. Kussmaul's sign.

D. Pulsus alternans.

E. Pulsus bisferiens.

21. The pulmonary valve M-mode in Figure 16-6 is most likely associated with which of the following clinical scenarios?

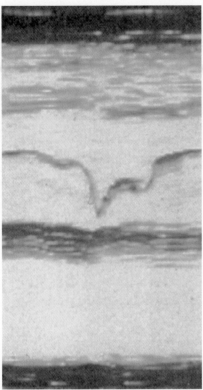

Fig. 16-6

A. Endocarditis of the pulmonary valve.
B. Infundibular pulmonic stenosis in a young man with prior repair of tetralogy of Fallot.
C. A young woman with primary pulmonary hypertension being considered for therapeutic intervention.
D. A retained PA catheter remnant in an elderly man with a prolonged hospital course.
E. Severe pulmonic insufficiency.

22. Which of the following statements concerning the condition shown in the image of the tricuspid valve in Figure 16-7 is correct?
A. It may require tricuspid valve replacement.
B. It does not respond to medical therapy.
C. The prognosis is excellent.
D. It frequently involves left-sided valves but rarely the pulmonic valve.
E. Infection is a major predisposing cause.

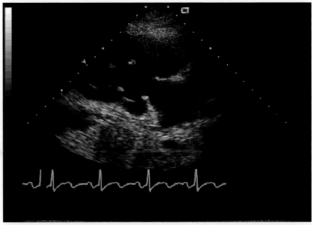

Fig. 16-7

23. The Doppler velocity in Figure 16-8 is through the pulmonary valve in the parasternal short-axis view of an 18-year-old man with chest pain. Which of the following statements is correct?

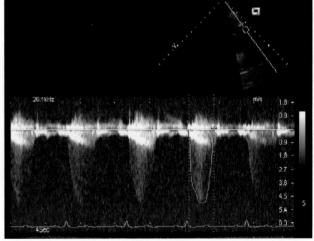

Fig. 16-8

A. In the absence of chest pain, there is no indication for any intervention.
B. He will likely benefit from a balloon valvuloplasty.
C. Based on the Doppler profile, he has associated subvalvular stenosis.
D. He most likely has a bicuspid pulmonic valve.
E. His chest pain is unrelated to the valve lesion.

24. Figure 16-9 illustrates a TEE transgastric view of the right atrium and right ventricle with the tricuspid valve open in diastole. The patient has been recently admitted with fevers 6 weeks after permanent pacemaker implantation with a DDD system. No obvious infection is evident at the site of the pacemaker insertion. Mild central TR is present. Which of the following statements is true about this case?

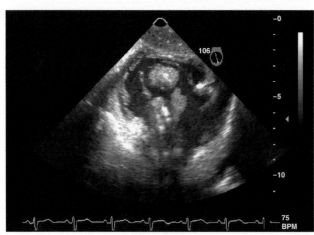

Fig. 16-9

A. The tricuspid valve will need to be replaced.
B. Only antibiotic therapy is required.
C. Surgical removal of the pacing wires followed by antibiotics is all that is required.
D. Percutaneous removal of the pacing wires and antibiotic therapy is required.
E. The patient will most likely require antibiotic treatment as well as surgical removal of the pacemaker wires and the pacemaker system including the generator.

25. A 22-year-old man is transferred from an outside hospital with endocarditis involving the tricuspid valve. A representative image of the tricuspid valve lesion as seen on TEE is shown in Figure 16-10. Based on the findings, which of the following is correct?
A. He requires immediate surgery because of the size of vegetation.
B. He may do well with medical therapy.
C. The most likely cause of the infection is *Enterococcus.*
D. The lesion represents a fungal infection.
E. The most likely complication is systemic embolization.

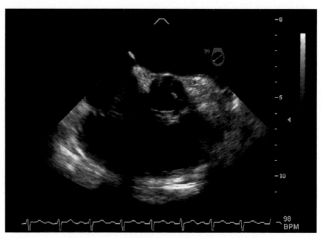

Fig. 16-10

CASE 1:

A 30-year-old woman presents with right-sided heart failure but without clubbing or cyanosis. She has had a murmur since childhood but has only recently complained of fatigue and ankle edema. On admission, she developed a wide complex tachycardia at a fast rate and required immediate cardioversion. An apical four-chamber view of her heart is shown in Video 16-1 and Figure 16-11.

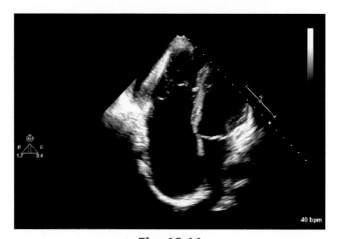

Fig. 16-11

26. What is the most likely cause of her heart failure symptoms?
A. Tachycardia-mediated cardiomyopathy.
B. Severe TR.
C. Severe pulmonary hypertension.
D. Recent endocarditis.
E. Right-to-left shunt at the atrial level.

27. Which of the following statements about treatment of this patient is true?
A. There is no indication for an electrophysiological study as surgical correction of the condition will also eradicate the arrhythmia.

B. Medical therapy is of little value in this condition and recourse to surgery is indicated.

C. Tricuspid valve replacement is the surgical therapy of choice.

D. The anterior leaflet is the most abnormal in this condition and should be removed if possible.

E. The size of the functional right ventricle is important in defining the likelihood and type of surgery.

CASE 2:

A 65-year-old man is readmitted 8 weeks following tricuspid and mitral valve repair for myxomatous disease of both valves. He has been feeling unwell and is anemic but has had no significant febrile illness. He has a white blood cell count of 12,000, with a leftward shift. A transesophageal echocardiogram is performed, an image of which is shown in Video 16-2 and Figure 16-12. He has no significant mitral regurgitation or TR.

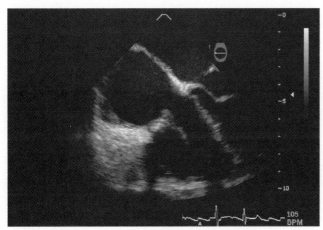

Fig. 16-12

28. The most likely cause of this scenario is:
A. Staphylococcal infection.
B. Thrombus formation at the valve ring.
C. Ring dehiscence.
D. Embolus in transit.
E. Fungal infection.

29. The best course of treatment for this patient now is:
A. Immediate surgical exploration and removal of the mass.
B. Intravenous thrombolysis.
C. Culture, broad-spectrum coverage pending cultures, and close monitoring of the valves by echocardiography.
D. Replacement of both mitral and tricuspid valves.
E. Heparin treatment followed by transition to warfarin (Coumadin).

CASE 3:

A color Doppler image of the RV outflow tract in an asymptomatic young man found to have a murmur on routine physical examination is shown in Figure 16-13 and Video 16-3. He has a right parasternal heave, an ejection click, and a loud ejection systolic murmur with a soft P2 heard on auscultation.

30. Based on these findings, select the correct statement from the following.

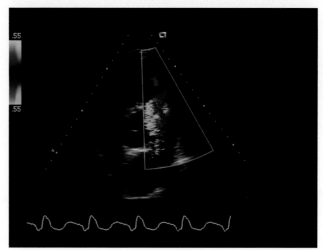

Fig. 16-13

A. He has a patent ductus arteriosus with Eisenmenger physiology.

B. He has an ASD with Eisenmenger physiology.

C. He has pulmonic stenosis, possibly severe, with mild pulmonic insufficiency.

D. He has a high outflow state with a flow murmur.

E. He has infundibular pulmonic stenosis.

31. The most appropriate next step in the management of this patient is to:
A. Perform balloon valvuloplasty of the pulmonic valve.
B. Establish the pulmonic valve area by continuity.
C. Measure the velocity and thus pressure across the RV outflow tract by continuous-wave Doppler.
D. Assess the PA systolic pressure.
E. Perform contrast echocardiography to define the presence and site of shunting.

CASE 4:

A 42-year-old woman who is an immigrant from India presents to a cardiology clinic with new onset right-sided heart failure. She has peripheral cyanosis, regular rhythm, a loud first heart sound, and an apical diastolic murmur. Her jugular venous pulse shows prominent pulsations that precede systole. She has an RV heave but normal P2. She has a prominent abdomen and a tender liver edge. A four-chamber image of her findings is shown in Video 16-4.

32. Based on this and her physical findings, what is the most likely diagnosis giving rise to her symptoms?
    A. Mitral stenosis and TR due to severe pulmonary hypertension.
    B. Tricuspid stenosis and regurgitation without significant mitral stenosis.
    C. Mitral stenosis and regurgitation.
    D. Tricuspid stenosis and mitral stenosis.
    E. Constrictive pericarditis.

33. What is the most appropriate treatment of this patient?
    A. Medical therapy only.
    B. Balloon valvuloplasty of the mitral and tricuspid valve.
    C. Surgical replacement of both mitral and tricuspid valve.
    D. Surgical commissurotomy of both mitral and tricuspid valve.
    E. Balloon valvuloplasty of the mitral valve.

CASE 5:

A 50-year-old man presents with heart failure. His physical examination is remarkable for jugular venous distention and abdominal distention. A soft systolic murmur is heard over the precordium but is soft and hard to elicit.

Apical images of his heart are shown in Video 16-5 and Figure 16-14.

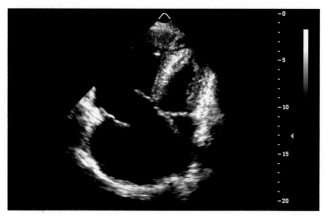

Fig. 16-14

34. The most likely cause of his presentation is:
    A. Flail anterior leaflet of the tricuspid valve with severe TR.
    B. Cor triatriatum dexter.
    C. Ebstein's anomaly.
    D. Perforation of the tricuspid valve with severe regurgitation and a vegetation.
    E. Carcinoid syndrome.

35. Which of the following scenarios is most likely to have had a role in the causation?
    A. Presence since birth.
    B. Marfan syndrome.
    C. Recent immobilization in a plaster cast.
    D. Placement of PA catheter a few months ago.
    E. Blunt trauma to the chest in the past.

ANSWERS

1. ANSWER: C. Right-sided valve lesions are usually well identified by transthoracic imaging as these structures lie anterior in the chest and in the near field of the chest wall transducer. However, better resolution of pulmonary valve endocarditis or mass, embolus in transit in the right heart, and of vegetations involving a pacer wire have been reported with transesophageal echocardiography (TEE) than with transthoracic echocardiography (TTE) alone. TEE is not usually indicated in the assessment of pulmonary artery (PA) pressures in primary pulmonary hypertension. When the tricuspid regurgitant velocity is difficult to measure by TTE, injection of agitated saline contrast has been shown to improve the spectral display of the regurgitant jet and is more likely to be helpful than a TEE in this situation.

2. ANSWER: B. A flail tricuspid valve is common with repeated endomyocardial biopsies following transplantation and leads to severe tricuspid regurgitation (TR) often with laminar rather than turbulent flow. McConnell's sign or apical sparing of right ventricular (RV) function is seen in acute pulmonary embolism but is not characteristic of this patient's scenario. Pulmonary insufficiency, tricuspid stenosis, and atrial septal defect (ASD) are usually not seen in transplanted hearts.

3. ANSWER: E. In the presence of severe TR with laminar flow through the valve, the right atrium and right ventricle operate more as a common chamber and Bernoulli's equation ($4 \times velocity^2$) is not operational. Severe TR, such as that due to a flail valve, is one of the few instances where Bernoulli's equation may not be used to accurately estimate the RV systolic pressure. If RV systolic pressure is required, recourse to invasive pressure recording may be needed.

4. ANSWER: A. His PA systolic pressure is normal. The estimated RV systolic pressure from his tricuspid regurgitant velocity is 36 mm Hg + 5 mm Hg = 41 mm Hg assuming a normal right atrial (RA) pressure (a reasonable assumption given normal RA size and inferior vena cava [IVC] size). The peak systolic pressure across the pulmonary valve is 20 mm Hg. Therefore, the PA systolic pressure is approximately 41 mm Hg− 20 mm Hg = 21 mm Hg or normal. PA systolic pressure can be estimated in pulmonary stenosis as long as the pressure gradient across the pulmonary valve is known.

5. ANSWER: B. Using TTE, the anterior leaflet and either the septal or posterior leaflet are imaged in the parasternal long-axis (RV inflow) view depending on the plane and the presence of the septum in the image. The posterior leaflet is imaged in the parasternal short-axis view at the level of the aortic valve, and is the leaflet adjacent to the RV free wall. The leaflet imaged adjacent to the aortic root can be either the septal or the anterior leaflet. The anterior and septal leaflets are also imaged in the apical four-chamber view, with the anterior leaflet adjacent to the RV free wall and the septal leaflet adjacent to the interventricular septum.

6. ANSWER: D. A Gerbode defect is a communication between the right atrium and left ventricle, often iatrogenic after surgery on the AV valves or following endocarditis of these valves. As the tricuspid valve is more apically situated under normal conditions in the heart than the mitral valve, the right atrium abuts the left ventricle over a small area. If a defect develops in this area, communication occurs between the right atrium and left ventricle.

7. ANSWER: C. The constant used to estimate the valve area in tricuspid stenosis is 190 not 220. Doming of the valve is seen in tricuspid stenosis but this is seen in diastole not systole. The mean gradient expected across the tricuspid valve in severe stenosis may be 5 mm Hg. Planimetry of the valve is difficult in tricuspid stenosis as it is difficult to get a true short-axis view of the valve. Although rheumatic involvement of the tricuspid valve occurs with some frequency, hemodynamic significant stenosis is relatively uncommon and is reported in about 5% of patients with rheumatic involvement of the mitral valve.

8. ANSWER: B. The severity of TR is assessed with a semiquantitative approach. Jet area, proximal flow acceleration, and the width of the vena contracta are used to quantify the severity of TR. If the tricuspid regurgitant jet is central, the Nyquist limit should be set at 50–60 cm/sec. A jet area of <5 cm² suggests mild TR, 5–10 cm² suggests moderate TR, and >10 cm²

suggests severe TR. An effective regurgitant orifice (ERO) of ≥0.40 cm² is a criterion of severe regurgitation in both TR and mitral regurgitation. A vena contracta dimension of >0.7 cm is diagnostic of severe TR.

9. ANSWER: D. Secondary pulmonary hypertension and/or RV dilatation is the most common cause of significant TR. All of the other conditions may lead to significant TR.

10. ANSWER: A. Normal RV systolic pressure should not occur with severe pulmonic stenosis as the RV systolic pressure will exceed the PA systolic pressure by the gradient across the pulmonary valve. RV hypertrophy (wall thickness of >0.4 cm) and post-stenotic dilatation are common in severe pulmonic stenosis. Severe pulmonic stenosis is defined by Doppler echocardiography as a peak velocity across the valve of 4 m/sec or higher. PA systolic pressure is usually normal in the setting of severe pulmonic stenosis.

11. ANSWER: D. Mild stenosis is considered present when the Doppler velocity is <3 m/sec or pressure of 36 mm Hg. The prognosis is excellent and intervention is rarely necessary. It is appropriate to follow with yearly echocardiography, but cardiac catheterization or TEE is not indicated. Doming of the valve in systole is a common echocardiographic feature of pulmonic stenosis.

12. ANSWER: C. Severe pulmonary insufficiency is usually seen in the setting of prior surgery on the RV outflow tract or pulmonary valve as part of the treatment of a congenital heart lesion. Pulmonary insufficiency is detected to be a trivial or mild degree normally. Severe pulmonary insufficiency is associated with a high end-diastolic pressure and a reduced pressure gradient across the pulmonic valve thus is more often associated with laminar rather than turbulent velocity. The pulmonary end-diastolic velocity (V) may be used to estimate the PA diastolic pressure as $4V^2$ + estimated RA pressure but is not used to estimate the PA systolic pressure.

13. ANSWER: B. A fibroelastoma is the most common cause of a mobile mass on the tricuspid valve among the choices provided. Myxoma and sarcoma of the valve are much less common. Chiari network is a fenestrated membranous structure, which originates at the orifice of the IVC and is an embryological remnant. It may rarely float through the tricuspid valve but is usually confined to the right atrium. It is not attached to the tricuspid valve. Carcinoid syndrome causes immobility of the valve leaflets such that they may remain in a partially open condition throughout the cardiac cycle.

14. ANSWER: D. Ebstein's anomaly involves the apical displacement of the septal leaflet of the tricuspid valve but does not involve the pulmonary valve. Carcinoid syndrome, staphylococcal endocarditis, and rheumatic involvement may involve both the tricuspid and pulmonic valve. Rheumatic involvement may be primary or more commonly secondary to pulmonary hypertension from left-sided valve lesions that produce tricuspid and pulmonary regurgitation.

15. ANSWER: B. Infundibular stenosis may give rise to a high-velocity jet that causes damage to the pulmonary valve leaflets and pulmonary insufficiency in a manner similar to subaortic stenosis. Infundibular stenosis may be either congenital or acquired. It occurs in congenital heart disease syndromes such as tetralogy of Fallot but also in hypertrophic cardiomyopathy, in tumors of the RV outflow tract or in infiltrative disorders. It may be discrete or consist of a more extensive region of fibromuscular thickening. It is often best imaged and evaluated from a parasternal short-axis view or from the subcostal window. Pressure gradients measured by Doppler across the infundibular stenosis are reasonably accurate. When concomitant pulmonic valvar stenosis is present, it is usually impossible to isolate the precise contribution of the pulmonic valve and infundibulum to the total gradient measured by continuous-wave Doppler across the RV outflow tract.

16. ANSWER: C. The image is characteristic of Ebstein's anomaly of the tricuspid valve with displacement of the septal leaflet into the right ventricle so that a portion of the right ventricle is "atrialized." Ebstein's anomaly is associated with accelerated conduction, severe TR but not with a parchment-like RV wall. This is seen in dysplastic RV or Uhl syndrome, which may be associated with ventricular arrhythmias.

17. ANSWER: C. This is severe pulmonary regurgitation with evidence of a proximal flow convergence on the PA side of the valve. It is consistent with RV dilatation and RV dysfunction. The most common cause of severe pulmonary regurgitation is prior surgery for congenital heart disease involving the pulmonary valve or RV outflow tract. Patent ductus arteriosus will give rise to continuous flow into the PA above the valve. A homograft is usually the valve replacement of choice at the pulmonic position. Mechanical valves are associated with higher rates of thrombosis at right-sided valve positions because of the lesser pressure gradient across them and are usually avoided.

18. ANSWER: C. There is severe TR present with a flow convergence area and dilatation of the right atrium. Intraoperative TEE is more likely to underestimate the degree of regurgitation compared with the ambulatory setting due to optimization of intravascular volume and change in loading consequent to anesthesia and mechanical ventilation. Severe TR occurs in mitral valve prolapse as a result of prolapse of the tricuspid valve or

secondary to pulmonary hypertension from severe mitral regurgitation but rarely due to flail of the tricuspid valve leaflet. Severe pulmonary hypertension is not necessary to cause this degree of TR; prolapse or secondary changes in the tricuspid annulus or valve may alone cause it. TR may improve after surgical repair of the mitral valve especially if the pulmonary pressures fall but this is less likely when the TR is severe preoperatively as here and concomitant tricuspid valve repair should be considered. This adds relatively little to the operative risk or the duration of the case in experienced centers.

19. ANSWER: D. This patient has a thickened pulmonary valve and pleuritic symptoms. Either endocarditis of the pulmonary valve or a pulmonary fibroelastoma is possible. The pleuritic symptoms suggest embolization to the lungs. A chest CT scan to look for septic emboli is the test of choice now. A chest CT scan was performed in this patient and showed abscess formation in the pulmonary parenchyma. Blood cultures were negative as the patient took oral antibiotics early in the course of treatment. Endocarditis was diagnosed and it transpired that the patient had an occult IV drug abuse habit.

20. ANSWER: A. High-velocity systolic reversal in the hepatic veins is seen in severe TR which also gives rise to large "v" waves in the jugular venous profile (Fig. 16-15). Pulsus paradoxus, a reduction in systolic blood pressure on respiration, is most characteristic of cardiac tamponade. Kussmaul's sign with an increase in the venous pressure on inspiration is most characteristic of constrictive pericarditis. Pulsus alternans, alternating strong and weak peripheral pulses, is seen in end-stage LV systolic dysfunction. Pulsus bisferiens is a characteristic pulse felt in the setting of both significant aortic stenosis and regurgitation.

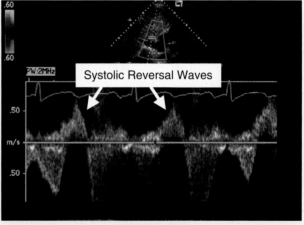

Fig. 16-15

21. ANSWER: C. Pulmonary hypertension is associated with abrupt midsystolic closure of the pulmonary valve in about 50% of cases especially when severe. The appearance is thought to occur from transient reversal of the PA–RV outflow tract gradient due to impaired PA compliance. This appearance is occasionally seen in severe TR and with a dilated PA. It is not associated with the other lesions previously described.

22. ANSWER: A. The condition illustrated is carcinoid, manifested by thickening and shortening of the tricuspid leaflets. Severe TR may result requiring tricuspid valve replacement. Carcinoid is thought to be due to the production of serotonin by a tumor that is inactivated in the lungs so that in the absence of right-to-left shunting, left-sided lesions are uncommon. The pulmonary valve is frequently involved. Medication to reduce the production of serotonin may be helpful in reducing the symptoms of flushing. However, survival is usually significantly reduced with carcinoid and thus prognosis is guarded.

23. ANSWER: B. The ACC/AHA guidelines suggest that balloon valvuloplasty is indicated when the peak pressure gradient across the pulmonary valve is >30 mm Hg with symptoms or 40 mm Hg in the absence of symptoms. Subvalvular stenosis may be present but is not evident on the Doppler profile. Two systolic velocity spectral displays are evident. A low-velocity (~1 m/sec) jet with a dense spectral pattern is consistent with flow in the RV outflow tract. This suggests a relatively low velocity in the RV outflow tract but does not entirely exclude some degree of subvalvar stenosis. The high-velocity (~4.5 m/sec) jet reflects the stenosis at the valve itself. Dysplastic unicuspid or trileaflet valves are a more common cause of pulmonic stenosis than a bicuspid valve. Chest pain is common in severe pulmonic stenosis and likely reflects reduced cardiac outflow and flow to the coronaries and/or subendocardial ischemia in the hypertrophied right ventricle.

24. ANSWER: E. The patient has large mass lesions consistent with vegetations involving the pacing wires, although sparing the tricuspid valve in this view. Given the size of the apparent vegetations, the risk of pulmonary embolism is high and an open surgical approach will likely be needed. Antibiotic coverage will be required and removal of the whole system including the generator is indicated to remove all potential sources of infection. Unless the tricuspid valve has been destroyed in the infective process, tricuspid valve replacement is not indicated.

25. ANSWER: B. There is a large vegetation on the septal leaflet of the tricuspid valve. The size of the vegetation and embolic risk is less of a consideration with tricuspid endocarditis where embolization to the lungs rather than the systemic vasculature is the norm. The exception is when a right-to-left shunt exists. The initial therapy should be appropriate antibiotic therapy and watchful management. If blood cultures fail to clear or there is evidence of severe tricuspid valve destruction, then tricuspid valve surgery may be necessary. Fungal infection may give rise to very large vegetations but staphylococcal infection is by far the most common cause of this particular scenario.

26. ANSWER: B. This is Ebstein's anomaly. The usual cause of right-sided heart failure at least with a later presentation is TR. ASD occurs in many patients with Ebstein's anomaly but would have been expected to present somewhat earlier if associated with significant shunting. Severe pulmonary hypertension is relatively rare. There is no evidence of endocarditis; and although tachycardia may occur in this condition, there is no evidence of cardiomyopathy on the images.

27. ANSWER: E. An electrophysiological study is indicated in the setting of suspected accessory pathway tachycardia, which occurs in about 10%–25% of these patients and especially if surgery is being contemplated. Medical therapy is often sufficient in many patients with mild to moderate lesions for the effective control of symptoms. Tricuspid repair is the initial surgical treatment of choice. Its feasibility depends on the degree of tethering of the leaflets and the size of the functional right ventricle. The smaller the functional right ventricle, the less likely tricuspid repair is to be successful. The septal leaflet is usually the one most tethered and the anterior leaflet is the least likely to be affected. It may have a sail-like configuration and float into the RV outflow tract causing obstruction in some individuals.

KEY POINTS:
- Ebstein's anomaly of the tricuspid valve is associated with TR, right-sided heart failure, accessory pathways, and ASDs.
- When tricuspid repair is required, it is dependent on the degree of septal leaflet tethering and the size and functionality of the right ventricle.

28. ANSWER: A. The patient has all the appearances of endocarditis except fever, and fever occasionally does not supervene in this setting. The most likely cause of infection here is staphylococcal perhaps from the time of implantation. Both thrombus formation and ring dehiscence are also possibilities, although somewhat less likely. Dehiscence is also less likely in the absence of associated regurgitation. The lesion is obviously attached to the tricuspid valve and thus is unlikely to be an embolus in transit.

29. ANSWER: C.

KEY POINTS:
- *Staphylococcus* is a common cause of early onset prosthetic valve endocarditis.
- Tricuspid valve endocarditis is usually amenable to antibiotic treatment.

30. ANSWER: C. The physical examination suggests valvular pulmonic stenosis with an ejection click and ejection murmur associated with RV hypertrophy. With more severe stenosis, the P2 becomes softer. The Doppler shows turbulent flow just beyond the pulmonary valve with mild pulmonary insufficiency. Patent ductus arteriosus usually leads to continuous flow in the PA, but this may be attenuated in Eisenmenger physiology. Pulmonary hypertension as part of Eisenmenger syndrome will lead to a loud P2. Infundibular pulmonic stenosis will not have the ejection click of a mobile but dysplastic valve and the turbulent velocity will be proximal to the valve.

31. ANSWER: C. The next step is to assess how severe the stenosis is by continuous-wave Doppler. Doppler measurements correlate well with those made by cardiac catheterization. Balloon valvuloplasty is considered in an asymptomatic patient who has at least a moderate increase in gradient (>30 mm Hg). Although the pulmonic valve area may be assessed by continuity, in practice this is not usually performed. The various guidelines on which decisions concerning intervention are based use the pressure gradient rather than the area. Although PA pressure should be measured, it is usually low in this setting. Contrast injection is reasonable, if a shunt is suspected. Most often valvular pulmonic stenosis is an isolated abnormality.

KEY POINTS:

■ Valvular pulmonary stenosis is generally graded on the basis of the gradient through the valve.

■ Valvular pulmonary stenosis when presenting as an isolated lesion is usually amenable to balloon valvuloplasty.

32. ANSWER: D. Both mitral stenosis and tricuspid stenosis are present on the image. The physical findings of an apical diastolic murmur and loud S1 suggest mitral stenosis, whereas the accentuated venous pulse in presystole is consistent with a large "a" wave seen with tricuspid stenosis. Absence of a loud P2 suggests that pulmonary hypertension has not occurred. Significant tricuspid stenosis when it complicates mitral stenosis may give rise to right-sided heart failure and ascites that may simulate constrictive pericarditis.

33. ANSWER: B. Assuming significant stenosis of both valves that is suggested by the images and physical examination, balloon valvuloplasty of both valves is the ideal approach if the lesions are suitable. Otherwise, surgical commissurotomy is appropriate given the symptomatic state.

KEY POINTS:

■ Mitral and tricuspid stenosis may coexist especially in patients with rheumatic heart disease and simulate constrictive pericarditis.

■ Both mitral and tricuspid stenosis may be amenable to balloon valvuloplasty in many patients.

34. ANSWER: A. The anterior tricuspid leaflet is flail with resultant severe TR. Cor triatriatum dexter is a rare condition in which a membrane septates the right atrium and presents with findings similar to tricuspid stenosis. Perforation of a tricuspid valve leaflet with an associated vegetation could give this appearance but the whole anterior leaflet is obviously flail in this example. Perforation is difficult to detect on two-dimensional imaging and is usually apparent by detecting an eccentric jet apparently coming through a leaflet on color Doppler examination. Ebstein's anomaly leads to apical displacement and tethering of the tricuspid leaflets—most often the septal leaflet. Carcinoid leads to thickening and reduced motion of the leaflet rather than excess motion as seen here.

35. ANSWER: E. Flail tricuspid valve may occur with blunt chest trauma and not be apparent at the time. Myxomatous changes may also give rise to a flail leaflet as may severing of a tricuspid chord at the time of endomyocardial biopsy especially after heart transplantation. Placement of a PA catheter is unlikely to cause this finding. Although Marfan syndrome can cause multivalvular prolapse, it is unlikely to be confined to the tricuspid valve. Congenital flail valve and flail in the setting of pulmonary thromboembolism are both very unlikely.

KEY POINT:

■ A flail tricuspid valve may be due to chest trauma, myxomatous changes, or endomyocardial biopsy.

SUGGESTED READINGS

Baumgartner H, Hung J, Bermejo J, et al. Echocardiographic assessment of valve stenosis EAE/ASE recommendations for clinical practice. *J Am Soc Echocardiogr.* 2009;22:1–23.

Bonow RO, Carabello BA, Chatterjee K, et al. 2008 focused update incorporated into the ACC/AHA 2006 guidelines for the management of patients with valvular heart disease: a report of the American College of Cardiology/American Heart Association Task Force on Practice Guidelines (Writing Committee to revise the 1998 guidelines for the management of patients with valvular heart disease). Endorsed by the Society of Cardiovascular Anesthesiologists, Society for Cardiovascular Angiography and Interventions, and Society of Thoracic Surgeons. *J Am Coll Cardiol.* 2008;52:e1–e142.

Bonow RO, Carabello BA, Kanu C, et al. ACC/AHA 2006 guidelines for the management of patients with valvular heart disease: a report of the American College of Cardiology/American Heart Association Task Force on Practice Guidelines (writing committee to revise the 1998 Guidelines for the Management of Patients With Valvular Heart Disease): developed in collaboration with the Society of Cardiovascular Anesthesiologists endorsed by the Society for Cardiovascular Angiography and Interventions and the Society of Thoracic Surgeons. *Circulation.* 2006;114:e84–e231.

Braunwald E, Zipes DP, Libby P. *Heart Disease: A Textbook of Cardiovascular Medicine.* 8th ed. Philadelphia: WB Sounders Company; 2007.

Griffin B, Rimmerman C, Topol E. *Intensive Review of Cardiovascular Medicine.* Philadelphia: Lippincott Williams &Wilkins; 2006.

Hayes CJ, Gersony WM, Driscoll DJ, et al. Second natural history study of congenital heart defects. Results of treatment of patients with pulmonary valvar stenosis. *Circulation.* 1993;87(2 Suppl):I28–I37.

Nair D, Griffin BP. Pulmonary and tricuspid and drug induced valve disease. In Griffin BP, Topol EJ, eds. *Manual of Cardiovascular Medicine.* 3rd ed. Philadelphia: Wolters Kluwer Health/Lippincott Williams & Wilkins; 2009:239–250.

Pellikka PA, Tajik AJ, Khandheria BK, et al. Carcinoid heart disease. Clinical and echocardiographic spectrum in 74 patients. *Circulation.* 1993;87:1188–1196.

Shah PM, Raney AA. Tricuspid valve disease. *Curr Probl Cardiol.* 2008;33:47–84.

Tribouilloy CM, Enriquez-Sarano M, Bailey KR, et al. Quantification of tricuspid regurgitation by measuring the width of the vena contracta with Doppler color flow imaging: a clinical study. *J Am Coll Cardiol.* 2000;36:472–478.

Weyman AE. *Principles and Practice of Echocardiography.* 2nd ed. Philadelphia: Lea and Febiger; 1994:824–900.

Zoghbi WA, Enriquez-Sarano M, Foster E, et al. Recommendations for evaluation of the severity of native valvular regurgitation with two-dimensional and Doppler echocardiography. *J Am Soc Echocardiogr.* 2003;16:777–802.

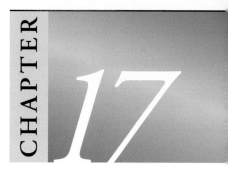

CHAPTER 17

Aortic and Mitral Valvular Disease

Sorin V. Pislaru and Maurice Enriquez-Sarano

1. A 72-year-old man is referred for a cardiology evaluation after his primary care physician noted presence of a loud ejection murmur. There is no history of angina, syncope, or exertional dyspnea. Clinical examination shows presence of a loud ejection murmur (3/6) over the aortic area, radiating to the neck vessels. There are no ejection clicks. The second heart sound is single. There are no other murmurs or gallops. Lung examination is unremarkable. Transthoracic echocardiogram shows normal left ventricular (LV) size with an ejection fraction (EF) of 65%. The left ventricular outflow tract time-velocity integral (LVOT TVI) is 15 cm with a velocity of 0.8 m/sec. The peak aortic velocity is 4.8 m/sec, and the aortic valve TVI is 100 cm. The LVOT area is 4 cm^2.

   Your interpretation of the echocardiogram is:
   A. Severe aortic stenosis because valve area is <1 cm^2.
   B. Severe aortic stenosis because the LVOT/aortic velocity ratio is <0.3.
   C. Severe aortic stenosis because peak aortic velocity is >3.5 m/sec.
   D. The severity of the aortic stenosis cannot be determined from the data presented.

2. In this asymptomatic patient, your further recommendation is:
   A. Inform patient that the chance of developing symptoms in the next 5 years is 20%.
   B. Recommend coronary angiography in anticipation of surgical intervention.
   C. Recommend transesophageal echocardiography (TEE).
   D. Recommend oxygen consumption treadmill test.
   E. Recommend repeat echocardiogram in 2 years.

3. A 60-year-old man with a history of chronic renal insufficiency, arterial hypertension, and history of moderate aortic stenosis is admitted to the hospital for worsening dyspnea on exertion. His previous echocardiogram obtained 2 years ago showed concentric LV hypertrophy with an EF of 55%. The aortic valve gradient was 30 mm Hg and the calculated valve area was 1.1 cm^2. Clinical examination shows a patient in mild respiratory distress. The apical impulse is laterally displaced. There is a 2/6 systolic ejection murmur over the aortic area, which does not radiate to the carotid vessels. The second heart sound is diminished in intensity. Peripheral arterial pulsations are reduced in volume. There is significant peripheral edema. Laboratory work-up shows a creatinine level of 3.2 mg/dl. Overnight, the patient is started on a furosemide infusion by the on-call resident, but this has to be stopped due to development of hypotension. Initial echocardiogram shows an enlarged left ventricle (64 mm) with severely reduced systolic function with an EF of 20% and global hypokinesis. The mean aortic gradient is 30 mm Hg, with an aortic valve TVI of 66 cm, and an LVOT TVI of 15 cm.

   Your recommendation is:
   A. Recommend adenosine sestamibi.
   B. Recommend exercise echocardiogram.
   C. Recommend full-dose dobutamine echocardiogram.
   D. Recommend low-dose dobutamine echocardiogram.

E. Findings are probably related to end-stage renal disease, no further cardiac workup is required. Initiate dialysis.

4. Which of the following statements referring to an echocardiographic evaluation of aortic stenosis is accurate?
   A. Echocardiographic assessment of maximum aortic gradient is usually higher than the pull-back gradient obtained during left heart catheterization. This is due to overestimation of the true gradient by echocardiography.
   B. Echocardiographic assessment of mean aortic gradient correlates well with the mean gradient obtained in the catheterization laboratory.
   C. The usual echocardiographic measurement of the mean aortic gradient cannot overestimate the true gradient.
   D. The assessment of mean aortic gradient with a nonimaging probe is more accurate because these probes allow for better Doppler software processing.

5. A patient is evaluated for aortic stenosis. Doppler measurements from all available windows show a highest peak aortic velocity of 5 m/sec and a TVI of 125 cm. The LVOT velocity is 2 m/sec, and the TVI is 25 cm. The LVOT diameter is 2 cm. Which of the following calculations is correct?
   A. Aortic valve area 0.78 cm^2, peak gradient 100 mm Hg.
   B. Aortic valve area 0.63 cm^2, peak gradient 100 mm Hg.
   C. Aortic valve area 0.78 cm^2, peak gradient 84 mm Hg.
   D. Aortic valve area 0.63 cm^2, peak gradient 84 mm Hg.

6. A 72-year-old woman is referred for surgical intervention for severe aortic stenosis. She has a long-standing history of dyspnea on exertion, which has recently worsened. She has hypertension requiring multiple medications, hyperlipidemia, and diabetes. She quit smoking last year after a 40 pack-year history. On clinical examination, there is a 2/6 systolic ejection murmur over the aortic area. The second heart sound is split at the base. Pulsations are 2/4 in the upper and lower extremities.

There is a left carotid artery bruit. Lung examination shows prolonged expiratory phase but is otherwise unremarkable. The echocardiographic report from the referring physician shows a normal LV size, EF of 70%, normal cardiac output, and severe aortic stenosis with a valve area of 0.68 cm^2 and a mean gradient of 30 mm Hg. The best recommendation at this stage is:
   A. Proceed with surgical intervention.
   B. Perform coronary angiography then proceed with surgical intervention.
   C. Repeat transthoracic echocardiogram.
   D. Perform transesophageal echocardiogram.
   E. Perform cardiac computed tomography (CT) for aortic valve calcium score.

7. A 30-year-old woman is referred for management of a newly diagnosed subaortic stenosis. She presented at an outside institution with complaints of mild dyspnea on exertion. Echocardiogram demonstrated a subaortic membrane with a gradient of 44 mm Hg and concomitant presence of moderate aortic valve regurgitation. The left ventricle is mildly enlarged, with an EF of 57%. At TEE, the aortic valve does not appear to be significantly calcified. Which of the following statements is correct?
   A. This type of lesion responds well to balloon dilatation.
   B. Presence of moderate aortic regurgitation is not an indication for surgical intervention.
   C. Careful inspection of the pulmonary artery should be carried out during TEE.
   D. Doppler interrogation of the abdominal aorta provides no information in this case.

8. Which of the following statements regarding aortic regurgitation is correct?
   A. A proximal isovelocity surface area (PISA) radius of 0.8 cm with an aliasing velocity of 40 cm/sec and a peak aortic regurgitant velocity of 4 m/sec is consistent with severe aortic regurgitation.
   B. A pressure halftime in excess of 250 milliseconds is consistent with severe aortic regurgitation.
   C. Vena contracta is best evaluated from the apical long-axis view.
   D. The use of the suprasternal notch window is not useful in the assessment of aortic regurgitation.

9. Which of the following echocardiographic findings is important in predicting the outcome of mitral balloon valvuloplasty?
   A. Presence of significant valvular calcification.
   B. Presence of significant valvular thickening.
   C. Presence of significant subvalvular calcifications.
   D. All.
   E. A and B.

10. During routine assessment of a patient with known valvular disease, the sonographer measures a mitral inflow deceleration time of 758 milliseconds. Which of the following is a reasonable estimate of the mitral valve area?
   A. 1 cm^2.
   B. 0.3 cm^2.
   C. 3 cm^2.
   D. 1.5 cm^2.
   E. 2 cm^2.

11. Which of the following mitral stenosis patients is likely to benefit from mitral balloon valvuloplasty?
   A. Asymptomatic 29-year-old woman with mitral gradient of 9 mm Hg and resting tricuspid regurgitation velocity of 4 m/sec.
   B. A 49-year-old man complaining of dyspnea and a mitral pressure halftime of 110 milliseconds.
   C. A 62-year-old woman complaining of dyspnea and evidence of heavily calcified mitral commissures and a mitral gradient of 12 mm Hg.
   D. Asymptomatic 35-year-old woman with a mitral valve gradient of 12 mm Hg and a loud apical systolic murmur.

12. A comprehensive echocardiogram is obtained for the assessment of mitral regurgitation. The mitral annulus measures 4 cm in diameter, and the TVI of the Doppler signal obtained from the plane of the mitral valve is 10 cm. The LVOT diameter is 2 cm, with a TVI of 25 cm. The mitral regurgitant volume is:
   A. 125 ml.
   B. 47 ml.
   C. 78.5 ml.
   D. 30 ml.
   E. The regurgitant volume cannot be calculated on the basis of presented data.

13. A cardiac surgeon calls you regarding an echocardiogram from an outside institution. He noticed the presence of significant mitral regurgitation by color Doppler and asks you to help with formal quantification of the degree of regurgitation. The study shows clips for mitral regurgitant PISA (aliasing velocity 40 cm/sec, PISA radius 1 cm), but there is no continuous wave (CW) Doppler interrogation of the mitral regurgitant signal. You tell him that an exact measurement cannot be done without knowing the exact mitral regurgitant velocity and TVI; however, with some reasonable assumptions you can say that:
   A. Mitral regurgitation is severe because mitral effective regurgitant area is approximately 0.50 cm^2.
   B. Mitral regurgitation is nearly severe because the effective regurgitant area is approximately 0.38 cm^2.
   C. Mitral regurgitation is severe because the regurgitant volume is approximately 75 ml.
   D. Mitral regurgitation cannot be quantified on the basis of existing data.
   E. A and C.

14. Mitral valve prolapse is best diagnosed from which of the following imaging planes?
   A. Apical four-chamber view.
   B. Apical two-chamber view.
   C. Apical long-axis view.
   D. Parasternal short-axis view.
   E. Parasternal long-axis view.

15. A 54-year-old man is hospitalized with an acute myocardial infarction. He is taken emergently to the catheterization laboratory, where a completely occluded right coronary artery is found. He undergoes successful stenting. On the third day of hospitalization, he becomes acutely dyspneic and appears diaphoretic. There are no murmurs on clinical examination. An emergency bedside echocardiogram shows hyperdynamic LV function; there is no pericardial effusion. The mitral CW interrogation shows a dense dagger-shaped signal in systole. The most likely explanation for the patient's symptoms is:
   A. LV free wall rupture.
   B. Ventricular septal rupture with large ventricular septal defect.
   C. Acute severe mitral regurgitation due to papillary muscle rupture.
   D. Acute thrombosis of the coronary stent.

16. A patient is referred for further evaluation of a systolic murmur. The echocardiographic finding in parasternal short axis in Figure 17-1 is most suggestive of:

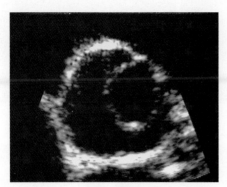

Fig. 17-1

A. Degenerative aortic stenosis.
B. Rheumatic aortic stenosis.
C. Bicuspid aortic stenosis.
D. Unicuspid aortic stenosis.

17. A 42-year-old woman presents with complaints of palpitations. She has no history of cardiac disease. She is otherwise completely asymptomatic. Clinical examination reveals presence of a moderate ejection murmur over the aortic area. There is a soft diastolic murmur along the left sternal border. Heart sounds are normal. A transthoracic echocardiogram is shown in Figure 17-2. The best answer regarding the patient's condition is:
A. Patient has an indication for surgery for severe aortic stenosis.
B. Patient's condition is benign, no further evaluation is necessary.
C. Patient's condition would be completely resolved with surgical intervention; there is no need for long-term follow-up.
D. TEE may be useful in deciding whether surgical intervention is required.

18. A 36-year-old man is referred for further evaluation of a cardiac murmur. He has noticed some decrease in his ability to exercise. He used to be an avid jogger but now is able to go only 15 minutes on a treadmill at moderate speed. Clinical examination shows a blood pressure of 164/68 mm Hg with a heart rate of 82 bpm. The cardiac impulse is laterally displaced. There is a loud diastolic murmur, and an ejection click is present. The echocardiogram is shown in Figure 17-3. The best statement regarding the patient's condition is:

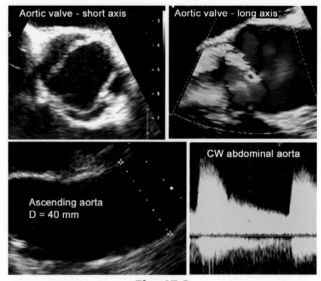

Fig. 17-3

A. The only surgical option is aortic valve replacement.
B. A valve sparing intervention is unlikely to be successful.
C. Ascending aortic graft repair is indicated only when the aortic diameter is >5.5–6 cm.
D. Chest CT will be required for surgical planning.

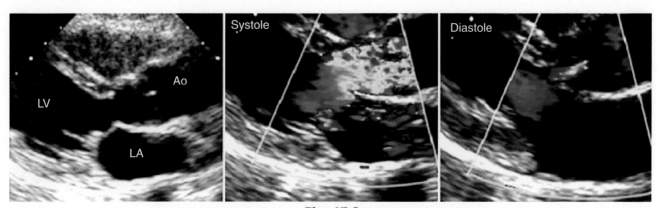

Fig. 17-2

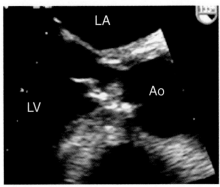
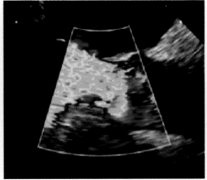
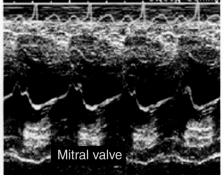

Fig. 17-4

19. A 45-year-old man is transferred for recurrent fevers, weight loss, and rapidly worsening dyspnea. The two-dimension and color Doppler echocardiographic diastolic frames and a mitral valve M mode are shown in Figure 17-4. The most likely clinical finding is:
   A. Marked v waves on the jugular venous contour.
   B. Loud continuous murmur over the left sternal border and in the back.
   C. Systolic click at the apex.
   D. Diastolic rumble at the apex.

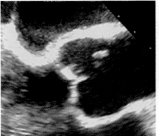
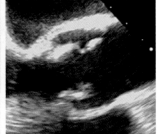

Fig. 17-5

20. A 60-year-old man without a history of cardiac disease presents with new complaints of palpitations and dyspnea on exertion for the last 10 days. The electrocardiogram demonstrates atrial fibrillation with rapid ventricular response. A TEE-guided cardioversion is performed; a mobile 1.5 cm echodensity is noted on the aortic valve (Fig. 17-5). Which of the following statements is correct?
   A. Patient should take lifelong anticoagulation.
   B. Surgical intervention may be required to reduce the risk of embolic events.
   C. Aortic valve replacement is the most recommended surgical intervention.

   D. If surgery is performed, there is no risk of recurrence.
   E. Aspirin has no role in this condition.

21. A 49-year-old woman presents with a history of progressively worsening dyspnea. She remembers having frequent throat infections as a child. Echocardiogram shows atrial fibrillation with an average heart rate of 85 bpm. An echocardiographic examination is performed (Fig. 17-6). Chest X-ray shows normal heart size. Clinical examination is most likely to show:
   A. Laterally displaced apical impulse.
   B. Opening snap occurring late after A2.
   C. Opening snap occurring early after A2.
   D. Apical diastolic rumble decreasing with leg exercise.

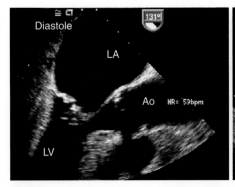
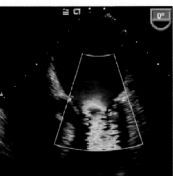
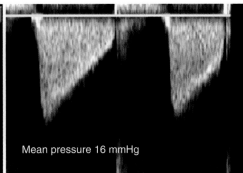

Fig. 17-6

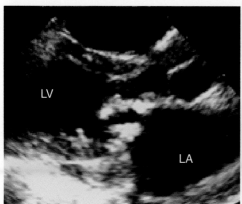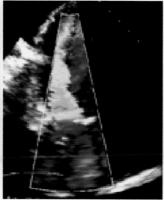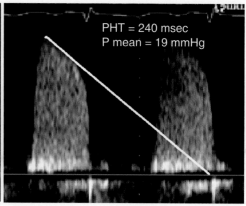

Fig. 17-7

22. A 67-year-old patient with a history of mitral valve repair 6 years ago for severe mitral regurgitation presents now with worsening dyspnea on exertion over the last 6 months. She also complains of cough with occasional blood-tinged sputum. An echocardiogram is performed and shown in Figure 17-7. Which of the following statements is correct?
    A. Patient's symptoms are likely due to development of secondary pulmonary hypertension.
    B. In this situation, accurate diagnosis can only be made by left and right heart catheterization.
    C. Supine bicycle echocardiography is the next step in evaluation.
    D. Mitral balloon valvuloplasty is likely to result in clinical improvement.
    E. All statements are correct.

23. A 39-year-old woman is referred for evaluation of mitral regurgitation due to a very eccentric jet. The TEE findings shown in Figure 17-8 are consistent with:
    A. Eccentric jets are not reliably quantified by PISA.
    B. The mitral regurgitation is moderate.
    C. The mitral regurgitation is severe.
    D. The regurgitant volume is <60 ml.
    E. The only definitive proof of severe regurgitation in the case of eccentric jets is a demonstration of systolic flow reversal in the pulmonary veins.

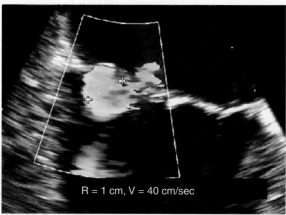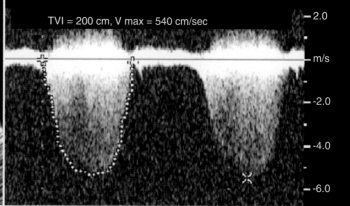

Fig. 17-8

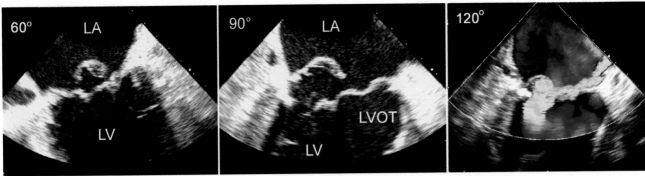

Fig. 17-9

24. The TEE images in Figure 17-9 are obtained for evaluation of a newly diagnosed mitral regurgitation. The imaging plane angles are provided. You advise the surgeon that:
   A. There is a flail segment in the P1 scallop.
   B. There is a flail segment in the P2 scallop.
   C. There is a flail segment in the P3 scallop.
   D. There is a flail segment in the A2 scallop.
   E. There is bileaflet prolapse.

25. You are called to assist with an intraoperative transesophageal echocardiogram. Images are shown in Figure 17-10. You advise the surgeon that:
   A. The mitral regurgitation is severe; he will need to perform a posterior leaflet repair.
   B. The mitral regurgitation is severe; he will need to perform an anterior leaflet repair.
   C. The mitral regurgitation is severe and the patient will need to be reassessed intraoperatively after coming off cardiac bypass.
   D. The mitral regurgitation is moderate and does not require intervention.
   E. Medical therapy is unlikely to have an effect on the mitral regurgitation in this type of disease.

CASE 1:

 A 65-year-old man presents for evaluation of chest pain. An echocardiogram is obtained (Video 17-1).

26. The echocardiographic images shown are suggestive of:
   A. Mitral regurgitation due to posterior leaflet prolapse.
   B. Mitral regurgitation due to ischemic tethering.
   C. Mitral regurgitation due to annular enlargement.
   D. Mitral regurgitation due to rheumatic valve disease.
   E. Mitral regurgitation due to ruptured posterior chord.

27. Which of the following statements is correct in this situation?
   A. An effective regurgitant orifice of only 0.25 cm^2 is associated with a good prognosis.
   B. Mitral valve ring annuloplasty is associated with excellent long-term results.
   C. Myocardial revascularization is likely to correct the mitral regurgitation; there is no need for an intervention on the mitral valve.
   D. The best surgical intervention for this type of mitral regurgitation is controversial.

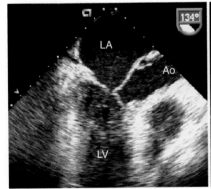
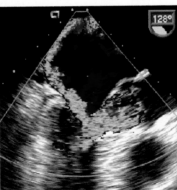
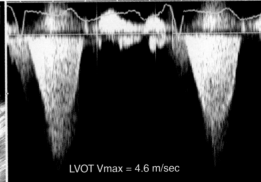

Fig. 17-10

CASE 2:

A 52-year-old man is referred for evaluation of a systolic murmur. He has no history of coronary or valvular disease. He is a nonsmoker and exercises regularly. Over the last few months, he noticed dizziness when lifting heavy weights but is otherwise completely asymptomatic. His only brother died at a young age of an unknown cause. An outside echocardiogram is available for review in Video 17-2.

28. The images shown are suggestive of:
    A. Mitral regurgitation due to posterior leaflet prolapse.
    B. Mitral regurgitation due to ischemic tethering.
    C. Mitral regurgitation due to annular enlargement
    D. Mitral regurgitation due to rheumatic valve disease.
    E. Mitral regurgitation due to LVOT obstruction.

29. Which of the following statements regarding this patient is correct?
    A. Treatment with angiotensin-converting enzyme inhibitors will reduce the degree of mitral regurgitation.
    B. The systolic murmur will decrease with Valsalva maneuver.
    C. The dizziness spells are not related to patient's condition; recommend neurologic evaluation.
    D. To correct the mitral regurgitation, the anterior mitral leaflet needs to be surgically repaired.
    E. Disopyramide can be used in this situation.

CASE 3:

A 60-year-old gentleman is referred for a cardiac consultation. He has had a known murmur for a long time; but during the most recent evaluation, his primary care physician noted that the murmur is more intense. The patient exercises regularly, alternating 20-mile bicycle rides with 3-mile walks. He has noted no change in his exercise ability. Physical examination shows presence of mild pectus excavatum, a 3/6 holosystolic murmur at the apex, but no systolic clicks and no peripheral edema. Lung examination is unremarkable. An echocardiogram is obtained (Video 17-3).

30. Which of the following statements is correct?
    A. There is evidence of bileaflet mitral valve prolapse.
    B. Afterload reduction is recommended even when normotensive.
    C. Screening of other family members is suggested.
    D. The calculated EF is 57%; reassure the patient.

E. There are no restrictions on physical activity in this type of disease.

31. In discussing surgical intervention with your patient, you tell him that:
    A. Surgery is contraindicated because the EF is normal and the patient is asymptomatic.
    B. The chance of repair is lower than if the lesion involved the other mitral leaflet.
    C. The chance of repair is >90% in experienced centers.
    D. Mortality rate for elective surgery is >2%, even in experienced centers.
    E. Presence of tricuspid valve regurgitant velocity of >4 m/sec has no bearing on the decision for surgical intervention.

CASE 4:

A 72-year-old gentleman is being evaluated for a murmur detected by the primary care physician. He denies any shortness of breath or chest discomfort. On clinical examination, he has a harsh systolic murmur over the aorta and a musical murmur best heard at the apex. Peripheral pulsations are of low volume. Echocardiographic study is shown in Video 17-4.

32. Which of the following statements is correct?
    A. Patient has a clear indication for surgical intervention; recommend preoperative coronary angiography.
    B. If surgery is performed, patient will need aortic and mitral valve replacement.
    C. If the aortic valve peak velocity is >4 m/sec, an exercise test is formally contraindicated.
    D. If the LVOT TVI is 15 cm and the aortic valve TVI is 75 cm, left heart catheterization is recommended to confirm the status of the aortic valve.
    E. If the aortic peak velocity is >4 m/sec, the chance of remaining asymptomatic at 5 years is <30%.

33. The patient tells you that he has decided against surgical intervention at this time. Which of the following statements is correct regarding future evaluation and treatment?
    A. Repeat echocardiogram will be required in the next 2–3 years.
    B. Antibiotic prophylaxis is recommended for periodontal procedures.
    C. Statins have a demonstrated effect in preventing progression of calcific aortic stenosis.
    D. Physical activity is recommended but the patient should avoid high levels of effort.
    E. Aortic balloon valvotomy is a reasonable alternative to aortic valve replacement in elderly patients.

CASE 5:

The echocardiographic study in Video 17-5 was performed at routine follow-up 6 months after septal myectomy.

34. The images show:
    A. A double-inlet ventricle.
    B. A ventricular septal defect as a complication after surgery.
    C. Cleft mitral valve.
    D. Repaired mitral valve.
    E. None of the above.

35. Which of the following statements is accurate?
    A. Antibiotic prophylaxis is recommended for a periodontal procedure.
    B. Recurrent mitral regurgitation after mitral valve repair occurs in more than 10% of patients 10 years after surgery.
    C. Increased mitral gradient requiring further surgical intervention can occur after this type of procedure.
    D. This is the preferred technique of repair for ischemic mitral regurgitation.

ANSWERS

1. ANSWER: A. The Doppler findings are consistent with severe aortic stenosis. Valve area can be calculated with the continuity equation. The basic formula is:

Left ventricular outflow tract (LVOT) flow = Aortic valve flow

LVOT area × LVOT time-velocity integral (TVI) = Aortic valve area (AVA) × Aortic TVI

$$4 \times 15 = AVA \times 100$$

In the example, the AVA is 0.6 cm². Answer B refers to the dimensionless index (LVOT/aortic TVI or velocity ratio), which has been shown to accurately predict presence of severe aortic stenosis when the ratio is <0.25 (rather than 0.3). This measurement avoids the use of LVOT diameter, which is the largest source of errors in AVA calculations. This is due to the inherent difficulty associated with the measurement in the presence of a heavily calcified valve; any error is further increased by using the squared value in the valve formula. Answer C is false; typical severe aortic stenosis has aortic velocities in excess of 4 m/sec. Echocardiographic criteria used in classification of the severity of valvular disease have been summarized in the latest AHA/ACC Guidelines (Table 17-1).

2. ANSWER: D. The evolution of completely asymptomatic aortic stenosis is not benign. Several studies have shown that once the stenosis is severe patients will inexorably develop symptoms. Rosenhek et al. have shown that among 128 patients with asymptomatic severe aortic stenosis, only 47% were free of death or aortic valve replacement after 2 years. Pellikka et al. have shown that among patients with asymptomatic aortic stenosis with aortic velocities >4 m/sec at baseline, only 33% remain free of symptoms after 5 years. Therefore, answer A is obviously false.

Available information in this question suggests presence of severe asymptomatic aortic stenosis. Although the patient is likely to require surgery, a decision cannot be made based solely on the information presented so far, and thus answer B is false.

Transesophageal echocardiography (TEE) can be used in the evaluation of aortic stenosis. Indeed, planimetry of the AVA at TEE correlates well with AVA by catheterization laboratory evaluation. However, this test is typically used as an incremental step only when the transthoracic study fails to establish disease severity (answer C is false).

Exercise studies are useful in clinical decision making for asymptomatic aortic stenosis. Current AHA/ACC guidelines for management of valvular heart disease suggest their use in asymptomatic aortic stenosis. Development of symptoms or a decrease in blood pressure at peak exercise would suggest a more advanced disease state, and aortic valve replacement should be considered. We are using the oxygen treadmill consumption test. In our experience, this test allows better quantification of patient's physical limitation; serial studies are also easier to compare to assess disease progression (answer D is correct). Current AHA guidelines recommend yearly echocardiographic evaluations in patients with severe asymptomatic aortic stenosis who are not undergoing aortic valve replacement (answer E is false).

3. ANSWER: D. Based on the Doppler data, the mean gradient is 30 mm Hg and the dimensionless index is less than 0.25. These findings are worrisome for severe aortic stenosis, low-gradient, low-output type. The hypotensive response to diuretics is also suggestive of severe aortic stenosis.

The substantial decrease in systolic function could represent end-stage valvular heart disease, but the question of an ischemic etiology is obvious. However, a vasodilator stress test is contraindicated when severe aortic stenosis is suspected (answer A is false); exercise and full-dose dobutamine stress echocardiogram are also contraindicated in the presence of acutely decompensated

TABLE 17-1 Echocardiographic Classification of the Severity of Valve Disease in Adults

Aortic Stenosis			
Indicator	Mild	Moderate	Severe
Jet velocity (m/sec)	<3.0	3.0–4.0	>4.0
Mean gradient (mm Hg)	<25	25–40	>40
Valve area (cm^2)	>1.5	1.0–1.5	<1.0
Valve area index (cm^2/m^2)			<0.6

Mitral Stenosis			
	Mild	Moderate	Severe
Mean gradient (mm Hg)	<5	5–10	>10
Pulmonary artery systolic pressure (mm Hg)	<30	30–50	>50
Valve area (cm^2)	>1.5	1.0–1.5	<1.0

Aortic Regurgitation			
	Mild	Moderate	Severe
Qualitative			
Color Doppler jet width	Central jet <25% LVOT	Greater than mild but no signs of severe AR	Central jet >65% LVOT
Doppler vena contracta (cm)	<0.3	0.3–0.6	≥0.6
Quantitative			
Regurgitant volume (ml per beat)	<30	30–59	≥60
Regurgitant fraction (%)	<30	30–49	≥50
Regurgitant orifice area (cm^2)	<0.10	0.10–0.29	≥0.30
Additional Essential Criteria			
Left ventricular size			Enlarged

Mitral Regurgitation			
	Mild	Moderate	Severe
Qualitative			
Color Doppler jet area	Small, central jet <4 cm^2 or <20% LA area		Large central jet >40% of LA area Wall impinging jet of any size, swirling in LA
Doppler vena contracta (cm)	<0.3	0.3–0.69	≥0.70
Quantitative			
Regurgitant volume (ml per beat)	<30	30–59	≥60
Regurgitant fraction (%)	<30	30–49	≥50
Regurgitant orifice area (cm^2)	<0.20	0.20–0.39	≥0.40
Additional Essential Criteria			
Left atrial size			Enlarged
Left ventricular size			Enlarged

(Modified with permission from the American College of Cardiology/American Heart Association Task Force on Practice Guidelines, Society of Cardiovascular Anesthesiologists, Society for Cardiovascular Angiography and Interventions, et al. ACC/AHA 2006 Guidelines for the management of patients with valvular heart disease. *Circulation*. 2006;114:e84–e231. ©2006, American Heart Association, Inc.)

heart failure (answers B and C are false). A low-dose dobutamine echocardiogram will allow assessment of aortic stenosis and provide prognostic information for surgical intervention. Indeed, in low-output, low-gradient aortic stenosis, the gradient is low because of the left ventricular (LV) systolic failure. With the inotropic support provided by low-dose dobutamine, one can distinguish between true severe aortic stenosis (gradient increases, similar valve area) and pseudo-severe aortic stenosis (the calculated valve area is low due to low stroke volume; with dobutamine, the mean gradient remains the same, but the calculated valve area increases). In addition, patients demonstrating presence of contractile reserve (defined as an increase in stroke volume of >20%) have better outcome after aortic valve replacement.

4. ANSWER: B. The peak-to-peak gradient typically evaluated at pullback in the catheterization laboratory does not reflect a true event, as the peak aortic pressure occurs after peak LV pressure when aortic stenosis is present. Echocardiographic estimation of the peak aortic gradient is more accurate as it reflects instantaneous pressure differences between the aorta and left ventricle (answer A is false). Statement B is correct in the vast majority of situations and established echocardiography is the main diagnostic tool in valvular disease. A number of assumptions are, however, made in echocardiographic assessment of valvular stenosis. If these are not accurate, Doppler-based estimations can be erroneously high (answer C is false). The simplified Bernoulli equation estimates the pressure gradient according to the formula $\Delta p = 4v^2$; this in turn is a simplification of the convective acceleration term $\frac{1}{2}\rho(v_2^2 - v_1^2)$ is the original Bernoulli equation. The number 4 in the simplified formula is the approximation of the $\frac{1}{2}\rho$ converted for expressing pressure in mm Hg units; it assumes a blood mass density of 1,060 kg/m^3. However, blood mass density is lower when significant anemia is present, which would lead to overestimation of the pressure gradient if the same formula is applied. In addition, conditions with increased cardiac output (anemia, fever, subvalvular aortic stenosis, and significant valvular regurgitation) will increase the inflow velocity v_1, which is usually considered negligible. This also leads to overestimation of pressure gradients (answer C is false).

The use of nonimaging probes is required in the assessment of aortic stenosis not because of hardware or software properties, but because the smaller footprint allows ultrasound interrogation from deeper position and better alignment of the Doppler signal with the direction of blood flow.

5. ANSWER: C. Based on the continuity equation, the aortic valve area is

$\pi \times$ LVOT diameter^2/4 $\times$ LVOT TVI/aortic TVI = 0.78 cm^2

Since the aortic valve inflow velocity (LVOT velocity) is 2 m/sec, the term v_1^2 cannot be ignored in the Bernoulli equation. The full formula ($\Delta p = 4(v_2^2 - v_1^2)$) has to be used. The pressure gradient is 84 mm Hg (answer C is correct).

6. ANSWER: C. Clinical examination argues against severe aortic stenosis (preserved A2 component, normal peripheral pulsations, and unimpressive murmur). On the echocardiographic report, there is a discrepancy between the estimated aortic valve gradient (consistent with moderate stenosis) and the calculated valve area (consistent with severe stenosis). This cannot represent a low-output, low-gradient aortic stenosis type, as the ejection fraction (EF) and cardiac index are normal. Obviously, a decision for surgery cannot be made immediately (answers A and B are false). Although both TEE (valve planimetry) and aortic valve calcium score can be useful in decision making, the most reasonable next step is to repeat the transthoracic study. The most common cause for the overestimation of the AVA is an erroneously low measurement of the LVOT diameter. Careful assessment at transthoracic echocardiography usually rectifies the mistake.

7. ANSWER: C. Subaortic stenosis does not respond to balloon dilatation. The only treatment is surgical resection (answer A is false). Presence of moderate aortic regurgitation is an indication for surgery, as further valve deterioration is expected because of the jet lesion from the subaortic acceleration (answer B is false). Associated lesions must be evaluated. The most common are patent ductus arteriosus and pulmonary valve stenosis (which both can be diagnosed during TEE examination of the pulmonary artery and bifurcation-answer C is correct); coarctation of the aorta (which can be diagnosed by pulsed Doppler of the abdominal aorta-answer D is false); and ventricular septal defect.

8. ANSWER: A. This question uses the proximal iso-velocity surface concept in calculating the effective regurgitant orifice (ERO). According to the continuity equation, the flow converging to the valve must be equal to the flow through the valve. As blood flow accelerates toward a narrowing orifice (in this case the regurgitant orifice), the spatial distribution of points in which the fluid has the same velocity (isovelocity surface) is approximated by a hemisphere.

Based on this concept, one can transcribe the continuity equation as

Isovelocity flow = regurgitant flow

Isovelocity area $\times$ aliasing velocity = ERO $\times$ regurgitant velocity

$2\pi R^2 \times$ aliasing velocity = ERO $\times$ regurgitant velocity

Replacing the numbers, this becomes

ERO = 2π (0.8 cm)$^2 \times$ 40 cm/sec/400 cm/sec
= 0.40 cm^2, consistent with severe aortic regurgitation
(answer A is correct).

A pressure halftime of <250 milliseconds is consistent with severe aortic regurgitation. The vena contracta is best measured on the parasternal long axis view (best axial resolution); in the apical long-axis view, the vena contracta will be typically perpendicular to the ultrasonic beam, reducing the spatial resolution (answer C is false).

TABLE 17-2 Determinants of the Echocardiographic Mitral Valve Score

	Leaflets			Subvalvular
Grade	Mobility	Thickening	Calcification	Thickening
1	Highly mobile, only leaflet tips restricted	Leaflets near normal in thickness (4–5 mm)	A single area of increased echo brightness	Minimal thickening just below the mitral leaflets
2	Leaflet mid and base portions have normal mobility	Midleaflets normal, thickening of margins (5–8 mm)	Scattered areas of brightness confined to leaflet margins	Thickening of chordal structures up to one-third of the chordal length
3	Valve moves forward in diastole, mainly from the base	Thickening extending through the entire leaflet (5–8 mm)	Brightness extending into the midportion of the leaflets	Thickening extending to the distal third of the chords
4	No or minimal forward movement of the leaflets in diastole	Thickening of all leaflet tissue (>8–10 mm)	Extensive brightness throughout much of the leaflet tissue	Thickening/shortening of all chordal structures extending down to the papillary muscles

(Modified from the American College of Cardiology/American Heart Association Task Force on Practice Guidelines, Society of Cardiovascular Anesthesiologists, Society for Cardiovascular Angiography and Interventions, et al. http://www.ncbi.nlm.nih.gov/pubmed?term=%22Society%20of%20Thoracic%20Surgeons%22%5BCorporate%20Author%5D ACC/AHA 2006 guidelines for the management of patients with valvular heart disease. *Circulation*. 2006;114:e84–e231 and Wilkins GT, Weyman AE, Abascal VM, et al. Percutaneous balloon dilatation of the mitral valve: an analysis of echocardiographic variables related to outcome and the mechanism of dilatation. *Br Heart J*. 1988;60:299–308.)

The suprasternal notch window allows Doppler evaluation of flow reversals in the descending thoracic aorta; holodiastolic flow reversals are suggestive of severe aortic regurgitation (answer D is false).

9. ANSWER: E. The score used for predicting the outcome of mitral balloon valvuloplasty takes into account valve leaflet mobility, thickness (answer B), calcification (answer A), and subvalvular thickening (7; Table 17-2). Each is given a score of 1 to 4. When the total score is 8 or less, the valve is considered amenable to balloon valvuloplasty. Subvalvular calcifications are not included in this score (answer C is false). The correct answer is E.

10. ANSWER: A. This question refers to mitral valve area (MVA) calculation based on the pressure halftime. Commonly in the echocardiography board examination, the candidate is not presented with the actual pressure halftime measurement, but rather with a still image of a continuous wave (CW) signal or in this case with the measured deceleration time. The relationship between pressure halftime and deceleration time is constant.

$$\text{Pressure halftime} = 0.29 \times \text{deceleration time}$$

Furthermore, the MVA is estimated according to the formula

$$\text{MVA} = 220/\text{pressure halftime}$$

Using the numbers provided, MVA is 220/0.29 × 758 milliseconds = 1 cm² (answer A).

11. ANSWER: A. This question addressed the indications and contraindications for mitral balloon valvuloplasty.

Case A is consistent with moderate mitral stenosis. Although asymptomatic, a tricuspid regurgitation velocity of 4 m/sec is suggestive of pulmonary artery systolic pressure in excess of 70 mm Hg; therefore, the patient has a clear indication for balloon valvuloplasty (correct answer). In case B, the MVA is estimated at 2 cm² (220/pressure halftime), and therefore the etiology of dyspnea must be sought elsewhere. The mechanism of successful mitral valvuloplasty is commissural separation; presence of heavy calcification is associated with lower procedural success and higher incidence of significant mitral regurgitation (answer C is false). Presence of significant mitral regurgitation (suggested by clinical examination) is a contraindication for valvuloplasty (answer D is false).

12. ANSWER: B. This question uses the continuity equation for estimating the mitral regurgitant volume (MRV). In the absence of significant aortic regurgitation, the net flow through the aortic valve must equal the net flow through the mitral valve:

Aortic flow = mitral forward flow − mitral regurgitant flow

Therefore, MRV can be estimated by the formula

MRV = mitral forward flow − aortic stroke volume

$$\text{MRV} = (\text{MVA} \times \text{mitral valve plane TVI}) - (\text{LVOT area} \times \text{LVOT TVI})$$

$$\text{MRV} = 3.14 \times (4/2)^2 \times 10 - 3.14 \times (2/2)^2 \times 25$$
$$= 125.6 - 78.5 = 47 \text{ ml (answer B)}$$

13. ANSWER: E. There are several simplified calculations that are commonly used in proximal isovelocity surface area (PISA) evaluation of mitral regurgitation. They are all based on some presumptions, but their simplicity makes them attractive for rapid calculations. Two simplified methods are commonly used for ERO calculation. In the first one, the aliasing velocity is set at 40 cm/sec. If the mitral regurgitant velocity is considered 500 cm/sec (a reasonable assumption when systemic blood pressure is normal), calculation of the ERO is:

$$\text{PISA surface} \times \text{aliasing velocity} = \text{ERO} \times \text{regurgitant velocity}$$

$$\text{ERO} = (2 \times 3.14 \times R^2 \times 40 \text{ cm/sec})/500 \text{ cm/sec}$$
$$= 251 \times R^2/500 = R^2/2$$

Using this simplification, the ERO is 0.5 cm^2.

A second simplification for ERO is using an aliasing velocity of 30 cm/sec and assuming again that the mitral regurgitant velocity is 500 cm/sec. With these numbers

$$\text{ERO} = 2 \times 3.14 \times R^2 \times 30/500 = 0.38 \times R^2$$

So that if PISA radius is more than 1 cm, the ERO is more than 0.38 cm^2, that is, the regurgitation is severe.

There is also a simplification for estimating the regurgitant volume (RV). This takes advantage of the observation that the ratio between mitral regurgitant TVI and velocity is relatively constant approximately 1/3.25.

$$\text{RV} = \text{ERO} \times \text{regurgitant TVI}$$

$$\text{RV} = (2 \times 3.14 \times R^2 \times \text{aliasing velocity}/ \text{mitral velocity}) \times \text{regurgitant TVI}$$

$$\text{RV} = 2 \times 3.14 \times R^2 \times \text{aliasing velocity}/3.25$$
$$= 1.9 \times R^2 \times \text{aliasing velocity}$$

Using the numbers provided, the RV is 75 ml (correct answer E)

14. ANSWER: E. Mitral valve annulus has a saddle shape. Mitral valve prolapse is considered to be present when a prolapse of 2 mm or more above the mitral annulus plane is found in the parasternal long-axis view of the mitral valve. Other views (especially the apical four-chamber view) can overestimate presence of prolapse.

15. ANSWER: C. Although all listed complications may occur early after a myocardial infarction and percutaneous intervention, the presence of a hyperdynamic ventricle excludes in-stent thrombosis. There is no evidence of pericardial effusion (free wall rupture). A ventricular septal defect is typically associated with a loud systolic murmur, even when acute. The murmur of acute severe mitral regurgitation due to papillary muscle rupture is unimpressive. This is due to rapid equalization of LV and atrial pressures, with little pressure gradient. The typical CW Doppler finding is a dagger-shaped mitral regurgitant signal (correct answer C).

16. ANSWER: D. The systolic frame is typical of the appearance of a unicuspid aortic valve. Unlike bicuspid valves, which typically have two commissures and a variable presence of a raphe, the unicuspid valves have only one commissure (Fig. 17-1) or even no commissure (central orifice).

17. ANSWER: D. The case is a typical presentation of subaortic stenosis, with flow acceleration visible well below the aortic valve plane. The diastolic frame also shows presence of aortic regurgitation. These can exist either as an isolated ridge/membrane in the LVOT, or as longer narrowing of the LVOT (tunnel). The status of the aortic valve is not certain at this stage, although significant stenosis can be suspected from the intense aliasing seen in the LVOT; however, no clear recommendation can be made in terms of surgical intervention (answer A is false). The condition is not benign, the status of the native valve must be established (answer B is false). Surgical intervention with resection of the ridge / membrane is usually successful but recurrence can be seen and regular follow up is recommended (answer C is false). TEE is ideal in imaging both the subaortic area and the native aortic valve (answer D is correct).

18. ANSWER: D. Echocardiographic images are diagnostic of a bicuspid aortic valve and severe aortic regurgitation. Valve repair techniques have become a reasonable alternative to valve replacement, especially in younger patients in whom the valve is not heavily calcified (answers A and B are false). Valve repair is suitable in patients who do not have restricted leaflet mobility; the freedom from reoperation is approximately 85% after 7 years. Patients with bicuspid aortic valve have a higher risk of progression of aortic aneurysm due to coexisting aortopathy, and therefore the current recommendation is to consider aortic repair when the diameter exceeds 4.5–5 cm (similar to patients with Marfan syndrome; answer D is false). The Doppler signal in the abdominal aorta is highly suggestive of coarctation of the aorta. A computed tomography (CT) scan will be required for further diagnosis and surgical planning (answer D is correct).

19. ANSWER: D. The echocardiographic pictures are diagnostic of severe aortic regurgitation, in this case, due to bacterial endocarditis. The mitral anterior leaflet is pushed by the aortic regurgitant jet. Note in the M mode that the anterior leaflet is displaced posteriorly, and the separation of the mitral valve leaflets is minimal. This will result in functional mitral stenosis and will be the cause of the diastolic apical rumble (Austin-Flint murmur; correct answer D). The other clinical findings would be consistent with severe tricuspid regurgitation (answer A), coarctation of the aorta or patent ductus arteriosus (B), and mitral valve prolapse (C).

20. ANSWER: B. This is the typical presentation of papillary fibroelastoma of the aortic valve. This benign tumor consists of a narrow stalk with numerous small frond-like excrescences. Anticoagulation is usually not recommended (answer A is false). The tumor is friable and has the potential for embolization, especially when larger than 10 mm or highly mobile; surgical intervention is usually recommended under these circumstances (answer B is correct). Surgery consists of shaving the tumor from the attachment point; sometime valve repair with pericardial patch is necessary (answer C is false). Recurrence is rare, but well described in the literature (answer D is false). Most authors would suggest use of an antiplatelet agent (answer E is false).

21. ANSWER: C. The echocardiographic images are diagnostic of rheumatic mitral stenosis. Note the hockey stick deformity of the anterior mitral leaflet and incomplete opening of the posterior leaflet. There is visible mitral inflow acceleration, and CW Doppler is consistent with severe mitral stenosis (pressure gradient is 16 mm Hg). This condition in isolation is associated with a normal LV size (answer A is false). The interval between the second heart sound A2 and the opening snap reflects the isovolumic relaxation time and is typically shorter with higher left atrial pressure (the shorter the A2-opening snap interval, the more severe is the stenosis; answer C is correct). The mitral gradient is significantly increased with increasing heart rates; presence of a diastolic rumble can be brought out with some physical activity at the time of examination (answer D is false).

22. ANSWER: A. The echocardiographic images show the hockey-stick deformity with limited excursion of the anterior mitral leaflet. In this case, this is occurring after surgical repair with a posterior reduction annuloplasty. Although uncommon, this is a known complication after mitral valve repair. The pathophysiologic mechanisms are similar to mitral stenosis of any other etiology, with left atrial hypertension leading to secondary pulmonary hypertension (answer A is correct); hemoptysis is in this case a direct reflection of elevated postcapillary pulmonary pressure. Estimation of the left atrial pressure (and indirectly of the mitral gradient) by catheterization with the use of pulmonary capillary wedge pressure is usually inaccurate. The echocardiographic assessment of the mitral gradient is the preferred technique. An accurate transmitral gradient can be obtained at catheterization only by transseptal approach with direct measurement of the left atrial and LV pressures (answer B is false). Patient has evidence of symptomatic severe mitral stenosis; an exercise echocardiogram will not provide additional information (answer C is false). Mitral balloon valvuloplasty cannot be used in patients who underwent mitral valve repair (answer D is false).

23. ANSWER: C. The PISA method is excellent in quantification of mitral regurgitation. The strength of the method is particularly important in eccentric jets, when the color Doppler aspect of the jet is less impres-

sive due to the loss of kinetic energy by contact with the atrial wall (Coanda effect). The concept is similar to the one described previously for aortic regurgitation.

Isovelocity area $\times$ aliasing velocity = effective regurgitant orifice $\times$ regurgitant velocity

RV = ERO $\times$ regurgitant TVI

Substituting the numbers, the ERO is 0.46 cm^2 and the RV 91 ml. Correct answer is C.

24. ANSWER: B. The echocardiographic images are typical of a flail P2 scallop. We typically start with the four-chamber view on TEE, which helps identify the location (anterior vs. posterior) based on 2D appearance and direction of the color jet (posteriorly directed for anterior flails and anteriorly directed for posterior flails). Imaging in the commissural view of the mitral valve (Fig. 17-9) helps further locate the scallop (lateral/central/medial). Real-time 3D TEE is rapidly emerging as an excellent tool in the assessment of mitral valvular disease.

25. ANSWER: C. Images are typical of mitral regurgitation secondary to systolic anterior motion. This is typically seen in dynamic LVOT obstruction in hypertrophic cardiomyopathy but can also occur in hypertensive heart disease with prominent basal septum, acute anterior infarcts with hyperdynamic compensatory function, or apical ballooning syndrome with hyperdynamic base. Usually surgical correction of the dynamic outflow obstruction with myectomy results in nearly complete resolution of the mitral regurgitation (answers A and B are false). This needs to be confirmed on postbypass images, when a decision can be made for additional mitral valve surgery (answer C is correct). Presence of an eccentric jet extending all the way to the posterior atrial wall is consistent with severe regurgitation (answer D is false). Agents with negative chronotropic and inotropic effects have been used for medical management (beta-blockers, calcium channel blockers, disopyramide); mitral valve replacement is usually not required (answer E is false).

26. ANSWER: B. There is no evidence of prolapse (answer A is false). The echocardiographic features are consistent with ischemic mitral regurgitation (answer B is correct). Note the tethered leaflets and stretched mitral chords. There is an override of the anterior leaflet with a posteriorly directed jet of mitral regurgitation. The annulus is of normal size and the valve does not have the appearance of rheumatic disease (answers C and D are false). A posterior chord rupture with a flail segment typically will result in an anteriorly directed jet of mitral regurgitation (answer E is false).

27. ANSWER: D. Presence of mitral regurgitation superimposed on ischemic LV dysfunction is of poor prognosis, even at lower degrees of regurgitation. Indeed, an ERO of more than 0.22 cm^2, and an RV in excess of 30 ml are associated with a poor prognosis (answer A is false). Surgical intervention for ischemic mitral regurgitation is a topic of intense debate; long-term results after classical reduction annuloplasty are clearly suboptimal (answer B is false). Although in theory positive LV remodeling with revascularization may occur, current recommendations are to correct significant mitral regurgitation at the time of coronary bypass surgery (answer C is false). Given the suboptimal results with reduction annuloplasty, there is an active search for alternative techniques (secondary chord resection, neochord implantation, papillary muscle repositioning, etc.). The optimal technique for repairing ischemic mitral regurgitation remains controversial at this time (answer D is correct).

KEY POINTS:

▨ "Ischemic" mitral regurgitation is typically central or posteriorly directed.

▨ Each grade of mitral regurgitation severity in patients with coronary artery disease (CAD) is associated with an increasingly poor prognosis.

▨ Although mitral regurgitation in patients with CAD is usually managed surgically with reduction annuloplasty, the results are suboptimal and alternative procedures are being sought.

28. ANSWER: E. The images are diagnostic of mitral regurgitation secondary to systolic anterior motion of the mitral valve. This is a common finding in severe dynamic LV outflow obstruction (answer E is correct) due to hypertrophic obstructive cardiomyopathy.

29. ANSWER: E. Afterload reduction will result in an increase in LVOT obstruction and is contraindicated (answer A is false). Medical management consists of agents with negative inotropic and chronotropic properties (beta-blockers, verapamil, disopyramide; answer E is correct). Valsalva maneuver typically increases the degree of LVOT obstruction and is associated with a louder murmur (answer B is false). It is also the most likely explanation for the patient's dizziness with heavy lifting (answer C is false). The mitral regurgitation is secondary to systolic anterior motion of the mitral valve and is typically resolved with septal reduction therapy alone (answer D is false).

KEY POINTS:

▨ Systolic anterior motion of the mitral valve is the cause of LVOT obstruction and mitral regurgitation in most patients with hypertrophic obstructive cardiomyopathy.

▨ Medical management of LVOT obstruction due to systolic anterior motion of the mitral valve should consist of agents with negative inotropic and chronotropic properties and vasodilators should be avoided.

30. ANSWER: C. The images show typical appearance of a flail P2 scallop of the mitral valve, with massive mitral regurgitation. The anterior leaflet is not prolapsing (answer A is false). There is no evidence of a beneficial effect of afterload-reducing agents in normotensive patients (answer B is false). There is a familial form of mitral valve prolapse, which is transmitted as an autosomal trait; screening of first-degree relatives is suggested (answer C is correct). An EF of <60% is likely to reflect LV dysfunction in patients with severe mitral regurgitation and is an indication for surgical intervention (answer D is false). Although a normal lifestyle and regular exercise are encouraged for most patients with mitral valve prolapse, restriction from competitive sports is recommended when moderate LV enlargement, LV dysfunction, uncontrolled tachyarrhythmias, unexplained syncope, or aortic root enlargement are present individually or in combination (answer E is false).

Transesophageal echocardiographic evaluation of the mitral valve is excellent in assessing mitral valve pathology. Although all views and windows need to be used for full interrogation, we find the commissural view (typically obtained from the esophageal window at an angle of approximately 60 degrees) very useful in defining which mitral scallop is involved. In this view, the imaged scallops from right to left are P1, A2, and P3 (see top row of Fig. 17-11). A diagram of the echocardiographic appearance of a flail posterior scallop is shown in the bottom row in Figure 17-11. Note the typical double contour appearance of the flail P2, which is the most common flail scallop.

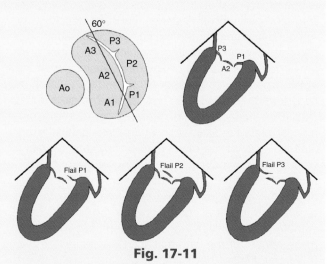

Fig. 17-11

31. ANSWER: C. Asymptomatic patients benefit from surgery even if the LV function is preserved, provided that the chance of repair is >90% (class IIa indication; answer A is false). The chance of repair is higher with posterior rather than anterior leaflet disease (answer B is false). The chance of repair is >90% in experienced hands (answer C is correct). Large centers have reported mortality rates below 1% in large series (answer D is false). Presence of pulmonary artery systolic pressure in excess of 50 mm Hg at rest is a class IIa indication to proceed with surgery in asymptomatic patients (answer E is false).

KEY POINTS:

◾ Mitral valve prolapse may be a familial trait transmitted as an autosomal trait.

◾ Valve repair of mitral valve prolapse and mitral regurgitation is considered acceptable in asymptomatic patients if the chance of repair is >90%.

◾ The likelihood of repair is higher for posterior compared with anterior leaflet pathology associated with mitral valve prolapse.

32. ANSWER: E. The echocardiographic images show a heavily calcified aortic valve, with concomitant presence of mild aortic regurgitation. Although 2D images are suggestive of severe aortic stenosis, no formal quantification is presented. In addition, there are no apparent symptoms from the presented data. Obviously, surgery cannot be recommended on these findings alone (answer A is false). There is no data to support the presence of mitral valve disease. Presence of a musical murmur at the apex with a harsh murmur over the aortic area is a typical description of the Gallavardin dissociation of aortic stenosis murmur into two components (answer B is false). Presence of severe aortic stenosis, as suggested by a velocity of >4 m/sec is not a formal contraindication for stress test. Current AHA/ACC guidelines give it a class IIb recommendation for exercise testing in apparently asymptomatic patients (answer C is false). With an LVOT TVI/aortic TVI ratio of 0.2, aortic stenosis is severe. If echocardiographic and clinical examinations are concordant, there is no indication for hemodynamic catheterization (answer D is false). Several studies have shown the poor prognosis of severe aortic stenosis in the absence of surgery (answer E is correct).

33. ANSWER: D. Severe aortic stenosis requires close follow-up; an echocardiogram is usually performed yearly (answer A is false). Antibiotic prophylaxis is no longer recommended for aortic stenosis (answer B is false). Although statins may have a beneficial effect in preventing progression of aortic valve stenosis, the only published randomized trial failed to demonstrate benefit. It was hypothesized that the patients included had heavily calcified valves, and under those circumstances, statin therapy could not influence the disease (answer C is false). Physical exercise in moderation is recommended, but caution must be taken to avoid high isometric or isotonic loads (answer D is correct). The only current recommendations for aortic balloon valvotomy are as a bridge to surgery in hemodynamically unstable patients, or as palliation in patients who have prohibitive surgical risk (answer E is false).

KEY POINTS:

◾ Even patients with severe aortic stenosis can be considered for exercise stress test, if they are asymptomatic to attempt to bring out symptoms or other poor prognostic variables such as arrhythmias, significant ST changes or hypotension.

◾ Patients with severe aortic stenosis managed medically should have yearly echocardiograms and avoid strenuous physical exertion.

34. ANSWER: D. Although mitral regurgitation secondary to systolic anterior motion (SAM) is usually corrected by surgical intervention on the LVOT obstruction, residual regurgitation can be seen on postbypass images. In this case, the surgeon performed an edge-to-edge (Alfieri) repair of the mitral valve. In this technique, the anterior and posterior leaflets are sutured together in the mid portion, giving the typical appearance of a double-orifice mitral valve (answer D is correct). The color jet that can be seen on the septal wall represents flow from a coronary-LV fistula. This is a common benign finding after septal myectomy procedures (answer B is false). Double inlet ventricle and cleft mitral valve are congenital diseases.

35. ANSWER: C. In this case, there is no evidence of an annuloplasty ring being placed. Since there is no prosthetic material, antibiotic prophylaxis is not recommended (answer A is false). In experienced centers, mitral valve repair is the procedure of choice for mitral regurgitation, with a success rate >90% at 10 years (answer B is false). Although rare, functional mitral stenosis requiring surgical intervention has been described after edge-to-edge repair (answer C is correct). The recurrence of significant regurgitation is high when the edge-to-edge technique is used in ischemic mitral regurgitation; this technique is currently best avoided in such situations (answer D is false).

KEY POINTS:

◾ Patients undergoing septal myectomy for hypertrophic obstructive cardiomyopathy may require concomitant repair of the mitral leaflets to minimize systolic anterior motion of the mitral valve and LVOT obstruction.

◾ The Alfieri edge-to-edge technique of mitral valve repair may reduce mitral regurgitation. A rare complication after this procedure is mitral stenosis. The Alfieri technique should not be used in ischemic mitral regurgitation.

SUGGESTED READINGS

American College of Cardiology/American Heart Association Task Force on Practice Guidelines, Society of Cardiovascular Anesthesiologists, Society for Cardiovascular Angiography and Interventions, et al. http://www.ncbi.nlm.nih.gov/pubmed?term=%22Society%20of%20Thoracic%20Surgeons%22%5BCorporate%20Author%5DACC/AHA 2006 guidelines for the management of patients with valvular heart disease. *Circulation.* 2006;114:e84–e231.

Cannan CR, Nishimura RA, Reeder GS, et al. Echocardiographic assessment of commissural calcium: a simple predictor of outcome after percutaneous mitral balloon valvotomy. *J Am Coll Cardiol.* 1997;29:175–180.

deFilippi CR, Willett DL, Brickner ME, et al. Usefulness of dobutamine echocardiography in distinguishing severe from nonsevere valvular aortic stenosis in patients with depressed left ventricular function and low transvalvular gradients. *Am J Cardiol.* 1995;75:191–194.

Enriquez-Sarano M, Miller FA Jr, Hayes SN, et al. Effective mitral regurgitant orifice area clinical use and pitfalls of the proximal isovelocity surface area method. *J Am Coll Cardiol.* 1995; 25:703–709.

Freed LA, Benjamin EJ, Levy D, et al. Mitral valve prolapse in the general population: the benign nature of echocardiographic features in the Framingham Heart Study. *J Am Coll Cardiol.* 2002; 40:1298–1304.

Grewal J, Mankad S, Freeman WK, et al. Real-time three-dimensional transesophageal echocardiography in the intraoperative assessment of mitral valve disease. *J Am Soc Echocardiogr.* 2009;22:34–41.

Klarich KW, Enriquez-Sarano M, Gura GM, et al. Papillary fibroelastoma: echocardiographic characteristics for diagnosis and pathologic correlation. *J Am Coll Cardiol.* 1997;30:784–790.

Minakata K, Schaff HV, Zehr KJ, et al. Is repair of aortic valve regurgitation a safe alternative to valve replacement? *J Thorac Cardiovasc Surg.* 2004;127:645–653.

Monin JL, Monchi M, Gest V, et al. Aortic stenosis with severe left ventricular dysfunction and low transvalvular pressure gradients: risk stratification by low-dose dobutamine echocardiography. *J Am Coll Cardiol.* 2001;37:2101–2107.

Oh J, Seward JB, Tajik AJ. Valvular heart disease. In: Oh J, Seward JB, Tajik AJ, eds. *The Echo Manual.* 3rd ed. Philadelphia, PA Wolters and Kulwers; 2006:186–225.

Pellikka PA, Sarano ME, Nishimura RA, et al. Outcome of 622 adults with asymptomatic, hemodynamically significant aortic stenosis during prolonged follow-up. *Circulation.* 2005;111: 3290–3295.

Rosenhek R, Binder T, Porenta G, et al. Predictors of outcome in severe, asymptomatic aortic stenosis. *N Engl J Med.* 2000;343:611–617.

Wilkins GT, Weyman AE, Abascal VM, et al. Percutaneous balloon dilatation of the mitral valve: an analysis of echocardiographic variables related to outcome and the mechanism of dilatation. *Br Heart J.* 1988;60:299–308.

Zoghbi WA, Enriquez-Sarano M, Foster E, et al. Recommendations for evaluation of the severity of native valvular regurgitation with two-dimensional and Doppler echocardiography. *J Am Soc Echocardiogr.* 2003;16:777–802.

Prosthetic Valves

Linda D. Gillam and Smriti Deshmukh

1. A diagnosis of patient prosthesis mismatch (PPM) is made in a 32-year-old woman with prior aortic valve replacement for a congenitally bicuspid aortic valve complicated by severe aortic regurgitation. The basis for this diagnosis is:
   A. A mechanical valve has been selected for a female patient in whom pregnancy is planned.
   B. A mechanical valve has been selected for a patient with a history of drug abuse.
   C. The valve implanted is too small for this patient.
   D. The valve implanted is too large for this patient.
   E. A bioprosthesis has been selected for a young patient.

2. A 55-year-old man with prior aortic valve replacement presents with dyspnea on exertion, which has been present since his surgery. PPM is suspected. Which of the following criteria is used to define this syndrome?
   Effective orifice area (EOA) corrected for body surface area:
   A. ≤ 0.55 cm^2/m^2.
   B. ≤ 0.65 cm^2/m^2.
   C. ≤ 0.75 cm^2/m^2.
   D. ≤ 0.85 cm^2/m^2.
   E. ≤ 0.95 cm^2/m^2.

3. An 11-year-old boy had a 19-mm bileaflet mechanical aortic valve implanted for severe aortic stenosis on the basis of a congenitally bicuspid valve. On echocardiographic evaluation, the peak transvalvular velocity was 3.5 m/sec. However, at catheterization the left ventricle (reached by transseptal puncture) to aortic gradient was only 25 mm Hg. What is the most likely explanation for this discrepancy?
   A. At catheterization, the aortic valve gradient could not be measured by pullback.
   B. The cardiac output was higher at the time of catheterization than at the time of the echocardiogram.
   C. The pressure recovery phenomenon has resulted in overestimation of the aortic valve gradients by Doppler.
   D. The aortic valve gradients have been overestimated because a mitral regurgitant spectrum was confused with the aortic valve spectrum.
   E. The valve is too small for this patient.

4. A 72-year-old man who had a ball and cage (Starr-Edwards) mitral valve implanted 20 years ago is followed echocardiographically. In echocardiograms of patients with this type of prosthesis, the size of the ball is:
   A. Overestimated because of faster propagation of sound in the ball relative to that in tissue.
   B. Overestimated because of slower propagation of sound in the ball relative to that in tissue.
   C. Underestimated because of faster propagation of sound in the ball relative to that in tissue.
   D. Underestimated because of slower propagation of sound in the ball relative to that in tissue.
   E. Accurately represented.

5. A 55-year-old man with a recent aortic valve replacement undergoes postoperative echocardiography to establish baseline values for the valve. A peak velocity of 2.5 m/sec is recorded. This value is:
   A. Abnormally high suggesting PPM.
   B. Abnormally high suggesting prosthetic valve stenosis.
   C. May be normal depending on the size and type of the valve.
   D. Low suggesting that the valve is a homograft valve.
   E. Abnormally low suggesting that the patient has a reduced cardiac output.

6. A 63-year-old patient with prior bioprosthetic mitral valve replacement undergoes an echocardiographic evaluation. The mean transvalvular gradient is 10 mm Hg. To interpret this result, which of the following patient information is most important?
   A. Height.
   B. Weight.
   C. Heart rate.
   D. Blood pressure.
   E. Gender.

7. A 71-year-old patient with a bileaflet mitral valve prosthesis undergoes a transthoracic echocardiographic evaluation with harmonic imaging. In the apical views, microcavitations (spontaneous microbubbles) are seen in the left ventricle. This finding is most consistent with:
   A. Hemolysis.
   B. Paravalvular regurgitation.
   C. Imaging artifact.
   D. A patent foramen ovalis.
   E. Normal prosthetic function.

8. An 82-year-old man with a bioprosthetic aortic valve prosthesis undergoes an echocardiographic evaluation. Which of the following is the formula for calculating EOA?
   A. Stroke volume/prosthetic velocity-time integral (VTI).
   B. (Stroke volume × heart rate)/peak transvalvular velocity.
   C. Subvalvular VTI/prosthetic VTI.
   D. Subvalvular peak velocity/peak transvalvular velocity.
   E. (Subvalvular VTI × stroke volume)/prosthetic VTI

9. A 12-year-old boy with a history of aortic valve replacement undergoes an echocardiographic evaluation. The peak velocity across the prosthesis is 3.5 m/sec. In which of the following valves is pressure recovery most likely to be a consideration?
   A. Bileaflet.
   B. Tilting disc.
   C. Homograft.
   D. Bovine stented bioprosthesis.
   E. Stentless bioprosthesis.

10. A 15-year-old boy who had bioprosthetic aortic valve replacement for a congenitally bicuspid aortic valve undergoes an echocardiographic evaluation. The peak velocity across the prosthesis is 3.5 m/sec. Which of the following is most supportive of the diagnosis of prosthetic valve stenosis?
    A. The bioprosthetic cusps are thickened with reduced mobility.
    B. The size of the valve is 19 mm.
    C. The aortic root is dilated.
    D. The patient's hematocrit level is 45%.
    E. The patient's left ventricular ejection fraction is 32%.

11. A 72-year-old woman with a bioprosthetic mitral prosthesis undergoes an echocardiographic evaluation. Which of the following statements is true?
    A. EOA calculated as 220/pressure halftime provides the best single measurement of functional valve area.
    B. EOA calculated as 270/pressure halftime provides the best single measurement of functional valve area.
    C. EOA calculated as 1.5 × (220/pressure halftime) provides the best single measurement of functional valve area.
    D. EOA calculated as 150/pressure halftime provides the best single measurement of functional valve area.

E. EOA calculated by the pressure halftime method is inaccurate in patients with mitral prostheses.

12. A 63-year-old patient with prior mitral valve replacement undergoes an echocardiographic evaluation. In which of the following valves is a large central jet most consistent with normal valve function?
   A. Starr-Edwards ball and cage valve.
   B. St. Jude bileaflet valve.
   C. Medtronic-Hall single-disc valve.
   D. Bovine pericardial bioprosthesis.
   E. Porcine bioprosthesis.

13. A 63-year-old patient with prior aortic valve replacement undergoes an echocardiographic evaluation for new symptoms of dyspnea. In addition to recording peak and mean gradients, the dimensionless index is calculated as:
   A. (Stroke volume × heart rate)/peak transvalvular velocity.
   B. Subvalvular VTI/prosthetic VTI.
   C. (Subvalvular VTI × stroke volume)/prosthetic VTI.
   D. Calculated EOA/factory-specified normal EOA.

14. An 81-year-old woman with prior bioprosthetic mitral valve replacement is noted to have a new systolic murmur and evidence of congestive heart failure. Transthoracic echocardiographic evaluation reveals only trace central mitral regurgitation. Which of the following statements is correct?
   A. Transesophageal echocardiography (TEE) is essential to evaluate the patient for paravalvular regurgitation.
   B. A peak transmitral velocity of 2 m/sec argues against undetected paravalvular regurgitation.
   C. A mean transmitral gradient of 10 mm Hg argues against undetected paravalvular regurgitation.
   D. Normal (S dominant) pulmonary venous flow excludes the possibility of paravalvular regurgitation.
   E. Paravalvular regurgitation is best detected in the apical three-chamber view.

15. A 22-year-old man presents for echocardiographic follow-up 10 years after a Ross procedure. A 3/6 murmur is heard. What complication is the echocardiogram most likely to demonstrate?
   A. Aortic homograft stenosis.
   B. Aortic autograft stenosis.
   C. Aortic autograft regurgitation.
   D. Aortic homograft regurgitation.
   E. Pulmonary autograft regurgitation.

16. A 72-year-old woman with prior mitral valve replacement is noted to have a new systolic murmur. An echocardiogram is obtained. Based on Figure 18-1, what is the diagnosis?

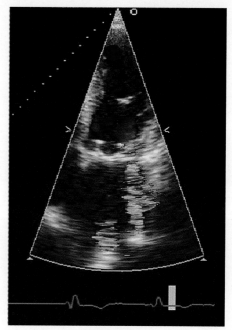

Fig. 18-1

   A. Bioprosthesis with paravalvular mitral regurgitation.
   B. Bileaflet prosthesis with paravalvular mitral regurgitation.
   C. Bioprosthesis with valvular mitral regurgitation.
   D. Bileaflet prosthesis with normal closure jets.
   E. Bileaflet prosthesis with valvular regurgitation.

17. A patient with recent bioprosthetic mitral valve replacement for endocarditis undergoes echocardiographic evaluation because of persistent fatigue and a loud murmur. Based on these parasternal (A) and apical long-axis views (B and C) in Figure 18-2, what is the most likely diagnosis?

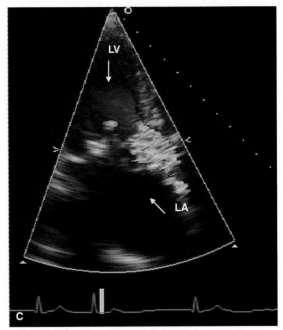

Fig. 18-2C

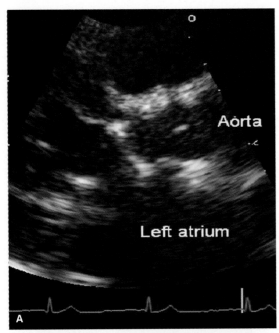

Fig. 18-2A

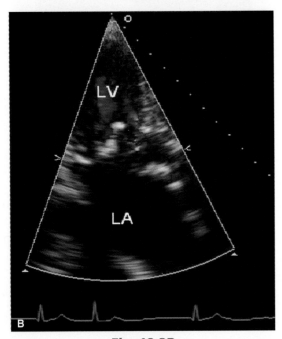

Fig. 18-2B

A. Severe paravalvular mitral regurgitation.
B. Severe valvular mitral regurgitation.
C. Left ventricular outflow tract (LVOT) obstruction due to mitral systolic anterior motion.
D. LVOT obstruction due to malalignment of the prosthesis.
E. Prosthetic mitral stenosis.

18. A 65-year-old woman underwent tricuspid valve replacement for traumatic flail tricuspid valve caused by acceleration-deceleration injury in a car accident. Two years later, she presented with peripheral edema. Transthoracic echocardiography was performed. The images in Figure 18-3 were recorded at a heart rate of 55 bpm and a blood pressure of 120/75 mm Hg. With which of the following diagnoses are these most consistent?

A. Normal tricuspid prosthetic function: high output state.
B. Normal tricuspid prosthetic function: pressure recovery.
C. Mild tricuspid prosthetic stenosis.
D. Moderate tricuspid prosthetic stenosis.
E. Severe tricuspid prosthetic stenosis.

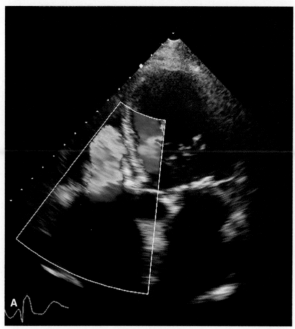

Fig. 18-3A

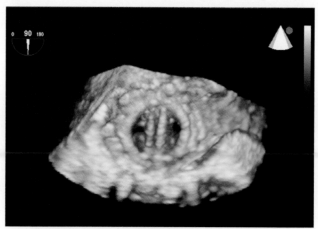

Fig. 18-4

A. Mitral ring annuloplasty.
B. Alfieri stitch valvuloplasty.
C. Tilting disc mitral valve replacement.
D. Bileaflet mitral valve replacement.
E. Mitral homograft replacement.

20. A 67-year-old man has undergone prior valve surgery. Based on the echocardiogram in Figure 18-5, what is the most likely diagnosis?

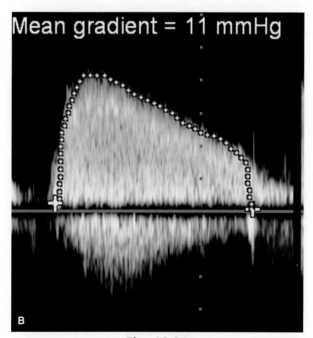

Mean gradient = 11 mmHg

Fig. 18-3B

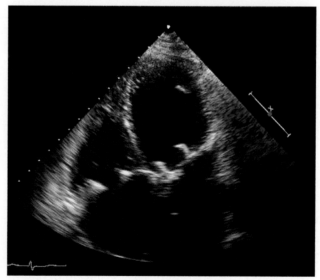

Fig. 18-5

19. A 52-year-old man with prior mitral valve surgery undergoes three-dimensional (3D) TEE following a suspected neuroembolic event (Fig. 18-4). What type of procedure has the patient undergone?

A. Normal mitral and tricuspid ring repair.
B. Normal mitral bioprosthesis, tricuspid ring dehiscence.
C. Normal mitral bioprosthesis and tricuspid ring.
D. Normal mitral bioprosthesis, pacer lead in the right ventricle.
E. Normal mitral bioprosthesis, tricuspid vegetation.

21. A 21-year-old man with recent aortic homograft valve replacement experiences a headache preceded by visual field deficits and undergoes TEE to rule out a cardiac source of embolus. He has been afebrile and Doppler evaluation reveals only trace aortic regurgitation. Based on the echocardiographic image in Figure 18-6, what would be an appropriate next step in management?

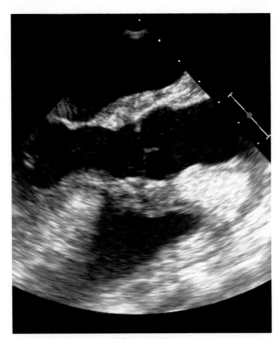

Fig. 18-6

A. Initiate broad-spectrum antibiotics.
B. Urgent reoperation.
C. Refer for computed tomography evaluation.
D. Refer for coronary angiography.
E. Provide reassurance that the appearance of the valve is normal.

22. A 62-year-old woman undergoes mitral valve surgery. What type of prosthesis is shown on the perioperative transesophageal echocardiogram in Figure 18-7?
A. Tilting disc.
B. Bileaflet.
C. Trileaflet.
D. Ball and cage.
E. Disc and cage.

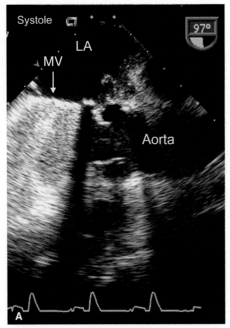

Fig. 18-7A

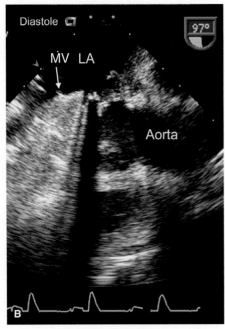

Fig. 18-7B

23. A 75-year-old man with prior aortic valve replacement undergoes an echocardiographic evaluation because of dyspnea on exertion (Fig. 18-8). The pulsed Doppler spectrum recorded in the LVOT yields a peak modal velocity of 1.1 m/sec. Continuous-wave Doppler recorded across the LVOT (and valve) yields a peak velocity of 3.3 m/sec. The LVOT diameter is 2.0 cm. The calculated dimensionless index is?

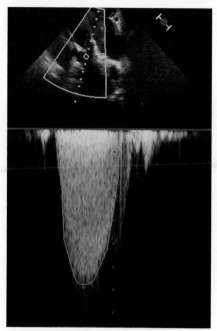

Fig. 18-8

A. 3.0.
B. 1.05.
C. 0.75.
D. 0.5.
E. 0.33.

24. A 32-year-old man with a prior history of aortic valve surgery undergoes TEE because of suspected aortic dissection. Based on the echocardiographic image in Figure 18-9, what type of procedure was performed?

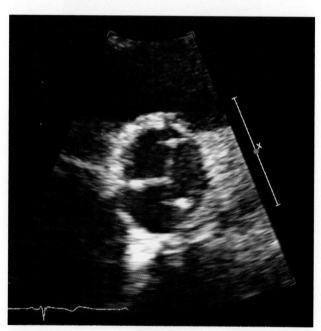

Fig. 18-9

A. Stentless bioprosthesis replacement.
B. Aortic homograft replacement.
C. Aortic autograft replacement.
D. Stented bioprosthesis replacement.
E. Aortic valve repair.

25. A 66-year-old woman undergoes a resting transthoracic echocardiographic evaluation following an episode of chest pain. What is the most likely explanation for the echodensity identified by the arrow in Figure 18-10?

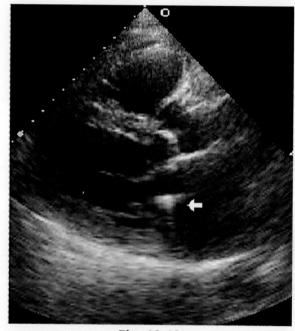

Fig. 18-10

A. Aortic prosthesis reverberation artifact.
B. Aneurysm of the interatrial septum.
C. Biventricular pacing lead.
D. Alfieri stitch.
E. Dehisced mitral ring.

CASE 1:

A 62-year-old female patient with prior mechanical mitral and aortic valve replacement is admitted with acute onset dyspnea. She is afebrile and the results of blood cultures are negative. A transesophageal echocardiogram is obtained.

26. Based on Figure 18-11, what is the most likely diagnosis? (See also Videos 18-1A and B.)

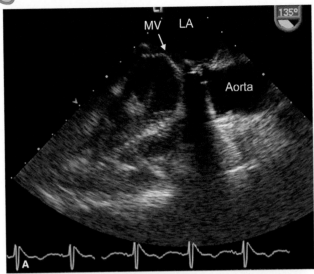

Fig. 18-11A

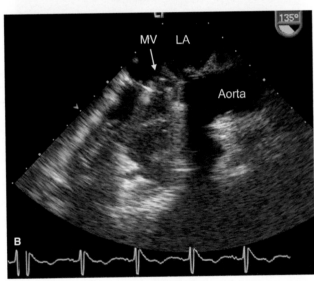

Fig. 18-11B

A. Mitral prosthetic endocarditis.
B. Mitral prosthetic thrombosis.
C. Mitral pannus ingrowth.
D. Normal Medtronic Hall mitral prosthesis.
E. Normal St. Jude mitral prosthesis.

CASE 2:

An 88-year-old woman with prior mitral valve replacement is referred for echocardiographic evaluation following a transient ischemic attack (Fig. 18-12 and Videos 18-2A and B.).

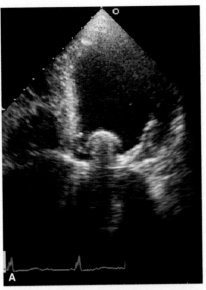

Fig. 18-12A

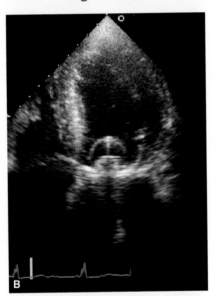

Fig. 18-12B

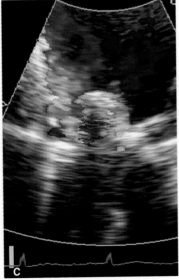

Fig. 18-12C

27. What type of prosthesis had been implanted?
  A. Starr-Edwards (ball and cage).
  B. Medtronic-Hall (tilting disc).
  C. St. Jude (bileaflet).
  D. Bovine pericardial bioprosthesis.
  E. Porcine bioprosthesis.

CASE 3:

A 36-year-old man with prior aortic valve replacement presents with a painful left toe. A transesophageal echocardiogram is obtained to rule out a cardiac source of embolus.

28. Based on the images in Figure 18-13 and Videos 18-3A–F, what is the most appropriate next step in management?

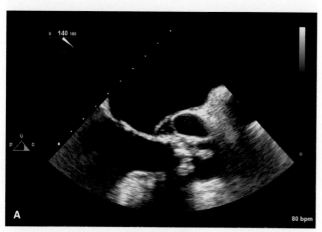

Fig. 18-13A

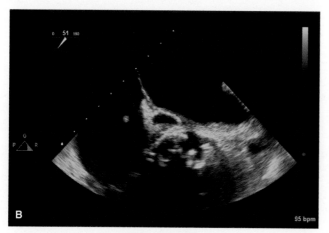

Fig. 18-13B

  A. Initiate anticoagulation.
  B. Initiate antibiotics.
  C. Perform coronary angiography.
  D. Perform femoral arteriography.
  E. Schedule urgent cardiac surgery.

CASE 4:

A 77-year-old woman is referred for an echocardiographic evaluation.

29. Based on the echocardiographic images in Figure 18-14 and Videos 18-4A–E, what is the most likely diagnosis?
  A. Isolated mitral ring annuloplasty.
  B. Bileaflet mitral valve replacement.
  C. Tilting disc mitral valve replacement.
  D. Bioprosthetic mitral valve replacement.
  E. Mitral Alfieri stitch repair with ring.

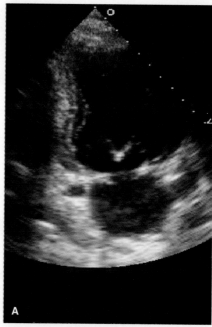

Fig. 18-14A

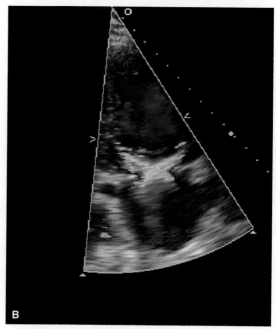

Fig. 18-14B

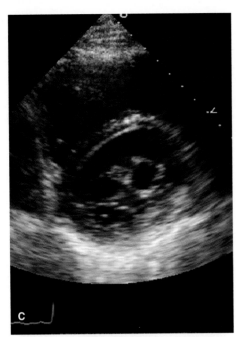

Fig. 18-14C

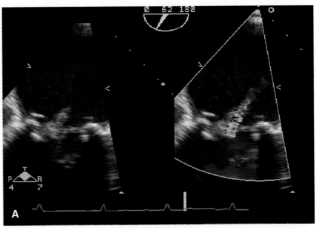

Fig. 18-15A

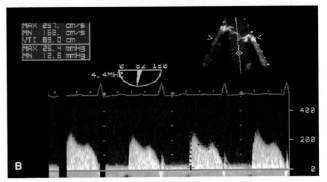

Fig. 18-15B

CASE 5:

A 42-year-old man with a prior history of mitral valve replacement presents with fever and dyspnea. Blood cultures are positive for methicillin-sensitive *Staphylococcus aureus*. A transesophageal echocardiogram is obtained.

30. Based on the findings shown in the images in Figure 18-15 and Videos 18-5A and B, what is the most likely basis for the patient's dyspnea?

A. Left ventricular systolic dysfunction.
B. Left ventricular diastolic dysfunction.
C. Multiple septic pulmonary emboli.
D. Severe prosthetic mitral regurgitation.
E. Severe prosthetic mitral stenosis.

ANSWERS

1. ANSWER: C. The term patient prosthesis mismatch (PPM) refers to the situation in which the effective orifice area (EOA) of a prosthesis is too small relative to the patient's body size resulting in abnormally high postoperative gradients. Although bioprostheses rather than mechanical valves are generally selected for women anticipating pregnancy as well as for patients with a prior history of drug abuse, these situations are not considered PPM. Children with prosthetic valves may outgrow their valves and develop PPM but this may be unavoidable regardless of whether a mechanical versus a bioprosthetic valve is implanted.

2. ANSWER: D. PPM refers to the situation in which the EOA of a prosthesis is too small relative to the patient's body size resulting in abnormally high postoperative gradients. The cutoff for PPM has been established to be a body surface area (BSA)-indexed EOA of ≤0.85 cm²/m² on the basis of the observation that at smaller areas there is a rapid increase in transvalvular gradients. BSA-corrected EOA ≤0.65 cm²/m² is considered severe PPM. The major adverse outcomes associated with PPM are reduced short-term and long-term survival, particularly if associated with left ventricular (LV) dysfunction. The high gradients associated with PPM may be distinguished echocardiographically from prosthetic valve dysfunction by comparing the echo-calculated EOA with published normal values for individual valves and by excluding imaging evidence of valve dysfunction.

3. ANSWER: C. Pressure recovery refers to the situation in which there is a localized pressure drop at the central orifice of a bileaflet mechanical valve that is partially recovered distally as flow from the lateral two orifices merges with the central flow jet. Since Doppler records the maximal pressure drop, it will yield a gradient higher than that measured at catheterization with catheters placed proximal and distal to the valve. Clinically significant pressure recovery is most often encountered in the setting of small bileaflet valves in the aortic position particularly when the cardiac output is increased.

Answer A is incorrect because the direct measure of left ventricle to aorta gradients used in this patient is superior to the pullback approach. It would be dangerous to attempt to cross this valve retrograde.

Answer B is incorrect because a relatively higher cardiac output at catheterization would result in a relatively higher (not lower) transvalvular gradient.

Answer D: Although it is may be possible to mistake a mitral regurgitant for a transaortic Doppler spectrum, the peak MR velocities are typically much higher than 3.5 m/sec (49 mm Hg) reflecting large gradients from the left ventricle to left atrium.

Answer E: In the case of PPM, elevated gradients are noted both by echocardiography and by catheterization.

4. ANSWER: B. Echocardiographic displays are calibrated on the basis of the velocity of sound through tissue, assuming that only tissue will be encountered by the ultrasound beam. The speed of sound in a Starr-Edwards valve ball is slower than that in tissue. Consequently, the ball is misrepresented echocardiographically as being larger than it actually is.

5. ANSWER: C. Although there is significant variability in the normal values reported for aortic prosthetic valves depending on size and valve type, a peak velocity of 2.5 m/sec is well within the normal range for many valves, and as such, would not be helpful in determining the type of prosthesis that has been implanted. In general, velocities of >3.0 m/sec prompt concern about pathologic elevation due to a variety of causes including PPM and intrinsic valve pathology although velocities of >3 m/sec may be normal for some valves. Stroke volume as an index of cardiac output is measured by the velocity-time integral (VTI) of the pulsed Doppler spectrum of the left ventricular outflow tract (LVOT).

6. ANSWER: C. Gradients across mitral and tricuspid prostheses are very heart rate dependent. Although a mean gradient of 10 at a heart rate of 60 bpm would be abnormal, the same gradient at a heart rate of 120 bpm would be "normal" for most mitral prostheses. While height and weight (choices A and B) and calculated BSA are important in evaluating patients for PPM (BSA-indexed EOA <1.15 cm^2/m^2), this assessment requires the calculation of EOA, which is not possible with only mean gradient. It is important to record blood pressure (choice D) at the time of echocardiography for patients with mitral disease. However, its major impact is on regurgitation rather than stenosis. Gender has no direct impact on valve gradients.

7. ANSWER: E. With harmonic imaging, microcavitations are frequently seen with normally functioning mechanical valves. Although their origin is uncertain, they are not imaging artifacts. In the era of fundamental imaging, microcavitations were reported as markers of hemolysis, which may be a feature of paravalvular regurgitation. In the absence of intravenously injected microbubbles, a patent foramen ovalis and associated right-to-left shunt will not result in left-sided microbubbles.

8. ANSWER: A. EOA is calculated using the continuity equation and is equivalent to the calculation of valve area in native valves. Thus

$$EOA = \frac{CSA_{LVOT} \times VTI_{LVOT}}{Prosthetic\ VTI} = \frac{Stroke\ volume}{Prosthetic\ VTI}$$

Choices B and C represent formulae that can be used to calculate the dimensionless index. By comparing calculated EOA with published norms, the diagnosis of prosthetic stenosis can be established.

9. ANSWER: A. See also discussion of question 3. Pressure recovery is typically encountered in small bileaflet or ball and cage valves.

10. ANSWER: A. Imaging features of restricted thickened cusps support the diagnosis of prosthetic stenosis as the basis for the elevated gradients. A small valve (19 mm Hg) as in choice B may be associated with elevated gradients even in a structurally normal valve if there is PPM (the valve is too small for the patient). The aortic root may be dilated (choice C) in patients with native aortic valve disease and does not regress following aortic valve replacement in the absence of aortic reconstructive surgery. Choice D: The normal hematocrit excludes anemia-associated high output, which may be associated with elevated gradients in structurally normal valves. Choice E: Reduced LV ejection fraction is typically associated with low gradients and provides no explanation for the elevated gradients noted here.

11. ANSWER: E. The pressure halftime should not be used to calculate EOA in patients with prosthetic valves.

12. ANSWER: B. All mechanical prosthetic valves have physiologic "regurgitation" that consists of a closing volume (a displacement of blood caused by the motion of the occluder) and leakage at the perimeter of or at hinge points of the occluders. Studies have shown bileaflet mechanical valves (St. Jude) to have the largest degree of physiologic regurgitation with central as well as peripheral jets. While Medtronic-Hall valves also have central and peripheral jets, the total amount of regurgitation is less compared to St. Jude valves.

13. ANSWER: B. The dimensionless index is defined as the ratio of subvalvular VTI or peak velocity to prosthetic VTI or peak velocity, respectively. It is particularly useful when image quality precludes accurate measurement of the LVOT as is needed to calculate EOA.

14. ANSWER: A. Because of acoustic shadowing and the eccentricity of paravalvular jets, transthoracic echocardiography is relatively insensitive for paravalvular regurgitation. Thus, transesophageal echocardiography (TEE) is indicated whenever paravalvular regurgitation is suspected. Elevated mitral gradients B and C favor mitral regurgitation. When jets are eccentric, normal (S dominant) flow may be preserved in pulmonary veins remote from the jet. All apical views should be used to assess for paravalvular regurgitation but no single view is ideal.

15. ANSWER: C. The Ross procedure consists of moving the patient's pulmonary valve to the aortic position (aortic autograft) and placing a homograft (cadaveric) valve in the pulmonic position (pulmonary homograft). Of the possible correct answers (aortic autograft stenosis or regurgitation), aortic regurgitation is the most common.

16. ANSWER: A. The prosthesis is identifiable as a stented bioprosthesis by the presence of clearly demarcated stents. There is a mitral regurgitant jet that clearly originates outside the sewing ring and extends to the back of the left atrium: this is paravalvular regurgitation. Although the image has not been optimized for proximal isovelocity surface area (PISA) based quantitation, note the clearly demarcated PISA shell. Although spontaneous valve dehiscence may occur, hemodynamically significant new paravalvular jets raise the possibility of endocarditis as the cause.

17. ANSWER: D. In the parasternal long-axis view and in the diastolic frame from the apical long axis, the mitral struts are seen abutting the interventricular septum. The systolic frame shows turbulent flow in the LVOT at the level of the mitral struts. Although rare, such malpositioning of high-profile mitral prostheses may cause significant LVOT obstruction. Patients at greatest risk are those with small hypertrophied ventricles. Mitral systolic anterior motion and LVOT obstruction may be a complication of mitral repair but not mitral valve replacement. Notably in patients with mitral valve replacement for active endocarditis, the mitral chords and leaflets are typically not preserved. Mitral stenosis would be associated with high-velocity flow in diastole not systole. There is no evidence of mitral regurgitation (high-velocity flow is in the LVOT not left atrium).

18. ANSWER: E. Although there are no large series of published normal values for tricuspid prosthetic gradients, the existing literature supports the diagnosis of prosthetic tricuspid stenosis whenever the mean gradients are more than 6 mm Hg. The mean gradient of 11 mm Hg at a slow heart rate is consistent with severe prosthetic stenosis. It is unlikely that this patient has a high output state with a heart rate of 55 bpm and even a significantly elevated cardiac output would unlikely be associated with gradient elevation of this degree.

Pressure recovery does not occur with large bioprosthetic valves in the tricuspid position. Note that the pressure halftime method has not been validated for prosthetic tricuspid valves and should not be used.

19. ANSWER: D. This is the typical three-dimensional (3D) view of a bileaflet mechanical mitral prosthesis as seen from the left atrial perspective. Two orifices are identified in this diastolic frame with the occluders in the open position. For 3D images of other prosthesis see the study of Sugeng et al as shown in the Suggesting Readings at the end of this chapter.

20. ANSWER: B. Mitral struts are clearly seen, identifying this valve as a bioprosthesis. On the right side, the septal leaflet of the tricuspid valve is seen in the open position with the dehisced portion of a tricuspid ring seen floating in the tricuspid inlet. The ring is appropriately attached laterally, identifying the normally attached portion of the ring. This helps prevent mistaking the dehisced portion for either a vegetation or pacer lead. This patient had severe tricuspid regurgitation.

21. ANSWER: E. Aortic homografts are treated cadaveric aortic roots and valves to which the native coronary arteries are implanted. The native aorta may be used to wrap the homograft aorta (the inclusion technique) or resected. Particularly when the inclusion technique is used, the normal postoperative appearance is one of a variably thickened root that may in part be due to hematoma. Over time, this resorbs and the appearance of the valve resembles that of the native aortic valve. In a clinical scenario suggestive of endocarditis, it may be impossible to differentiate a normal homograft from abscess. However, postimplantation perioperative TEE can be very helpful in resolving this dilemma. In the absence of clinical features of infection, the appearance shown here can be interpreted as normal.

22. ANSWER: A. This is a typical appearance for a tilting disc mechanical mitral prosthesis. The disc pivots from an eccentric pivot point and closure is associated with a prominent central jet. This valve should not be confused with bileaflet or ball/disc and cage valves examples of which are provided elsewhere in this chapter. There are no trileaflet mechanical valves.

23. ANSWER: E. The dimensionless index is the ratio of subvalvular VTI or peak velocity to prosthetic VTI or peak velocities respectively (= 1.1/3.3). It is easily performed and an alternative to EOA when the LVOT diameter is difficult to measure.

24. ANSWER: D. This short-axis image shows three stents and cusps in the closed position. This appearance is typical of a stented bioprosthesis. Stents are not elements of homografts or autografts, which are human valves or stentless heterograft bioprostheses. Aortic repairs are also not associated with stents. Stented valves are the most common type of bioprosthesis.

25. *ANSWER: E.* The arrow indicates a dehisced mitral ring. The anterior rim of the ring is seen in a normal position adjacent to the aortic root. This patient had severe posteriorly directed mitral regurgitation. Alfieri stitches are seen in the left ventricle, tying together the A2 and P2 scallops. The LV lead of biventricular pacing is placed in the coronary sinus. The aortic valve in this patient is a native valve. Although atrial septal aneurysms may project into the left atrium and be visible from this window, they do not appear as discrete echodensities as is seen here.

26. *ANSWER: B.* This patient has a mitral bileaflet (St. Jude) mechanical prosthesis in which one of the discs does not move and is stuck in the closed position. As in this case, this is associated with severe prosthetic stenosis. Although this may occur on the basis of either pannus ingrowth or thrombus, the acuity of the symptoms in this case favors thrombus. Vegetations may also interfere with disc function but the clinical information (absence of fever and negative blood cultures) argues against active endocarditis. Medtronic Hall valves are single tilting disc valves.

KEY POINTS:

- Bileaflet disc valves incorporate symmetrically positioned discs that normally open synchronously (a delay of one to two frames between discs can be normal).
- Immobility of one or both discs results in severe stenosis and/or regurgitation.
- Immobility is occasionally intermittent so it is important to record multibeat clips and look carefully for Doppler evidence of valve dysfunction.
- Suspicion of occluder malfunction is an indication for urgent echocardiography since thrombosis may be progressive and fatal.

27. *ANSWER: A.* This appearance is typical for a ball and cage valve. Note that the ball appears larger than its actual size due to slower transmission of sound through the ball as opposed to tissue. Transmitral flow emerges from around the ball. Spontaneous microcavitations are frequently seen as is evident in this case.

KEY POINTS:

- Although ball and cage valves are no longer implanted, there are still many patients with this type of valve.
- Understanding the physics of sound transmission and the artifactually large appearance of the ball on echocardiography is important.
- Microcavitations are frequently seen in the left ventricle in the presence of mechanical valves in the mitral position and may be a normal finding.

28. *ANSWER: E.* These images show valvular vegetations as well as a large root abscess. Root abscess is an indication for urgent surgery. There is no indication for anticoagulation as the painful toe can be attributed to a septic embolus. Coronary arteriography is contraindicated in the presence of large aortic valve vegetations and a friable root. Since the source of embolus has been identified, there is no need for femoral arteriography.

Another common manifestation of root abscess is heart block, which may progress to complete heart block. It occurs because of extension of the abscess into the upper septum where it involves the conduction system. Heart block in the presence of known or suspected endocarditis is an indication for TEE, the best way to diagnose abscess.

KEY POINTS:

- Abscess is a serious complication of endocarditis recognized by the presence of irregular spaces with variable sonolucency surrounding the valve.
- Flow into abscess cavities may be observed but is not necessary to establish the diagnosis.
- Abscess may occur without detectable vegetation on the valve.
- Abscesses can expand quickly and result in catastrophic intracardiac or extracardiac rupture. Urgent surgery is therefore indicated.

29. *ANSWER: E.* These images demonstrate the double orifice that is typical of an Alfieri stitch mitral repair. The supplemental image C is pathognomonic for this form of repair in which the A2 and P2 scallops are stitched together to create a double-orifice valve that mimics a congenitally double orifice mitral valve. Transcatheter mitral valve repair with the mitral clip is patterned on this type of repair.

KEY POINTS:

- Alfieri stitch repair (usually in combination with ring angioplasty) may be used for mitral repair in patients with functional mitral regurgitation.
- This approach is rarely associated with significant stenosis although residual regurgitation may be present.

30. *ANSWER: E.* At a heart rate of 73 bpm, a mean gradient of 12.6 mm Hg is severely elevated consistent with severe prosthetic stenosis attributable to obstruction of the prosthesis by vegetations. Color flow Doppler shows only trace mitral regurgitation. Although prosthetic mitral endocarditis is associated with peripheral emboli, pulmonary emboli are not a

6. In native valve IE, which of the following clinical scenarios carries the worst prognosis?
   A. A vegetation of 10 mm of the aortic valve.
   B. A vegetation of 10 mm of the mitral valve.
   C. A vegetation of 10 mm of the tricuspid valve.
   D. A vegetation of 15 mm of the tricuspid valve.

7. What is the most frequent location of an abscess in patients presenting with IE?
   A. Mitral valve annulus.
   B. Tricuspid valve annulus.
   C. Aortic root.
   D. Myocardium.
   E. Pericardial space.

8. Which of the following is more likely to be confused with a mitral abscess on a transthoracic echocardiogram?
   A. Caseous calcification of mitral annulus.
   B. Dilated coronary sinus.
   C. Descending thoracic aorta.
   D. Epicardial fat.

9. By TEE, which of the following is the best view to determine the location and extent of an aortic root abscess?
   A. Midesophageal five-chamber view at 0–15 degrees.
   B. Midesophageal short-axis view at 45–60 degrees.
   C. Midesophageal long-axis view at 120–140 degrees.
   D. Deep transgastric five-chamber view at 0–10 degrees.

10. Which of the following represents an early sign of aortic root abscess in the setting of native aortic valve IE?
    A. Abnormal flow between aorta and right atrium.
    B. An echolucent space at the aortic root without drainage into the aortic lumen.
    C. Abnormal thickness of the aortic root (>10 mm).
    D. Abnormal aortic root dilatation (>42 mm).

11. A patient has been found to have a vegetation on the left ventricular aspect of the anterior mitral valve leaflet (AMVL) with a leaflet aneurysm. What other structure should be sought for the presence of vegetation?

A. Aortic valve.
B. Posterior mitral valve leaflet.
C. Tricuspid subvalvular apparatus.
D. Left atrium (LA).
E. Myocardium.

12. A 49-year-old man presents with IE. The TEE shows a 10 mm × 15 mm vegetation on the left atrial aspect of the posterior mitral valve leaflet. The patient has been given IV antibiotics. He remains stable during his 4 weeks course of therapy. A repeat TEE reveals a persistent vegetation on the mitral valve with similar dimension but without significant mitral regurgitation.
    If the size of the vegetation remained the same after 4 weeks of antibiotics, which of the following statements is true regarding the short-term prognosis of the patient?
    A. After 4 weeks of therapy, the size of the vegetation usually remains unchanged.
    B. After 4 weeks of therapy, an increase in echo brightness of vegetations is associated with an increased risk of complications related to endocarditis.
    C. After 4 weeks of therapy, persistence of vegetations in the absence of significant valvular regurgitation is associated with no increased risk of complications related to endocarditis.
    D. After 4 weeks of therapy, rapid reduction of vegetation size has been shown to correlate with an increased risk of embolic events.

13. After complete resolution of a vegetation, what proportion of the affected valves retains normal structure and function?
    A. 10%.
    B. 15%.
    C. 20%.
    D. 25%.
    E. 30%.

14. IE involving the Eustachian valve is a rare entity. Its incidence has been reported as low as 3% in the setting of right-sided endocarditis. Unfortunately, the Eustachian valve is not routinely examined to rule out vegetation.
    What are the best views to visualize the Eustachian valve during a transthoracic echocardiographic study?

A. Right ventricular (RV) inflow view/parasternal short-axis view.

B. Apical four-chamber view/subcostal view.

C. Parasternal long-axis view/apical four-chamber view.

D. Subcostal view/parasternal long-axis view.

15. What are the two features that distinguish a vegetation on the Eustachian valve from the normal Eustachian valve?

A. Abnormal thickness of >2 mm and high-frequency motion independent of the underlying structure.

B. Abnormal thickness of >2 mm and high-frequency motion similar to the underlying structure.

C. Abnormal thickness of >5 mm and high-frequency motion independent of the underlying structure.

D. Abnormal thickness of >5 mm and high-frequency motion similar to the underlying structure.

16. What is the negative predictive value of multiplane TEE?

A. 50%.

B. 60%.

C. 70%.

D. 80%.

E. >85%.

17. A mitral valve aneurysm has the following characteristics:

A. A localized bulging of mitral leaflet toward the LA with expansion throughout the cardiac cycle.

B. A localized bulging of mitral leaflet toward the LA with systolic expansion and diastolic collapse.

C. A localized bulging of mitral leaflet toward the left ventricle (LV) with expansion throughout the cardiac cycle.

D. A localized bulging of mitral leaflet toward the LV with systolic expansion and diastolic collapse.

18. What condition is most likely to be confused with a mitral valve aneurysm?

A. Mitral valve prolapse.

B. Mitral valve blood cyst.

C. Mitral valve flail leaflet.

D. Mitral valve repair with Alfieri stitch.

19. Which abnormality is the result of a satellite lesion in this patient with endocarditis (Fig. 19-1 and Video 19-1)?

A. Aortic root abscess.

B. Anterior mitral valve aneurysm.

C. Aortic cusp perforation.

D. Aorta to right ventricular outflow tract (RVOT) fistula.

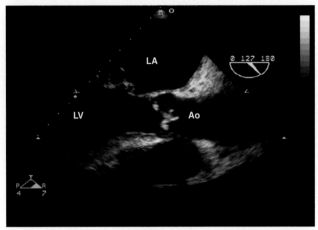

Fig. 19-1

20. You suspect severe aortic regurgitation. To confirm your suspicion in this patient, you demonstrate significant diastolic flow reversal by:

A. Pulsed wave (PW) Doppler through the LVOT in its deep transgastric five-chamber view.

B. PW Doppler through the descending aorta in its long-axis view.

C. PW Doppler through the ascending aorta in its long-axis view.

D. PW Doppler through the abdominal aorta in its long-axis view.

E. Continuous wave (CW) Doppler through the abdominal aorta in its long-axis view.

21. Based on the TEE image, (Fig. 19-1 and Video 19-1) the vegetation on the aortic valve appears to affect more than one cusp. What is the best view to assess the extent of the lesion on the aortic valve?

A. Short-axis view of the aortic valve (40–60 degrees).

B. Short-axis view of the LVOT (40–60 degrees).

C. Long-axis view of the LVOT and aortic valve (110–140 degrees).

D. Five-chamber view of the LVOT and aortic valve (0 degree).

E. Deep transgastric five-chamber view (0 degree).

22. Based on the TEE findings, what is the prognosis of the patient?
   A. Low risk of embolic event, low risk of mortality, high risk of valve replacement.
   B. High risk of embolic event, low risk of mortality, high risk of valve replacement.
   C. High risk of embolic event, high risk of mortality, high risk of valve replacement.
   D. High risk of embolic event, high risk of mortality, low risk of valve replacement.
   E. High risk of embolic event, low risk of mortality, high risk of valve replacement.

23. A 25-year-old man, injection drug user, presents with fever and shortness of breath. Two sets of blood culture grew Gram positive cocci in clusters. An echocardiogram is performed and showed a vegetation of 2.5 cm × 3.5 cm on the tricuspid valve (Fig. 19-2 and Video 19-2).

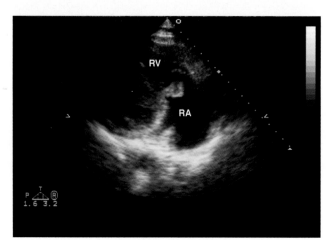

Fig. 19-2

   Which leaflet of the tricuspid valve is the vegetation attached to?
   A. Anterior leaflet.
   B. Septal leaflet.
   C. Posterior leaflet.

24. What is the prognosis of this patient based on the vegetation size?
   A. High risk of embolic event, high risk of valve replacement, high risk of mortality.
   B. Low risk of embolic event, low risk of valve replacement, low risk of mortality.
   C. High risk of embolic event, high risk of valve replacement, low risk of mortality.
   D. Low risk of embolic event, high risk of valve replacement, low risk of mortality.

25. Where should the presence of a satellite lesion be sought?
   A. Vegetation on the right atrial wall.
   B. Vegetation on the pulmonic valve.
   C. Vegetation on the tricuspid papillary muscle.
   D. Vegetation on the RV wall.

26. A 50-year-old man admitted for aortic valve endocarditis develops a new murmur and becomes more short of breath. A repeat echocardiogram with Doppler is performed.

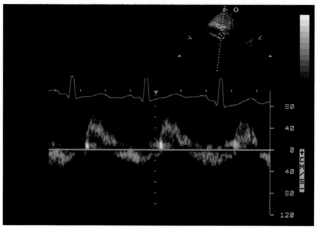

Fig. 19-3

   A Doppler tracing is illustrated in Figure 19-3; where is it obtained?
   A. PW Doppler in the sinus of Valsalva.
   B. PW Doppler in the descending or abdominal aorta.
   C. PW Doppler in VSD.
   D. PW Doppler in the LVOT.
   E. CW Doppler of the descending or abdominal aorta.

27. Based on Figure 19-3, what does it represent?
   A. Rupture of the sinus of Valsalva.
   B. VSD shunt.
   C. Severe aortic regurgitation.
   D. Aortic valve cusp rupture.

28. A 65-year-old man presents with fever and transient loss of right eye vision. He has had a previous valve replacement. Four weeks ago, he had a dental extraction and received prophylactic antibiotic therapy. An echocardiogram is performed and shows vegetations on the aortic valve (Fig. 19-4 and Video 19-3).

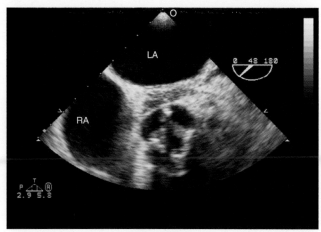

Fig. 19-4

What is the type of prosthesis that the patient has?
A. Aortic homograft.
B. Aortic bioprosthesis.
C. Aortic stentless prosthesis.
D. Aortic mechanical prosthesis.

29. What is the other complication related to the endocarditis?
A. Aortic cusp rupture.
B. Aortic root abscess.
C. Aortic root pseudoaneurysm.
D. Aortic root-LVOT fistula.

30. Where is it located?
A. Anterior and medial.
B. Medial.
C. Lateral.
D. Posterior and lateral.

31. In the same patient as in question 4, color Doppler of the aortic prosthesis is performed (Fig. 19-5 and Video 19-4).

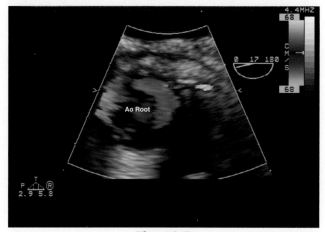

Fig. 19-5

What is the additional complication?
A. Severe aortic regurgitation.
B. Left main compression by the abscess.
C. Aortic root to RVOT fistula.
D. Rupture of sinus of Valsalva.

32. A patient presented with mitral valve endocarditis. He had been treated with antibiotics for 4 weeks. Figure 19-6 shows parasternal long- and short-axis views of the mitral valve (Video 19-5).

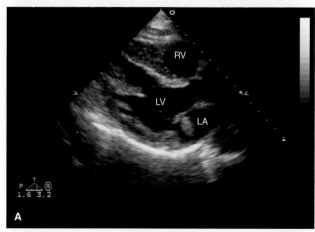

Fig. 19-6A

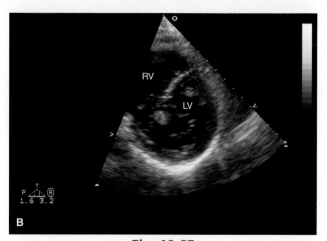

Fig. 19-6B

What is the site of the attachment of the vegetation on the mitral valve?
A. A1.
B. A2.
C. A3.
D. P3.

33. A patient with a previous mitral valve replacement is admitted for jaundice and shortness of breath. A zoomed apical four-chamber view is shown in Figure 19-7 and Video 19-6.

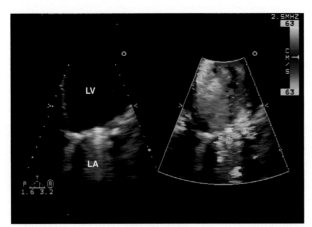

Fig. 19-7

What is abnormal about the mitral prosthesis?
A. Large left atrial mass.
B. Dehiscence of the prosthesis.
C. Fistula between LA and aorta.
D. There is no abnormality.

34. What are the mean and peak pressure gradients of the prosthesis?
A. Normal for its type and size.
B. Both are increased to a similar degree.
C. Both are decreased.
D. The peak gradient is increased more than the mean gradient.

35. A patient with a previous aortic valve replacement is admitted for increased dyspnea. A TEE is performed and the long-axis view of the LVOT is shown in diastole (Fig. 19-8A) and systole (Fig. 19-8B; Video 19-7).

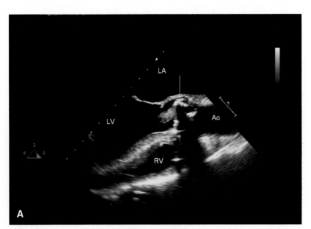

Fig. 19-8A

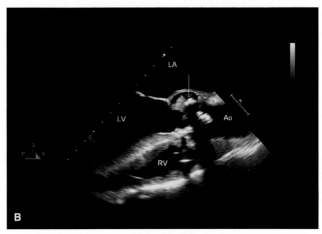

Fig. 19-8B

The primary abnormality seen in this image is?
A. Dehiscence of the aortic prosthesis.
B. Severe mitral regurgitation.
C. Flail prosthetic leaflet.
D. Severe aortic stenosis.

36. What other lesion is also present?
A. Abscess of the aortic root.
B. Pseudoaneurysm of the aortic root.
C. Localized aortic dissection.
D. No other lesion is noted.

37. A 65-year-old man has been treated with 4 weeks of antibiotics for endocarditis in the aortic position. A repeated TEE was performed prior to discontinuation of antibiotics.

Based on the images shown in Figure 19-9, and Videos 19-8A and B, which of the following is true about the mitral valve?

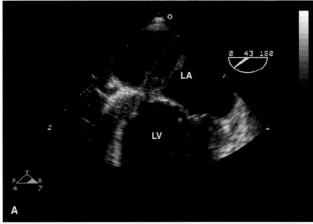

Fig. 19-9A

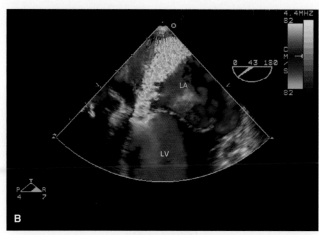

Fig. 19-9B

A. There are two long vegetations on the posterior mitral valve leaflet.

B. There is a mitral valve aneurysm on the posterior mitral valve leaflet.

C. There is a fistula between LV and LA.

D. There is a rupture of the mitral papillary muscle.

---

38. A 78-year-old woman is admitted for endocarditis. A TEE is performed and confirms a vegetation, measuring 2.5 cm × 0.5 cm (Fig. 19-10 and Video 19-9).

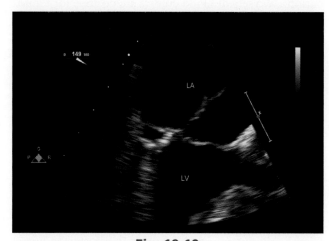

Fig. 19-10

What is the site of attachment of the vegetation?

A. Left atrial aspect of the posterior mitral valve leaflet.

B. Left atrial aspect of the AMVL.

C. Left atrial aspect of A1 of mitral valve.

D. Left atrial aspect of P1 of mitral valve.

E. Left atrial aspect of A2 of mitral valve.

39. What other finding present on the TEE is associated with a worsening prognosis?

A. Echolucent nature of the vegetation.

B. Highly mobile vegetation.

C. Mitral annulus calcification.

D. Mitral annulus abscess.

CASE 1:

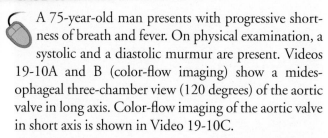

A 75-year-old man presents with progressive shortness of breath and fever. On physical examination, a systolic and a diastolic murmur are present. Videos 19-10A and B (color-flow imaging) show a midesophageal three-chamber view (120 degrees) of the aortic valve in long axis. Color-flow imaging of the aortic valve in short axis is shown in Video 19-10C.

40. Which of the following statements about the aortic valve is correct?

A. There are vegetations on the right coronary cusp (RCC) and noncoronary cusp (NCC) of the aortic valve. There is severe prolapse of the RCC.

B. There is a perforation of the RCC of the aortic valve.

C. There are vegetations on the RCC and NCC of the aortic valve. There is severe prolapse of the RCC and a perforation of the NCC.

D. There is prolapse of the NCC of the aortic valve.

41. In addition to aortic regurgitation, what is the other finding on the color-flow imaging or the short-axis view of the aortic valve?

A. A fistula between left sinus of Valsalva and LA.

B. A fistula between right sinus of Valsalva and RA.

C. A fistula between left sinus of Valsalva and RA.

D. A fistula between right sinus of Valsalva and LA.

E. A fistula between left sinus of Valsalva and RV.

42. Which of the following statements regarding the aortic regurgitation is correct?

A. There is severe aortic regurgitation.

B. There is moderate aortic regurgitation.

C. There is mild aortic regurgitation.

D. Cannot exclude severe aortic regurgitation.

43. Which of the following PW Doppler tracings belongs to this patient?

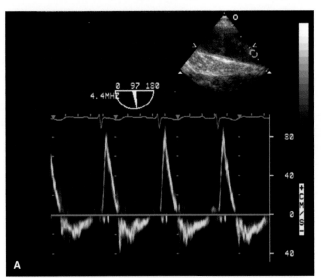

Fig. 19-11A

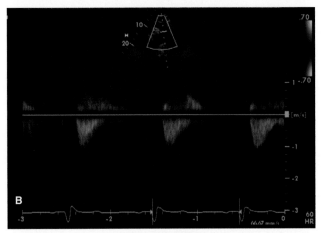

Fig. 19-11B

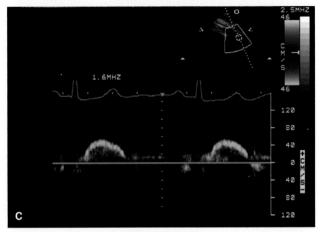

Fig. 19-11C

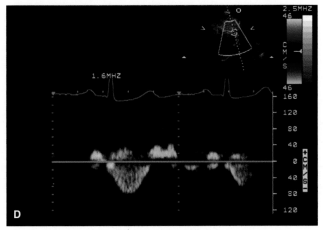

Fig. 19-11D

A. Figure 19-11A.
B. Figure 19-11B.
C. Figure 19-11C.
D. Figure 19-11D.

CASE 2:

A 42-year-old man has previously been treated as an outpatient for pneumonia. After 3 days of antibiotics, he remains febrile and becomes progressively weak. At presentation, the patient appears toxic. A systolic murmur is present on physical examination. Two sets of blood culture are positive for Gram-positive cocci. A transthoracic echocardiogram and TEE are performed. Videos 19-11A and B show a midesophageal 65-degree view of the mitral valve and the same view with color-flow imaging, respectively. Video 19-11C shows a midesophageal four-chamber view.

44. What lesion is being illustrated in Videos 19-11A and B?
A. There is a vegetation on the AMVL.
B. There is an aneurysm on the AMVL, which is perforated.
C. There is a vegetation on the posterior mitral valve leaflet.
D. There is an aneurysm on the posterior mitral valve leaflet, which is perforated.

45. What other lesion is shown in Video 19-11C?

   A. There is a mural thrombus attached to the lateral wall.
   B. There is a mural vegetation attached to the lateral wall.
   C. There is an abscess attached to the lateral wall.
   D. There is a mural vegetation attached to the posterior wall.

CASE 3:

A 65-year-old woman presents with progressive shortness of breath. Four weeks ago, she had been diagnosed to have endocarditis and is being treated with antibiotics. Videos 19-12A and B represent TTE parasternal long axis views of the mitral valve and the same view with color-flow imaging, respectively. Video 19-12C illustrates TTE parasternal short-axis view of the mitral valve with color-flow imaging.

46. After complete resolution of the vegetation, what proportion of affected valves will have normal structure and function?
   A. 10%.
   B. 20%.
   C. 30%.
   D. 50%.
   E. 80%.

47. Which of the following statements is true about the mitral valve?
   A. A vegetation is present on the mitral valve.
   B. There is anterior mitral leaflet perforation associated with significant mitral regurgitation.
   C. The mitral valve leaflets appear abnormal.
   D. There is a cleft of the anterior mitral leaflet with significant mitral regurgitation.

48. The cardiac surgeon asks you: where is the mitral regurgitant jet located?
   A. The regurgitant jet is located at P1.
   B. The regurgitant jet is located at A1.
   C. The regurgitant jet is located at A2.
   D. The regurgitant jet is located at the junction of P2.

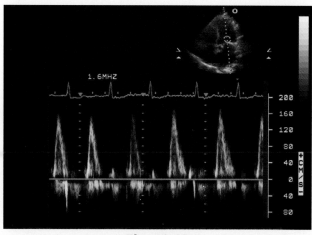

Fig. 19-12

49. What is the mitral valve abnormality?
   A. A calcified vegetation on the posterior mitral valve leaflet with valve disruption, leading to a coaptation defect.
   B. A fistula of the posterior mitral valve annulus between the LV and LA.
   C. An abscess of the posterior mitral valve annulus with a posterior mitral valve perforation.
   D. A ruptured chordae with flail of the posterior mitral leaflet.

50. PW Doppler tracing of the pulmonary veins do not show systolic flow reversal. The E velocity of mitral valve inflow is illustrated in Figure 19-12 Based on the images, how would you grade the mitral regurgitation?
   A. Mild mitral regurgitation.
   B. Moderate mitral regurgitation.
   C. Severe mitral regurgitation.
   D. Cannot comment.

51. The absence of the systolic flow reversal in the pulmonary veins despite the presence of severe mitral regurgitation is least likely explained by the following:
   A. High left atrial compliance.
   B. Inadequate sampling of the pulmonary veins.
   C. Severe enlargement of the left atrial.
   D. Low left atrial compliance.

CASE 4:

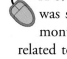

A 67-year-old man with a history of endocarditis was successfully treated with antibiotic therapy 6 months ago. He has no known complications related to endocarditis. His family physician orders a routine echocardiogram for follow-up. TTE shows severe mitral regurgitation. A TEE is then performed. See Videos 19-13A and B, and Figure 19-12.

CASE 5:

A 24-year-old woman with history of intravenous drug abuse, presents with fever, fatigue, and shortness of breath. Two sets of blood cultures grew Gram positive cocci within 24 hours. A chest X-ray shows multiple small infiltrates in both lungs, highly suggestive of septic emboli. An initial TTE revealed two echogenic masses; one is on the tricuspid valve and the other is ill defined and is in the LA. A TEE is then performed. See Videos 19-14A–D.

52. What is the involvement on the tricuspid valve?
    A. There are vegetations on the anterior and posterior leaflets of the tricuspid valve.
    B. There are vegetations on the anterior and septal leaflets of the tricuspid valve.
    C. There are vegetations on all three tricuspid leaflets.
    D. There is an annular abscess.

53. How severe is the tricuspid regurgitation?
    A. Mild tricuspid regurgitation.
    B. Moderate tricuspid regurgitation.
    C. Severe tricuspid regurgitation.
    D. Cannot comment.

54. Which of the following is the PW Doppler tracing of the hepatic vein flow in this patient?

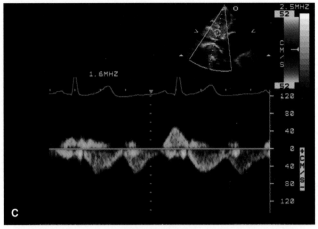

Fig. 19-13C

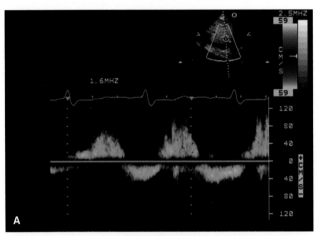

Fig. 19-13A

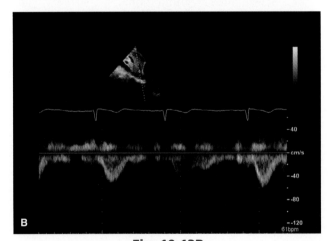

Fig. 19-13B

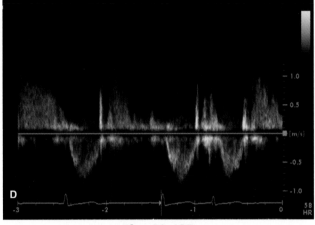

Fig. 19-13D

    A. Figure 19-13A.
    B. Figure 19-13B.
    C. Figure 19-13C.
    D. Figure 19-13D.

55. There is a large mobile left atrial mass attached to the posterior left atrial wall. This mass is likely:
    A. A vegetation.
    B. A thrombus.
    C. An angiosarcoma.
    D. A myxoma.

ANSWERS

1. ANSWER: C. Studies comparing transthoracic echocardiography (TTE) with transesophageal echocardiography (TEE) for the detection of vegetations with TEE as gold standard have shown that the sensitivity of TTE is dependent on vegetation size. It varies from 0% to 25% for vegetations of <5 mm and from 84% to 100% for vegetations of >10 mm. Therefore, vegetations of <5 mm can easily be missed by TTE even with the application of harmonic imaging. The resolution of echocardiography is affected by image quality. A recent meta-analysis showed that the sensitivities of TTE and TEE in detecting vegetations in native valve endocarditis were 62% and 92%, respectively.

2. ANSWER: A. TEE provides high spatial resolution of cardiac structures due to its close proximity to the heart and the high frequency of the transducer. Sachdev et al. showed that TEE can depict a structure as small as 1 mm in diameter.

3. ANSWER: D. Initially, M-mode was used to detect vegetations. With 2D TTE, better spatial definition of vegetations can now be obtained. An active vegetation is an echolucent mass with an irregular shape. It is usually located at the upstream side and near the tips of leaflets with high-frequency motion independent of the underlying cardiac structure. The mass can be associated with valve dysfunction. Chronic healed vegetations become echo-dense masses due to fibrin, collagen, and calcium deposition. According to the modified Duke's criteria, a vegetation is "an oscillating intracardiac mass on valves or supporting structures, or in the path of regurgitant jets, or on implanted material, in the absence of an alternative anatomical explanation." Compared with infective vegetations, noninfective vegetations from marantic or Libman-Sacks endocarditis have similar morphologic features and can only be differentiated from infective vegetations on the basis of the clinical findings.

4. ANSWER: C. Because of its close proximity to the ventricular septal defect (VSD) jet, the septal leaflet of the tricuspid valve is usually affected. However, right ventricular outflow tract (RVOT) and subpulmonic vegetation have also been described in patients with VSD presenting with infective endocarditis.

5. ANSWER: B. Dehiscence of a prosthetic valve is defined as a rocking motion of the prosthetic valve with an excursion of >15 degrees in at least one direction throughout the cardiac cycle. Studies show that only valves with ring dehiscence more than 40% of their annular circumference exhibit excessive rocking motion. Thus, absence of rocking motion does not exclude dehiscence.

6. ANSWER: A. Studies have shown that vegetations of >10 mm in the aortic position are associated with a higher risk of mortality, abscess formation, and valve replacement when compared with mitral valve vegetations; although in the study by Mugge et al., mitral valve vegetations of >10 mm were associated with a higher embolic risk. Tricuspid valve endocarditis carries the best prognosis because the affected patients are usually young. However, the prognosis seems to be worse with bulky tricuspid valve vegetation of >20 mm. No head-to-head comparison study has been reported between right-sided and left-sided endocarditis with respect to short-term and long-term prognosis.

7. ANSWER: C. On echocardiography, an abscess is identified as localized abnormal thickening of the perivalvular tissue or echolucent space within the perivalvular tissue that does not communicate with surrounding cardiac chambers. It is predominantly located at the aortic root and mitral-aortic intervalvular fibrosa. Myocardial abscesses are associated with very high mortality. The development of heart block in this setting is an indication of abscess formation involving the ventricular septum. A pericardial abscess usually represents a fistula formation between an annular abscess and the pericardial space.

8. ANSWER: A. Caseous calcification of the mitral annulus can present as an echolucent space within the calcification of the mitral annulus, simulating a mitral valve annular abscess. To differentiate from an abscess, other echocardiographic features need to be sought, such as a vegetation, perforation of the leaflet, or valve dysfunction.

A dilated coronary sinus, thoracic descending aorta, and epicardial fat can be easily distinguished from an abscess in the presence of normal mitral valve anatomy and function.

9. ANSWER: B. On TEE or TTE, the short-axis view of the aortic valve allows better visualization of the location and extent of an aortic root abscess. This view provides a 360-degree spatial orientation of the aortic root and aortic valve leaflet.

10. ANSWER: C. Abnormal thickness of the aortic wall of >10 mm is suspicious for an aortic root abscess in native aortic valve endocarditis. If present, serial echocardiograms can follow the evolution of this thickening and identify formation of an echolucent space over time. This criterion cannot be used in patients with recent aortic valve or aortic root replacement, as postoperative inflammation can contribute to thickening of the aortic wall. Prosthetic valvular thrombosis and pannus formation can be differentiated from an abscess by their predilection to involve the sewing ring encroaching onto the prosthetic orifice instead of the surrounding annulus. A pseudoaneurysm can be recognized by the presence of an echolucent cavity with communication with a neighboring cardiac chamber.

11. ANSWER: A. Aortic valve endocarditis usually leads to valve disruption and aortic regurgitation. The regurgitant jet can either be directed anteriorly against the anterior septum or posteriorly against the anterior mitral valve leaflet (AMVL). If aortic regurgitation is directed posteriorly, the jet lesion can seed the AMVL. This localized infection destroys the endothelium and fibrosa of the valve. If the infection is not controlled, aneurysm (diverticulum formation) and perforation of the AMVL ensue.

12. ANSWER: C. Vegetations evolve during successful antibiotic treatment. Reduction in vegetation size and increase in density are common. Persistence of vegetations alone does not predict a worse outcome. Rohmann et al. reported that the lack of regression of vegetation size after 4–6 weeks of antibiotic therapy is associated with an increased risk of mortality and complications related to endocarditis. However, this occurs only in patients with progressive valve disruption and dysfunction. In contrast, in patients with endocarditis but without significant valve dysfunction, the mortality and morbidity rate is not increased despite the lack of reduction in the vegetation size.

13. ANSWER: A. Rohmann et al. have shown that after healing from endocarditis, <10% of affected valves regain their normal structure. The majority of affected valves show nodular changes, thickening, or disruption of the leaflet after healing. No reliable predictors for complete healing have been identified.

14. ANSWER: A. Right ventricular (RV) inflow and parasternal short-axis views are the best views to appreciate the anatomy of the Eustachian valve. Sometimes, the apical four-chamber view and the subcostal views can also be used to assess the extent of vegetation, but the Eustachian valve is usually not well seen because of the increased image depth necessary for these views. The Eustachian valve is an embryonic remnant from the incomplete resolution of the membranous partition between the smooth posterior venous chamber and the anterior trabeculated primitive atrium. When the membranous embryonic remnant is extensive and weblike with attachment to multiple sites, it is referred to as Chiari network.

15. ANSWER: C. San Roman et al. found two specific features of the normal Eustachian valve: the valve is thin with a width of <3 mm, and it has predictable oscillating motion. They suggested that abnormal thickness (>5 mm) of a Eustachian valve leaflet and a mass with chaotic high-frequency motion are suspicious for an Eustachian valve vegetation.

16. ANSWER: E. Multiplane TEE has been reported as a highly diagnostic tool with a negative predictive value varying from 87% to 98% in IE, depending on the clinical setting and the criteria used to define IE (native valve vs. prosthetic valve, modified Duke criteria vs. pathological confirmation). The negative predictive value of TEE can be further increased if a repeat TEE 7–10 days later remains negative.

17. ANSWER: B. Mitral valve aneurysms are usually due to endocarditis. Surgical repair is frequently indicated because of the concomitant presence of perforation involving the aneurysm resulting in significant mitral regurgitation.

18. ANSWER: A. Mitral valve prolapse can sometimes mimic mitral valve aneurysm because of the systolic bulging of the mitral valve leaflet toward the left atrium. However, the absence of vegetation and valve disruption favor the diagnosis of prolapse.

Mitral valve blood cyst is a very rare condition that can present as an immobile echogenic mass on the mitral valve leaflet.

Flail of mitral valve leaflet is usually associated with ruptured chordae that can be identified by the typical "snake-tongue" appearance of the corresponding mitral leaflet into the LA during systole.

Mitral valve repair with Alfieri stitch presents as a double orifice mitral valve on the parasternal short-axis view. On the parasternal long-axis view, the mitral valve leaflets appear thickened and restricted.

19. ANSWER: B. Aortic valve endocarditis usually leads to valve disruption and aortic regurgitation. The regurgitant jet can either be directed anteriorly against the septum or posteriorly against the AMVL. If aortic regurgitation is directed posteriorly, a satellite vegetation may form on the AMVL. This localized infection destroys the endothelium and fibrosa of the valve. If the infection is not controlled, aneurysm (diverticulum) formation and perforation of the AMVL ensue.

20. ANSWER: D. The abdominal aorta is easily imaged by turning the probe to either direction when it is in the stomach. Pulsed-wave (PW) Doppler in the long axis can be obtained by rotating the probe to 90 degrees. Diastolic reversal in the abdominal aorta, if present, suggests severe aortic regurgitation. Diastolic reversal in the ascending aorta but not in the abdominal aorta probably suggests moderate to severe aortic regurgitation.

21. ANSWER: A. On TEE, the short-axis view of the aortic valve allows better visualization of the location of a vegetation on its three cusps. This view provides a 360-degree spatial orientation of the aortic root and aortic valve leaflet on the aorta aspect. To better assess the LVOT aspect of the aortic valve, real-time 3D imaging may be very helpful.

22. ANSWER: C. The patient has double valve lesions, multiple mobile aortic vegetations, and severe aortic valve disruption with severe aortic regurgitation. These findings suggest a poor outcome and high likelihood for surgical intervention and embolic events.

23. ANSWER: B. This is an RV inflow view. We normally see the anterior leaflet (anterior on the screen) and posterior leaflet (posterior on the screen) of the tricuspid valve. However, because of the shallow angle of the transducer, the interventricular septum instead of the RV posterior wall is imaged and thus, the leaflet is in fact the septal leaflet (not the posterior leaflet).

24. *ANSWER: C.* Studies have shown that vegetations of >2.5 cm on the tricuspid position is significantly associated with an increase risk of an embolic event and a need for valve replacement. However, the mortality rate remains low because most of these patients are young and are without serious comorbidities.

25. *ANSWER: A.* The tricuspid regurgitation jet, if present can be directed against the right atrial wall. The resultant jet can "seed" the infection on the right atrial wall as a satellite lesion.

26. *ANSWER: B.* This tracing is a PW Doppler with systolic and diastolic flows that are in opposite directions. This helps to eliminate the possibility of a VSD shunt (mainly systolic component), rupture of sinus of Valsalva (continuous flow in one direction), and LVOT flow (high-velocity turbulent diastolic flow).

27. *ANSWER: C.* This tracing represent a diastolic reversal in the abdominal aorta, which suggests severe aortic regurgitation. One cannot distinguish the mechanism of the aortic regurgitation. Two-dimensional imaging is necessary to determine the underlying mechanism.

28. *ANSWER: B.* The detection of biologic leaflets excludes a mechanical prosthesis. Because of the presence of struts (stents), it is a bioprosthesis. A homograft or stentless prosthesis does not have struts on its sewing ring.

29. *ANSWER: B.* In the setting of aortic bioprosthesis endocarditis, the thickening of the aortic root is highly suggestive of an aortic root abscess. The thickening seems to have several ill-defined echolucent areas that further support this diagnosis.

30. *ANSWER: D.* The abscess is located posteriorly as it is close to the LA and laterally as it is away from the interatrial septum. The anterior aspect of the sewing ring is shadowed and not well seen.

31. *ANSWER: B.* As shown by the color Doppler, there is high-velocity flow in the left main coronary artery during diastole and evidence of extrinsic compression of by the abscess.

32. *ANSWER: C.* The scallops of the mitral leaflet can be classified as lateral (A1), middle (A2), and medial (A3) of the anterior mitral leaflet, and lateral (P1), middle (P2), and medial (P3) of the posterior mitral leaflet.

The vegetation is attached to the medial aspect of the AMVL, which is the A3 scallop.

33. *ANSWER: B.* Dehiscence of a prosthetic valve is present as there is a large perivalvular regurgitation jet at the lateral sewing ring indicated by the large flow convergence. Most valvular dehiscences are due to

infection. A mechanical mitral valve can produce a reverberation artifact in the LA simulating a mass.

34. *ANSWER: D.* In the setting of severe prosthetic mitral regurgitation and normal LV function, the peak early diastolic velocity (pressure gradient) is more significantly increased than the mean gradient. It should be noted that a small amount of regurgitation is normal for many types of mechanical prosthesis, particularly the bileaflet type. The normal mitral prosthetic regurgitant flow has a regurgitant jet area of <2 cm² and jet length of <2.5 cm. However, with TTE it is usually difficult to detect mitral regurgitation by color-flow imaging because of shielding of the LA by the mitral prosthesis.

35. *ANSWER: A.* The posterior sewing ring (arrow) of the aortic prosthesis is dehisced from the aortic annulus and demonstrates rocking motion, which is not well appreciated in these still images. Severe aortic regurgitation is expected when there is dehiscence of the prosthesis. A large pedunculated vegetation is present. No definite flail prosthetic leaflet is detected.

36. *ANSWER: B.* The pseudoaneurysm is demonstrated by the localized bulging at the posterior aortic root that is better seen in systole (Fig. 19-8B) and is a sequela of an aortic root abscess.

37. *ANSWER: B.* After 4 weeks of antibiotic therapy and a favorable clinical response, it is unlikely to still have large vegetations. The two linear "vegetations" move in unison, and the mitral regurgitant jet is confined within these linear masses, which are in fact the walls of the mitral valve aneurysm. This aneurysm is defined as a localized bulging of mitral leaflet toward the LA with expansion during systole. In addition to mitral valve endocarditis, this condition can be encountered in the setting of aortic valve endocarditis with an aortic regurgitant jet impinging on the AMVL leading to satellite infection. Acquired mitral valve aneurysm is invariably due to endocarditis. Congenital mitral valve aneurysm is rare.

38. *ANSWER: A.* The vegetation is attached to the posterior mitral valve leaflet. However, it is unclear which scallop the vegetation is attached to. Other views are necessary to determine its exact attachment site; the best view to localize the specific scallop is the transgastric short-axis view of the mitral valve at 0 degree.

39. *ANSWER: D.* As shown in Figure 19-10, there is an echolucent space located posteriorly just under the mitral annulus. This echolucent space is probably communicating with the left ventricular cavity represents an abscess or pseudoaneurysm of the mitral annulus. Studies have shown that the abscess or pseudoaneurysm associated with a mitral valve vegetation carries a worse prognosis as compared to patients without abscess.

40. *ANSWER: C.* There are vegetations on the right coronary cusp (RCC) and noncoronary cusp (NCC) of the aortic valve. There is severe prolapse of the RCC.

The midesophageal long-axis view of the aortic valve usually shows the RCC (anterior) and NCC (posterior) in patients with a tricuspid aortic valve. The two cusps are embedded by vegetations. There is severe prolapse of the RCC. Color-flow imaging shows that the posterior aortic regurgitant jet arises from the base of the NCC, which is consistent with a perforation.

41. ANSWER: B. Vegetations of the aortic valve are frequently associated with aortic root abscesses. The abscess erodes the aortic root wall and eventually ruptures. This results in a communication with other chambers. If the abscess has communication with the aortic lumen, it is called a pseudoaneurysm. If the abscess has communication with two chambers, it is then called a fistula. As illustrated by the color-flow imaging, there is a diastolic flow from the right coronary sinus of Valsalva (at 7 o'clock) to the right atrium (the flow is above the tricuspid valve). This flow results from a fistula between these two chambers.

42. ANSWER: A. Based on the 2D image, the severe prolapse of the RCC of the aortic valve leads to a severe coaptation defect, resulting in severe valvular insufficiency even if there is no other color-flow imaging or Doppler interrogation.

43. ANSWER: A. In the setting of the severe aortic regurgitation, PW Doppler usually shows diastolic flow reversal in the descending aorta (3+) and in the abdominal aorta (4+). To obtain an adequate tracing, the Doppler beam must be as parallel as possible to the aorta. The diastolic flow is considered significant if it is >20 cm/sec at the end of diastole. Some authors suggest 40 cm/sec as a cutoff threshold, which increases the specificity but decreases the sensitivity.

KEY POINTS:

- Endocarditis can cause valvular regurgitation by different mechanisms including leaflet erosion, leaflet retraction, flail leaflet, and perforation of the leaflet.
- Leaflet perforation should be suspected when the origin of the regurgitant jet is located away from the site of leaflet coaptation.
- Perivalvular complications, including abscess and fistula formation, are more common in aortic valve endocarditis.

44. ANSWER: D. Vegetations are not detected on either the anterior or posterior mitral valve leaflet. An aneurysm is seen on the posterior mitral valve leaflet. Color-flow imaging shows systolic flow traversing the aneurysm into the LA, consistent with perforation at the base of the aneurysm.

An aneurysm of the mitral valve leaflet is usually a rare condition. Its incidence has been reported as low as 0.29%. It is almost always associated with IE, but rare cases can occur in patients with connective tissue disease without endocarditis. It is mostly located on the AMVL, which is frequently impinged on by the aortic regurgitant jet. The size of the aneurysm varies—as large as 30 mm has been reported. Perforation of the aneurysm can occur and is the main mechanism of the mitral regurgitation.

45. ANSWER: B. In the setting of a mitral valve aneurysm, a satellite lesion should be sought after. The mass attached to the lateral wall of the LV is most likely a vegetation, which is probably "seeded" from the mitral valve vegetation.

KEY POINTS:

- Endocarditis is the most common cause of valvular diverticula or aneurysms.
- Leaflet perforation frequently coexists with valvular diverticula or aneurysms.
- Satellite vegetations should be sought along the path of the "infected" flow jet.

46. ANSWER: A. After complete resolution of endocarditis, most affected valves remain abnormal in structure and in function. The valve leaflet can appear thickened, retracted, perforated, or flail. It is not unusual that a vegetation becomes calcified and persists over time on the affected valve.

47. ANSWER: B. The mitral leaflet appears normal, but color-flow imaging shows a perforation at the lateral scallop (A1) of the AMVL.

The regurgitant jet does not originate from the coaptation site but rather from the leaflet suggesting a perforation. The perforation is not well seen on the 2D imaging. Based on the jet size with color-flow imaging, the mitral regurgitation is significant. No mitral valve cleft is present.

48. ANSWER: B. The regurgitant jet is located at the A1 segment of the mitral leaflet.

The parasternal short-axis view with color-flow imaging clearly demonstrated that the jet is located laterally at the A1 scallop and is directed posteriorly.

KEY POINTS:

- The short-axis view of the mitral valve allows precise localization of the abnormality involving the individual scallop of the mitral leaflets responsible for the mitral regurgitation.
- Valvular dysfunction is common even after successful medical treatment of endocarditis.

49. ANSWER: B. There is a fistula at the posterior mitral valve annulus between the LV and LA.

The vegetation induces a cascade of structural complications including abscess, pseudoaneurysm, and fistula formation. The extension of necrosis forms an abscess. Drainage of the abscess into one chamber is called a pseudoaneurysm. A fistula is formed as a result of communication of abscess with two chambers. In this case, the mitral annular abscess leads to formation of a fistula between the LV and LA and causes paravalvular mitral regurgitation. Infrequently in patients with an annular abscess, the infection may respond to antibiotic therapy alone.

50. ANSWER: C. The dimension of the fistula on 2D images, the size of the color jet, and the mitral valve inflow E velocity suggest that there is severe paravalvular mitral regurgitation.

51. ANSWER: D. Systolic flow reversal in the pulmonary vein may not be present in the setting of severe mitral regurgitation when the LA is severely dilated or highly compliant, and when the regurgitant jet is highly eccentric and directed away from the pulmonary veins.

The systolic flow reversal in the pulmonary veins is highly indicative of severe mitral regurgitation but its absence does not exclude severe mitral regurgitation.

KEY POINTS:
- Perivalvular abscess is a dynamic process and can lead to long-term sequelae such as fistula and pseudoaneurysm formation.
- Color-flow imaging can demonstrate the path of the fistula.

52. ANSWER: C. There are vegetations on all three leaflets of the tricuspid valve. The anterior and the septal leaflets are retracted, causing a coaptation defect.

53. ANSWER: C. The lack of leaflet coaptation results in severe tricuspid regurgitation. The color-flow imaging is only confirmatory.

54. ANSWER: A. Systolic retrograde flow in the hepatic vein is demonstrated.

55. ANSWER: A. In this clinical setting, it is likely a vegetation. In many injection drug users, vegetations can be present on the left-sided valves and can be seen in unusual locations, such as in this patient. Tumor (myxoma or angiosarcoma) is less likely in this case.

KEY POINTS:
- Intravenous drug users are at risk to develop right-sided and left-sided endocarditis, although the presence of right-sided endocarditis strongly suggests intravenous drug use.
- Isolated right-sided endocarditis has a better prognosis compared with left-sided endocarditis.
- Vegetations in right-sided endocarditis are frequently large regardless of the etiologic agent.
- TTE is usually adequate to detect vegetations in right-sided endocarditis.

SUGGESTED READINGS

Bashore TM, Cabell C, Fowler V. Update on infective endocarditis. *Curr Probl Cardiol.* 2006;31:274–352.

Chan K. Early clinical course and long-term outcome of patients with infective endocarditis complicated by perivalvular abscess. *CMAJ.* 2002;167:19–24.

Erbel R, Liu F, Ge J, Rohmann S, et al. Identification of high-risk subgroups in infective endocarditis and the role of echocardiography. *Eur Heart J.* 1995;16:588–602.

Erbel R, Rohmann S, Drexler M, et al. Improved diagnostic of echocardiography in patients with infective endocarditis by transesophageal approach: a prospective study. *Eur Heart J.* 1988;9:43–53.

Hecht SR, Berger M. Right-sided endocarditis in intravenous drug users. Prognostic features in 102 episodes. *Ann Intern Med.* 1992;117:560–566.

Jaffe WM, Morgan DE, Pearlman AS, et al. Infective endocarditis, 1983–1988: echocardiographic findings and factors influencing morbidity and mortality. *JACC.* 1990;15:1227–1233.

Johnson C, Chan KL. Role of transthoracic and transesophageal echocardiography in the management of endocarditis. In: Chan KL, Embil JM, eds. *Endocarditis, Diagnosis and Management.* London: Springer: 2006:79–103.

Law A, Honos G, Huynh T. Negative predictive value of multiplane transesophageal echocardiography in the diagnosis of infective endocarditis. *Eur J Echocardiogr.* 2004;5:416–421.

Mugge A, Daniel WG, Frank G, et al. Echocardiography in infective endocarditis: reassessment of prognostic implications of vegetation size determined by the transthoracic and the transesophageal approach. *J Am Coll Cardiol.* 1989;14:631–638.

Reynolds HR, Jagen MA, Tunick PA, et al. Sensitivity of transthoracic versus transesophageal echocardiography for the detection of native valve vegetation in modern era. *JASE.* 2003;16:67–70.

Rohmann S, Erbel R, Darius H, et al. Prediction of rapid versus prolonged healing of infective endocarditis by monitoring vegetation size. *JASE.* 1991;4:465–474.

Sachdev M, Peterson GE, Jollis JG. Imaging techniques for diagnosis of infective endocarditis. *Cardiol Clin.* 2003;21:185–195.

San Roman SA, Vilacosta I, Sarria C, et al. Eustachian valve endocarditis: is it worth searching for? *Am Heart J.* 2001;142:1037–1040.

Stewart JA, Silimperi D, Harris P, et al. Echocardiographic documentation of vegetation lesions in infective endocarditis: clinical implications. *Circulation.* 1980;61:374–380.

Tingleff J, Egeblad H, Gotzsche C-O, et al. Perivalvular cavities in endocarditis: abscess versus pseudoaneurysm? A transesophageal Doppler echocardiographic study in 118 patients with endocarditis. *Am Heart J.* 1995;103:93–100.

Vilacosta I, San Roman JA, Sarria C, et al. Clinical, anatomic, and echocardiographic characteristic of aneurysms of the mitral valve. *AJC.* 1999;84:110–113.

Vuille C, Nidorf M, Weyman AE, et al. Natural history of vegetations during successful medical treatment of endocarditis. *Am Heart J.* 1994;128:1200–1209.

Cardiomyopathies

Marianela Areces and Craig R. Asher

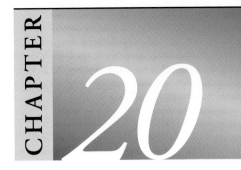

CHAPTER 20

1. Which statement regarding idiopathic dilated cardiomyopathy is correct?
   A. Segmental wall motion abnormalities are predictors of worse outcome in idiopathic dilated cardiomyopathy.
   B. Atrial dilatation is uncommon; biventricular dilatation is common.
   C. Improvement in sphericity index in response to dobutamine is a predictor of late recovery of left ventricular (LV) systolic function.
   D. The finding of significant coronary artery disease is common.
   E. Routine endomyocardial biopsy is recommended for adequate diagnosis.

2. A 48-year-old woman presents to the emergency department complaining of shortness of breath and recurrent palpitations. Initial electrocardiography (EKG) showed atrial flutter at a rate of 150 bpm with 2:1 atrioventricular conduction. A transthoracic echocardiogram is obtained and it revealed four-chamber dilatation and moderate to severe biventricular systolic dysfunction. Which of the following statements is correct regarding this patient's cardiomyopathy?
   A. This cardiomyopathy is most likely irreversible.
   B. The ventricular systolic dysfunction may be improved by radiofrequency ablation of the atrial flutter.
   C. Idiopathic dilated cardiomyopathy is not in the differential diagnosis in this patient.

   D. Electrical cardioversion is not helpful in these type of patients.

3. Which of the following statements is true about peripartum cardiomyopathy?
   A. If the patient's ejection fraction (EF) normalizes after the initial cardiomyopathy episode, there is no recurrence of LV systolic dysfunction in subsequent pregnancies.
   B. Up to 25% of patients have marked improvement in LV systolic function and clinical symptoms after the initial episode.
   C. Most women initially present with symptoms and echocardiographic abnormalities between 3 and 6 months postpartum.
   D. An elevated E/e' ratio is uncommon in these patients.
   E. Marked inotropic contractile reserve measured during dobutamine stress echocardiography may serve as a predictor of the likelihood of recurrence of cardiomyopathy with subsequent pregnancy.

4. A 49-year-old man comes in for an evaluation of syncopal episodes. As part of the initial evaluation, he had a 12-lead EKG that revealed complete atrioventricular block. A transthoracic echocardiogram showed an overall EF of 55% with thinning of the basal septum and moderate to severe mitral regurgitation (MR). Which of the following statements is true regarding this patient's condition?

A. The initial presentation is expected to be a dilated cardiomyopathy.

B. This patient's MR is likely to improve after a course of high-dose steroids.

C. The correct diagnosis is usually made by endomyocardial biopsy.

D. Other areas of the left ventricle (besides the basal septum) and right ventricle are rarely involved in this disorder.

5. A 52-year-old man presents for evaluation of dyspnea on exertion and lower extremity edema. He has a history of lymphoma and has completed chemotherapy treatment 5 months ago. He received a total cumulative lifetime dose of doxorubicin of 450 mg/m^2. Transthoracic echocardiogram reveals four-chamber dilatation and reduced LV systolic function. Which of the following statements regarding doxorubicin-induced cardiomyopathy is true?

A. The probability of developing doxorubicin-induced cardiomyopathy only increases after total cumulative doses of 600 mg/m^2 or more.

B. Inflammatory infiltrates are commonly seen in histological examination.

C. Doppler-derived diastolic parameters are sensitive measures to detect early onset doxorubicin-induced cardiomyopathy.

D. Patients with doxorubicin-induced cardiomyopathy have a better 4-year survival compared with patients with idiopathic dilated cardiomyopathy.

E. Echocardiographic-derived LV systolic parameters demonstrate abnormalities before LV diastolic parameters.

6. When differentiating athlete's heart from hypertensive LV hypertrophy (LVH), which echocardiographic parameter is most consistent with athlete's heart?

A. Reduced peak annular early diastolic filling velocity (e′)

B. Increased E/e′ ratio

C. Normal longitudinal strain and peak systolic strain rates

D. LV systolic dysfunction

7. Which of the following echocardiographic parameters has been demonstrated to be the best independent predictor of development of future congestive heart failure (CHF) symptoms?

A. Myocardial performance index (Tei Index)

B. Left ventricular ejection fraction (LVEF)

C. LV wall motion score

D. E/A ratio

E. Pulmonary artery pressure

8. Which of the following statements best describes the cardiac findings in patients with Friedreich's ataxia?

A. In patients with the asymmetric septal hypertrophy form, provocable LV outflow obstruction is consistently seen, similar to classical hypertrophic obstructive cardiomyopathy (HOCM).

B. Patients with the concentric hypertrophy form have a worse prognosis than patients with HOCM.

C. There is a direct relationship between the degree of neurologic involvement and the degree of cardiac abnormalities.

D. Prolonged isovolumic relaxation period, decreased E/A ratio, increased LV mass index, and normal LV cavity dimensions are initial echocardiographic findings in these patients.

E. Patients with global hypokinesis and the dilated cardiomyopathy form usually have the best prognosis of the three types of cardiac involvement.

9. Which of the following statements is correct regarding cardiac involvement in primary hemochromatosis?

A. Cardiac chamber dilatation is uncommon in this disease.

B. Iron deposition is consistent with an infiltrative cardiomyopathy.

C. Cardiac involvement leads to a restrictive filling pattern with severe increase in wall thickness and overall preserved LV systolic function.

D. With treatment, the cardiomyopathy may be reversible.

10. Based on echocardiographic criteria, which asymptomatic athlete should be allowed to participate in competitive sports without further testing?
    A. A 20-year-old American football player with an LVEF of 65%, left ventricular end-diastolic diameter (LVEDD) of 5.3 cm, septal wall thickness of 1.9 cm, posterior wall thickness of 1.3 cm, lateral e' (by tissue Doppler imaging) of 6 cm/sec.
    B. A 21-year-old basketball player with an LVEDD of 5.9 cm, left ventricular end-systolic diameter (LVESD) of 3.6 cm, septal wall thickness of 1.3 cm, posterior wall thickness of 1.3 cm, left atrial area of 22 cm², lateral e' (by tissue Doppler) of 18 cm/sec.
    C. A 26-year-old soccer player with an LVEF of 55%, LVEDD of 5.2 cm, right ventricular (RV) outflow tract measurement in diastole of 3.2 cm, RV apical hypokinesis.
    D. A 24-year-old basketball player with an LVEF of 60%, LVEDD of 5.3 cm, mitral valve prolapse with mild to moderate MR, aortic diameter at the sinuses of 4.2 cm, and at the ST junction of 4.1 cm.

11. Which of the following descriptions helps differentiate cardiomyopathy related to Duchenne muscular dystrophy from cardiomyopathy related to Becker muscular dystrophy?
    A. Four-chamber dilatation and LV systolic dysfunction.
    B. Mitral valve prolapse and MR.
    C. Predilection for involvement of the posterobasal and posterolateral LV walls.
    D. The severity of cardiac involvement does not correlate with the extent of skeletal muscle weakness.

12. A 32-year-old man presents to the emergency department with angina. Pertinent findings on the physical examination include an audible S4. As part of his cardiac evaluation, a transthoracic echocardiogram is obtained. It shows an apical thickness of 19 mm, interventricular septal thickness of 11 mm, and posterior wall thickness of 10 mm. Which of the following is most likely found in this patient?
    A. A normal 12-lead electrocardiogram.
    B. LV outflow tract (LVOT) peak velocity by continuous-wave Doppler of 1 m/sec after amyl nitrite administration.
    C. Systolic anterior motion of the mitral valve.
    D. A malignant clinical course.

13. Which of the following echocardiographic findings are consistent with noncompaction cardiomyopathy?
    A. Three layers should be identifiable: epicardial, myocardial, and endocardial layers with the endocardial layer representing the noncompacted region.
    B. The ratio of the noncompacted to compacted layers should be >1.5:1.
    C. The most commonly affected regions are the midventricular lateral, inferior, and anterior walls.
    D. Deep recesses filled with blood from the ventricular cavity should be seen by contrast echocardiography or color Doppler.

14. Which of the following measures of diastolic function is most likely found in a patient with restrictive cardiomyopathy?
    A. Propagation velocity V_p of 60 cm/sec.
    B. Peak early diastolic filling velocity of 115 cm/sec; tissue Doppler e' lateral velocity of 6 cm/sec.
    C. Mitral E deceleration time of 165 milliseconds.
    D. Mitral filling velocity ratio (E/A ratio) of 1.1.
    E. Pulmonary vein Doppler pattern: systolic velocity > diastolic velocity.

15. Which of the following serves as a predictor of mortality in patients with primary (AL) amyloidosis with cardiac involvement?
    A. LV end-diastolic dimension.
    B. LV wall thickness.
    C. Pericardial effusion.
    D. Increased myocardial echogenicity.

16. Based on Figure 20-1, which of the following statements is true about this patient's condition?

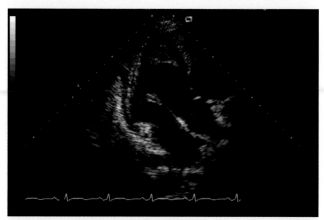

Fig. 20-1

A. The right ventricle is usually spared from this abnormality.
B. MR is an uncommon finding.
C. Eosinophil granule proteins could be responsible for the development of this disease.
D. LV systolic function is usually reduced.

17. A 44-year-old man presents for evaluation of worsening dyspnea and palpitations. He has a family history of sudden cardiac death in a male cousin. A transthoracic echocardiogram is obtained and is shown in Figure 20-2. EF is calculated at 65%. The

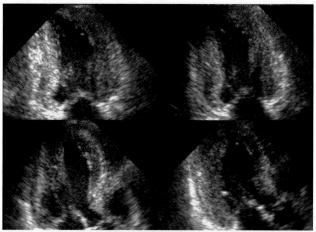

Fig. 20-2

Doppler analysis including tissue Doppler imaging revealed prolonged mitral early filling (E) deceleration time, reduced systolic and diastolic tissue Doppler velocities, and increased E/e' ratio. Which of the following parameters would indicate that enzyme replacement therapy may be beneficial in this patient?

A. Normal EF.
B. Increased LV septal wall thickness.
C. Increased echodensity and thickness of the subendocardial border.
D. Reduced tissue Doppler velocities and increased E/e' ratio.

18. Figure 20-3 is most consistent with which type of cardiomyopathy?

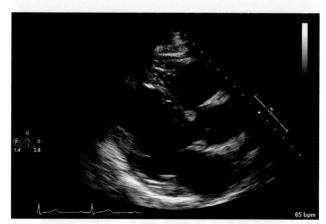

Fig. 20-3

A. Idiopathic restrictive.
B. Hemochromatosis.
C. Primary (AL) type amyloidosis.
D. Duchenne muscular dystrophy.

24. Which of the following statements is correct regarding the images shown in Figure 20-9 of two patients with hypertrophic cardiomyopathy (HCM)?

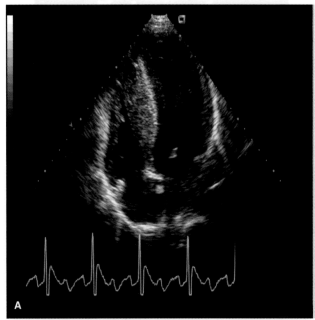

Fig. 20-9A

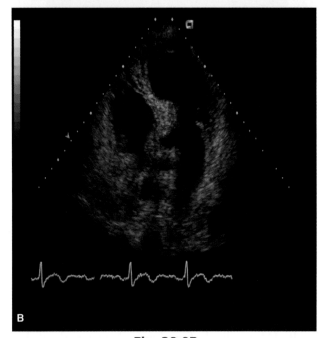

Fig. 20-9B

A. Figure 20-9B panel demonstrates reversed septal curvature that is typically seen in elderly patients with HCM.

B. Figure 20-9B demonstrates proximal septal hypertrophy (septal bulge) that is mostly seen in elderly patients and commonly associated with a sarcomeric mutation.

C. Figure 20-9A demonstrates severe asymmetric septal hypertrophy and is commonly associated with RV hypertrophy.

D. The elderly form of HCM as seen in Figure 20-9B is commonly associated with LVOT obstruction, symptoms, and sudden cardiac death.

25. A 79-year-old woman presents to the hospital with worsening shortness of breath. Physical examination reveals a dyspneic patient with a BP of 184/90 mm Hg and a heart rate of 82 bpm. She is afebrile with an O_2 saturation on room air of 93%. There are bilateral rales and a regular rhythm is present on auscultation. A transthoracic echocardiogram is obtained revealing normal ventricular size, normal right atrial size, and mild left atrial enlargement. Measurement include interventricular septum of 1.4 cm and posterior wall of 1.4 cm, and the myocardium and pericardium appear normal. The pulmonary artery pressure is estimated at 42 mm Hg. The calculated EF and wall motion are normal. There is trace mitral and tricuspid regurgitation. Doppler images are shown in Figure 20-10.

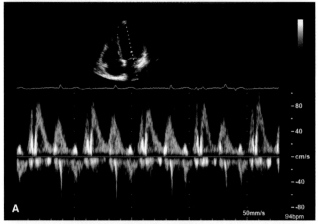

Fig. 20-10A

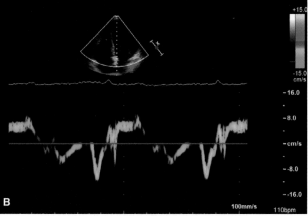

Fig. 20-10B

Which of the following is the most likely diagnosis?

A. Diastolic heart failure due to hypertension.
B. Diastolic heart failure due to amyloidosis.
C. Noncardiac pulmonary edema.
D. Diastolic heart failure due to an acute coronary syndrome.

CASE 1:

A 50-year-old man presents to the cardiology clinic for evaluation of progressive dyspnea on exertion. He has also been referred to the nephrology clinic as his basic laboratory work showed decreased glomerular filtration rate and proteinuria. A transthoracic echocardiogram is obtained as part of his initial evaluation and is shown in Figure 20-11 and Video 20-1.

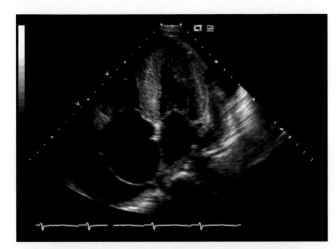

Fig. 20-11

26. Which of the following statements is true about this patient's condition?
    A. These patients usually have a normal EKG.
    B. There is severe biventricular hypertrophy.
    C. There is severe LVH.
    D. Atrioventricular valves are usually affected.
    E. An impaired relaxation pattern is expected.

27. Which of the following parameters has been shown to be useful in early detection of the disease?
    A. LV wall thickening.
    B. Strain and strain rate measurements.
    C. Pulmonary artery pressure.
    D. LV ejection fraction.

CASE 2:

A 72-year-old woman, with a history of hypertension presents to the emergency department complaining of substernal chest pain. Her 12-lead EKG shows ST elevations in the precordial leads. Initial troponin measurement was slightly elevated. She was taken emergently to the cardiac catheterization laboratory. Her cardiac catheterization showed minimal (30%) coronary artery stenosis in the right and circumflex coronary arteries. She underwent a transthoracic echocardiogram for further evaluation. (Fig. 20-12 and Videos 20-2A and B).

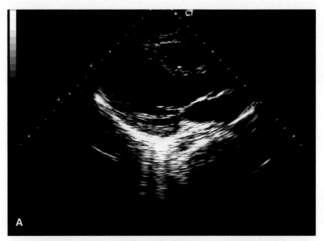

Fig. 20-12A

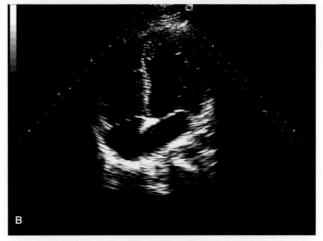

Fig. 20-12B

28. Based on the echocardiogram shown in Figure 20-12, which is the most likely diagnosis?
    A. Coronary spasm of the left anterior descending artery.
    B. Acute pericarditis.
    C. Acute myocarditis.
    D. Apical ballooning syndrome.

29. Which of these findings could also be found in this patient's echocardiogram?
   A. Normal diastolic function.
   B. Systolic anterior motion of the mitral valve.
   C. Hypokinesis of the basal segments.
   D. Wall motion abnormalities confined to one coronary artery distribution.

CASE 3:

A 24-year-old asymptomatic female patient presents to the cardiology clinic for evaluation. Her father has a history of HCM, which was diagnosed when he was 54 years old. He is status post–implantable cardioverter defibrillator placement for primary prevention. Cardiovascular examination in this patient was normal including no murmur at rest or after the Valsalva maneuver. Her EKG is normal. A transthoracic echocardiogram is obtained for further evaluation (Fig. 20-13 and Video 20-3).

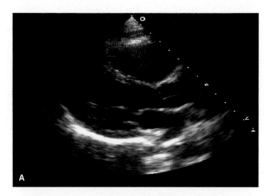

Fig. 20-13A

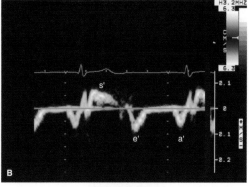

e' lateral-8 cm/s
a' lateral-5 cm/s
s' lateral-9 cm/s

Fig. 20-13B

30. Which of the following would be the best recommendation for this patient?
   A. It appears that the patient did not inherit the mutation from her father, as her LV wall thickness and systolic function are normal.

B. There are no signs in this echocardiogram to suggest that the patient could develop HCM in the future.
   C. She should obtain a repeat echocardiogram in 3–5 years.
   D. She should not undergo further testing unless symptoms develop.

31. Which of the following statements is correct regarding echocardiographic findings in HCM?
   A. There is delayed closure of the aortic valve.
   B. Continuous-wave Doppler through the LVOT has a characteristic early-peaking velocity profile.
   C. The duration of contact between the mitral leaflet and the septum during systole directly correlates with the magnitude of the LVOT pressure gradient.
   D. The left ventricular end diastolic dimension is usually increased.

CASE 4:

A 26-year-old woman presents to the office for evaluation of dyspnea on exertion and lower extremity edema. She has been told in the past that her "heart function is normal" but her symptoms continue to worsen. The EKG reveals an intraventricular conduction delay. As part of her evaluation, a transthoracic echocardiogram is ordered and is shown in Figure 20-14 and Videos 20-4A and B.

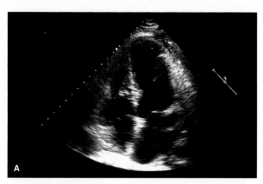

Fig. 20-14A

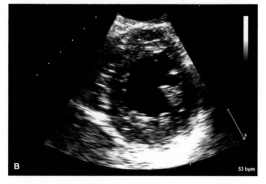

Fig. 20-14B

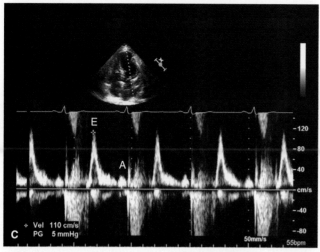

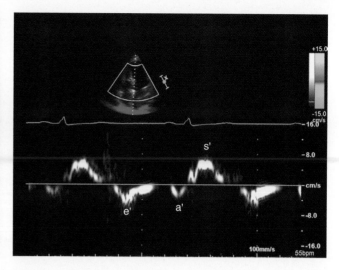

Measurements:

LVEDD-4.4 cm, LVESD-2.9 cm.
Mitral inflow deceleration time 120 ms, E/e' 22, and s' 6 cm/s.

Fig. 20-14C

32. Which is the most likely diagnosis in this patient?
    A. Idiopathic restrictive cardiomyopathy.
    B. Noncardiac etiology for her symptoms.
    C. Constrictive pericarditis.
    D. HCM, early stage.

33. Which of the following statements is correct regarding this patient's condition?
    A. Histology examination will show myocyte disarray.
    B. Atrial enlargement is uncommon.
    C. Marked diastolic dysfunction is the hallmark of this condition.
    D. Endomyocardial biopsy is necessary for diagnosis.
    E. LVEF is usually reduced.

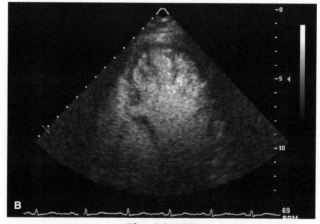

Fig. 20-15A

CASE 5:

A 42-year-old man presents for evaluation of dyspnea on exertion and palpitations worsening for the past year. His shortness of breath is now present with mild exertion and the patient denies chest pain. His EKG shows normal sinus rhythm and LBBB. A transthoracic echocardiogram is obtained for further evaluation (Fig. 20-15 and Videos 20-5A and B).

Fig. 20-15B

34. Which is the most likely diagnosis in this patient?
    A. Idiopathic dilated cardiomyopathy.
    B. HCM.
    C. LV noncompaction.
    D. Infiltrative cardiomyopathy with restrictive physiology.

35. Which of the following is true regarding this condition?
    A. The predominant segmental location of the abnormality is usually found in the midventricular and apical regions of both the inferior and lateral walls.
    B. These patients usually have a favorable prognosis.
    C. Contrast echocardiography offers little help in facilitating the diagnosis.
    D. RV involvement is common.
    E. LV systolic function is usually within normal limits on presentation.

ANSWERS

1. ANSWER: C. Improvement in left ventricular (LV) geometry as expressed by the sphericity index and improvement in LV contractile response to dobutamine predicted late recovery of LV function in idiopathic dilated cardiomyopathy, as demonstrated by several studies. The left ventricular sphericity index is the ratio of the long axis (apex to mitral annulus) to short axis dimension and represents the extent of chamber remodeling. Segmental wall motion abnormalities are present in up to 65% of patients with idiopathic dilated cardiomyopathy and actually predicted a more favorable prognosis than global hypokinesis. Four-chamber dilatation, including atrial and ventricular chamber dilatation, is present in idiopathic dilated cardiomyopathy. The coronary arteries are typically normal in autopsy studies. The routine use of ventricular endomyocardial biopsy is not recommended because of its low yield.

2. ANSWER: B. Tachycardia-induced cardiomyopathy is an often underrecognized, reversible dilated cardiomyopathy that occurs secondary to prolonged periods of supraventricular and ventricular tachycardia. The most important treatment goal is heart rate control. In this patient with atrial flutter, radiofrequency ablation could be potentially curative. Electrical cardioversion is the initial treatment option for heart rate/arrhythmia control in these patients. There are primary and secondary forms of tachycardia-induced cardiomyopathy, with the primary form occurring in otherwise normal subjects. The secondary form occurs in patients with underlying cardiac disease. An arrhythmia could be the initial presentation of any cardiomyopathy.

3. ANSWER: E. Peripartum cardiomyopathy is a disorder of uncertain etiology characterized by the development of heart failure symptoms during the last trimester of pregnancy or during the first 5 months postpartum in the absence of any other identifiable cause of heart failure, and an ejection fraction (EF) of <40%. Up to 50% of patients fully recover with normalization of EF and resolution of congestive heart failure (CHF) symptoms.

There is a significant rate of recurrence during subsequent pregnancies, most commonly in patients with persistent LV dysfunction, but there is also a chance of recurrence in patients with normalization of the left ventricular ejection fraction (LVEF). For those women having a recurrent pregnancy despite persistent cardiomyopathy, the risks of mortality and heart failure are high. Most women present with symptoms during the first month of the postpartum period. It is very common to have markedly elevated LV filling pressures, which would be demonstrated as an abnormally elevated E/e' ratio by echocardiography. It has been demonstrated in small series of patients who have recovered from peripartum cardiomyopathy that dobutamine stress echocardiography is a useful tool to predict the safety of a recurrent pregnancy. Those women who have recovery of function to normal and normal contractile reserve with dobutamine have a lower risk of recurrence.

4. ANSWER: B. This is a description of a patient with cardiac sarcoidosis. Although only approximately 5% of patients with sarcoidosis have apparent cardiac manifestations, nearly 50% of patients have confirmed disease at autopsy. The presence of conduction disease and a regional cardiomyopathy with preserved LV function suggests this disorder. With sarcoidosis, there is granulomatous infiltration of the myocardium and subsequent healing and scar formation in various areas that may manifest as segmental wall thinning, regional wall motion abnormalities, dilation of the left ventricle, and apical LV aneurysm formation in some cases. In addition, patients may have findings consistent with cor pulmonale. The mechanism for mitral regurgitation (MR) in this patient is likely due to granulomatous infiltration of the papillary muscles resulting in restriction of leaflet motion and may improve after a course of high-dose steroids. The systolic function may remain normal initially, progressing to systolic dysfunction later in the disease. Many other areas of the left ventricle besides the basal septum and also the right ventricle have been involved with cardiac sarcoidosis. Endomyocardial biopsy has a low sensitivity in detecting sarcoid granulomas and is not routinely performed to make the diagnosis. Gadolinium-enhanced cardiac magnetic resonance imaging is a useful tool for the diagnosis of cardiac sarcoidosis.

5. ANSWER: C. The incidence of doxorubicin-induced cardiomyopathy is closely related to the total lifetime cumulative dose that the patient receives. The probability of developing this cardiomyopathy greatly increases after cumulative doses above 400 to 500 mg/m². Characteristic changes in electron microscopy include vacuolar degeneration and then progressive myofibrillar loss; inflammatory infiltrates are not usually seen in this cardiomyopathy. Patients with doxorubicin-induced cardiomyopathy have a worse prognosis at 4 years compared with patients with idiopathic-dilated cardiomyopathy and ischemic cardiomyopathy.

Echocardiography is a very important tool in the follow-up of these patients and usually LVEF is used to help guide possible future doses. However, abnormalities in diastolic echocardiographic parameters usually precede systolic abnormalities and serve as a sensitive tool to detect early cases when the systolic parameters still remain normal.

6. ANSWER: C. In athlete's heart, most diastolic parameters including those obtained via tissue Doppler imaging are very similar to normal controls. Athletes have normal diastolic e' velocities and normal E/e' ratio consistent with normal LV filling pressures. Athletes most commonly have normal LV systolic function and they also have normal or exaggerated values when measuring systolic and diastolic strain/strain rate parameters, which are usually abnormal in hypertensive patients with LV hypertrophy (LVH). These strain parameters help differentiate an athlete's heart from a patient with hypertensive LVH.

7. ANSWER: A. The myocardial performance index (MPI or Tei index) is a measurement that incorporates both systolic and diastolic parameters and it is defined as the sum of the isovolumic contraction time and isovolumic relaxation time divided by the ejection time. This Doppler-derived index has been shown to closely correlate to $+dP/dt$ and $-dP/dt$ measurements directly obtained via cardiac catheterization. Other echocardiographic parameters such as LVEF, LV wall motion score, E/A ratio, and E deceleration time, also serve as predictors of future heart failure morbidity. MPI is believed to have strong independent predictive value due to the fact that MPI reflects both systolic and diastolic function.

8. ANSWER: D. Up to 90% of patients with Friedreich's ataxia may demonstrate various cardiac abnormalities. There are two types of cardiac involvement: the most common, the hypertrophic form that is subdivided into asymmetric septal hypertrophy and concentric LVH. The other type of cardiomyopathy is the dilated form with global hypokinesis. Abnormalities in diastolic parameters like isovolumic relaxation time (IVRT) and LV filling pattern may be the first signs of cardiac involvement in patients with this disease entity. Interestingly, in patients who develop the asymmetric septal hypertrophy form, a provocable significant left ventricular outflow tract (LVOT) gradient is rarely seen in contrast to patients with HOCM. Patients with the concentric hypertrophy form have a better prognosis than patients with HOCM. Patients who develop the dilated cardiomyopathy form have the worse prognosis. There is no relationship between the degree of neurologic and cardiac involvement.

9. ANSWER: D. Hemochromatosis is a form of iron-storage disease with deposition in various organs including the sarcoplasmic reticulum of myocardial cells in the heart. By the proposed American Heart Association (AHA) classification of cardiomyopathies, it is characterized as a secondary cardiomyopathy since it is part of a systemic disease. It is not an infiltrative disorder, and wall thickness is generally normal (Fig. 20-16 and Table 20-1). The atrium, ventricles, and atrioventricular conduction system may be involved. Cardiac involvement in hemochromatosis leads to cavity enlargement in approximately one-third of patients with normal wall thickness. The earliest form may manifest as a restrictive cardiomyopathy, although subsequently mixed or dilated forms may occur. As the disease progresses, there may be a decrease in LV systolic function, significant cavity dilation, and biatrial enlargement. Identification of cardiac hemochromatosis is important since treatment with chelating agents or phlebotomies may improve cardiac function.

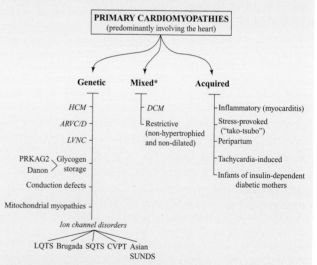

(Reprinted with permission from Maron BJ, Towbin JA, Thiene G, et al. Contemporary definitions and classification of the cardiomyopathies: an American Heart Association Scientific Statement from the Council on Clinical Cardiology, Heart Failure and Transplantation Committee Quality of Care and Outcomes Research and Functional Genomics and Translational Biology Interdisciplinary Working Groups and Council on Epidemiology and Prevention. *Circulation.* 2006;113:1807–1816.)

Fig. 20-16

TABLE 20-1 Secondary Cardiomyopathies

- Infiltrative
- Storage
- Toxicity
- Endomyocardial
- Endomyocardial fibrosis
- Hypereosinophilic syndrome (Löeffler endocarditis)
- Inflammatory (granulomatous)
- Cardiofacial
- Neuromuscular/neurological
- Nutritional deficiencies
- Autoimmune/collagen
- Electrolyte imbalance
- Consequence of cancer therapy

(*Adapted with permission from* Maron BJ, Towbin JA, Thiene G, et al. Contemporary definitions and classification of the cardiomyopathies an American Heart Association Scientific Statement from the Council on Clinical Cardiology, Heart Failure and Transplantation Committee Quality of Care and Outcomes Research and Functional Genomics and Translational Biology Interdisciplinary Working Groups and Council on Epidemiology and Prevention. *Circulation.* 2006;1131807–1816.)

10. ANSWER: B. In athlete's heart, there is usually an increase in LV cavity size (rarely beyond 6.0 cm); and in a small group of athletes, there may be a symmetric increase in wall thickness (between 1.2 and 1.5 cm—"the gray zone"). There is normal LV systolic and diastolic function. Mild atrial enlargement can be seen. Choice A is suggestive of hypertrophic cardiomyopathy (HCM). In HCM, there is often an asymmetric increase in LV wall thickness, typically >15 mm, and LV cavity size remains normal (Table 20-2).

Choice C is suggestive of arrhythmogenic RV dysplasia, and choice D could be consistent with a patient with Marfan syndrome.

11. ANSWER: C. In the cardiomyopathy related to Duchenne muscular dystrophy, there is usually predilection for involvement of the posterobasal and posterolateral walls. This is thought to be related to the increased stress that cardiac myocytes encounter in the posterior wall. In Becker muscular dystrophy cardiomyopathy, perfusion defects have been observed in the anterior and septal walls. Four-chamber dilatation, LV dysfunction, mitral valve prolapse, and MR are usually seen in both disease entities. The degree of cardiac involvement is not necessarily related to the degree of skeletal muscle weakness in both etiologies.

12. ANSWER: B. This patient presents with features consistent with apical HCM. Most commonly, these patients complain of angina or atypical chest pain between the ages of 20 and 59 years. Most patients have a characteristic pattern on their electrocardiography (EKG), showing "giant negative T waves" in the precordial leads. They typically do not present with systolic anterior motion (SAM) of the mitral valve or LV

TABLE 20-2 Typical Echocardiographic Features of Athlete's Heart Versus Hypertrophic Cardiomyopathy

	Athlete's Heart	HCM
LVIDd	Normal or ↑ (<6.0 cm)	↓ or normal
LV wall thickness	Normal or ↑ (≤15 mm)	↑ (≥15 mm)
IVS/LVIDd	<0.48	≥0.48
LV mass	↑	↑
LV mass index (g/m^2)	Normal or ↑	↑
LVEF	Normal	Normal or ↑
RVIDd	Normal or ↑	Normal
RV wall thickness	Normal	Normal or ↑
LA size	Normal or ↑	Normal or ↑
RA size	Normal or ↑	Normal
Diastolic function	Normal	Abnormal
e' annular (TDI)	>9 cm/sec	<9 cm/sec
Systolic annular (TDI)	>9 cm/sec	<9 cm/sec
Longitudinal strain	>20%	<20%

LVIDd, left ventricular internal dimension in diastole; LV, left ventricular; IVS, interventricular septum; PW, posterior wall; LVEF, left ventricular ejection fraction; RVIDd, right ventricular internal dimension in diastole; RV, right ventricular; LA, left atrial; RA, right atrial; TDI, tissue Doppler imaging.

outflow obstruction either at rest or after provocative maneuvers. They usually have a more benign clinical course, especially when compared to the classic patients with HCM, although atrial fibrillation and stroke are not uncommon.

13. ANSWER: D. Noncompaction cardiomyopathy may occur as an isolated cardiomyopathy when no associated congenital abnormalities are present. It is classified as a primary genetic cardiomyopathy according to the AHA proposed classification scheme (Fig. 20-16). It results from a failure of the normal embryologic process of compaction of myocardial fibers in the endocardial layer. Various echocardiographic and cardiac magnetic resonance imaging criteria have been proposed. The criteria by Oechslin et al. require that (1) the ratio of noncompacted to compacted layer is ≥2; (2) there are prominent and excessive trabeculations; and (3) deep recesses are present that fill with blood from the LV cavity as seen by color Doppler (or contrast echocardiography). The most commonly involved region of noncompaction is the apex followed by the midventricular lateral, inferior, and anterior walls.

14. ANSWER: B. In restrictive cardiomyopathy, the main abnormality is diastolic dysfunction that is usually advanced. The LV filling pressure is usually elevated. LV systolic function is usually preserved, and LV size is usually normal. Choice B describes a patient with rapid transmitral early filling, decreased mitral annular tissue Doppler velocities, and an E/e' ratio of >15 suggestive of elevated LV filling pressures. The other choices describe normal diastolic function parameters.

15. *ANSWER: B.* Amyloid cardiomyopathy is the most common infiltrative cardiomyopathy and it has been reported to account for 10% of all nonischemic cardiomyopathies. There is abnormal deposition of fibrils of various precursor proteins, which lead to this restrictive cardiomyopathy. A direct relationship between LV wall thickness and mortality has been established with worsening survival as LV thickness increases above 15 mm. There is also a correlation between increased LV wall thickness and the occurrence of heart failure symptoms. Diastolic parameters such as decreased deceleration time, increased transmitral inflow velocity ratio (E/A ratio), and an elevated Tei index are also strong predictors of survival. Other prognostic echocardiographic variables include LV dysfunction and RV enlargement. LV cavity size usually remains normal and does not give significant prognostic information. The finding of a pericardial effusion is common and is usually not clinically significant. One of the distinguishing features of cardiac amyloid infiltration is the increased echogenicity and "speckled" appearance of the LV wall on 2D echocardiography; however, this finding does not offer specific prognostic information.

16. *ANSWER: C.* This echocardiographic image is from a patient with endomyocardial fibrosis. This disorder is a restrictive cardiomyopathy and it is characterized by marked endocardial fibrotic thickening of the apex and subvalvular regions of one or both ventricles. Classically, two variants of this disease have been described: tropical endomyocardial fibrosis and hypereosinophilic (Loffler's) endomyocardial fibrosis. There is debate on whether these are distinct disease entities. The tropical variant is not related to hypereosinophilia, and dietary and environmental factors are thought to be responsible. In hypereosinophilic endomyocardial fibrosis, the intracytoplasmic granular content of the eosinophil is considered to cause toxic endomyocardial damage. Both variants usually present very similarly in echocardiography and obliteration of the apex by thrombus/fibrosis is characteristic. LV systolic function is usually preserved and biatrial enlargement is typical. There is involvement of the right ventricle in up to 50% of cases. The fibrosis also typically involves the subvalvular regions and papillary muscles making mitral and tricuspid regurgitation a common finding.

17. *ANSWER: C.* This echocardiogram is from a patient diagnosed with Fabry's cardiomyopathy. Fabry's disease is an X-linked lysosomal enzyme deficiency (alpha-galactosidase A) that results in progressive intracellular glycosphingolipid accumulation affecting various organs including the heart. Characteristic features of cardiac involvement include progressive LVH, preserved LV systolic function, normal LV dimensions, impaired diastolic function, abnormal tissue Doppler parameters, and MR. All these features could also be found in HCM, thus Fabry's cardiomyopathy can be misdiagnosed as HCM. Correct diagnosis is very important as enzyme replacement therapy in patients with Fabry's disease has proven to reduce glycosphingolipid accumulation and improve cardiac function.

One characteristic that has been suggested to differentiate Fabry's cardiomyopathy from HCM is a binary appearance of the LV wall by 2D echocardiography. There is increased thickness and echodensity in the subendocardial layer representing the glycosphingolipid-rich layer, paralleled by a less affected myocardial middle layer.

18. *ANSWER: D.* This echocardiogram depicts thinning of the basal posterior wall. This is a more typical presentation of Duchenne cardiomyopathy. In the cardiomyopathy related to Duchenne muscular dystrophy, there is usually predilection for involvement of the posterobasal and posterolateral walls. This is thought to be related to the increased stress that cardiac myocytes encounter in the posterior wall. The other cardiomyopathies listed do not usually result in segmental thinning. However, there are other diseases with cardiac involvement not listed where similar findings may occur including sarcoidosis, Fabry's disease, and coronary artery disease.

19. *ANSWER: B.* This is a case of arrhythmogenic RV dysplasia, which is a myocardial disease characterized by fibrofatty ventricular replacement and ventricular arrhythmias. This patient presents with syncope, an abnormal EKG, and frequent ventricular ectopy. He has a family history of sudden cardiac death. Transthoracic echocardiograms are likely to show RV dilatation with global or regional systolic dysfunction, with instances of localized RV aneurysms (as seen in this patient) or diastolic sacculations. This is one of the major criteria for the diagnosis of this disease. The left ventricle is often involved as well with up to 75% of cases having some degree of LV fibrofatty replacement. Sports activity increases the risk of sudden death up to fivefold. The development of heart failure symptoms is not a guide for treatment as many young patients present with sudden cardiac death as their initial manifestation without previous symptoms. Ventricular tachycardia arises from the right ventricle and therefore is typically of LBBB morphology with a superior axis. See Table 20-3.

TABLE 20-3 Typical Echocardiographic Features of RV Cardiomyopathy

- RV cavity dilation (rest or stress)
- RV outflow tract dilation (in isolation or associated with cavity dilation)
- RV dysfunction (rest or stress)
- RV regional abnormalities
- Prominent trabeculations/moderator band hypertrophy
- Aneurysms (systolic) in the "triangle of dysplasia"
- Sacculations (diastolic) outpouchings in the "triangle of dysplasia"

Triangle of dysplasia consists of the basal right ventricular inflow, right ventricular outflow segment, and apex.

20. *ANSWER: A.* This patient has HCM with asymmetric septal hypertrophy and LVOT obstruction. The LVOT gradient appears to be close to 60 mm Hg, derived from the Bernoulli equation using peak LVOT velocity at 3.8 m/sec. Choice B is incorrect as it is measuring the peak velocity of the MR jet, not the LVOT jet. The MR jet can be distinguished as higher velocity, with a rapid increase in velocity starting at the onset of ventricular contraction. It also extends beyond aortic valve closure. The LVOT profile is characterized by a dagger shape with a late systolic peak velocity. Diastolic dysfunction parameters are initial markers of this disease even before the appearance of hypertrophy. Therefore, diastolic dysfunction would be seen in this patient. With SAM of the mitral valve and LVOT obstruction, premature closure of the aortic valve is expected.

21. *ANSWER: D.* This echocardiogram is from a patient diagnosed with familial (TTR) amyloidosis. There are several subtypes of amyloidosis differing in the types of proteins that are deposited in different organs. Table 20-4 illustrates their similarities and differences.

The most common type in the United States is the AL type or primary amyloidosis. Cardiac involvement is common in this subtype and prognosis is usually poor on presentation. Secondary or AA subtype, is characterized by tissue deposition of protein A and cardiac involvement (and CHF) is actually rare. Familial or TTR amyloidosis is usually an autosomal dominant disorder with frequent cardiac involvement. The SSA or senile systemic amyloidosis is not uncommon in patients older than 80 years of age and usually has a good prognosis but is manifested by recurrent heart failure symptoms.

22. *ANSWER: C.* This is the case of a patient with a dilated cardiomyopathy. Transthoracic echocardiogram shows four-chamber dilatation, normal wall thickness, increased LV volumes, and a decreased EF (calculated to be 23%). There are several possible etiologies that could explain this patient's findings. In general, dilated cardiomyopathy is considered to be a common and usually irreversible form of myocardial disease. It is the most frequent cause of cardiac transplantation worldwide. Dilated cardiomyopathy can be secondary to infectious agents, particularly viral (coxsackievirus, adenovirus, parvovirus, HIV), but also bacterial and parasitic. A myocarditis can develop often preceding the development of the dilated cardiomyopathy. Other causes include toxins, alcohol, and chemotherapeutic agents. Another common etiology is genetic mutations and up to 20%–35% of these cases have been reported as familial. An additional group of patients are reported to have idiopathic dilated cardiomyopathy. Medical therapy with angiotensin-converting enzyme inhibitors and beta-blockers has been proven beneficial with improvement in EF and prognosis.

23. *ANSWER: C.* Hypertrophic cardiomyopathy is a genetically determined cardiac disorder that is defined by a hypertrophied, nondilated ventricle in the absence of another disease capable of producing the degree of hypertrophy noted (i.e., hypertension, aortic stenosis). LV systolic function is usually normal or hyperdynamic. Asymmetric hypertrophy affecting the interventricular

TABLE 20-4 Four Common Subtypes of Amyloidosis

Type	Protein	Cardiac Involvement	Other Organs	Prognosis	Major Cardiac Manifestation
AL (1°)	Immunoglobulin light chain	Common	Liver, kidney, GI tract, skin, CNS	Poor	CHF, bradyarrhythmias, AF
AA (2°)	Nonimmunoglobulin	Rare	Kidney, liver, spleen	Variable	Rare
TTR (familial)	Transthyretin (mutant)	Common	CNS, liver	Variable	CHF
SSA (senile)	Transthyretin (wild-type)	Common	Uncommon	Good	CHF, AF

GI, gastrointestinal; CNS, central nervous system; CHF, congestive heart failure; AF, atrial fibrillation; SSA, senile systemic amyloidosis.

septum is the most common form. However, asymmetry can affect any region including the apex, lateral, posterior, or inferior walls. A pattern of concentric hypertrophy occurs less often. About 25% of patients have a resting gradient between the LVOT and the aorta at rest. Mitral regurgitation is seen in most patients with LVOT obstruction. The LVOT gradient is nearly always associated with a forward movement of the anterior mitral valve leaflet or SAM. The severity of this outflow tract gradient correlates with the time of onset and duration of contact between the mitral valve and the septum. This creates the midsystolic deceleration in the aortic flow profile that coincides with mitral valve-septal contact.

24. ANSWER: C. Figure 20-9A is consistent with a young patient and Figure 20-9B is consistent with an older patient with HCM. There are age-related differences seen in patients with HCM. Young patients typically have asymmetric hypertrophy involving the septum with reversed septal curvature and RV hypertrophy. Reversed septal curvature means that the shape of the LV cavity is crescent shaped with the hypertrophy convex toward the LV cavity. Elderly patients more often have a localized proximal septal hypertrophy that is due in part to geometric changes in the heart with aging. The LV cavity is ovoid shaped, the septal curvature is normal (concave toward the cavity), and RV hypertrophy is not present (Fig. 20-17). The elderly form of HCM is associated with a sarcomeric mutation

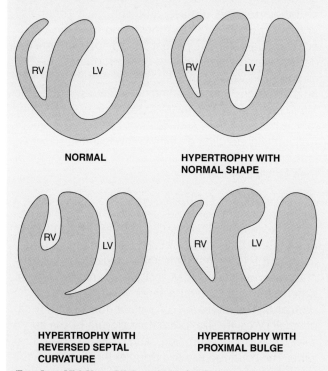

NORMAL

HYPERTROPHY WITH NORMAL SHAPE

HYPERTROPHY WITH REVERSED SEPTAL CURVATURE

HYPERTROPHY WITH PROXIMAL BULGE

(From Lever HM, Karam RF, Currie PJ, Healy BP. Hypertrophic cardiomyopathy in the elderly: distinctions from the young based on cardiac shape. *Circulation.* 1989;79:580–589. With permission of Lippincott Williams & Wilkins.)

Fig. 20-17

in approximately 8% of patients. Most patients present with symptoms due to LVOT obstruction, although sudden cardiac death is uncommon.

25. ANSWER: A. This elderly female patient is presenting with diastolic heart failure due to accelerated hypertension. Diastolic heart failure is characterized by (1) clinical manifestations of heart failure; (2) normal or near normal LV function; and (3) diastolic dysfunction with evidence of elevated filling pressures, compliance, or relaxation abnormalities. In this patient the E/e' is approximately 20 consistent with a high filling pressure and there is pseudonormal mitral filling with a relaxation abnormality evident on tissue Doppler imaging of the mitral annulus. Common etiologies include hypertension, diabetes, coronary artery disease, and advanced age. There should be no evidence of pericardial and valvular etiologies of heart failure. Amyloidosis is unlikely given normal cavity dimensions including only mild left atrial enlargement. In addition, in most patients with amyloidosis, the BP normalizes and pulmonary artery pressures are >50 mm Hg. An acute coronary syndrome is excluded because of normal wall motion.

26. ANSWER: D. This patient has cardiac primary (AL type) amyloidosis with cardiac and renal involvement. (See answer to question 15 for further details.) In cardiac amyloid, there is infiltration of the heart by various proteins (including the ventricles, atria, atrioventricular valves, and interatrial septum). The atrioventricular valves appear thickened when infiltrated by amyloid particles. A thickened interatrial septum (from amyloid infiltration) is less common but a specific finding for cardiac amyloid. The increased wall thickening is not due to hypertrophy in primary (AL type) amyloidosis but rather infiltration. If there is uncertainty about the diagnosis, the findings should be described as increased wall thickness and a differential diagnosis should be provided on the basis of the available echocardiographic, electrocardiographic, and clinical data.

The prognosis in these patients is usually poor, especially after they present with CHF symptoms. Median survival after diagnosis is 1 year, but only 6 months after onset of CHF symptoms. Their EKGs are frequently abnormal classically showing low voltage that is out of proportion to the degree of ventricular wall thickening ("mass voltage mismatch"). They can also show a pseudoinfarct pattern and atrial fibrillation among other abnormalities. This is a secondary restrictive cardiomyopathy (Table 20-1); therefore, diastolic parameters are mostly abnormal. In the early stage of the disease, an impaired relaxation abnormality may be present; but once heart failure has occurred, a more advanced stage of diastolic impairment is expected.

27. ANSWER: B. The evaluation and diagnosis of cardiac amyloid by conventional echocardiographic methods usually detect amyloid-related abnormalities once the disease is in a more advanced stage. The early detection of amyloid deposition is very important as initiating therapy early on before the development of overt heart failure is beneficial to the patient. The use of tissue Doppler imaging and strain rate imaging has been proven successful in identifying early abnormalities in diastolic and systolic function even in the absence of ventricular wall thickening.

KEY POINTS:

■ Amyloid cardiomyopathy is the most common infiltrative cardiomyopathy, which leads to a restrictive cardiomyopathy. The classic findings include, increased LV and RV wall thickness, a "speckled" or "sparkling granular" appearance by echocardiography (most notably without harmonic imaging), thickening of the atrioventricular valves and atrial septum, biatrial dilation, pulmonary hypertension, and advanced stages of diastolic dysfunction. These points distinguish this condition from hypertensive heart disease.

■ Tissue Doppler and strain imaging can be used to detect early cardiac involvement even when LV systolic function and LV wall thickness are normal.

28. ANSWER: D. This elderly woman presented with chest pain, EKG abnormalities with ST elevation, and positive cardiac enzymes. The initial working diagnosis has to be ST segment elevation myocardial infarction (STEMI), which would be more common in this hypertensive, postmenopausal female patient. However, her cardiac catheterization did not reveal significant obstructive coronary artery disease, spasm, or ruptured plaque. The transthoracic echocardiogram reveals LV dysfunction with severe hypokinesis of the mid and apical ventricular segments and hyperdynamic basal segments. This syndrome characteristically affects postmenopausal females usually after an episode of acute emotional or physiologic stress. In most cases, LV systolic dysfunction and regional abnormalities are transient due to catecholamine release and patients completely recover after days or weeks. The clinical syndrome described is not consistent with coronary spasm, acute pericarditis, or acute myocarditis.

29. ANSWER: B. Typical echocardiographic findings in ABS (also called stress cardiomyopathy or Takotsubo cardiomyopathy) include marked LV systolic dysfunction with reduced EF. The mid to apical segments of all regions have severe hypokinesis, akinesis, or dyskinesis, with preserved or hyperdynamic basal segment function. These hyperdynamic basal segments can lead to SAM of the mitral valve and significant MR. Diastolic function parameters usually reveal diastolic impairment.

One of the distinguishing features between ABS and acute STEMI is that the regional dysfunction in ABS extends beyond the distribution of a single epicardial coronary artery.

KEY POINTS:

■ ABS usually affects postmenopausal females and results in transient LV dysfunction. Patients present with chest pain, ST elevation on their EKGs, abnormal cardiac enzymes, and show no obstructive coronary artery disease.

■ ABS has a characteristic segmental dysfunction of the LV, with mid and apical akinesis or dyskinesis extending beyond a single epicardial coronary artery territory.

■ Due to hyperkinetic basal segments, SAM of the mitral valve and MR may occur.

■ The LV systolic dysfunction usually normalizes within days or weeks.

30. ANSWER: C. This young, asymptomatic patient with a family history of HCM presents for a screening evaluation. The 2D transthoracic echocardiogram reveals normal LV size and systolic function with normal wall thickness. However, her tissue Doppler imaging reveals decreased systolic annular velocities (s') as well as decreased early and late diastolic mitral annular velocities (e', a'). These tissue Doppler parameters have been shown to identify subjects that have a genetic mutation for the disease, but still have otherwise normal structure, wall thickness, and function by 2D echocardiography. The patient should not wait until the development of symptoms to obtain further evaluation as advanced disease may already be present. The recommendations for screening in adult asymptomatic family members of patients with HCM are with transthoracic echocardiogram and EKG every 3–5 years or more frequently depending on activity levels of the screened individual, age of onset, and severity of the disease in their family members.

31. ANSWER: C. There is a direct correlation between the time of onset and duration of the contact between the mitral leaflet and the interventricular septum and the degree of LVOT obstruction as measured by the LVOT gradient. Other typical echocardiographic findings in HCM include asymmetric septal hypertrophy (septum to posterior wall ratio of ≥1.3:1), normal or hyperdynamic LV systolic function, normal or small LV cavity size, premature closure of the aortic valve, diastolic dysfunction, and SAM of the mitral valve. The continuous-wave Doppler through the LVOT has a characteristic late-peaking, "dagger-shaped" velocity profile.

KEY POINTS:

- Familial HCM is an autosomal dominant disease caused by a variety of mutant genes encoding for cardiac sarcomeric components. Patients harboring the genetic defect do not necessarily show the hallmark echocardiographic and clinical markers for the disease, especially early in the course of the disease.

- Tissue Doppler velocities serve an accurate method for identifying subjects with the mutations independent of LVH (phenotype negative, genotype positive individuals).

- Typical echocardiographic features of HCM are asymmetric septal hypertrophy, SAM of the mitral valve, early aortic valve closure, LVOT obstruction with characteristic late-peaking, "dagger-shaped" velocity profile, and diastolic dysfunction. LV size and function are usually normal.

32. *ANSWER: A.* This case description is consistent with an idiopathic restrictive cardiomyopathy. In this type of cardiomyopathy, patients present with heart failure symptoms like dyspnea and lower extremity edema and may have several EKG abnormalities. Mean age at presentation is usually between 20 and 30 years. Echocardiographically, there is normal LV size and systolic function, characteristic biatrial enlargement, and the primary abnormality is advanced diastolic dysfunction as seen in this case. Most notably, the wall thickness in this form of primary restrictive cardiomyopathy is usually normal or mildly increased. The mitral inflow velocities show rapid early filling of the LV with a short deceleration time, E/A >2, low systolic and diastolic mitral annular velocities, and an elevated E/e' ratio of >15—all consistent with a restrictive filling pattern or advanced diastolic dysfunction and elevated LV filling pressures.

33. *ANSWER: C.* The hallmark of restrictive cardiomyopathies is advanced diastolic dysfunction. Diastolic function parameters in this patient reveal a restrictive filling pattern consistent with advanced diastolic dysfunction including an abnormality of relaxation. Tissue Doppler velocities, particularly the e' velocity help differentiate restrictive cardiomyopathy from constrictive pericarditis. In the latter, normal mitral annular tissue velocities (e' >8 cm/sec) would be expected. Histology will reveal marked interstitial fibrosis; myocyte disarray is not seen in these cases as seen in HCM. As mentioned above, biatrial enlargement is common together with a normal-sized left ventricle with normal LVEF. Idiopathic restrictive cardiomyopathy is usually a diagnosis of exclusion after other etiologies for restrictive cardiomyopathy, which include cardiac amyloidosis hemochromatosis, sarcoidosis, endomyocardial fibrosis,

and pericardial disease. Endomyocardial biopsy is helpful in this regard, although not absolutely required.

KEY POINTS:

- Idiopathic restrictive cardiomyopathy is characterized by abnormal diastolic function with elevated ventricular filling pressures; normal LV internal dimensions; and absence of pericardial, endomyocardial disease, and infiltrative cardiomyopathy.

- Typical echocardiographic findings include normal LV size and systolic function, normal or mildly increased wall thickness, biatrial enlargement, advanced diastolic dysfunction parameters with a restrictive filling pattern, and evidence of elevated LV filling pressures.

34. *ANSWER: C.* The clinical presentation and echocardiographic images demonstrate LV noncompaction cardiomyopathy. This disorder is characterized by the presence of deep intertrabecular recesses with communication with the LV cavity and prominent trabeculations in the noncompacted myocardium. The noncompacted myocardium is hypokinetic and consists of a thick noncompacted endocardial layer and a thin compacted epicardial layer and with a ratio of ≥2. The other choices are incorrect diagnoses.

35. *ANSWER: A.* In ventricular noncompaction cardiomyopathy, the predominant location of the hypokinetic noncompacted segments is in the mid and apical ventricular segments, most commonly of the inferior and lateral LV walls. These patients usually have a poor prognosis with the usual cause of death being sudden cardiac death or heart failure. Common arrhythmias include atrial fibrillation and ventricular tachyarrhythmias. Thromboembolic events are common in these patients and the recommendation is for anticoagulation. Contrast echocardiography is a valuable tool in the delineation of the noncompacted, hypokinetic segments. LV systolic dysfunction is common, with a reported mean EF of 33% in a cohort of patients with this condition.

KEY POINTS:

- Left ventricular noncompaction is characterized by the presence of deep intertrabecular recesses, prominent trabeculations in hypertrophied and hypokinetic segments of the left ventricle. These segments consist of a thick noncompacted endocardial layer and a thin compact epicardial layer (≥2).

- The common presentation is heart failure symptoms, arrhythmias, and thromboembolic events. The prognosis is poor.

SUGGESTED READINGS

Arnlov J, Ingelsson E, Riserus U, et al. Myocardial performance index, a Doppler-derived index of global left ventricular function, predicts congestive heart failure in elderly men. *Eur Heart J.* 2004;25:2220–2225.

Asher CR, Lever HM. Echocardiographic profiles of diseases associated with sudden cardiac death in young athletes. In: Williams RA, ed. *The Athlete and Heart Disease: Diagnosis, Evaluation and Management.* Philadelphia: Lippincott Williams & Wilkins; 1999:155–172.

Bart BA, Shaw LK, McCants CB Jr, et al. Clinical determinants of mortality in patients with angiographically diagnosed ischemic or nonischemic cardiomyopathy. *J Am Coll Cardiol.* 1997;30:1002–1008.

Basso C, Corrado D, Marcus FI, et al. Arrhythmogenic right ventricular cardiomyopathy. *Lancet.* 2009;373:1289–1300.

Dorbala S, Brozena S, Zeb S, et al. Risk stratification of women with peripartum cardiomyopathy at initial presentation: a dobutamine stress echocardiography study. *J Am Soc Echocardiogr.* 2005;18:45–48.

Eriksson MJ, Sonnenberg B, Woo A, et al. Long-term outcome in patients with apical hypertrophic cardiomyopathy. *J Am Coll Cardiol.* 2002;39:638–645.

Felker GM, Thompson RE, Hare JM, et al. Underlying causes and long-term survival in patients with initially unexplained cardiomyopathy. *N Engl J Med.* 2000;342:1077–1084.

Gianni M, Dentali F, Grandi AM, et al. Apical ballooning syndrome or takotsubo cardiomyopathy: a systematic review. *Eur Heart J.* 2006;27:1523–1529.

Hyodo E, Hozumi T, Takemoto Y, et al. Early detection of cardiac involvement in patients with sarcoidosis by a non-invasive method with ultrasonic tissue characterization. *Heart.* 2004;90:1275–1280.

Jenni R, Oechslin EN, van der Loo B. Isolated ventricular noncompaction of the myocardium in adults. *Heart.* 2007;93:11–15.

Lever HM, Karam RF, Currie PJ, et al. Hypertrophic cardiomyopathy in the elderly: distinctions from the young based on cardiac shape. *Circulation.* 1989;79:580–589.

Lindqvist P, Olofsson BO, Backman C, et al. Pulsed tissue Doppler and strain imaging discloses early signs of infiltrative cardiac disease: a study on patients with familial amyloidotic polyneuropathy. *Eur J Echocardiogr.* 2006;7:22–30.

Marron BJ, Seidman JG, Seidman CE. Proposal for contemporary screening strategies in families with hypertrophic cardiomyopathy. *J Am Coll Cardiol.* 2004;44:2125–2132.

Maron BJ, Towbin JA, Thiene G, et al. Contemporary definitions and classification of the cardiomyopathies. an American Heart Association Scientific Statement from the Council on Clinical Cardiology, Heart Failure and Transplantation Committee Quality of Care and Outcomes Research and Functional Genomics and Translational Biology Interdisciplinary Working Groups and Council on Epidemiology and Prevention. *Circulation.* 2006;113:1807–1816.

Maron BJ, Zipes DP. The 36th Bethesda Conference, eligibility recommendations for competitive athletes with cardiovascular abnormalities. *J Am Coll Cardiol.* 2005;45:1318–1345.

Mason JW, O'Connell JB. Clinical merit of endomyocardial biopsy. *Circulation.* 1989;79:971–979.

Nagueh SF, Bachinski LL, Meyer D, et al. Tissue Doppler imaging consistently detects myocardial abnormalities in patients with hypertrophic cardiomyopathy and provides a novel means for an early diagnosis before and independently of hypertrophy. *Circulation.* 2001;104:128–130.

Naqvi TZ, Goel RK, Forrester JS, et al. Myocardial contractile reserve on dobutamine echocardiography predicts late spontaneous improvement in cardiac function in patients with recent onset idiopathic dilated cardiomyopathy. *J Am Coll Cardiol.* 1999;34:1537–1544.

Oechslin EN, Attenhofer Jost CH, Rojas JR, et al. Long-term follow-up of 34 adults with isolated left ventricular noncompaction: a distinct cardiomyopathy with poor prognosis. *J Am Coll Cardiol.* 2000;36:493–500.

Pereira NL, Dec GW. Restrictive and infiltrative cardiomyopathies. In: Crawford MH et al, eds. *Cardiology.* 2nd ed. Philadelphia: Mosby and Elsevier Limited. 2004:983–992.

Pieroni M, Chimenti C, De Cobelli F, et al. Fabry's disease cardiomyopathy, echocardiographic detection of endomyocardial glycosphingolipid compartmentalization. *J Am Coll Cardiol.* 2006;47:1663–1671.

Saghir M, Areces M, Makan M. Strain rate imaging differentiates hypertensive cardiac hypertrophy from physiologic cardiac hypertrophy (athlete's heart). *J Am Soc Echocardiogr.* 2007;20:151–157.

Sallach JA, Klein AL. Tissue Doppler imaging in the evaluation of patients with cardiac amyloidosis. *Curr Opin Cardiol.* 2004;19:464–471.

Schmitt K, Tulzer G, Merl M, et al. Early detection of doxorubicin and daunorubicin cardiotoxicity by echocardiography: diastolic vs. systolic parameters. *Eur J Pediatr.* 1995;154:201–204.

Sokol L, Vincelj J, Saric M. Echocardiographic assessment of diagnosis and prognosis of biopsy-proven amyloid cardiomyopathy. *Med Arh.* 2005;59:388–390.

Wynne J, Braunwald E. The cardiomyopathies and myocarditides. In: Zipes DP et al, eds. *Braunwalds's Heart Disease: A Textbook of Cardiovascular Medicine.* 7th. ed. Philadelphia: Elsevier Saunders. 2005:1751–1806.

Systemic Disease

Imran S. Syed, Charles J. Bruce, and Heidi M. Connolly

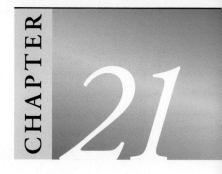

1. A 56-year-old homeless man with a body mass index of 17 kg/m^2 and recently diagnosed cardiomyopathy undergoes echocardiography. The following Doppler variables are obtained. Left ventricular outflow tract time velocity integral (LVOT TVI) = 36 cm; aortic valve TVI = 40 cm; LVOT diameter = 2.2 cm, heart rate = 86 bpm, body surface area = 1.9 m^2. No significant valvular heart disease is identified. Which nutritional deficiency is most likely?
   A. Selenium deficiency.
   B. Thiamine deficiency.
   C. Carnitine deficiency.
   D. Folate deficiency.
   E. Vitamin B$_{12}$ deficiency.

2. Cardiac involvement in hereditary hemochromatosis typically manifests as:
   A. Dilated left ventricle and systolic dysfunction.
   B. Increased left ventricular (LV) wall thickness.
   C. Regional wall motion abnormalities.
   D. Pulmonary hypertension.
   E. Pericardial effusion.

3. Which of the following nutritional deficiencies is associated with development of a dilated cardiomyopathy?
   A. Vitamin B$_{12}$.
   B. Selenium.
   C. Folic acid.
   D. L-lysine.

4. In chronic Chagas disease, echocardiography may demonstrate:
   A. Cardiac granulomas.
   B. Intracavitary cystic lesions.
   C. An apical aneurysm.
   D. Libman-Sacks endocarditis.

5. A 22-year-old man presents with 1 week of increasing shortness of breath associated with bilateral lower extremity swelling. Three months ago he underwent treatment of Hodgkin's lymphoma. The mitral inflow wave E and mitral annular e' velocities are 110 cm/sec and 3 cm/sec, respectively. There are no significant valvular abnormalities. A small circumferential pericardial effusion is present. The most likely explanation for these findings is:
   A. Noncardiac etiology.
   B. Severe anemia.
   C. Early doxorubicin cardiotoxicity.
   D. Radiation-induced heart disease.

6. A 15-year-old boy with severe ataxia is referred for an echocardiogram. Which of the following constellation of echocardiographic findings is most characteristic of Friedreich ataxia?
   A. Dilated cardiomyopathy.
   B. Severe LV hypertrophy mimicking hypertrophic cardiomyopathy.
   C. Normal LV dimensions, preserved LV systolic function with isolated severe diastolic dysfunction.
   D. Regional wall motion abnormalities in a noncoronary distribution.

7. A patient with longstanding poorly controlled hypertension and chronic renal failure on maintenance hemodialysis undergoes an echocardiogram. LV size and systolic function are normal. There is increased concentric wall thickening. There is severe left atrial enlargement. The E/A ratio is 2.0, and the E/e′ ratio is 25. The aortic and mitral valves are thickened and calcified and associated with moderate aortic, mitral, and tricuspid regurgitation. There is severe mitral annular calcification. The right ventricular (RV) systolic pressure is 60 mm Hg. A small pericardial effusion is present. Which of the following tests should be reviewed at the time of the echocardiogram to exclude cardiac involvement with amyloid?
A. Complete blood cell count.
B. Serum creatinine level.
C. Serum brain natriuretic peptide.
D. Chest X-ray.
E. Electrocardiogram (ECG).

8. Which of the following echocardiographic findings is most likely to be encountered in a patient with Wegener granulomatosis?
A. Regional wall motion abnormalities not confined to a specific coronary artery territory.
B. Concentric increased wall thickness and restrictive physiology consistent with an infiltrative cardiomyopathy.
C. Aortic cusp perforation with severe aortic regurgitation.
D. Large pericardial effusion with cardiac tamponade.

9. Reduced systolic function with normal LV dimension is noted on a transthoracic echocardiogram. Which of the following conditions that can cause reduction in ejection fraction is most often associated with normal LV cavity dimension?
A. Amyloidosis.
B. Sarcoidosis.
C. Hemochromatosis.
D. Human immunodeficiency virus (HIV).
E. Excess alcohol.

10. A 45-year-old man with symptoms of heart failure is referred for a transthoracic echocardiogram. Which of the following echocardiographic features suggests that the heart failure may be related to sarcoidosis?
A. LV dysfunction with apical dyskinesis and preserved basal cardiac function.
B. Enlarged left ventricle with hypokinesis involving the anterior ventricular septum and inferior lateral wall.
C. Normal LV cavity size with increased LV wall thickness and LVOT obstruction.
D. Right atrial and ventricular enlargement with reduced systolic function and normal left ventricular systolic function.

11. A 20-year-old Caucasian woman presents with findings of progressive dyspnea and edema 3 weeks after delivering twins. During pregnancy and at the follow-up visit, the blood pressure was approximately 100 mm Hg systolic. An echocardiogram demonstrates mild LV enlargement with severe reduction in global systolic function. Which of the patient's clinical characteristics is a risk factor for her cardiovascular condition?
A. Age.
B. First pregnancy.
C. Race.
D. Twin pregnancy.
E. Blood pressure.

12. A 45-year-old woman presents with dyspnea. She has a remote history of Hodgkin's lymphoma and received mantle radiation many years ago. An echocardiogram is requested. Which of the following echocardiographic findings would suggest radiation-related cardiovascular disease in this patient?
A. LV hypertrophy.
B. Multivalve thickening and regurgitation.
C. Ascending aortic dilatation.
D. Pericardial effusion.

13. Which of the following is a typical cardiovascular manifestation of HIV disease?
A. Atrial myxoma.
B. Hypertrophic cardiomyopathy.
C. Pericardial effusion.
D. Rhabdomyoma.

14. A 60-year-old woman has a history of labile hypertension. She complains of a severe headache, diaphoresis, central chest pain, and profound shortness of breath, lasting 20 minutes, shortly after total abdominal hysterectomy. The blood pressure is 130/85 mm Hg in the right arm and 140/90 mm Hg in the left arm. Additional findings are a fourth heart sound and bibasilar crackles.

The chest X-ray demonstrates pulmonary edema. The ECG demonstrates sinus tachycardia, LV hypertrophy, and widespread ST segment depression. An echocardiogram demonstrates akinesis of the mid and apical LV segments. The LV ejection fraction is 25%. A coronary angiography is performed and is normal. The most likely explanation for these findings is:

A. Coronary artery vasospasm.

B. Coronary artery thromboembolism.

C. Pheochromocytoma.

D. Cushing syndrome.

15. A 61-year-old woman has longstanding rheumatoid arthritis and is referred for an echocardiogram to evaluate dyspnea. Which of the following echocardiographic features is a manifestation of rheumatoid cardiac involvement?

A. Bileaflet mitral valve prolapse with mitral regurgitation.

B. Thickened and fixed tricuspid valve leaflets with tricuspid regurgitation.

C. Pericardial effusion with tamponade physiology.

D. Regional wall motion abnormalities and diastolic dysfunction.

16. A 67-year-old woman with no prior history of cardiac disease presents with severe chest pain and dyspnea over the past 24 hours. Initial ECG demonstrates ST elevation in the anterior precordial leads and she is taken emergently to the cardiac catheterization laboratory. Coronary angiography demonstrates only mild epicardial coronary artery disease. Echocardiography is performed and representative end-diastolic and end-systolic four-chamber images are shown in Figure 21-1.

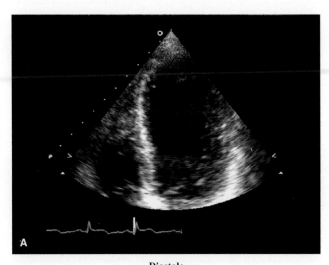

Diastole

Fig. 21-1A

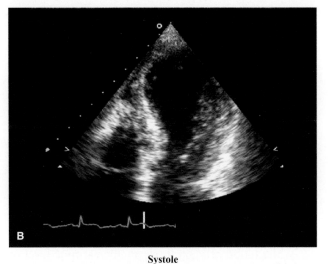

Systole

Fig. 21-1B

Which of the following may be present in this patient?

A. Persistent LV systolic dysfunction at 1 year.

B. Dynamic LVOT obstruction.

C. Markedly increased cardiac biomarkers.

D. Increased urinary 5-hydroxyindole acetic acid.

17. A 66-year-old woman who appears younger than her stated age presents with complaints of dyspnea, arthralgias, and swelling of her hands and feet. Echocardiography is performed and a short-axis view is provided in Figure 21-2.

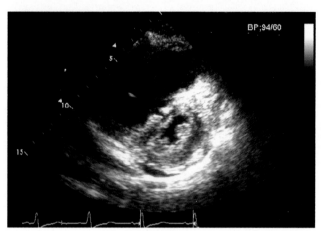

Fig. 21-2

What is the most likely diagnosis?
A. Cardiac amyloidosis.
B. Scleroderma.
C. Hemochromatosis.
D. Rheumatoid arthritis.

18. A transesophageal echocardiogram (TEE) is obtained in a 29-year-old woman who presents with symptoms of arthralgias, low-grade fever, chest pain, skin rash, and photosensitivity. There is no history of illicit drug use. Chest X-ray demonstrates small bilateral pleural effusions. Initial laboratory tests demonstrate a mildly elevated white blood cell count, elevated creatinine level of 1.5 mg/dl, and an elevated erythrocyte sedimentation rate of 45 mm/hr. Based on the TEE image (120 degrees) shown in Figure 21-3, the most likely diagnosis is:
A. Ergot-alkaloid use.
B. Infective endocarditis.
C. Libman-Sacks endocarditis.
D. Rheumatic mitral valve disease.

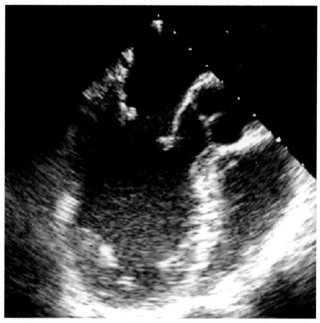

Fig. 21-3

19. A 20-year-old man is being evaluated for palpitations. The physical examination is unremarkable except for red skin lesions involving the groin. The ECG demonstrates LV hypertrophy and the echocardiogram demonstrates increased concentric wall thickness measuring 18 mm. The skin lesions are shown in Figure 21-4.

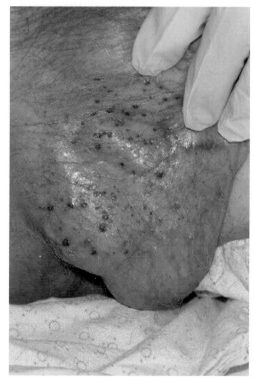

Fig. 21-4

Which of the following conditions most likely accounts for the echocardiographic findings in this patient?

A. Acromegaly.

B. Amyloid.

→ C. Fabry disease.

D. Hypertrophic cardiomyopathy.

---

20. A 1-year-old boy has a history of seizures. His mother remembers that a prenatal echocardiogram was abnormal, but she was reassured and told that follow-up echocardiography was all that was needed. He is an active child and has no cardiovascular symptoms. The physical examination is unremarkable except for the skin lesion shown (Fig. 21-5A). A transthoracic echocardiogram is obtained (Fig. 21-5B). Which statement below describes the best course of management for this patient?

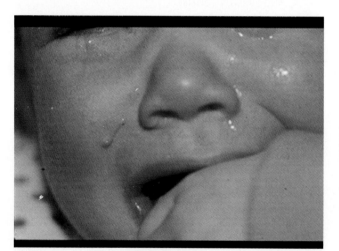

Fig. 21-5A

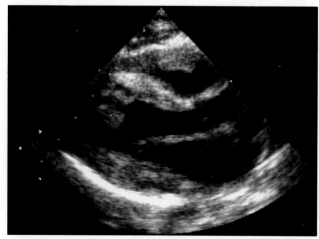

Fig. 21-5B

A. Reassurance and follow-up echocardiography is recommended in 1 year.

B. Whole body computed tomography is indicated to identify the primary tumor.

C. Prognosis is poor and thus surgical resection is not recommended.

D. Surgical resection is indicated now to prevent further growth and potential damage to sensitive cardiac structures.

---

21. A 23-year-old man is sent for an echocardiogram because of a widened mediastinum appreciated on chest X-ray performed during a routine pre-employment physical examination. He has a history of lens dislocation as a child. His grandfather died suddenly of unknown cause. The pertinent echocardiographic images are shown in Figure 21-6.

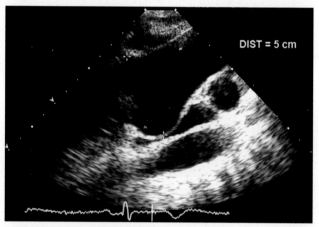

DIST = 5 cm

High parasternal long axis view

Fig. 21-6

Which of the following is the best course of action?

A. TEE to better evaluate the aorta and aortic valve.

B. Cardiac surgical consultation for elective aortic root replacement.

C. Treatment with beta-blockers, avoid heavy lifting, and reassessment in 6 months.

D. Treatment with losartan, avoid heavy lifting, and reassessment in 1 year.

22. A 29-year-old Asian woman is referred to echocardiography for assessment of fatigue and a murmur noted on physical examination. Pertinent features on physical examination include inability to measure a blood pressure in the left arm, a left carotid and subclavian bruit, and a long decrescendo diastolic murmur. An abdominal bruit is also noted.

Laboratory testing is remarkable for mild normocytic anemia and increased erythrocyte sedimentation rate and C-reactive protein. An echocardiogram is obtained. The ascending aorta is dilated measuring 45 mm at the mid-ascending level; the sinus dimension is normal. Other pertinent images are demonstrated in Figure 21-7.

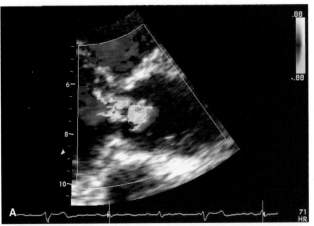

Parasternal long axis with color-Doppler and zoom of the aortic valve

Fig. 21-7A

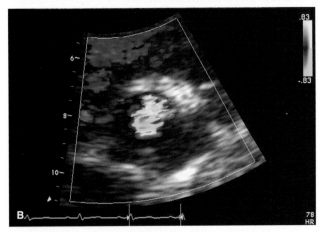

Parasternal short axis with color Doppler and zoom of the aortic valve

Fig. 21-7B

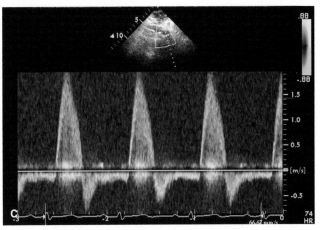

Pulsed wave Doppler from abdominal aorta

Fig. 21-7C

Which of the following diagnoses is most likely in this patient?
A. Marfan syndrome.
B. Takayasu arteritis.
C. Familial thoracic aortic aneurysmal disease.
D. Ankylosing spondylitis.

23. A patient with a diagnosis of metastatic carcinoid presents to the echocardiographic laboratory for evaluation. She has features of right heart enlargement with associated dysfunction and tricuspid valve regurgitation. Additional echo-Doppler images of the RV outflow tract are obtained.

What do the echo-Doppler images in Figure 21-8 demonstrate?

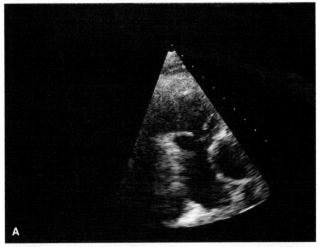

Fig. 21-8A

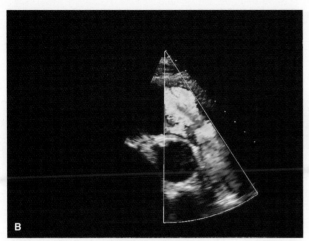
Fig. 21-8B

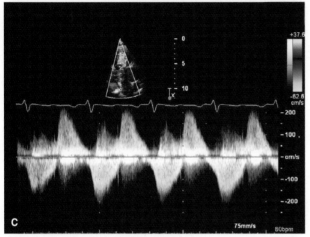
Fig. 21-8C

A. Severe pulmonary valve regurgitation.
B. Severe pulmonary valve stenosis.
C. Severe pulmonary hypertension.
D. Patent ductus arteriosus.

24. A patient with a history of flushing, diarrhea, and weight loss presents for echocardiographic evaluation. The finding in Figure 21-9 is noted (see arrow).

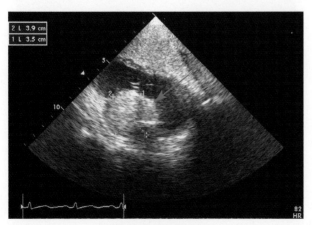
Subcostal long axis view
Fig. 21-9

What is the most likely cause of this finding?
A. Extra-adrenal catecholamine-secreting paraganglioma (extra-adrenal pheochromocytoma).
B. Thrombus.
C. Metastatic carcinoid.
D. Coronary artery aneurysm.

25. The LV M-mode, mitral inflow pulsed wave (PW) Doppler, mitral annulus tissue Doppler, and hepatic vein Doppler in Figure 21-10 were obtained in a 56-year-old man with prior history of non-Hodgkin's disease and radiation therapy. What radiation-associated complication is present?
A. Pericardial effusion.
B. Constrictive pericarditis.
C. LV hypertrophy.
D. Restrictive cardiomyopathy.

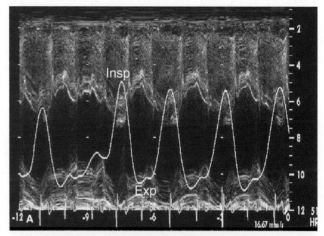
M-mode of the left ventricle with respirometer
Fig. 21-10A

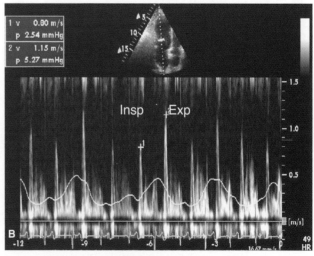
Mitral inflow pulse wave Doppler with respirometer
Fig. 21-10B

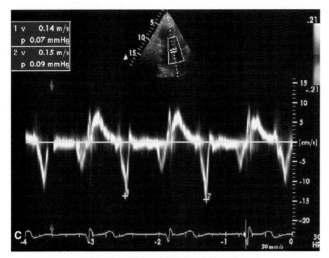

Mitral medial annulus tissue Doppler
Fig. 21-10C

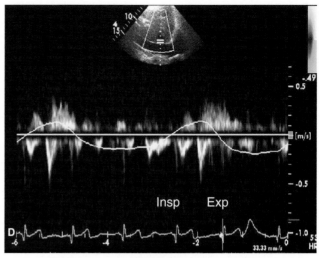

Hepatic vein pulse wave Doppler with respirometer
Fig. 21-10D

CASE 1:

A 54-year-old man presents with progressive dyspnea. Physical examination is consistent with congestive heart failure and also reveals an apical III/VI holosystolic murmur. ECG demonstrates sinus tachycardia and no other abnormalities. Echocardiography is performed without and with the aid of contrast. See Videos 21-1A and B of the four-chamber view without and with contrast and Figure 21-11 of the mitral inflow PW Doppler.

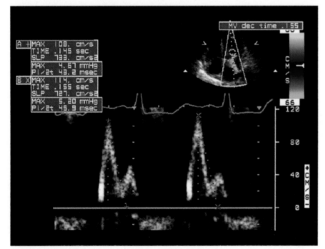

Fig. 21-11

26. What is the most likely diagnosis?
    A. Apical hypertrophic cardiomyopathy.
    B. Gaucher disease.
    C. Fabry disease.
    D. Eosinophilic endomyocardial disease.

27. Which of the following is typically associated with this condition?
    A. Aortic regurgitation.
    B. Isolated LV involvement.
    C. LVOT obstruction.
    D. Restrictive cardiomyopathy.

CASE 2:

A 72-year-old woman with chest pain and ST elevation on ECG undergoes coronary angiography that demonstrates minimal coronary atherosclerosis. Left ventriculography is performed and an end-systolic frame is shown in Figure 21-12.

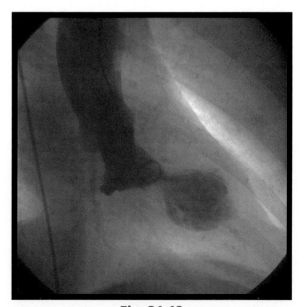

Fig. 21-12

The patient is transferred to the ICU where she becomes hypotensive and develops a systolic heart murmur. Urgent echocardiography is performed.

28. Based on the echocardiographic images in Videos 21-2A and B, the cause of hypotension is:
   A. Papillary muscle rupture.
   B. LVOT obstruction.
   C. Ventricular septal defect.
   D. Acute severe aortic regurgitation.

29. What is the most appropriate course of action?
   A. Dobutamine.
   B. Phenylephrine, cautious beta-blockade, and fluid administration.
   C. Urgent surgery for papillary muscle repair.
   D. Percutaneous closure with an Amplatzer occluder device.

CASE 3:

A 68-year-old man who is an ex-competitive cyclist presents with gradually progressive dyspnea and lightheadedness. ECG demonstrates small Q waves in the inferior leads and normal voltages. Initial laboratory evaluations including blood count and serum chemistries are normal. Echocardiography is performed (see Videos 21-3A and B and Fig. 21-13).

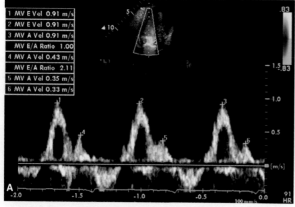

Mitral inflow pulsed wave Doppler
Fig. 21-13A

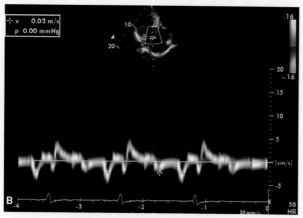

Mitral medial annulus tissue Doppler
Fig. 21-13B

30. What is the most likely diagnosis?
   A. Cardiac amyloidosis.
   B. Hypertrophic cardiomyopathy.
   C. Athlete's heart.
   D. Hypertensive heart disease.
   E. Hemochromatosis.

31. Which of the following is most helpful in distinguishing this diagnosis from other causes of increased LV wall thickness?
   A. Restrictive filling physiology.
   B. Systolic anterior motion of the mitral apparatus.
   C. Normal e′ velocity.
   D. Inverse relationship between LV mass and ECG voltage.

CASE 4:

A 46-year-old woman presents to her physician with lightheadedness and presyncope for 2 days on a background of increasing shortness of breath with exertion for 1 month. The examination is notable for jugular venous distention, soft heart sounds, and bilateral non–pitting pedal edema. The ECG demonstrates sinus bradycardia and low-voltage QRS complexes.

An echocardiogram is obtained and the pertinent 2D images are shown in Videos 21-4A–C. The mitral annular e′ velocity is 80 cm/sec.

32. The most likely explanation for the constellation of findings in this patient is:
   A. Breast cancer.
   B. Cardiac amyloid.
   C. Hypothyroidism.
   D. Renal failure.
   E. Systemic lupus erythematosus.

33. The next best course of action is:
   A. Observation until a specific etiology is identified and treat underlying disorder.
   B. Nonsteroidal anti-inflammatories.
   C. High-dose oral steroids.
   D. Echocardiographic-guided pericardiocentesis.

34. With appropriate therapy, which of the following echocardiographic parameters would most likely decrease?
   A. Isovolumic contraction interval.
   B. LVOT time-velocity integral.
   C. Mitral annular diastolic velocity.
   D. Mitral annular systolic velocity.

CASE 5:

A 50-year-old man is admitted with palpitations, dyspnea, recurrent syncope, and transient left arm weakness. The physical examination is remarkable for a bounding pulse, cyanosis, and clubbing. A computed tomography scan of the head is normal. A TEE is performed and agitated saline is administered via a left antecubital vein. A Valsalva maneuver is not performed. Representative transesophageal images are shown in Videos 21-5A–C.

35. The most likely explanation for the echocardiographic findings is:
    A. Persistent left superior vena cava.
    B. Intrapulmonary shunt.
    C. Patent foramen ovale.
    D. Sinus venosus atrial septal defect.

36. The best treatment for this condition is:
    A. Liver transplantation.
    B. Percutaneous closure.
    C. Surgical closure.
    D. Warfarin anticoagulation.

CASE 6:

A 25-year-old woman with a history of bilateral adrenalectomy for Cushing syndrome undergoes a transthoracic echocardiogram for palpitations and shortness of breath. The physical examination is unremarkable except for pigmented lip lesions. The lip lesions are shown in Figure 21-14, and representative echocardiographic images are shown in Videos 21-6A and B.

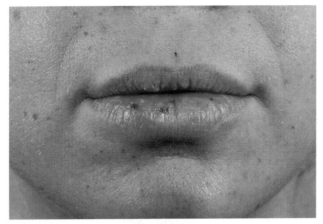

Fig. 21-14

37. The most likely diagnosis of the abnormality seen on the echocardiogram is:
    A. Angiosarcoma.
    B. Fungal endocarditis.
    C. Myxoma.
    D. Renal cell carcinoma.
    E. Thrombus.

38. The patient undergoes surgical exploration and removal of the mass. The postoperative course is uneventful and the patient is asymptomatic. An echocardiogram is performed 3 months postoperatively; four-chamber and RV images are demonstrated in Videos 21-7A–C.

    The most likely explanation for the finding shown in the follow-up echocardiogram is:
    A. CAT (calcified amorphous tumor).
    B. Metastatic disease.
    C. Recurrent thrombus.
    D. Synchronous lesion missed at the time of the first surgery.

CASE 7:

A 52-year-old woman is referred to the echocardiographic laboratory for further evaluation of symptoms of fatigue, exertional dyspnea, and lower extremity edema.

She had her appendix removed many years ago and was told that there was a tumor in the appendix. No additional information is available.

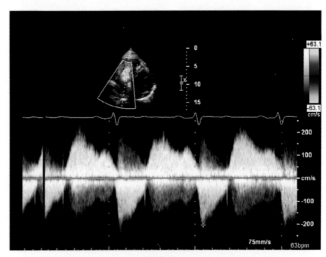

Tricuspid valve continuous wave Doppler signal
Fig. 21-15

39. Based on the echocardiographic images in Figure 21-15 and Videos 21-8A and B, what is the cause of this patient's symptoms?

A. Carcinoid heart disease.

B. Arrhythmogenic RV dysplasia.

C. Drug-related valve disease.

D. Ebstein's anomaly.

40. Which of the following tests would help confirm the suspected clinical diagnosis?
    A. Serum angiotensin-converting enzyme (ACE) level.
    B. Subcutaneous fat aspirate.
    C. Complete blood cell count with differential white blood cell count and smear.
    D. Urinary 5-hydroxyindole acetic acid.

CASE 8:

A 40-year-old woman with fatigue and dyspnea has a systolic and diastolic murmur on examination. Her past history is remarkable for two miscarriages and a remote history of deep venous thrombosis. She is undergoing evaluation including echocardiography (see Video 21-9A–C).

41. Which of the following statements about the color-flow Doppler imaging in patients with aortic valve regurgitation is correct?
    A. The color-flow Doppler scale alters the subjective assessment of regurgitation.
    B. Measurement of vena contracta should not be used to assess the degree of regurgitation in the presence of both aortic and mitral regurgitation.
    C. Normal LV chamber dimension excludes severe aortic regurgitation.
    D. Echocardiographic contrast aids in the assessment of aortic regurgitation severity.

42. Based on the clinical and echocardiographic features shown, which of the following is the most likely diagnosis?
    A. Rheumatic heart disease.
    B. Radiation-related valve disease.
    C. Drug-related valve disease.
    D. Antiphospholipid antibody syndrome.

ANSWERS

1. ANSWER: B. Selenium, thiamine, and carnitine deficiency are all associated with development of a reversible cardiomyopathy that responds to repletion of the deficient vitamin/mineral. Folate and B_{12} deficiency are not usually associated with cardiomyopathy. Thiamine deficiency or beriberi is usually seen in alcoholic patients with poor nutrition and produces a clinical syndrome that is characterized by high-output cardiac failure. Selenium deficiency, also called Keshan disease, is usually seen in patients undergoing total parenteral nutrition or in patients from areas where food is grown in selenium-deficient soil and results in cardiac enlargement and systolic heart failure. Carnitine deficiency may be primary due to a genetic defect or secondary as a result of total parenteral nutrition or liver or renal disease. Carnitine is required for normal energy metabolism and contractile function in the heart and its deficiency can result in systolic impairment.

The description of a homeless man with a low body mass index and cardiomyopathy is suspicious for nutritional deficiency as a potential etiology. The Doppler variables shown in this question can be used to calculate the cardiac output and index. Cardiac output = Stroke volume (cross-sectional area × left ventricular outflow tract time velocity integral [LVOT TVI]) × heart rate = 3.14 × (LVOT diameter)^2/4 × 36 × 86 = 11.8 l/min. Cardiac index = cardiac output/body surface area = 6.2 l/min/m^2. Although selenium and carnitine deficiency can also cause cardiomyopathy, only thiamine deficiency causes high cardiac output failure. The correct answer is therefore (B) thiamine deficiency.

2. ANSWER: A. Hereditary hemochromatosis is an autosomal recessive iron-storage disease associated with mutations in the HLA-linked *HFE* gene and is seen almost entirely in people of northern European descent. There is accumulation of iron in the heart, liver, pancreas, skin, and gonads. When cardiac involvement is present, the disease is usually in the advanced stage with multiorgan involvement (diabetes, cirrhosis, arthritis, and impotence). The severity of myocardial dysfunction is proportional to the extent of myocardial iron deposition. Cardiac manifestations include congestive heart failure, arrhythmias, and conduction abnormalities.

Echocardiographic findings usually consist of mild left ventricular (LV) dilatation, LV systolic dysfunction, normal or mildly increased wall thickness, relatively normal cardiac valves, and biatrial enlargement. The LV diastolic filling pattern is usually restrictive and morphologic 2D features are essentially those of dilated cardiomyopathy.

The correct answer is (A) dilated LV and systolic dysfunction. LV wall thickness may be mildly increased but is frequently normal. Regional wall motion abnormalities are not typically present. Although secondary pulmonary hypertension may be present due to restrictive LV physiology, this is not a prominent finding. Pericardial effusion is not typical.

3. ANSWER: B. Selenium deficiency, also called Keshan disease, is associated with a reversible dilated cardiomyopathy that responds to selenium replacement. Selenium deficiency can be seen in patients receiving total parenteral nutrition and in patients from regions where food is grown in selenium-deficient soil (it was originally described in China). In the acute form, it can result in cardiogenic shock, pulmonary edema, and arrhythmias. In the chronic form, it presents as LV dilatation and systolic dysfunction. Vitamin B_{12}, folic acid, and L-lysine deficiency are not usually associated with cardiomyopathy.

4. ANSWER: C. Chagas disease (American trypanosomiasis) is endemic in Latin America. In infected patients, the heart muscle is invaded by the protozoan parasite *Trypanosoma cruzi*. Echocardiographic abnormalities include biventricular enlargement, ventricular wall thinning, mural thrombi, and a characteristic apical aneurysm.

Noncaseating cardiac granulomas are a feature of sarcoidosis. Intracavitary cardiac cystic lesions or hydatid cysts are a feature of a parasitic infection with *Echinococcus granulosus*. Libman-Sacks endocarditis refers to a nonbacterial endocarditis with verrucous valvular lesions that are typically found on the mitral valve in patients with autoimmune disorders and some malignancies.

5. ANSWER: C. In this patient, the E/e' ratio is 37 consistent with marked elevation in LV filling pressures. This observation points to either anthracycline cardiotoxicity or radiation-induced myocardial disease since both of these conditions can be associated with severe diastolic dysfunction. Manifestations of radiation-induced heart disease usually occur years after therapy. Thus, the most likely explanation for these findings is early doxorubicin toxicity. In view of the severe diastolic dysfunction, a cardiac explanation for this patient's symptoms is most likely. The mitral annular velocity should not be affected by anemia per se, although anemia in addition to diastolic dysfunction in this particular patient is a possibility. Anemia causes the mitral inflow velocity to increase secondary to a generalized high flow state.

Doxorubicin is an anthracycline, and the incidence of cardiotoxicity is related to the cumulative dose administered. The risk is increased in patients with underlying heart disease, when anthracyclines are used concurrently with other cardiotoxic agents or radiation, and in patients undergoing subsequent hematopoietic cell transplantation. Cardiotoxicity may occur early (usually around 3 months after treatment) or may occur late (sometimes decades after treatment is completed) presenting as a nonischemic dilated cardiomyopathy.

6. ANSWER: B. Friedreich ataxia, an autosomal recessive degenerative disorder, is the most common hereditary ataxia and is manifested clinically by neurologic dysfunction, cardiomyopathy, and diabetes mellitus. Echocardiographic abnormalities are common, reported in 86% of patients, and are useful in confirming a diagnosis of Friedreich ataxia since cardiac involvement is not present in other ataxic disorders. The most common echocardiographic abnormality is concentric increased wall thickness occasionally mimicking hypertrophic cardiomyopathy. Asymmetric septal thickening and dilated cardiomyopathy are uncommon. Other findings include globally decreased LV function and decreased LV end-diastolic diameter. Regional wall motion abnormalities in a noncoronary distribution are typically seen in infiltrative disorders, such as Wegener granulomatosis and sarcoidosis.

7. ANSWER: E. This patient has many of the typical cardiac manifestations of chronic renal failure. These include significant diastolic dysfunction (manifested by left atrial enlargement and restrictive filling Doppler hemodynamics), generalized valve thickening, and pericardial effusion, which is usually of no hemodynamic significance if unrelated to acute uremic pericarditis. Calcification of the valves results in both regurgitant and stenotic lesions. Mitral annular calcification is also common and is caused by derangements in calcium and phosphorous metabolism. Other findings that may be seen include regional wall motion abnormalities secondary to underlying coronary artery disease. Concentric wall thickening is often seen in patients with chronic renal failure and is usually secondary to longstanding hypertension; however, another important complication of longstanding renal failure is amyloidosis. An important distinguishing feature between wall thickening secondary to hypertension versus amyloid is the low or inappropriately normal voltage seen on the electrocardiogram (ECG) in amyloid. Thus, it is important to review the ECG when concentric wall thickening is appreciated in this clinical setting.

8. ANSWER: A. Wegener granulomatosis is a systemic necrotizing small vessel vasculitis characterized by granulomatous lesions with predilection for pulmonary and renal involvement. Recent research has identified a high frequency of echocardiographic abnormalities that appear related to Wegener granulomatosis and are associated with increased mortality even though cardiac involvement is often clinically silent. Regional wall motion abnormalities that are not confined to a typical coronary artery distribution are a typical finding seen in infiltrative disorders, such as Wegener granulomatosis, sarcoidosis, and cardiac amyloid. When present in younger patients with a low cardiovascular risk profile, Wegener granulomatosis and sarcoid should be considered. In patients with Wegener granulomatosis, the granulomatous inflammation may resolve with treatment including resolution of the regional wall motion abnormalities. Although pericardial effusions are common, they are usually small and hemodynamically insignificant. The aortic and mitral valves may be involved but valvular regurgitation is seldom severe. Wegener granulomatosis may manifest as a cardiomyopathy but this is usually an isolated dilated cardiomyopathy.

9. ANSWER: A. Amyloid cardiac disease is caused by extracellular deposition of proteins in the myocardium. Characteristic echocardiographic features of amyloid include LV wall thickening with evidence of diastolic dysfunction. In advanced disease, wall thickening progresses resulting in a restrictive cardiomyopathy with a nondilated or small LV cavity.

Sarcoidosis is a noncaseating granulomatous disorder. Granulomatous infiltration of the myocardium can cause both systolic and diastolic dysfunction. Cardiac sarcoidosis may present as a dilated cardiomyopathy. Hemochromatosis can lead to a dilated cardiomyopathy characterized by heart failure and conduction disturbances, due to excess deposition of iron within the myocardium. Cardiac involvement in hemochromatosis can be diagnosed on the basis of clinical evaluation, specialized laboratory testing, and cardiac imaging. Human immunodeficiency virus (HIV) causes dilated cardiomyopathy in approximately 1%–3% of patients with acquired immunodeficiency virus. The causes of cardiac damage include drug toxicity, secondary infection, myocardial damage by HIV, and an autoimmune process induced by HIV or other cardiotropic viruses, such as coxsackie virus, cytomegalovirus, or Epstein-Barr virus. Excessive alcohol consumption can lead to myocardial dysfunction. Alcohol is believed to be toxic to cardiac myocytes via oxygen-free radical damage and abnormal cardiac protein synthesis. Abstinence can lead to a dramatic improvement in cardiac function if the disease is diagnosed early.

10. ANSWER: B. Sarcoidosis is a noncaseating granulomatous disorder. Patients with sarcoid cardiac disease may have a known history of sarcoidosis, or cardiac involvement may be the first identification of the disease. The characteristic echocardiographic features seen in sarcoid heart disease include LV systolic dysfunction with regional wall motion abnormalities that do not follow a usual coronary artery distribution. Additional findings in sarcoid heart disease include atrioventricular block, abnormal wall thickness, and perfusion defects affecting the anteroseptal and apical regions.

LV dysfunction with apical dyskinesis and preserved basal cardiac function suggests stress-induced cardiomyopathy. In this disorder, typically the contractile function of the mid and apical segments of the left ventricle are depressed, and there is compensatory hyperkinesis of the basal walls, producing ballooning of the apex with systole. Stress-induced cardiomyopathy (Takostsubo syndrome) is much more common in women than in men and is frequently, but not always, triggered by an acute illness or by emotional or physical stress. Normal LV cavity size with increased LV wall thickness and LVOT obstruction suggests hypertrophic cardiomyopathy. Hypertrophic cardiomyopathy has an autosomal dominant pattern of inheritance, characterized by hypertrophy of the left ventricle, with variable clinical manifestations and morphologic and hemodynamic abnormalities. In a subset of patients, the site and extent of cardiac hypertrophy results in obstruction to LV outflow. Less commonly, LV outflow obstruction can be seen with infiltrative cardiomyopathy such as amyloid. Right atrial and ventricular enlargement with reduced systolic function as an isolated finding would be uncommon in patients with sarcoidosis. This finding would suggest a left-to-right shunt at atrial or pulmonary vein level. Alternatively, this could be seen in patients with arrhythmogenic RV cardiomyopathy.

11. ANSWER: D. The patient presents with symptoms of heart failure shortly after delivery. The clinical history is consistent with peripartum cardiomyopathy. Although the etiology of peripartum cardiomyopathy remains unclear, a number of factors have been associated with increased risk. These risk factors include age >30 years, multiparity, African descent, pregnancy with multiple fetuses, history of preeclampsia, eclampsia, postpartum hypertension, and oral tocolytic therapy.

12. ANSWER: B. Chest radiation can cause late cardiovascular disease, which can manifest as dyspnea. Possible causes include conduction system disease, coronary artery disease, pericardial constriction, myocardial disease, which manifests as restrictive cardiomyopathy, or endocardial disease. The endocardial disease causes valve thickening, typically affecting the aortic-mitral intervalvular fibrosa with calcification and associated valve dysfunction. The right-sided valves are affected less commonly. A comprehensive echo-Doppler examination is an excellent test to determine whether there is a structural cardiac cause of dyspnea in a patient with prior radiation.

LV hypertrophy would not be expected after cardiac radiation. This finding would suggest systemic hypertension or outflow tract obstruction. Ascending aortic dilatation is not noted in patients with radiation-induced heart disease. Pericardial effusion can occur during chest radiation or early after completion but would not be expected as a late complication of chest irradiation.

13. ANSWER: C. A range of cardiac abnormalities is associated with HIV infection. Cardiac complications of HIV disease tend to occur late in the disease and are becoming more prevalent as longevity improves. The most common clinical manifestation of cardiac disease in patients with HIV disease is pericardial effusion, occurring in up to 40%. Additional findings include dilated cardiomyopathy, lymphocytic myocarditis, infective endocarditis, nonbacterial thrombotic endocarditis, cardiac tumors, primary pulmonary hypertension, and RV dysfunction.

Atrial myxomas are the most common benign cardiac tumor in adults, and rhabdomyomas are the most common benign cardiac tumor in children but neither is associated with HIV-related cardiac disease. If present, cardiac tumors tend to be lymphomas or Kaposi sarcoma. Hypertrophic cardiomyopathy is not associated with HIV-related cardiac disease.

14. ANSWER: C. Coronary vasospasm and atherosclerotic coronary artery disease are unlikely to cause the distribution of regional wall motion abnormalities seen in this patient. Apical ballooning syndrome, subarachnoid hemorrhage, and pheochromocytoma result in catecholamine-mediated severe subendocardial myocardial ischemia that can occur in the absence of epicardial coronary artery disease. The clue to the diagnosis in this patient is the prior history of labile hypertension and acute chest pain episode associated with severe headache occurring shortly after abdominal surgery. Pheochromocytoma typically presents with paroxysms of severe hypertension with associated headache, diaphoresis, and chest pain sometimes precipitated by abdominal surgery or even tumor palpation. Cardiac manifestations of pheochromocytoma include hypertensive heart disease, reversible regional wall motion abnormalities, and a dilated cardiomyopathy. The diagnosis is confirmed by measuring plasma and urinary catecholamines as well as computed tomography identification of the adrenal tumor. Rarely, an extra-adrenal cardiac pheochromocytoma may present as a cardiac mass characteristically located in the atrioventricular groove. Cushing syndrome is due to excess glucocorticoid. The cardiac manifestations include moderate chronic diastolic hypertension rather than paroxysms of systolic hypertension and acute symptoms around the time of stress.

15. ANSWER: D. Rheumatoid arthritis may involve the heart in many ways. Coronary artery disease as well as diastolic heart failure is commonly seen in patients with rheumatoid arthritis. Antimalarial therapy used in the treatment may result in a reversible cardiomyopathy.

Despite small pericardial effusions being common, acute pericarditis and large pericardial effusions with tamponade are rare. Nevertheless, occult constrictive pericarditis may occur and, if unrecognized, can result in significant morbidity and mortality. Rheumatic nodules may involve all cardiac structures including valves but infrequently result in significant valve dysfunction. An important complication of longstanding rheumatoid arthritis is cardiac amyloid. Mitral valve prolapse is not generally associated with rheumatoid arthritis. Thickened and fixed tricuspid valve leaflets with tricuspid regurgitation would be expected in patients with carcinoid and drug-related valve disease.

16. ANSWER: B. The echocardiogram demonstrates significant apical and midventricular akinesis. The patient is a postmenopausal woman with a presentation that simulates acute myocardial infarction. These features are all consistent with apical ballooning syndrome.

Transient LV apical ballooning syndrome (also known as Takotsubo cardiomyopathy or stress-induced cardiomyopathy) is a reversible cardiomyopathy triggered by profound psychological or physical stress and has a clinical presentation that is similar to acute myocardial infarction. Most patients are postmenopausal women. Proposed criteria for the diagnosis of apical ballooning require all four of the following characteristics: (1) electrocardiographic abnormalities (usually ST elevations followed by T wave inversion), (2) transient apical and midventricular wall motion abnormalities, (3) absence of obstructive coronary artery disease or acute plaque rupture, and (4) absence of other conditions, such as significant head trauma, intracranial hemorrhage, pheochromocytoma, or another etiology of myocardial dysfunction.

Catecholamine-induced microvascular dysfunction is currently postulated as a likely mechanism. According to recent reports, RV apical dysfunction may be present in 30%–40% of cases. Dynamic LVOT obstruction, which is due to basal hyperkinesis, is a well-described complication of apical ballooning syndrome and may result in hypotension.

Persistent LV systolic dysfunction is not an expected complication in stress-induced cardiomyopathy. Although cardiac biomarkers are always elevated, the elevation is usually mild and disproportionate to the degree of cardiac compromise. Increased urinary 5-hydroxyindole acetic acid is seen in carcinoid patients.

It is important to remember that apical ballooning syndrome is a diagnosis of exclusion and can only be diagnosed once obstructive coronary disease and acute plaque rupture have been excluded. Similar wall motion abnormalities can also result from myocardial infarction due to occlusion of a large wraparound left anterior descending artery. Hence, coronary angiography is required for the diagnosis even in the setting of typical regional wall motion abnormalities.

17. ANSWER: B. The 2D echocardiographic findings of a pericardial effusion and an enlarged right ventricle with a D-shaped LV cavity due to pulmonary hypertension are suspicious for scleroderma. The clinical presentation of a patient who appears younger than her stated age, likely due to taut facial skin, dyspnea, arthralgias, and swelling of the hands and feet is also consistent with a diagnosis of scleroderma.

The most common primary cardiac abnormality associated with scleroderma is a pericardial effusion, often small. The myocardium may be involved by fibrosis or sclerosis and systolic and diastolic dysfunction may be present. Systemic and pulmonary hypertensions are prominent secondary complications of scleroderma.

Cardiac amyloidosis is an infiltrative cardiomyopathy that results in a restrictive disease and is characterized by increased biventricular wall thickness. Hemochromatosis can lead to a dilated cardiomyopathy due to excess deposition of iron within the myocardium. Finally, cardiac manifestations of rheumatoid arthritis include pericarditis and less commonly dilated cardiomyopathy with congestive heart failure.

18. ANSWER: C. The transesophageal echocardiogram (TEE) image demonstrates small verrucous valvular lesions on the tips of the mitral valve leaflets. In the clinical setting of a young woman with arthralgias, low-grade fever, skin rash, photosensitivity, elevated white blood cell count, pleural effusion, and no history of illicit drug use, the most likely diagnosis is systemic lupus erythematosus (SLE) with Libman-Sacks endocarditis.

Libman-Sacks endocarditis (also known as nonbacterial thrombotic endocarditis, or marantic endocarditis) refers to a characteristic verrucous valvular lesion that usually affects the mitral valve in patients with SLE. The lesion is typically present on the ventricular aspect of the mitral leaflets and may extend to the chordal and papillary structures.

Ergot-alkaloid use is associated with valvulopathy and valvular regurgitation usually affecting the aortic and mitral valves. Echocardiographic features of infective endocarditis are an oscillating intracardiac mass on a valve or other cardiac structure, abscesses, and dehiscence of a prosthetic valve. The vegetations are typically on the "upstream" surface of the affected valve. Rheumatic mitral valve disease is associated with thickened and calcified mitral leaflets and subvalvular apparatus, "hockey-stick" deformity of the anterior leaflet and relative immobility of the posterior leaflet, and associated stenosis or regurgitation.

19. ANSWER: C. The clue to the correct diagnosis in this case lies in the dermatologic findings. The skin lesions are angiokeratomas, which occur commonly in the groin, hip, and periumbilical areas. They are characteristically seen in patients with Fabry disease. Fabry disease is a rare X-linked inborn error of the glycosphingolipid metabolic pathway that results in accumulation of globotriaosylceramide in several organs including the skin, kidney, nervous system, cornea, and the heart leading to the clinical manifestations that usually begin in childhood or adolescence. The prominent features include severe neuropathic pain, telangiectasias and angiokeratomas, heat and exercise intolerance, and gastrointestinal symptoms, such as abdominal pain and diarrhea. Renal manifestations include proteinuria and renal failure. Cardiac involvement is usually manifest by concentric LV hypertrophy, myocardial dysfunction, aortic and mitral valve abnormalities, and conduction abnormalities. In some patients, LV hyper-

trophy may be the only overt manifestation of the disease. Fabry disease may be present in up to 4% of patients suspected to have hypertrophic cardiomyopathy. Thus, in patients presenting with unexplained LV hypertrophy, Fabry disease should be included in the differential diagnosis. The diagnosis is usually confirmed by demonstrating decreased leukocyte or plasma alpha-Gal A activity but can also be made histologically on endomyocardial biopsy.

Acromegaly, cardiac amyloid, and Fabry disease can all result in increased LV wall thickness, and rarely asymmetric wall involvement that can mimic hypertrophic cardiomyopathy. Moreover, dynamic LVOT obstruction, typically seen in hypertrophic obstructive cardiomyopathy with systolic anterior motion of the anterior mitral leaflet may be present. In cardiac amyloid, the ECG voltage would be expected to be normal or even reduced and is thus an unlikely diagnosis in this case. This case illustrates the importance of integrating the clinical and echocardiographic findings to make an accurate diagnosis.

20. ANSWER: A. The skin lesion is an angiofibroma, which is a typical skin lesion seen in patients with tuberous sclerosis. Tuberous sclerosis is an inherited autosomal dominant neurocutaneous disorder that is characterized by multiorgan system involvement, including multiple benign hamartomas of the brain, eyes, heart, lung, liver, kidney, as well as skin. The diagnosis of tuberous sclerosis is made clinically. The characteristic cardiac feature of tuberous sclerosis is a rhabdomyoma, the most frequent cardiac neoplasm of childhood representing 60% of pediatric cardiac tumors. Rhabdomyomas are benign tumors that almost always present as multiple lesions. Although they are often associated with tuberous sclerosis, they can occur as an isolated finding. They typically develop in utero and are often detected on prenatal ultrasound. They occur with equal frequency in both ventricles growing in the ventricular walls or on the atrioventricular valves. They vary in size from a few millimeters to a few centimeters and may be pedunculated often obstructing ventricular inflow or outflow. The morbidity and mortality associated with these tumors reflect the potential for flow abnormalities, if they grow to sufficient size to restrict blood flow. Although many are asymptomatic, some present with heart failure, a cardiac murmur, or arrhythmia. A unique and peculiar feature of cardiac rhabdomyomas is that they usually undergo spontaneous regression in the first few years of life. There is no evidence that these tumors undergo malignant transformation and no treatment is necessary for asymptomatic tumors. Thus, the most appropriate management strategy in this patient is reassurance with follow-up echocardiography in 1 year as well as family screening for affected siblings.

21. ANSWER: B. This young man has Marfan syndrome. The characteristic pear-shaped dilatation of the aortic root (aortic sinuses) is characteristic and a major diagnostic criterion of this autosomal dominant inherited condition usually resulting from a fibrillin 1 gene mutation. An additional major Ghent diagnostic criterion is the history of lens dislocation. Since there is an increased risk of aortic dissection or rupture when the aortic caliber reaches a dimension of 50 mm, elective aortic root replacement is indicated.

A TEE is not indicated at this time since the patient is asymptomatic and there is no suspicion of a dissection flap on the image shown. Although beta-blockers are indicated in patients with Marfan syndrome to delay progression of aortic root dilatation and losartan may be beneficial in patients with coexisting hypertension, this patient should undergo surgery in the near future.

22. ANSWER: B. Takayasu arteritis is a chronic vasculitis of unknown etiology affecting primarily the aorta and its primary branches. The inflammation may be localized or may involve the entire vessel. The initial vascular lesions frequently occur in the middle or proximal subclavian artery. As the disease progresses, the carotids, vertebrals, brachiocephalic, right middle or proximal subclavian artery, and aorta may also be affected. The abdominal aorta and pulmonary arteries are involved in approximately 50% of patients. The inflammatory process causes thickening of the walls of the affected arteries or involved segment of the aorta. The proximal aorta may become dilated secondary to inflammatory injury. Aortic valve regurgitation may be present and is usually caused by dilatation of the proximal ascending aorta.

Marfan syndrome is associated with aortic root enlargement, with or without aortic regurgitation, but is not associated with carotid, subclavian, or abdominal bruits and loss of pulses in the absence of dissection. Isolated mid-ascending aortic enlargement is not typically seen in patients with Marfan disease. Abnormal phase reactants would not be expected in these patients. Familial thoracic aortic aneurysmal disease is an aneurysmal disorder that occurs in the absence of syndromic features. It is inherited in an autosomal dominant manner with decreased penetrance and variable expression. Aneurysms can affect the ascending or descending thoracic or abdominal aorta and also the intracranial vascular system. Ankylosing spondylitis is a chronic inflammatory disease of the axial skeleton manifested by back pain and progressive stiffness of the spine. Asymptomatic cardiovascular disease secondary to ankylosing spondylitis is not uncommon, especially aortic regurgitation. This is caused by scar tissues in the aortic valve cusps and neighboring aorta.

23. ANSWER: A. The echocardiographic images demonstrate the RV outflow tract. Two-dimensional images demonstrate thickening of the pulmonary valve cusps, and the color-flow images demonstrate a broad-based regurgitant jet of pulmonary regurgitation. The continuous-wave Doppler signal is dense and demonstrates a diastolic signal that decelerates rapidly to baseline. All of these features are consistent with severe pulmonary valve regurgitation related to carcinoid involvement of the pulmonary valve.

Severe pulmonary valve stenosis is characterized by a high systolic antegrade signal across the pulmonary valve, and systolic doming of the pulmonary valve cusps is usually also noted. Carcinoid heart disease can cause severe pulmonary valve stenosis, but pulmonary regurgitation is more common. The antegrade signal across the pulmonary valve in this patient is of low velocity (<2 m/sec), which is not consistent with severe pulmonary valve stenosis.

Severe pulmonary hypertension is characterized by a low-antegrade systolic continuous-wave Doppler signal across the pulmonary valve. However, in severe pulmonary hypertension, the diastolic Doppler signal is of high velocity. An estimate of the pulmonary artery end-diastolic pressure can be made by measuring an elevated pulmonary regurgitant end-diastolic velocity. Patent ductus arteriosus is a communication between the main pulmonary artery and the descending thoracic aorta, which persists from fetal life. Color-flow Doppler echocardiography will demonstrate continuous flow from the descending thoracic aorta to the pulmonary artery, in the absence of severe pulmonary hypertension. This signal originates in the region of the proximal left pulmonary artery. The continuous-wave Doppler profile will demonstrate a high systolic signal with persistent flow throughout the cardiac cycle in the absence of pulmonary hypertension.

24. ANSWER: C. Metastatic carcinoid to the heart affects less than 5% of patients with metastatic carcinoid disease. This usually occurs in conjunction with valve disease. The echocardiographic appearance of metastatic carcinoid tumor appears as a homogeneous, circumscribed, noninfiltrating mass, which can affect the left or right ventricular myocardium. The history of flushing, diarrhea, and weight loss are consistent with the clinical features of carcinoid syndrome.

Extra-adrenal catecholamine-secreting paraganglioma (extra-adrenal pheochromocytoma) should be suspected when the patient presents with a clinical triad of headache, sweating, and tachycardia. The diagnosis can be confirmed biochemically by measuring 24-hour urinary fractionated metanephrines and catecholamines. Radiologic evaluation is performed to locate the tumor after biochemical confirmation. About 10% of the tumors are extra-adrenal. Thrombus would not be expected in the right atrioventricular groove. Thrombus usually occurs in the left atrium in patients with atrial fibrillation or mitral stenosis, in the left ventricle in the setting of a myocardial infarction with resultant regional wall motion abnormality or in the right heart chambers in patients with atrial fibrillation, or a venous thrombosis in transit. Coronary artery aneurysm can be seen in the right atrioventricular groove. Commonly, there is flow noted in the atrioventricular groove mass by echocardiography, differentiating it from solid masses.

25. ANSWER: B. The M-mode demonstrates prominent inspiratory leftward motion of the ventricular septum. The mitral inflow pulsed wave (PW) Doppler demonstrates significant (>25%) respiratory variation with increased expiratory E velocity and decreased inspiratory E velocity. The mitral annulus tissue Doppler demonstrates a normal e' of >0.08 m/sec (0.14 m/sec). Finally, the hepatic vein Doppler demonstrates expiratory diastolic reversals. These findings are consistent with a diagnosis of constrictive pericarditis. A history of radiation therapy is the third most common cause of constrictive pericarditis, after idiopathic causes and prior cardiac surgery.

Radiation therapy may also result in a restrictive cardiomyopathy. Mitral annulus e' velocity is especially helpful in distinguishing between restrictive cardiomyopathy and constrictive pericarditis. A value >8 cm/sec (this patient had e' of 14 cm/sec) strongly favors constrictive pericarditis. Although hepatic vein diastolic reversals may be seen with restrictive cardiomyopathy, these are typically inspiratory rather than expiratory. Finally, respiratory variation in mitral inflow and ventricular septal shift would not be expected with restrictive cardiomyopathy. A pericardial effusion can occur during or early after completion of chest radiation but would not be expected as a late complication. LV hypertrophy would not be expected as a complication of radiation therapy. The M-mode does not show evidence of pericardial effusion or LV hypertrophy.

26. ANSWER: D. The echocardiogram demonstrates LV apical thickening and obliteration and biatrial enlargement, which is suspicious for either apical hypertrophic cardiomyopathy or eosinophilic endomyocardial disease. Contrast images demonstrate a layer of nonperfusing thrombus in the apex, consistent with eosinophilic endomyocardial disease. Mitral inflow PW Doppler demonstrates restrictive filling physiology, which is also consistent with eosinophilic endomyocardial disease.

Cardiac involvement occurs in most patients with the hypereosinophilic syndrome defined as unexplained eosinophilia with >1,500 eosinophils per cubic mm for more than 6 months, associated with organ involvement. Cardiac manifestations include biventricular apical thrombotic-fibrotic endocardial obliteration, limited motion of the posterior mitral leaflet with mitral regurgitation due to thickening of the inferobasal wall, and restrictive ventricular diastolic filling physiology.

Apical hypertrophic cardiomyopathy can be differentiated from eosinophilic endomyocardial disease by the use of myocardial contrast, which demonstrates apical perfusion with a slit-like cavity within the hyperdynamic myocardium. It is typically associated with giant T wave inversions on ECG. Gaucher disease is a lysosomal storage disease and cardiac manifestations include LV thickening, left-sided valvular thickening, diastolic dysfunction, and pericardial effusion. Fabry disease is a glycosphingolipid-storage disease and cardiac manifestations include LV thickening, left-sided valvular thickening, mitral regurgitation, and myocardial dysfunction.

27. ANSWER: D. Mitral rather than aortic regurgitation and biventricular involvement are typically seen in patients with eosinophilic endomyocardial disease. LVOT obstruction is not associated with this condition.

KEY POINTS:

■ Cardiac involvement occurs in most patients with hypereosinophilic syndrome.

■ Eosinophilic endomyocardial disease is characterized by biventricular apical thrombotic-fibrotic obliteration, mitral regurgitation due to restriction of posterior mitral leaflet motion from inferobasal endocardial thickening, and restrictive physiology.

■ Myocardial contrast is helpful in distinguishing eosinophilic endomyocardial disease from apical hypertrophic cardiomyopathy.

28. ANSWER: B. The clinical presentation and left ventriculogram is consistent with apical ballooning syndrome. The echocardiogram demonstrates apical and midventricular akinesis and basal hyperkinesis with dynamic outflow tract obstruction, systolic anterior motion of the mitral leaflets, and associated posteriorly directed mitral regurgitation. LVOT obstruction is an important complication of apical ballooning syndrome and may result in clinically significant hypotension. Mitral regurgitation, either in association with mitral systolic anterior motion or due to papillary muscle displacement/dysfunction has also been described as a potential complication of apical ballooning syndrome.

Papillary muscle rupture, ventricular septal defect, and severe aortic regurgitation are not recognized complications of apical ballooning syndrome, and are not present in this case.

29. ANSWER: B. The dynamic LVOT obstruction with associated mitral systolic anterior motion and mitral regurgitation is the result of basal LV hyperkinesis. The most appropriate remedy is to increase LV afterload with phenylephrine and to reduce basal hyperkinesis with gradual initiation of beta-blockade. Cautious fluid administration may also be helpful, unless significant mitral regurgitation is present. Dobutamine would exacerbate the dynamic outflow tract obstruction. Percutaneous or surgical management is not indicated.

KEY POINTS:

▓ Dynamic LVOT obstruction is a possible complication of apical ballooning syndrome and may result in clinically significant hypotension/ shock. It is the result of basal LV hyperkinesis.

▓ Other possible causes of shock in patients with apical ballooning syndrome include profound LV systolic dysfunction and severe mitral regurgitation, either in association with mitral systolic anterior motion or due to displacement/dysfunction of the papillary muscles.

30. ANSWER: A. The echocardiogram demonstrates severe concentric thickening of the left ventricle, a granular myocardial echotexture, and biatrial enlargement and thickened cardiac valves. The subcostal view also shows a thickened RV free wall (10 mm) and a small posterior pericardial effusion. These 2D features are highly suggestive of cardiac amyloidosis. Mitral inflow PW Doppler demonstrates a restrictive filling pattern (E/A ratio of 3 and deceleration time of <160 milliseconds) and tissue Doppler demonstrates severely reduced annular é velocity of 0.03. The mitral E/é ratio is 30, which is consistent with severely increased LV filling pressures. The ECG findings of normal voltages despite severely increased wall thickness and pseudoinfarct are also consistent with amyloidosis. Overall, the 2D and Doppler features are classic for cardiac amyloidosis.

Hypertrophic cardiomyopathy is less likely given the diffuse nature of increased LV thickness (although this can sometimes be present), increased RV thickness, valvular thickening, and pericardial effusion as well as the ECG findings. Athlete's heart may be associated with increased LV thickness and enters the differential because of the history of the patient being an ex-competitive cyclist but notably this entity is associated with a normal mitral E' velocity. Hypertensive heart disease may be associated with increased LV thickness, reduced mitral é velocity, and increased mitral E/é velocity but would not be associated with the other abnormalities described. Finally, echocardiographic findings of hemochromatosis are those of a dilated cardiomyopathy with normal or mildly increased LV wall thickness.

31. ANSWER: D. Cardiac amyloidosis is associated with an inverse relationship between LV mass and ECG voltage since the increased wall thickness is due to interstitial amyloid fibril deposition rather than LV hypertrophy. ECG features may include low limb lead (<5 mm) or precordial lead (<10 mm) voltages and a

pseudoinfarct pattern. Fairly good sensitivity and specificity for the diagnosis of cardiac amyloidosis have been described using various combinations of increased LV wall thickness and low ECG voltages or LV mass/ECG voltage ratios. In contrast, hypertensive heart disease, hypertrophic cardiomyopathy, and athlete's heart—where wall thickness is increased due to LV hypertrophy—are associated with a proportional relationship between LV mass and ECG voltage. Restrictive filling physiology is not unique to cardiac amyloidosis and may also be seen in other conditions where LV wall thickness is increased such as hypertrophic cardiomyopathy or hypertension. Systolic anterior motion of the mitral apparatus is a typical feature of obstructive hypertrophic cardiomyopathy but can also be seen in other conditions such as hypertensive heart disease in the elderly (when sigmoid basal septal hypertrophy is present) or occasionally in cardiac amyloidosis. A normal é velocity helps to distinguish athlete's heart from pathologic causes of increased LV wall thickness (such as hypertensive heart disease, cardiac amyloidosis, or hypertrophic cardiomyopathy).

KEY POINTS:

▓ Cardiac amyloidosis is an infiltrative cardiomyopathy.

▓ Echocardiographic findings include increased biventricular and atrial wall thickness, valvular thickening, pan-valvular regurgitation, pericardial effusion, and restrictive physiology.

▓ Cardiac amyloidosis is associated with an inverse relationship between LV mass and ECG voltage.

32. ANSWER: C. This patient has hypothyroidism. Although the echocardiogram demonstrates a large pericardial effusion with RV collapse suggesting cardiac tamponade a definitive etiology cannot be made on the basis of the echocardiogram alone. In this case, all of the conditions above can result in a pericardial effusion and should be included in the differential diagnosis.

Cardiac tamponade is an unlikely consequence in patients with cardiac amyloid, renal failure, SLE, as well as hypothyroidism. Nevertheless, cardiac tamponade can rarely occur in all of these conditions. The clue to the correct answer lies in the physical examination that reveals non–pitting pedal edema (pretibial myxedema secondary to interstitial accumulation of glycosaminoglycans) and bradycardia in the setting of cardiac tamponade making hypothyroidism the most likely explanation for the clinical and echocardiographic findings in this patient.

The low voltage on the ECG is unhelpful to distinguish a cause since the findings may reflect attenuation of the ECG signal by the large pericardial effusion. Furthermore, although we would expect a higher mitral annular velocity in a middle-aged woman, diastolic dysfunction can be present in all of these conditions except in a patient with breast cancer who otherwise has no cardiac disease. The incidence of pericardial effusion in hypothyroidism varies depending on the severity of the disease and occurs in 30%–80% of patients with advanced severe disease.

33. ANSWER: D. Since the patient is symptomatic, experiencing lightheadedness and presyncope, and there is evidence of collapse of the right-sided chambers, therapeutic echocardiographic-guided pericardiocentesis is indicated at this time. Had the effusion been smaller and without associated hemodynamic compromise, it would have been reasonable to re-evaluate the effusion after confirming the diagnosis and restoring a euthyroid state.

34. ANSWER: A. Overt hypothyroidism can result in impaired ventricular systolic and diastolic performance manifested by prolongation of the isovolumic contraction and relaxation intervals as well as a frank dilated cardiomyopathy and congestive heart failure. Thus, in this patient with hypothyroidism, the only echocardiographic parameter that would be expected to decrease with thyroid supplementation is the isovolumic contraction interval since this is a measure of cardiac contractility—the shorter the interval, the better the myocardial contractility. Both systolic and diastolic mitral annular velocities are likely to increase as systolic and diastolic function improves and the LVOT time-velocity integral will also increase since the cardiac output will likely increase with treatment. Apart from pericardial effusion and reduced cardiac output (related to a reduction in heart rate and contractility) and diastolic function, other cardiac manifestations of hypothyroidism include increased LV mass and LV wall thickness, which may rarely be asymmetric.

KEY POINTS:

- Pericardial effusion is a common cardiac manifestation of hypothyroidism.
- Reversible systolic and diastolic dysfunction can occur in patients with hypothyroidism.

35. ANSWER: B; 36. ANSWER: A. The echocardiographic contrast entering the left atrium is delayed appearing after more than three cardiac cycles subsequent to agitated saline contrast administration. This finding suggests an intrapulmonary shunt. All of the options other than persistent left superior vena cava can result in right-to-left shunting at the atrial level since they all involve a defect in the atrial septum. Chronic liver failure is a common cause of intrapulmonary shunting resulting from diffuse or localized dilated pulmonary capillaries and, less commonly, pleural and pulmonary arteriovenous communications. This is referred to as the hepatopulmonary syndrome. Contrast-enhanced echocardiography with agitated saline is the most practical method to detect pulmonary vascular shunting. After administration of agitated saline in a peripheral vein in the arm, microbubble opacification of the left atrium within three to six cardiac cycles after right atrial opacification indicates microbubble passage through an abnormally dilated vascular bed.

KEY POINTS:

- Not all right-to-left shunts with agitated saline contrast opacification of both atria are atrial in origin.
- Delayed appearance (more than three cardiac cycles) of agitated saline in the left atrium suggests an intrapulmonary shunt.
- Direct visualization of the atrial septum and fossa ovalis membrane and evaluation of each pulmonary vein to visualize microbubble passage confirm the site of shunt.

37. ANSWER: C; 38. ANSWER: D. This patient has Carney syndrome. The Carney complex is an inherited, autosomal dominant disorder characterized by multiple tumors, including atrial and extracardiac myxomas, schwannomas, and various endocrine tumors. The cardiac myxomas generally are diagnosed at an earlier age than sporadic myxomas and have a higher tendency to recur. In addition, patients have a variety of pigmentation abnormalities, including pigmented lentigines and blue nevi on the face, neck, and trunk. The skin lesions present in this young woman are lentigines, which are characteristically seen in patients with Carney syndrome. This finding, combined with the history of adrenal tumors, makes it the most likely diagnosis. Therefore, the mass seen in the right atrium is most likely a myxoma. Even though myxomas (the most common benign primary cardiac tumor) typically arise in the left atrium and are most often attached to the fossa ovalis membrane by a thin stalk, the "atypical" location is characteristic of this syndrome. Furthermore, it is imperative that careful scrutiny for other lesions is undertaken since multiple synchronous lesions are commonly present. In this instance, the RV lesion was missed during the initial assessment. These tumors are benign but recurrent tumors can occur mandating careful lifelong echocardiographic follow-up.

Angiosarcoma is a malignant tumor with a dismal prognosis (rarely exceeding 6 months) and often presents as a broad-based right atrial mass near the inferior vena cava. Epicardial, endocardial, and intracavitary extensions are common. They may be associated with a pericardial effusion, presenting with cardiac tamponade. Fungal endocarditis may mimic a right-sided mass lesion when tricuspid valve involvement is present, even resulting in tricuspid valve obstruction. The clinical setting is usually intravenous drug abuse or indwelling intravenous infusion catheter in patients with renal failure or undergoing chemotherapy. Valve destruction is usually present with valvular regurgitation. Renal cell carcinoma, which characteristically metastasizes to the right-sided cardiac chambers as a tumor/thrombus via the inferior vena cava as well as thrombi in transit from the deep venous system may also present as right-sided masses and therefore should be included in the differential diagnosis. A CAT is an acronym describing a calcified amorphous tumor that probably represents a calcified thrombus. This is a benign finding and would not be expected in this patient.

KEY POINTS:

■ It is important to integrate the history and physical examination findings when making an echocardiographic diagnosis.

■ When atrial myxomas arise in unusual locations and multiple tumors are present, think Carney syndrome.

■ Do not focus on one abnormality at the exclusion of other synchronous lesions or abnormalities!

39. ANSWER: A. The patient presents with symptoms of right heart failure and the echocardiographic images demonstrate thickening and malcoaptation of the tricuspid valve leaflets with severe tricuspid regurgitation. There is a laminar jet of tricuspid regurgitation noted in the left atrium, and the continuous wave Doppler signal demonstrates a dense systolic signal with a cutoff sign consistent with rapid equalization of pressures between the right atrium and right ventricle.

Arrhythmogenic RV dysplasia is characterized by ventricular arrhythmias and fatty replacement of the RV free wall. The fibrofatty replacement of the RV myocardium initially produces regional wall motion abnormalities and eventual RV dilation. Drug-related valve disease has been reported to occur with ergot alkaloid derivatives, anorexigens, and pergolide. These agents cause primarily left-sided valve disease but tricuspid valve disease can also occur. The echocardiographic appearance of drug-related valve disease includes thickening of the valve leaflets or cusps with reduced mobility. Echocardiographic images are similar to those seen in carcinoid valve disease. However, the patient history is consistent with carcinoid rather than drug-related valve disease. Ebstein's anomaly is a congenital cardiac disorder, which involves apical displacement of the septal and posterior tricuspid leaflets and variable tethering of the anterior leaflet. Tricuspid regurgitation is a common finding in patients with Ebstein's anomaly. Additional echocardiographic features include right heart enlargement with dysfunction and atrial septal defect or patent foramen ovale.

40. ANSWER: D. Urinary 5-hydroxyindole acetic acid is a breakdown product of serotonin and is measured using a 24-hour urine collection. Patients with carcinoid heart disease have increased levels of circulating serotonin related to metastatic disease. Serotonin is produced by the primary tumor and metastases. Increased serotonin levels have been demonstrated to cause tricuspid and pulmonary valve thickening and associated regurgitation. The mechanism is thought to be activation of the 5HT 2B receptors on the valves. The diagnosis of carcinoid can be confirmed by pathologic examination of the primary tumor or metastases, increased 24-hour urine 5-hydroxyindole acetic acid and/or by Octreoscan.

Serum angiotensin-converting enzyme (ACE) level is often elevated in patients with sarcoidosis. Subcutaneous fat aspirate is used to help confirm suspected primary amyloid. Complete blood cell count with differential white blood cell count and smear is performed when hypereosinophilic syndrome is suspected. Eosinophilic endomyocardial disease affects primarily the endocardium and valves.

KEY POINTS:

■ Patients with carcinoid syndrome usually present with flushing and diarrhea.

■ Carcinoid heart disease is characterized by thickening and regurgitation of the right-sided cardiac valves.

■ Serotonin is responsible for the valve damage that occurs in patients with carcinoid syndrome.

41. ANSWER: A. Alteration of the color Doppler scale affects the degree of regurgitation appreciated by color-flow imaging. The color scale should always be checked when assessing the degree of regurgitation by color-flow Doppler and the scale should be maximized. When the color velocity scale is low, the degree of regurgitation appreciated by color-flow imaging may be overestimated. Ideally, a comprehensive assessment of the degree of regurgitation should be performed using multiple echo-Doppler modalities.

Measurement of vena contracta is one of the methods used to assess valvular regurgitation by Doppler echocardiography and can be used in the presence of both aortic and mitral regurgitation. The lack of LV enlargement does not exclude the possibility of severe aortic regurgitation. In patients with acute severe aortic regurgitation or mixed aortic stenosis and regurgitation, LV dilatation may not be present. Injection of echo contrast does not aid in the assessment of the degree of aortic regurgitation. Echo contrast material is generally administered to opacify the LV cavity, which permits improved endocardial border detection and is used to assess wall motion at rest and during stress echo imaging. In addition, echo contrast may be used to assess myocardial perfusion.

42. ANSWER: D. The clinical history and echocardiographic features suggest antiphospholipid antibody syndrome. This diagnosis is supported by the presence of at least one type of autoantibody known as an antiphospholipid antibody in the serum. Patients with antiphospholipid antibody syndrome commonly have valvular thickening, valve nodules, and nonbacterial vegetations causing valve regurgitation. Pathologic findings on explanted valves include platelet-rich fibrin deposits on the coapting surfaces of the valves.

Patients with rheumatic heart disease usually have a history of rheumatic or scarlet fever. Deep venous thrombosis and miscarriage are not characteristic clinical features. Although either can occur, valve stenosis is more common in rheumatic valve disease than regurgitation. Chest radiation can cause late cardiovascular disease, which can manifest as dyspnea. Endocardial disease causes valve thickening and affects left-sided valves more commonly than right-sided valves. Drug-related valve disease has been reported to occur with ergot alkaloid derivatives, anorexigens, and pergolide. These agents cause primarily left-sided valve disease but tricuspid valve disease can also occur. The echocardiographic appearance of drug-related valve disease includes thickening of the valve leaflets or cusps with reduced mobility. The clinical history makes the diagnosis of antiphospholipid antibody syndrome the most likely cause for these otherwise nonspecific echocardiographic findings.

KEY POINTS:

- Patients with antiphospholipid antibody syndrome commonly have valvular thickening, valve nodules, and nonbacterial vegetations causing valve regurgitation.
- Pathologic findings on explanted valves include platelet-rich fibrin deposits on the coapting surfaces of the valves.
- Additional clinical features include a personal or family history of thromboembolism or recurrent miscarriages.

SUGGESTED READINGS

Alizad A, Seward JB. Echocardiographic features of genetic diseases: part 2. Storage disease. *J Am Soc Echocardiogr*. 2000;13:164–170.

Andrews J, Al-Nahhas A, Pennell DJ, et al. Non-invasive imaging in the diagnosis and management of Takayasu's arteritis. *Ann Rheum Dis*. 2004;63:995.

Barbaro G, Klatt EC. HIV infection and the cardiovascular system. *AIDS Rev*. 2002;4:93–103.

Bargout R, Kelly RF. Sarcoid heart disease: clinical course and treatment. *Int J Cardiol*. 2004;97:173–182.

Bouillanne O, Millaire A, de Groote P. Prevalence and clinical significance of antiphospholipid antibodies in heart valve disease: a case-control study. *Am Heart J*. 1996;132:790–795.

Click RL, Olson LJ, Edwards WD, et al. Echocardiography and systemic diseases. *J Am Soc Echocardiogr*. 1994;7:201–216.

Edwards A, Bermudez C, Piwonka G, et al. Carney's syndrome: complex myxomas. Report of four cases and review of the literature. *Cardiovasc Surg*. 2002;10:264–275.

Falk RH. Diagnosis and management of the cardiac amyloidoses. *Circulation*. 2005;112:2047.

Kerber RE, Sherman B. Echocardiographic evaluation of pericardial effusion in myxedema. Incidence and biochemical and clinical correlations. *Circ*. 1975;52:823–827.

Klein AL, Hatle, LK, Taliercio CP, et al. Prognostic significance of Doppler measures of diastolic function in cardiac amyloidosis. A Doppler echocardiography study. *Circulation*. 1991;83:808–816.

Moller JE, Connolly HM, Rubin JR, et al. Carcinoid heart disease: factors associated with progression. *N Eng J Med*. 2003;348:1005–1015.

Møller JE, Pellikka PA, Bernheim AM, et al. Prognosis of carcinoid heart disease: analysis of 200 cases over two decades. *Circulation*. 2005;112:3320–3327.

Nir A, Tajik AJ, Freeman WK, et al. Tuberous sclerosis and cardiac rhabdomyoma. *Am J Cardiol*. 1995;76:419–421.

Ommen SR, Seward JB, Tajik AJ. Clinical and echocardiographic features of hypereosinophilic syndromes. *Am J Cardiol*. 2000;86:110–113.

Oliveira GH, Seward JB, Tsang TSM, et al. Echocardiographic findings in patients with Wegener granulomatosis. *Mayo Clin Proc*. 2005;80(11):1435–1440.

O'Neill TW, King G, Graham IM, et al. Echocardiographic abnormalities in ankylosing spondylitis. *Ann Rheum Dis*. 1992;51:652–654.

Pearson GD, Veille JC, Rahimtoola S, et al. Peripartum cardiomyopathy: National Heart, Lung, and Blood Institute and Office of Rare Diseases (National Institutes of Health) workshop recommendations and review. *JAMA*. 2000;283:1183–1188.

Rodriguez-Roisin R, Krowka MJ. Hepatopulmonary syndrome—a liver-induced lung vascular disorder. *N Eng J Med*. 2008;358:2378–2387.

Sliwa K, Fett J, Elkayam U. Peripartum cardiomyopathy. *Lancet*. 2006;368:687.

Smedema JP, Snoep G, van Kroonenburgh MP, et al. Cardiac involvement in patients with pulmonary sarcoidosis assessed at two university medical centers in the Netherlands. *Chest*. 2005; 128:30.

Sudano I, Spieker LE, Noll G, et al. Cardiovascular disease in HIV infection. *Am Heart J*. 2006;151:1147.

CHAPTER 22

Pericardial Diseases

Partho P. Sengupta and James B. Seward

1. According to the 2003 task force of the American College of Cardiology (ACC), the American Heart Association (AHA), and the American Society of Echocardiography (ASE), which of the following is a class I recommendation for the use of echocardiography in known or suspected pericardial disease?
   A. Pericardial friction rub in early uncomplicated myocardial infarction or in the early postoperative period after cardiac surgery.
   B. Pericardial friction rub developing in acute myocardial infarction accompanied by symptoms such as persistent pain, hypotension, and nausea.
   C. Postsurgical pericardial disease, including postpericardiotomy syndrome, with potential for hemodynamic impairment.
   D. Routine follow-up of small pericardial effusion in clinically stable patients.

2. Which of the following points will differentiate a left-sided pleural effusion from pericardial effusion?
   A. In the parasternal long-axis view, pleural effusions are located posterior to the descending aorta, whereas pericardial effusions are located anterior to the aorta.
   B. Pleural effusion can be recognized because they appear as very large anterior space without any posterior component.
   C. Pericardium is reflected from the pulmonary veins as they enter the left atrium. Thus, any collection posterior to this space has to be a pericardial effusion.
   D. The motion of the heart is reduced in the presence of pericardial effusion and remains normal or excessive in pleural effusion.

3. Which of the following is the single most important parameter to assess in terms of avoiding major diagnostic errors in assessing the hemodynamic importance of pericardial disease?
   A. Right atrial collapse.
   B. Right ventricular free wall inversion.
   C. Transmitral flow Doppler respiratory variation.
   D. Inferior vena cava size.

4. Two-dimensional (2D) echocardiographic features of congenital complete absence of the pericardium resemble which of the following conditions?
   A. Mitral stenosis.
   B. Aortic stenosis.
   C. Ventricular septal defect.
   D. Atrial septal defect.

5. Which of the following echocardiographic techniques is best for evaluating pericardial thickness?
   A. M-mode transthoracic echocardiography.
   B. B-mode speckle tracking echocardiography.
   C. Tissue Doppler echocardiography.
   D. Transesophageal echocardiography.

6. Which of the following can unmask the characteristic respiratory variation in early mitral inflow velocity in patients with constrictive pericarditis (CP) and high left atrial pressures?
   A. Valsalva.
   B. Head-up tilting.
   C. Amyl nitrite inhalation.
   D. Squatting.

7. Which of the following conditions is characterized by marked diastolic flow reversal in hepatic veins that increases in expiration compared with inspiration?
   A. CP.
   B. Restrictive cardiomyopathy.
   C. Chronic obstructive lung disease.
   D. Pericardial effusion.

8. What is the suggested cut off value of longitudinal early diastolic annular velocities for differentiating CP from restrictive cardiomyopathy?
   A. 8 cm/sec.
   B. 15 cm/sec.
   C. 4 cm/sec.
   D. 12 cm/sec.

9. Enhanced respiratory variation of ventricular filling represents which pathophysiological feature of pericardial disease?
   A. Enhanced interventricular interdependence.
   B. Elevated ventricular filling pressure.
   C. Equalization of intrathoracic and extrathoracic pressures.
   D. Intrathoracic and extrathoracic dissociation.

10. Which of the following is frequently seen in CP but is not necessarily a specific sign for constriction?
    A. B bump.
    B. Abnormal interventricular septal motion.
    C. Pulmonary hypertension.
    D. Dilated coronary sinus.

11. Demonstration of which of the following is obligatory for the diagnosis of CP?
    A. Abnormal hemodynamics.
    B. Pericardial thickening/calcification.
    C. Pulmonary hypertension.
    D. Biatrial enlargement.

12. Which of the following differentiates echocardiographic features of CP from chronic obstructive pulmonary disease (COPD)?
    A. In COPD, the mitral inflow pattern is not restrictive.
    B. In COPD, the highest mitral E velocity occurs toward the beginning of inspiration, whereas in CP it occurs immediately after the onset of expiration.
    C. In COPD, the superior vena cava flow velocities are markedly attenuated during respiration.
    D. Hepatic vein Doppler signals are useful for differentiating COPD from CP provided that tricuspid regurgitation is severe.

13. Which of the following is the most common primary neoplasm of the heart associated with a pericardial effusion?
    A. Myxoma.
    B. Hemangioma.
    C. Angiosarcoma.
    D. Rhabdomyoma.

14. Which of the following is an echocardiographic feature of a pericardial cyst?
    A. It is commonly located behind the atrium.
    B. It is usually located at the cardiophrenic angle.
    C. It is usually located near the left ventricular (LV) apex.
    D. It is usually located near the transverse sinus.

15. Which of the following statements related to pericardial disease is true?
    A. Loculated pericardial effusions can cause significant hemodynamic compromise.
    B. Features of pericardial constriction are always persistent.
    C. Cardiac tamponade is dependent upon the volume of pericardial fluid collection.
    D. Chronic calcific CP is never associated with myocardial diseases.

16. A 43-year-old patient presented in the emergency department with chest pain. His unusual 2D echocardiographic images, shown in Figure 22-1, are consistent with:

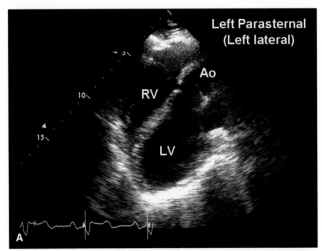

Fig. 22-1A

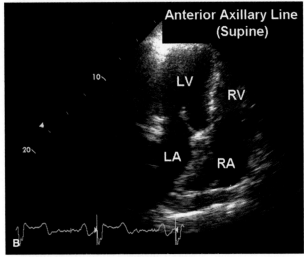

Fig. 22-1B

A. CP.
B. Acute pericarditis.
C. Absent pericardium.
D. Pericardial cyst.

17. The labeled portion (white arrow) of the 2D echocardiographic image in Figure 22-2 is consistent with:

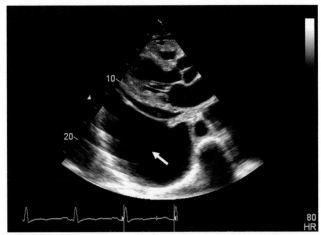

Fig. 22-2

A. Pleural effusion.
B. Pericardial effusion.
C. Pericardial cyst.
D. Mediastinal cyst.

18. The labeled portion (white arrow) of the 2D echocardiographic image in Figure 22-3 is consistent with:

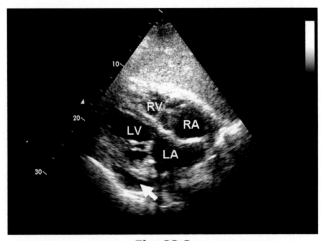

Fig. 22-3

A. Pericardial cyst.
B. Loculated pericardial effusion.
C. Pericardial metastasis.
D. CP.

19. The labeled portion (white arrow) of the 2D echocardiographic image in Figure 22-4 is consistent with:

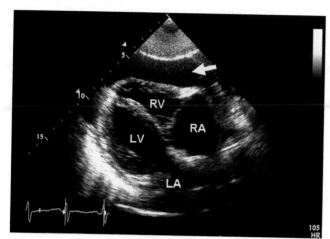

Fig. 22-4

A. Epicardial fat.
B. Mediastinal hemorrhage.
C. Pericardial effusion.
D. Pleural effusion.

20. The M-mode echocardiographic features shown in Figure 22-5 are suggestive of:
A. Pleural effusion.
B. CP.
C. Large pericardial effusion.
D. Cardiac tamponade.

21. Transmitral and transtricuspid flow profiles shown in Figure 22-6 in a patient with a large pericardial effusion is suggestive of:

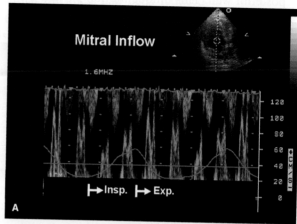

Fig. 22-6A

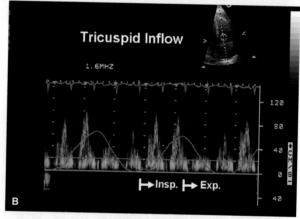

Fig. 22-6B

A. Cardiac tamponade.
B. CP.
C. Normal pattern.
D. Accompanying pulmonary hypertension.

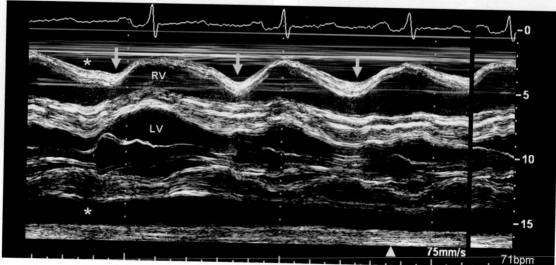

Fig. 22-5

CASE 3:

A 35-year-old woman presented with shortness of breath for 1 week. Chest X-ray showed cardiomegaly (cardiac-thoracic ratio of 65%) and a left-sided pleural effusion. Her echocardiogram revealed a large pericardial effusion.

30. She underwent an echo-guided pericardiocentesis. Part of the procedure is shown in the echo in Video 22-2. What is the echo consistent with?
    A. Identification of blood coagulum in the peri-cardial cavity.
    B. Spontaneous echo contrast in the pericardial cavity.
    C. Identification of a pericardial-pleural fistula.
    D. Injection of agitated saline contrast.

31. Which of the following describes the best position of the echocardiography transducer in relation to the needle used for pericardiocentesis?
    A. Needle and transducer are best aligned close and parallel to each other.
    B. Needle and transducer are best placed close and orthogonal to one another.
    C. Needle and transducer are best placed remote and orthogonal to each other.
    D. Needle and transducer should be remote and parallel to each other.

CASE 4:

A 38-year-old man presented with a 1-year history of bilateral leg edema and shortness of breath. Previous medical evaluations investigated the possibility of inferior vena cava thrombosis. The review of systems was positive for significant weight gain over the last month. His medical history was unremarkable other than a documented episode of viral pericarditis 4 years prior that resolved with nonsteroidal anti-inflammatory medication. Laboratory data revealed moderate hypoalbuminemia, a slight elevation in total bilirubin, and a low platelet count. A nephrology evaluation showed no kidney disease. As part of a cardiac evaluation, 2-D echocardiography was performed. The transhepatic and transmitral flow tracings are shown in Figure 22-13.

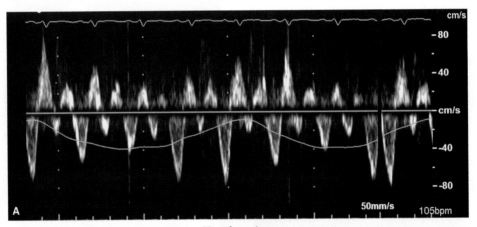

Transhepatic
Fig. 22-13A

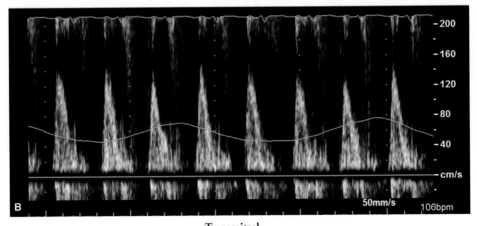

Transmitral
Fig. 22-13B

32. The maneuver that will help confirm the diagnosis is:
   A. Valsalva.
   B. Leg raising.
   C. Head up tilt.
   D. Hand grip.

33. The pathophysiological basis of the maneuver is:
   A. Preload increase.
   B. Preload reduction.
   C. Afterload increase.
   D. Afterload reduction.

CASE 5:

A 46-year-old woman with a history of Hodgkin's lymphoma as a child requiring radiation therapy presented with congestive heart failure. This was presumed to be secondary to mitral and tricuspid valve insufficiency. She underwent a mitral valve replacement with a St. Jude mechanical valve and a tricuspid valve repair. She was readmitted a few months later with bilateral pleural effusions requiring thoracentesis. The patient was also noted to have abdominal ascites. A diagnosis of CP was made by echocardiogram. To differentiate the extent of pericardial versus myocardial disease related to radiation, myocardial function was analyzed by speckle tracking strain echocardiography (Videos 22-3A and B of speckle tracking strain imaging performed in apical four-chamber and LV apical short-axis views)

34. Which of the following would be consistent with radiation-induced CP?
   A. Reduced longitudinal and circumferential strains.
   B. Relatively normal longitudinal strain and reduced circumferential strain.
   C. Reduced longitudinal and normal circumferential strain.
   D. Normal longitudinal and circumferential strains.

35. Which of the following component of LV mechanics when reduced will suggest pericardial tethering in CP?
   A. Longitudinal strain.
   B. Radial strain.
   C. LV rotation.
   D. All of the above.

ANSWERS

1. ANSWER: B. A 2003 task force of the American College of Cardiology (ACC), the American Heart Association (AHA), and the American Society of Echocardiography (ASE) gave class I recommendations for the following uses of echocardiography in known or suspected pericardial disease [Available at: www.acc.org/qualityandscience/clinical/statements.htm].
a) Patients with suspected pericardial disease, including effusion, constriction, or effusive-constrictive process.
b) Patients with suspected bleeding in the pericardial space (e.g., trauma, perforation).
c) Follow-up study to evaluate recurrence of effusion or to diagnose early constriction. Repeat studies may be goal directed to answer a specific clinical question.
d) Pericardial friction rub developing in acute myocardial infarction accompanied by symptoms such as persistent pain, hypotension, and nausea.

2. ANSWER: A. Left pleural effusions can present as large echo-free spaces that resemble pericardial effusions. These can be recognized because they appear as very large posterior spaces without an anterior component. Generally, in the parasternal long-axis view, pleural effusions are located posterior to the descending aorta, whereas pericardial effusions are located anterior to the aorta (arrow, Fig. 22-14; Ao, descending thoracic aorta).

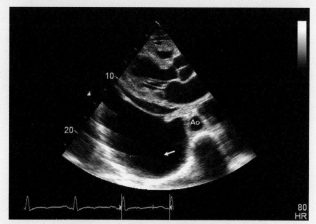

Fig. 22-14

3. ANSWER: D. A plethoric inferior vena cava is a specific marker of raised central venous pressure. Although this sign may not manifest if the patient has undergone brisk diuresis or is severely dehydrated, its absence usually makes the diagnosis of advanced or hemodynamically significant pericardial diseases unlikely.

4. ANSWER: D. Congenital complete absence of the pericardium is associated with the enlargement of the right ventricle, excessive motion of the posterior left ventricular (LV) wall, and shift of the heart to the left, resulting in more of the right ventricle being seen on the routine left parasternal echocardiogram; these changes may result in paradoxical motion of the interventricular septum. All of these findings mimic right ventricular volume overload as seen in atrial septal defect.

5. ANSWER: D. Pericardial thickness of ≥3 mm on transesophageal echocardiography has 95% sensitivity and 86% specificity for the detection of thickened pericardium. Figure 22-15 shows a transesophageal echocardiogram (four-chamber transverse plane view) and the corresponding transaxial electron beam computed tomographic scan from a patient with a markedly thickened pericardium (up to 18 mm) over the right side of the heart (reproduced from http://circ.ahajournals.org/cgi/content/full/95/6/1686#SEC6 accessed on Sep 14, 2010).

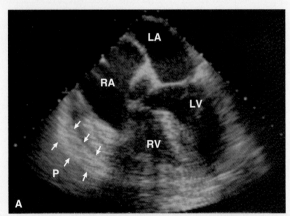

Fig. 22-15A

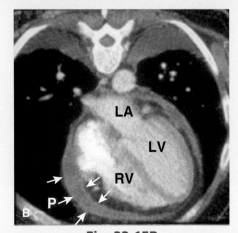

Fig. 22-15B

6. ANSWER: B. In a subset of patients with constrictive pericarditis (CP), the typical respiratory variation (≥25%) of mitral E velocity may not be present. This most likely is related to a marked increase in left atrial pressure. Reduction of preload by head-up tilt, upright position, or diuresis may augment or unmask the typical respiratory variation. Valsalva does not permit visualization of respiratory changes. Both amyl nitrite inhalation and squatting can theoretically reduce cardiac preload; however, these have not been specifically studied in patients with CP.

7. ANSWER: A. Hepatic vein diastolic flow reversal, which increases with expiration, is a classical feature of CP. There is reversal of forward flow during expiration, since the right ventricular cavity size is reduced due to right-sided shift of the interventricular septum, becoming less compliant as the left ventricle fills more. In contrast, reversal of hepatic vein flow occurs during inspiration in restrictive cardiomyopathy.

8. ANSWER: A. e' of >8 cm/sec has approximately 95% sensitivity and 96% specificity for the diagnosis of CP. In normal subjects, mitral lateral e' velocity is higher than the medial e' velocity. The presence of relatively normal lateral and/or septal corner mitral annular velocities suggests the presence of CP. However, the lateral e' velocity is usually lower than the medial e' velocity, resulting in annulus reversal. This finding is likely due to the tethering of the adjacent fibrotic and scarred pericardium, which influences the lateral mitral annulus of patients with CP.

9. ANSWER: A. In patients with CP, the pulmonary capillary wedge pressure (PCWP) is influenced by the inspiratory fall in thoracic pressure, whereas the LV pressure is shielded from respiratory pressure variations by the pericardial scar. Thus, inspiration lowers the PCWP and presumably left atrial pressure, but not LV diastolic pressure, thereby decreasing the pressure gradient for ventricular filling. The less favorable filling pressure gradient during inspiration explains the decline in filling velocity. Reciprocal changes occur in the velocity of right ventricular filling. These changes are mediated by the ventricular septum, not by increased systemic venous return and represent features of exaggerated interventricular interdependence.

10. ANSWER: B. In CP, total cardiac volume is fixed by the noncompliant pericardium. The septum is not involved and can therefore bulge toward the left ventricle (Fig. 22-16, arrow 1), when LV volume is less than that on the right. As a result, ventricular interaction is greatly enhanced. This periodic bulging may be seen on echocardiography and represents an abnormal pattern of septal motion. In addition, the rapid filling in early diastole gives rise to additional brisk motion of the septum, which is also referred to as "septal shudder" (Fig. 22-16, arrow 2). Abnormal septal motion, however, is not specific for constriction and is also seen following cardiac surgery, in the presence of left bundle branch block or pulmonary hypertension.

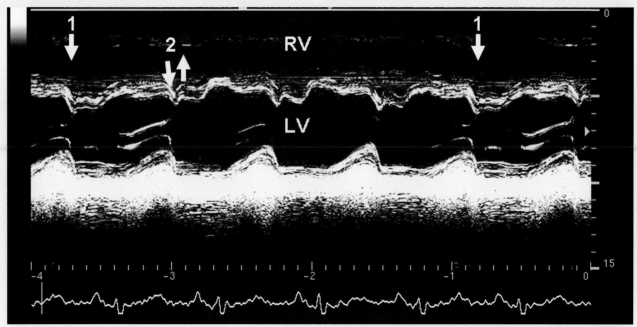

Fig. 22-16

11. ANSWER: A. Demonstration of constrictive physiology and elevated filling pressure is a key requisite for the diagnosis of CP and can occur in the absence of a thickened pericardium. Significant pulmonary hypertension and more than mild enlargement of atria are not usually features of CP.

12. ANSWER: A. Respiratory variation in mitral E velocity of ≥25% is the main diagnostic criterion for CP on Doppler echocardiography but it can also be present in patients with chronic obstructive pulmonary disease (COPD). However, transmitral filling is usually never restrictive in COPD. In an attempt to further distinguish between these disorders, the pulsed-wave Doppler recordings of mitral and superior vena cava flow velocities can be compared. Patients with pulmonary disease have a marked increase in inspiratory superior vena cava systolic flow velocity (Fig. 22-17A, arrows), which is not seen in those with CP (Fig. 22-17B). DR = diastolic reversal.

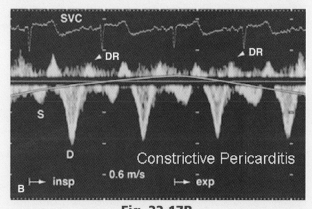

Fig. 22-17B

13. ANSWER: C. The most common primary neoplasm of the heart associated with pericardial effusion is angiosarcoma. Nearly 80% of cardiac angiosarcomas arise as mural masses in the right atrium. Typically, they completely replace the atrial wall and fill the entire cardiac chamber. They may invade adjacent structures (e.g., vena cava, tricuspid valve). These tumors are both symptomatic and rapidly fatal. Extensive pericardial spread and encasement of the heart often occur.

14. ANSWER: B. The most common location of a pericardial cyst is in the right cardiophrenic angle, where the cyst appears as a perfectly round fluid density, usually 2 to 4 cm in diameter, although some are much larger.

15. ANSWER: A. Loculated pericardial effusions can cause significant hemodynamic compromise, often when seen as a part of effusive-CP. Features of pericardial constriction can be transient and may resolve with the use of anti-inflammatory drugs. Features of cardiac tamponade are not dependent upon the volume of

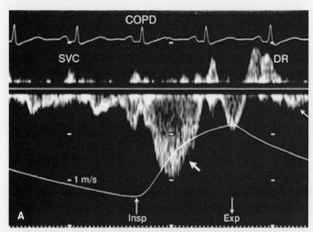

Fig. 22-17A

pericardial fluid collection but on rapidity of fluid collection. Rapid collection of small amounts of pericardial effusion can cause significant hemodynamic changes. Longstanding chronic CP may be associated with concomitant myocardial diseases or lead to epicardial fibrosis and myocardial atrophy.

16. *ANSWER: C.* Complete absence of the pericardium is associated with the enlargement of the right ventricle and shift of the heart to the left, resulting in more of the right ventricle being seen on the routine left parasternal echocardiogram. Unusual windows for obtaining traditional appearing images of the left ventricle are often needed.

17. *ANSWER: A.* Left pleural effusions can present as large echo-free spaces that resemble pericardial effusions. These can be recognized because they appear as very large posterior spaces without any anterior component. Generally, in the parasternal long-axis view, pleural effusions are located posterior to the descending aorta, whereas pericardial effusions are located anterior to the aorta.

18. *ANSWER: B.* Pericardial fluid can become loculated or compartmentalized. Loculated fluid in the pericardium or surrounding mediastinum under pressure may produce severe hemodynamic instability. Small effusions are generally confined to the region behind the left ventricle when the patient is in a supine position and may appear to vanish when the patient sits up, as they drain to the apical region.

19. *ANSWER: C.* This patient has a large loculated anterior pericardial effusion. Pericardial fat typically appears as anterior echo-free space on 2D echo. Pericardial fat usually can be distinguished from fluid because of subtle echogenicity resulting from the presence of fibrous material within the fat.

20. *ANSWER: D.* Figure 22-5 shows M-mode features of early diastolic collapse of the right ventricular free wall in cardiac tamponade. The yellow arrows point to right ventricular diastolic collapse. The * denotes the pericardial effusion. The primary abnormality is compression of all cardiac chambers due to increased pericardial pressure. The pericardium has some degree of elasticity; but once the elastic limit is reached, the heart must compete with the intrapericardial fluid for the fixed intrapericardial volume.

21. *ANSWER: A.* The respiratory variation of mitral and tricuspid flow velocities in cardiac tamponade is greatly increased and out of phase, reflecting the increased ventricular interdependence in which the hemodynamics of the left and right heart chambers are directly influenced by each other to a much greater degree than normal. In addition, patients with cardiac tamponade exhibit predominant systolic inflow through the hepatic vein or superior vena cava (with a

predominant X descent with little or no Y descent). In CP, the pattern of transmitral flow variation is comparable to that observed in cardiac tamponade; however, a prominent Y descent is often observed on a hepatic vein or superior vena cava flow Doppler study.

22. *ANSWER: C.* In CP, when intracardiac volume is less than that defined by the stiff pericardium, diastolic filling is unimpeded, and early diastolic filling occurs abnormally rapidly because venous pressure is elevated. The rapid early diastolic filling, which is halted abruptly when intracardiac volume reaches the limit set by the noncompliant pericardium, is reflected by the abrupt displacement of the interventricular septum into the left ventricle during early diastole (i.e., the septal bounce).

23. *ANSWER: B.* Paradoxical to the positive correlation between E/e' and PCWP in patients with myocardial disease, an inverse relationship is seen in patients with CP (Fig. 22-18). The likely explanation for this finding is the exaggerated longitudinal motion of the mitral annulus, despite high filling pressures in patients with CP. This is because the lateral expansion of the entire heart is limited by the constricting pericardium. The more severe the constriction with a higher filling pressure, the more accentuated is the longitudinal motion of the mitral annulus.

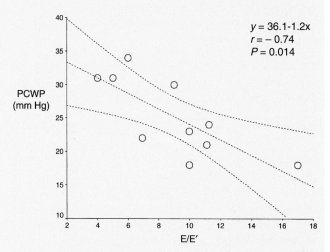

$y = 36.1-1.2x$
$r = -0.74$
$P = 0.014$

(From Ha, JW, Oh JK, Ling LH, et al. Annulus paradoxus: transmitral flow velocity to mitral annular velocity ratio is inversely proportional to pulmonary capillary wedge pressure in patients with constrictive pericarditis. *Circulation.* 2001;104:976, with permission.)

Fig. 22-18

24. *ANSWER: C.* Hepatic vein diastolic flow reversal with expiration suggests CP, even when the transmitral flow velocity pattern may not be diagnostic. Typical respiratory flow velocity changes in transmitral flow should not exclude the diagnosis, because up to 50% of patients with constriction may not meet these criteria. In such a situation, hepatic vein flow reversal that increases with expiration may still be seen and reflect the ventricular interaction and dissociation of intracardiac and intrathoracic pressures. The white arrow in Fig. 22-9 refers to hepatic vein diastolic reversal.

25. ANSWER: B. Although a pericardial effusion generally appears as echo-free space encircling the heart, sometimes echogenic materials such as fibrinous strands and shaggy exudative coating are found in pericardial effusion. Tuberculous pericardial effusion shows the highest prevalence of echogenic pericardial effusion, followed by malignant and idiopathic pericardial effusions.

26. ANSWER: A. Figure 22-11 shows respiratory variations in mitral E velocity and hepatic veins that are consistent with the diagnostic criterion for CP on Doppler echocardiography. The clinical presentation in this patient implies the presence of acute inflammatory pericarditis with constriction. CP in such a situation may resolve either spontaneously or in response to various combinations of nonsteroidal anti-inflammatory agents, steroids, and antibiotics. Specific antibiotic (e.g., antituberculous) therapy should be initiated in presence of a confirmed tubercular etiology. Diuretics can be used sparingly with the goal of reducing, not eliminating, elevated jugular pressure, edema, and ascites. The central venous pressure may take weeks to months to return to normal.

27. ANSWER: B. The resolution of edema and pleural effusion with documentation of reduction in pericardial thickening on computed tomography scan is consistent with the diagnosis of transient pericardial constriction.

KEY POINT:

■ In the absence of symptoms that suggest chronicity of disease (e.g., cachexia, atrial fibrillation, hepatic dysfunction, or pericardial calcification), patients with newly diagnosed CP who are hemodynamically stable may be given a trial of conservative management for 2 to 3 months before pericardiectomy is recommended.

28. ANSWER: B. Apical two-chamber and short-axis views of the left ventricle in Videos 22-1A and B show marked thickening of the parietal and visceral pericardium with a small loculated pericardial effusion. The Video 2-1C shows increased respiratory variation of transmitral flow. Both these features suggest presence of occult effusive-CP.

29. ANSWER: A. Significant pericardial disease can exist without overt manifestations. Occult constrictive pericardial disease is identified by normal baseline hemodynamics and normal LV systolic function with a characteristic response to rapid volume infusion. Following the intravenous administration of 1,000 ml of normal saline over 6–8 minutes, striking elevations of filling pressures are seen during cardiac catheterization.

KEY POINT:

■ In some patients, physical and hemodynamic features of constriction are not apparent in their baseline state; but when rapidly fluid challenged, they will present a typical hemodynamic CP pattern. This subgroup is called occult CP.

30. ANSWER: D. A cross-sectional contrast echocardiogram showing pericardial space containing a cloud of echogenic microbubbles is seen. Although pericardiocentesis is a relatively safe procedure, there are some hazards, particularly when hemorrhagic fluid is aspirated. Having the opportunity to outline the space from which the fluid is withdrawn is of particular interest in this situation. A current technique of echocardiography with contrast enhancement involves injection of a few milliliters of agitated saline solution. In the pericardium, contrast movement is slow and swirling and has a longer half-life. Performing this procedure helps in ensuring that the needle is within the pericardial cavity and not within the cardiac chambers.

31. ANSWER: C. During pericardiocentesis, a proposed entry point is marked on the patient's skin where the percutaneous needle should penetrate the chest wall. The transducer angle is noted as this will need to be replicated by the pericardiocentesis needle. The distance from the chest wall to the effusion and the distance to the nearest cardiac structure are determined as this will determine the maximum distance that the pericardial needle can be safely advanced. It is best to locate an acoustic window remote to the proposed puncture site. The transducer, if possible, is held in a direction orthogonal so that needle puncture can be directly visualized. If not, the imaging probe should be covered with a sterile cover and available for the physician performing the procedure to use if needed.

KEY POINT:

■ Contrast echocardiography is a simple, effective technique that aids localization of needle position during pericardiocentesis.

32. ANSWER: C. The upper panel in Figure 22-13 shows the respiratory changes in hepatic vein flow Doppler velocity profile. Presence of exaggerated diastolic flow reversals suggests possible CP. The lower panel in Figure 22-13 shows lack of significant respiratory changes (>25% variation) in transmitral flow velocities. In patients with symptoms and signs of right ventricular failure, Doppler echocardiography can be diagnostic for constriction if mitral inflow and hepatic vein flow velocities show characteristic respiratory changes. However, in the absence of significant respiratory changes, Doppler echocardiographic study should be repeated with maneuvers such as tilting, sitting, or diuresis.

33. ANSWER: B. Tilting, sitting, or diuresis helps in reducing preload in an effort to determine whether the characteristic Doppler velocity changes with respiration can be demonstrated.

KEY POINT:

◼ A lack of typical respiratory flow velocity changes should not exclude the diagnosis of CP because up to 50% of patients with CP may not meet these criteria.

34. ANSWER: B. Video 22-3A shows the apical four-chamber view of the left ventricle with a region of interest depicting longitudinal strain values obtained by speckle tracking imaging. With pericardial restraint and potential epicardial involvement, LV expansion in CP is limited in the circumferential rather than in the longitudinal direction. Accordingly, patients with CP have reduced circumferential strain. The mechanoelastic properties of the myocardium are relatively preserved in the longitudinal direction resulting in relatively preserved longitudinal early diastolic velocities and longitudinal myocardial strains.

35. ANSWER: C. Video 22-3B shows the apical short-axis view of the left ventricle with a region of interest showing the extent of apical rotation. Patients with CP

have significantly reduced net LV twist and torsion compared with normal subjects and those with restrictive cardiomyopathy (RCM). Although the base and mid cardiac rotation was relatively preserved, apical rotation was markedly reduced, including the peak systolic and diastolic rotation rates. The relationship between different principal strains and myocardial rotation are presented in Table 22-1.

TABLE 22-1   Myocardial Mechanics in CP and RCM

Deformation Parameter	CP	RCM
Longitudinal strain	Normal[a]	Decreased
Longitudinal early diastolic velocity	Normal or increased	Decreased
Circumferential strain	Decreased	Decreased
Net twist angle	Decreased	Normal
Apical untwisting velocity	Decreased	Normal[b]

[a]Except apical and lateral wall segments.
[b]Although normal in magnitude, early diastolic apical untwisting velocities may be delayed in timing.

(Reprinted from Dal-Bianco JP, Sengupta PP, Mookadam F, et al. Role of echocardiography in the diagnosis of constrictive pericarditis. *J Am Soc Echocardiogr.* 2009;22:24–33, with permission from Elsevier.)

KEY POINT:

◼ Pericardial tethering in constriction limits rotational and circumferential mechanics of the left ventricle, whereas the longitudinal mechanics are relatively normal.

SUGGESTED READINGS

Armstrong WF, Schilt BF, Helper DJ, et al. Diastolic collapse of the right ventricle with cardiac tamponade: an echocardiographic study. *Circulation.* 1982;65:1491.

Boonyaratavej S, Oh JK, Tajik AJ, et al. Comparison of mitral inflow and superior vena cava Doppler velocities in chronic obstructive pulmonary disease and constrictive pericarditis. *J Am Coll Cardiol.* 1998;32:2043.

Cheitlin MD, Armstrong WF, Aurigemma GP, et al. ACC/AHA/ASE 2003 guideline for the clinical application of echocardiography. Available at: www.acc.org/qualityandscience/clinical/statements.htm.

Dal-Bianco JP, Sengupta PP, Mookadam F, et al. Role of echocardiography in the diagnosis of constrictive pericarditis. *J Am Soc Echocardiogr.* 2009;22:24–33.

Engel PJ, Fowler NO, Tei CW, et al. M-mode echocardiography in constrictive pericarditis. *J Am Coll Cardiol.* 1985;6:471.

Feigenbaum H, Zaky A, Waldhausen JA. Use of ultrasound in the diagnosis of pericardial effusion. *Ann Intern Med.* 1966;65:443.

Gillam LD, Guyer DE, Gibson TC, et al. Hydrodynamic compression of the right atrium: a new echocardiographic sign of cardiac tamponade. *Circulation.* 1983;68:294.

Ha JW, Oh JK, Ling LH, et al. Annulus paradoxus: transmitral flow velocity to mitral annular velocity ratio is inversely proportional to pulmonary capillary wedge pressure in patients with constrictive pericarditis. *Circulation.* 2001;104:976.

Himelman RB, Kircher B, Rockey DC, et al. Inferior vena cava plethora with blunted respiratory response: a sensitive echocardiographic sign of cardiac tamponade. *J Am Coll Cardiol.* 1988; 12:1470.

Horowitz MS, Schultz CS, Stinson EB, et al. Sensitivity and specificity of echocardiographic diagnosis of pericardial effusion. *Circulation.* 1974;50:239.

Hynes JK, Tajik AJ, Osborn MJ, et al. Two-dimensional echocardiographic diagnosis of pericardial cyst. *Mayo Clin Proc.* 1983; 58:60.

Ling LH, Oh JK, Tei C, et al. Pericardial thickness measured with transesophageal echocardiography: feasibility and potential clinical usefulness. *J Am Coll Cardiol.* 1997;29:1317.

Oh JK, Tajik AJ, Appleton CP, et al. Preload reduction to unmask the characteristic Doppler features of constrictive pericarditis. A new observation. *Circulation*. 1997;95:796.

Payvandi MN, Kerber RE. Echocardiography in congenital and acquired absence of the pericardium. An echocardiographic mimic of right ventricular volume overload. *Circulation*. 1976; 53:86.

Rajagopalan N, Garcia MJ, Rodriguez L, et al. Comparison of new Doppler echocardiographic methods to differentiate constrictive pericardial heart disease and restrictive cardiomyopathy. *Am J Cardiol*. 2001;87:86.

Schiller NB, Botvinick EH. Right ventricular compression as a sign of cardiac tamponade: an analysis of echocardiographic ventricular dimensions and their clinical implications. *Circulation*. 1977;56: 774.

Sengupta PP, Krishnamoorthy VK, Abhayaratna WP, et al. Disparate patterns of left ventricular mechanics differentiate constrictive pericarditis from restrictive cardiomyopathy. *JACC Cardiovasc Imaging*. 2008;1:29–38.

Sengupta PP, Mohan JC, Mehta V, et al. Accuracy and pitfalls of early diastolic motion of the mitral annulus for diagnosing constrictive pericarditis by tissue Doppler imaging. *Am J Cardiol*. 2004;93: 886–890.

Sengupta PP, Mohan JC, Mehta V, et al. Doppler tissue imaging improves assessment of abnormal interventricular septal and posterior wall motion in constrictive pericarditis. *J Am Soc Echocardiogr*. 2005;18: 226–230.

Singh S, Wann LS, Schuchard GH, et al. Right ventricular and right atrial collapse in patients with cardiac tamponade—a combined echocardiographic and hemodynamic study. *Circulation*. 1984; 70:966.

Tyberg TI, Goodyer AVN, Hurst VW III, et al. Left ventricular filling in differentiating restrictive amyloid cardiomyopathy and constrictive pericarditis. *Am J Cardiol*. 1981;47:791.

Aortic Diseases

Gian M. Novaro and Craig R. Asher

1. When considering the size of the ascending aorta, which of the following is the most accurate statement?
   A. The diameter measurement should be made during end-systole.
   B. The size of the aorta is influenced by an individual's height.
   C. It is not feasible to measure the ascending aorta from transthoracic windows.
   D. The size of the aorta is most influenced by an individual's weight.

2. Which of the following statements regarding aortic anomalies is correct?
   A. A bovine aorta is defined as a left subclavian artery arising from the brachiocephalic artery.
   B. A bovine aortic branching pattern is present in 1% of individuals.
   C. A bovine aorta is readily detectable from a standard parasternal long-axis image.
   D. A bovine aorta is defined as a left common carotid artery arising from a common origin along with the brachiocephalic artery.

3. By echocardiography, an aortic intramural hematoma may be difficult to distinguish from which of the following?
   A. A descending thoracic aortic aneurysm with mural thrombus.
   B. An ascending thoracic aortic dissection.
   C. A descending thoracic aortic saccular aneurysm.
   D. Protruding mobile atheroma in the aortic arch.

4. The so-called "blind spot," which occurs when imaging the distal ascending aorta by transesophageal echocardiography is most commonly created by acoustic interference from which of the following structures?
   A. Sliding hiatal hernia.
   B. Right main bronchus.
   C. Trachea.
   D. Azygous vein.

5. In trauma cases, transesophageal echocardiography is a highly accurate tool in the evaluation of aortic injury and rupture. Which of the following findings is most consistent with a traumatic aortic injury of the thoracic aorta?
   A. A sessile irregularly bordered echodensity in the mid descending thoracic aorta.
   B. A markedly dilated ascending aorta and aortic arch.
   C. A mobile linear flap located just distal to the aortic isthmus.
   D. A mural echodensity in a large descending thoracic aortic aneurysm.

6. By imaging from the suprasternal notch, a diagnosis of coarctation of the aorta based on continuous-wave Doppler findings is most suggested by which of the following?
   A. Peak systolic velocity of 1.6 m/sec below the baseline, and pandiastolic flow of 0.4 m/sec above the baseline.
   B. Peak systolic velocity of 1.8 m/sec below the baseline.

C. Peak systolic velocity of 4 m/sec above the baseline.

D. Peak systolic velocity of 3.2 m/sec below the baseline, and pandiastolic flow below the baseline.

7. A 38-year-old man is seen in consultation for a bicuspid aortic valve. He brings with him a recent outside report of an echocardiogram that reports a bicuspid aortic valve with right-left fusion of cusps with moderate aortic stenosis and moderate aortic regurgitation (AVA = 1.2 cm²; P/M gradient = 44/25 mm Hg). The left ventricular function is normal with no left ventricular hypertrophy. The M-mode reports an aortic root measurement of 4.0 cm. Which of the following statements is correct?

A. Approximately 20% of patients undergoing aortic valve surgery with a bicuspid aortic valve require aortic surgery.

B. Approximately 20% of patients with a bicuspid aortic valve have coarctation of the aorta.

C. Most patients with bicuspid aortic valves have predominantly enlargement of the aortic sinuses.

D. The aortopathy of bicuspid aortic valve rarely involves the aortic arch.

8. An aneurysm of the ascending thoracic aorta is best characterized by which of the following definitions?

A. Aortic dilation to at least 1.5 times its reference diameter.

B. Aortic dilation to at least 2.0 times its reference diameter.

C. Aortic dilation of >3.5 cm.

D. Aortic dilation of at least 2.0 times the size of the aortic root.

9. Which of the following statements is correct regarding Marfan syndrome–related aortic disease?

A. Usually aortic enlargement is primarily in the region above the aortic root.

B. Involvement of the descending thoracic aorta with an aortic aneurysm without ascending thoracic aortic disease is rare.

C. Abdominal aortic aneurysms are common.

D. An "onion-bulb" appearance with enlargement of the aortic root, sino-tubular junction effacement, and a relatively normal size tubular aorta are commonly seen.

10. Of the following echocardiographic characteristics, which of the following is most predictive of an adverse outcome in the presence of an aortic intramural hematoma?

A. Maximal hematoma thickness of >11 mm.

B. Hematoma location in the distal descending thoracic aorta.

C. Absence of a penetrating aortic ulcer.

D. Presence of echolucent areas in the hematoma.

11. A 68-year-old man undergoes a cardiac catheterization, which demonstrates no significant obstructive coronary artery disease. Within 1 hour after the catheterization, he complains of severe chest pain. The electrocardiogram is normal. An aortic dissection is diagnosed by a transesophageal echocardiogram. A cardiac surgeon is called. The cardiologist tells the surgeon that the dissection should be classified as a DeBakey type 2/Stanford A with a variant form limited, iatrogenic hematoma. Which of the following statements are correct?

A. There is an intramural aortic hematoma in the aortic arch.

B. There is likely severe aortic regurgitation.

C. The aortic dissection extends throughout the aorta to the femoral artery.

D. There is an intramural aortic hematoma in the ascending aorta.

12. Which of the following statements regarding a right-sided aortic arch is correct?

A. The aberrant right subclavian artery can compress the esophagus.

B. It can be diagnosed by the anterior compression of a barium-filled esophagus.

C. The nonmirror image type is rarely associated with congenital cardiac anomalies.

D. The mirror image type often occurs with normal cardiac structure.

13. Which of the following series of aortic dimensions would be considered pathologic for a 30-year-old woman (height—72 inches/183 cm) undergoing a transthoracic echocardiogram for chest pain?
    A. Annulus—2.6 cm; sinus—3.2 cm; ST junction—3.5 cm; tubular—3.6 cm.
    B. Annulus—2.0 cm; sinus—3.6 cm; ST junction—3.4 cm; tubular—3.4 cm.
    C. Annulus—2.2 cm; sinus—3.6 cm; ST junction— 3.3 cm; tubular—3.4 cm.
    D. Annulus—1.9 cm; sinus—3.7 cm; ST junction—3.4 cm; tubular—3.6 cm.

14. Which of the following pairings of aortic abnormalities and disease states or syndromes is correct?
    A. Supravalvular aortic stenosis–Turner syndrome.
    B. Aortic coarctation–Shone complex.
    C. Aortic coarctation–Noonan syndrome.
    D. Right aortic arch–Down syndrome.

15. Which of the following anatomic abnormalities of the aorta is most likely to be associated with cyanotic heart disease requiring corrective surgery during infancy?
    A. An aorta overriding the ventricular septum with a malalignment ventricular septal defect.
    B. An aorta that is anterior to the pulmonary artery associated with atrioventricular discordance and ventricular-arterial discordance.
    C. An aorta that is anterior to the pulmonary artery associated with atrioventricular concordance and ventricular-arterial discordance.
    D. A periductal aorta-pulmonary connection with normal pulmonary pressure.

16. A 67-year-old woman is admitted to the hospital with a 2-day history of hemianopsia. A head computed tomography scan reveals multiple ischemic infarcts suggestive of emboli and a transesophageal echocardiogram is obtained to evaluate a source of embolism.

    Based on Figure 23-1, showing the distal aortic arch, which of the following is most likely true about this patient's condition?

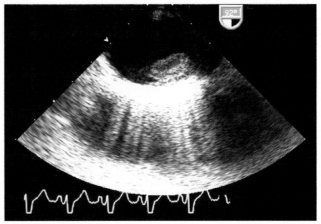

Fig. 23-1

A. There is a predisposition to aortic dissection.
B. The treatment of choice is systemic anticoagulation.
C. It is a common complication of aortic aneurysms.
D. It can be a complication of systemic bacteremia.

17. A 78-year-old man has undergone a transesophageal echocardiogram for chest pain and atrial fibrillation prior to cardioversion. Which of the following statements regarding Figure 23-2 is correct (the white arrow points to the structure of interest)?

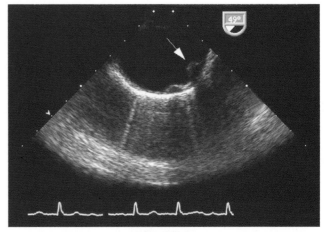

Fig. 23-2

A. The finding seen in this aorta can be graded as severe.
B. The finding seen in this aorta can be graded as mild.
C. The finding seen represents an intramural hematoma.
D. The finding seen is located in the ascending aorta.

18. Based on Figure 23-3, which of the following statements is true about this patient's abnormality?

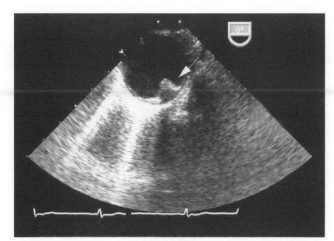

Fig. 23-3

A. The treatment of choice is endovascular stent grafting.
B. It is associated with an increased risk of stroke and cardiovascular events.
C. It may progress to a pseudoaneurysm.
D. It presents with fever, constitutional symptoms, and back pain.

19. A 42-year-old woman underwent a transthoracic echocardiogram due to an episode of congestive heart failure. The aortic valve was found to be bicuspid. Which of the following statements is true regarding the continuous-wave Doppler signal obtained from the suprasternal notch (Fig. 23-4)?

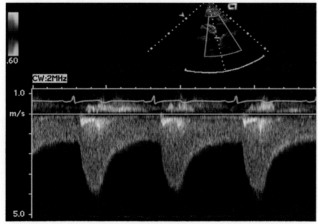

Fig. 23-4

A. It represents severe aortic regurgitation.
B. It suggests severe coarctation of the aorta.
C. It is consistent with mild coarctation of the aorta.
D. It can be seen in sinus of Valsalva rupture with fistula formation.

20. A 68-year-old man underwent a transthoracic echocardiogram because of poorly controlled hypertension. Based on Figure 23-5 (see structure noted by arrow) and Video 23-1, which of the following findings is most likely to be present?

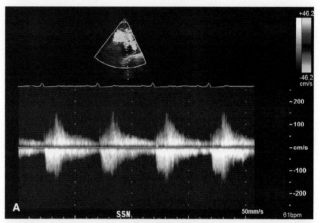

Fig. 23-5A

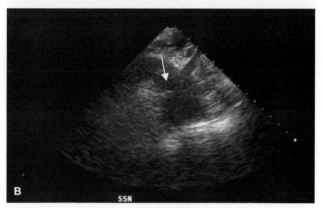

Fig. 23-5B

A. Rib notching on plain radiograph of the chest.
B. A redundant and tortuous distal aortic arch.
C. Right arm systemic hypertension.
D. An ascending thoracic aortic aneurysm.

21. A 37-year-old man is undergoing a routine out-patient transthoracic echocardiogram because of palpitations. His physical examination is unremarkable. An abnormality is noted, which prompts a transesophageal echocardiogram. From the short- and long-axis views in Figure 23-6, which of the following is true of the abnormality shown (see arrow)?

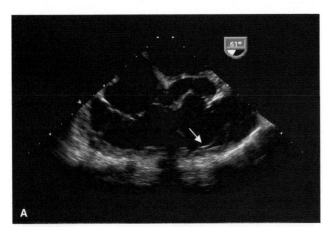

Fig. 23-6A

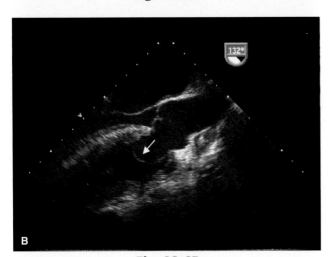

Fig. 23-6B

A. It is located on the left coronary sinus.
B. It can be the result of endocarditis.
C. It is more common in females.
D. It is rarely of congenital origin.

22. A 41-year-old man underwent echocardiography because of a heart murmur. On physical examination, he is 6 feet 10 inches tall, and weighs 249 pounds (body surface area is 2.56 m²). He was found to have a dilated ascending aorta as seen on the parasternal long-axis image in Figure 23-7. The maximum measured diameter of the aortic root at the sinuses of Valsalva was 4.3 cm (measured during end-diastole). Based on these findings, which of the following is most accurate?

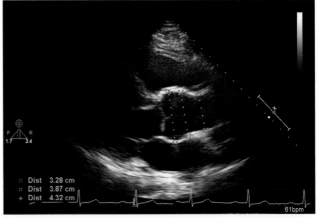

Fig. 23-7

A. The aortic size as measured is unreliable because transthoracic echocardiography of the ascending aorta is inaccurate.
B. He should be referred for elective prophylactic aortic repair given an aortic size of >4.0 cm.
C. Based on his height and body surface area, an aortic size of 4.3 cm is within the range of normal limits.
D. The aortic size is inaccurate because it was measured during end-diastole.

23. In the parasternal long-axis transthoracic image in Figure 23-8, which structure is denoted by the arrow?

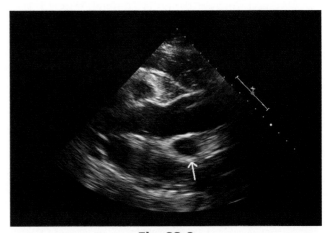

Fig. 23-8

A. The ascending thoracic aorta.
B. The superior vena cava.
C. The left pulmonary artery.
D. The right pulmonary artery.

24. A 54-year-old man underwent transthoracic echocardiography because of chest pain. On physical examination, he is 5 feet 8 inches tall, and weighs 213 pounds (body surface area is 2.15 m²). His aortic morphology, shown in Figure 23-9, is best described by which of the following? Note that the calibration on the left side of the image correspond to 1 cm each.

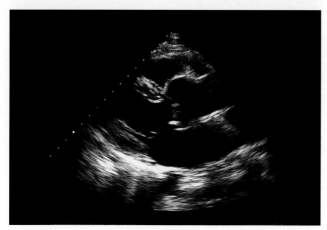

Fig. 23-9

A. Diffuse ascending aortic dilation.

B. Dilation of the sinuses of Valsalva and proximal tubular ascending aorta.

C. Dilation of the mid tubular ascending aorta.

D. Dilation of the sinuses of Valsalva with preserved sino-tubular junction.

E. Dilation of the sinuses of Valsalva with effacement of the sino-tubular junction.

25. An 80-year-old hypertensive man presents to the emergency department with the sudden onset of acute severe tearing back pain. Initial cardiac enzymes and electrocardiogram are normal. He has a history of chronic kidney disease stage III and therefore a transesophageal echocardiogram is obtained. Which of the following diagnoses is most accurate based on Figure 23-10?

A. A proximal type A aortic dissection with a thrombosed false lumen.

B. An aortic aneurysm with a prior elephant trunk surgery.

C. A distal type B aortic dissection with patent true and false lumen.

D. A proximal type A aortic dissection with patent true and false lumen.

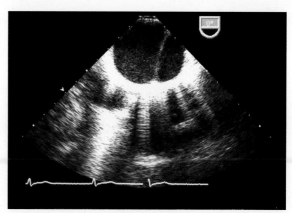

Fig. 23-10

CASE 1:

A 47-year-old man presented with intermittent substernal chest pain during the preceding week. His past medical history was significant for reactive arthritis for the past 15 years. On presentation, he was afebrile and nontoxic appearing. Cardiovascular examination disclosed a grade II/VI early peaking systolic ejection murmur at the base and a grade I/VI decrescendo diastolic murmur radiating to the left lower sternal border. Figures 23-11A and B from a transesophageal echocardiogram show the long-axis and apical four-chamber views, respectively. Arrowhead points to the finding of interest.

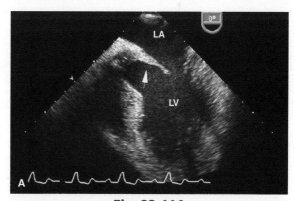

Fig. 23-11A

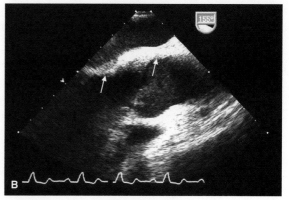

Fig. 23-11B

26. Which of the following statements about the abnormality shown is correct?

    A. It can be mistaken echocardiographically for a periaortic abscess.

    B. It commonly occurs in association with systemic lupus erythematosus.

    C. Intramural areas of echolucency are a common finding.

    D. Progression to an intramural dissection flap is imminent.

27. Regarding the related aortic valve abnormalities, which of the following is most likely to be true?

    A. Aortic valve vegetations are a common associated finding.

    B. Aortic regurgitation rarely develops and if present, is often trivial.

    C. Thickening of the aortic-mitral curtain aids in the diagnosis.

    D. Aortic valve perforations and leaflet dehiscence may occur.

CASE 2:

A 44-year-old woman with a history of severe aortic regurgitation underwent aortic valve replacement surgery with an aortic homograft. The postpump intraoperative transesophageal echocardiogram confirmed a normal functioning aortic homograft and an intact ascending aorta. Her postoperative course was uneventful. One month later during a baseline postoperative echocardiogram, an abnormality of the homograft was noted. She denied fevers, night sweats, or chest pain.

28. Based on Videos 23-2A–C, which of the following aortic abnormalities is most likely to be present?

    A. Typical postoperative changes related to homograft insertion.

    B. Proximal type A aortic dissection.

    C. Postoperative periaortic hematoma.

    D. Early prosthetic valve (homograft) endocarditis.

29. Which of the following flows would be considered to be pathological in a patient with an aortic homograft?

    A. Central aortic regurgitation with a vena contracta width of 0.3 cm.

    B. Eccentric aortic regurgitation with a vena contracta width of 0.2 cm.

    C. A high velocity systolic flow entering the left ventricular outflow tract.

    D. A 2.5 m/sec systolic flow through the aortic valve.

CASE 3:

A 58-year-old man with a history of Hodgkin's lymphoma presents with symptomatic coronary artery disease and calcific aortic stenosis. As part of his preoperative evaluation, transthoracic echocardiography is performed (Fig. 23-12).

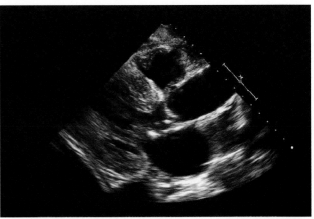

Fig. 23-12

30. Which of the following statements is most accurate regarding the abnormality affecting the aorta in this patient?

    A. The abnormality does not impact the risk of aortic valve surgery.

    B. The abnormality can be readily estimated on the basis of manual palpation.

    C. The abnormality can alter the surgical approach of aortic valve surgery.

    D. The abnormality is not related to the risk of perioperative stroke.

31. When attempting to detect atherosclerosis of the aorta, which of the following provides the most accurate information?

    A. Epiaortic echocardiography.

    B. Manual palpation by an experienced surgeon.

    C. Transthoracic echocardiography.

    D. Transesophageal echocardiography.

CASE 4:

A 73-year-old man presents with severe, sudden onset of back pain of 7-hour duration. The presence of a myocardial infarction is ruled out. He undergoes a transesophageal echocardiogram to evaluate the aorta given his persistent back pain. The images reveal an abnormality, which helps confirm the diagnosis.

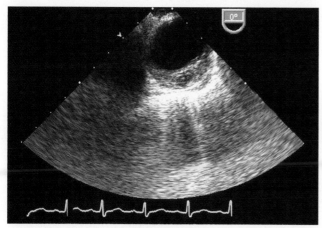

Fig. 23-13

32. Based on Figure 23-13, the most likely diagnosis is?
    A. A distal type B aortic dissection with thrombosed false lumen.
    B. Severe descending thoracic aortic atheromatous disease.
    C. A descending thoracic aortic rupture with a pseudoaneurysm.
    D. A descending thoracic aortic intramural hematoma.

33. Based on Figure 23-13, which of the following statements is true?
    A. The expected in-hospital mortality risk of this patient exceeds 30%.
    B. As opposed to classic aortic dissection, the mortality rates for type A and type B intramural hematoma are similar.
    C. The most likely long-term evolution for the abnormality shown is aortic aneurysm or pseudoaneurysm.

D. The treatment of choice for this condition in urgent aortic repair.

CASE 5:

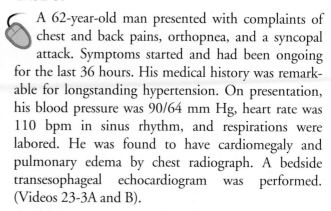

A 62-year-old man presented with complaints of chest and back pains, orthopnea, and a syncopal attack. Symptoms started and had been ongoing for the last 36 hours. His medical history was remarkable for longstanding hypertension. On presentation, his blood pressure was 90/64 mm Hg, heart rate was 110 bpm in sinus rhythm, and respirations were labored. He was found to have cardiomegaly and pulmonary edema by chest radiograph. A bedside transesophageal echocardiogram was performed. (Videos 23-3A and B).

34. After reviewing the echocardiographic Videos 23-3A and B, which of the following therapies is most appropriate in this patient's management?
    A. Emergent surgical repair.
    B. Urgent pericardiocentesis.
    C. High-dose intravenous hydrocortisone.
    D. Intravenous beta-blocker therapy.

35. Based on the clinical history and Videos 23-3A and B, which of the following statements is correct?
    A. Most patients with proximal aortic dissection are hypotensive upon presentation.
    B. Congestive heart failure is seen in half of acute type A aortic dissection cases.
    C. Syncope occurs in 1 out of 10 patients with type A aortic dissection.
    D. Pulse deficits are frequently occurring physical signs in proximal dissection.

ANSWERS

1. ANSWER: B. The size of the ascending aorta correlates with several anthropometric measures. Aortic size correlates most closely with body height and body surface area, and with increasing age. Aortic size correlates less well with body weight as an isolated factor. In a majority of patients, the proximal to mid portion of the ascending aorta can be adequately imaged from the transthoracic left parasternal window from various intercostal spaces. Because it is subject to pulsatile blood flow, its size varies between systole (expands) and diastole (recoil). Thus if the aorta can be imaged adequately throughout the cardiac cycle, it should be ideally imaged during diastole. By echocardiography, measurements should be made using the internal diameters, perpendicular to the axis of blood flow. For the aortic root at the sinus level, the widest diameter should be used.

2. ANSWER: D. The term "bovine aortic arch" refers to a common anatomic variant pattern of the aortic arch. Although a common misnomer (the human bovine aortic arch variant does not resemble the aortic arch pattern found in cattle), it remains a widely used descriptive term in the medical literature. In the common configurations referred to as bovine aortic arch, the innominate artery and the left common carotid artery have a common origin (Fig. 23-14) or the left common carotid artery originates directly from the innominate artery. In both of these variants, there are two great vessels that stem from the aortic arch. These aortic configurations occur in about 9%–13% of patients.

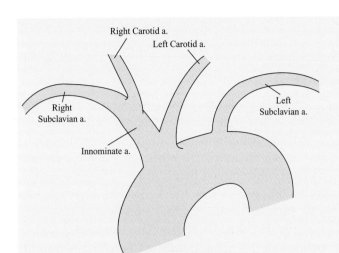

Fig. 23-14

In a true bovine aortic arch (seen in cattle), a single great vessel comes off the aortic arch as a large brachiocephalic trunk, from which both subclavian arteries and a bicarotid trunk originate. The bicarotid trunk divides into the left and right common carotid arteries.

The aortic arch and great vessels are not visualized from the standard parasternal window but can be best imaged from the suprasternal notch.

3. ANSWER: A. Aortic intramural hematoma is characterized by echocardiography as a circumferential or crescent-shaped smooth-margined thickening of the aortic wall without an intimal flap. The degree of aortic wall thickening should be >5–7 mm. Intimal calcium may be displaced by the accumulation of medial hematoma. Echolucent areas in the aortic wall may be seen suggestive of noncommunicating blood in the medial hematoma. An intramural hematoma is generally continuous over a relatively localized or extensive portion of the aorta.

Aortic atheromatous disease and aortic aneurysms with mural thrombus can be commonly encountered diagnostic challenges. Important distinguishing features of intramural hematoma are its smooth aortic wall contour, continuous nature, and its echogenic border due to displaced intimal calcium. In contrast, aneurysms with mural thrombus have irregular borders, and the thrombus is located above the calcified intima. Aortic atheromatous disease often has irregular borders with protruding and/or mobile components, scattered areas of calcification, and is not continuous.

4. ANSWER: C. A potential limitation of transesophageal echocardiography in the evaluation of the thoracic aorta is the so-called "blind spot." This area is the 3–6 cm portion of the distal ascending aorta and proximal arch. The blind spot is caused by the interposition of air, most commonly from the trachea or left main bronchus, causing acoustic interference between the transducer and the aorta. The blind spot is not caused by interference from the right main bronchus or azygous vein. Although a hiatal hernia may interfere with cardiac imaging from the mid to lower transesophageal windows, it is not the cause of the aortic blind spot. Despite the potential for the blind spot to interfere in aortic imaging, the diffuse processes of the aorta rarely render the blind spot a significant limitation.

5. ANSWER: C. Transesophageal echocardiographic imaging of the aorta is a highly accurate method of aortic evaluation in patients with deceleration and blunt chest trauma. Characteristic echocardiographic findings suggestive of aortic injury include the presence of an intraluminal flap located near or just distal to the aortic isthmus, or near the gastroesophageal junction. The intraluminal flap is usually mobile, may be extensive or localized to a short segment of the aorta, and usually occurs at points of attachment such as the sinuses of Valsalva, the isthmus, and the diaphragm. Alternatively, intraluminal masses suggestive of discrete thrombus formation can be seen and typically occur at the arch, isthmus, or near the diaphragm; in these cases, development of aortic thrombus occurs in areas overlying intimal tears or injury.

A sessile irregularly bordered echodensity located in the mid descending thoracic aorta is descriptive of aortic atheromatous disease. The presence of a dilated ascending aorta alone is not consistent with aortic injury. A mural echodensity in a large descending thoracic aortic aneurysm is most suggestive of mural thrombus.

6. ANSWER: D. Coarctation of the aorta can be best imaged echocardiographically from the suprasternal view. Doppler assessment can yield information on the severity of the aortic narrowing and the modified Bernoulli equation can be employed to estimate peak systolic pressure gradients. Imaging from the suprasternal notch, a Doppler pattern suggestive of coarctation shows elevated systolic velocities (generally >2.0 m/sec),

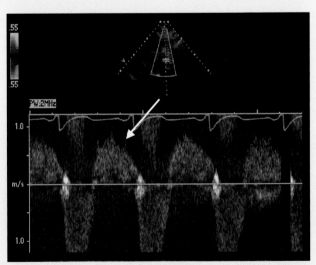

Fig. 23-15

seen as Doppler signals below the baseline. In cases of significant coarctation, persistent forward flow during diastole will be present in the descending aorta and detected by Doppler as diastolic flow velocity signals below the baseline. From the suprasternal notch, elevated Doppler flow velocities during diastole above the baseline would be suggestive of persistent diastolic flow reversals as seen in severe aortic regurgitation or sinus of Valsalva aneurysm rupture with aortic fistula formation (Fig. 23-15). The white arrow points to high velocity holodiastolic flow reversal consistent with severe aortic regurgitation as seen from the suprasternal notch.

7. ANSWER: A. Bicuspid aortic valves are associated with ascending aortic dilation with a prevalence ranging up to 50%–60%. The underlying predisposition is likely related to genetic abnormalities of connective tissue, along with tensile stresses, which render the aorta susceptible to dilation, aneurysm, and aortic instability. When presenting for aortic valve surgery, the ACC/AHA guidelines recommend elective aortic repair when the aortic size reaches >4.5 cm. On average, about 20% of bicuspid aortic valve patients undergoing cardiac surgery require concomitant aortic repair because of aortic dilation.

Although the connective tissue changes are poorly characterized and aortic alteration is heterogeneous, there are distinct patterns of ascending aortic dilation, which occur with bicuspid aortic valves. Pattern I involves the aortic root only; pattern II involves the aortic root and tubular ascending aorta; pattern III involves the tubular ascending and the aortic arch; and pattern IV involves the aortic root, tubular ascending, and aortic arch. The most commonly dilated portion of the ascending aorta is the tubular ascending aorta (present in 88% of dilated bicuspid aortas). Isolated aortic root dilation (pattern I) occurs in a minority of bicuspid aortas (~12%), whereas aortic arch involvement can occur in up to 73% of cases.

Coarctation of the aorta is a commonly associated congenital malformation, which develops in patients with bicuspid aortic valves. It occurs in ~5% of all bicuspid aortic valve patients. Conversely, in those with coarctation of the aorta, a bicuspid valve is present >50% of the time.

8. ANSWER: A. Aneurysmal dilatation of an artery, by definition, is a localized or diffuse dilation with a diameter at least 1.5 times greater than the normal reference size of the artery. That is, if the ascending aorta is normally 3.0 cm in diameter, an aortic aneurysm would be present if the maximal diameter was >4.5 cm. Dilation of 1.1 to 1.5 times the normal is referred to as ectasia.

9. ANSWER: D. Marfan syndrome is a systemic disorder of connective tissue characterized by a proximal aortic aneurysm and other cardiovascular, skeletal, and ocular abnormalities. The condition is caused by a genetic mutation in the matrix protein fibrillin 1 and affected by deregulation of transforming growth factor β. A principal manifestation (major criteria) of the disease is dilation/aneurysms of the ascending aorta involving at least the sinuses of Valsalva, the site generally of greatest dilation. This is in contrast to bicuspid aortic valves, where the tubular ascending aorta is the most common and greatest dilated segment. Dilation/aneurysms of the descending thoracoabdominal aorta are not uncommon, and represent one of the minor criteria in the diagnosis of Marfan syndrome. Notably, they can develop in the absence of coexisting ascending aortic aneurysms. Isolated true abdominal aortic aneurysms, however, are relatively rare.

10. ANSWER: A. Aortic location and imaging findings are important predictors of unfavorable clinical outcomes in patients with aortic intramural hematoma. A significant independent predictor of adverse outcomes in acute type A hematoma is an initial hematoma thickness of >11 mm. Location in the ascending thoracic aorta also identifies a greater risk as opposed to the descending aorta. For both ascending and descending locations, the presence of echolucent spaces in the hematoma is not a finding supportive of adverse outcome. The finding of an intramural hematoma associated with a penetrating aortic ulcer is significantly associated with a progressive disease course and adverse outcome.

11. ANSWER: D. Several classification systems have been developed to describe aortic dissections. There are three systems commonly in use and are based either on the location/extent of the dissection or on the type of aortic syndrome (Table 23-1). The DeBakey classification has types I, II, IIIa, and IIIb and is based on

TABLE 23-1 Classification Systems for Acute Aortic Dissection/Syndromes

DeBakey Classification	Region of Aorta Involved
Type I	Ascending, arch, descending
Type II	Ascending only
Type IIIa	Descending (above diaphragm)
Type IIIb	Descending (below diaphragm)

Stanford Classification	Region of Aorta Involved
Type A	Ascending (proximal to left subclavian artery)
Type B	Descending (distal to left subclavian artery)

Svensson Classification	Type of Aortic Syndrome
Class 1	Classic intimal flap (2 lumens)
Class 2	Intramural hematoma (no intimal flap)
Class 3	Localized intimal flap
Class 4	Penetrating aortic ulcer
Class 5	Iatrogenic/posttraumatic

the location/extent of aortic dissection. The Stanford classification has types A and B and is based on whether the dissection is in the proximal or distal aorta. The Svensson classification has classes 1–5 and is based on the type of aortic syndrome.

Our patient developed a DeBakey type 2/Stanford A with a variant form limited, iatrogenic hematoma. DeBakey type 2 refers to the ascending aortic location, Stanford A implies a proximal aortic location, and by Svensson classification there is a class 5 iatrogenic intramural hematoma.

12. ANSWER: C. There are two types of a right-sided aortic arch: mirror image and nonmirror image (aberrant left subclavian). The mirror image type is commonly associated with congenital heart disease (tetralogy of Fallot, pulmonary atresia with ventricular septal defect); whereas nonmirror image type (the most common form) is infrequently associated with other congenital cardiac malformations. In the mirror-image right arch (Fig. 23-16A), the left innominate artery originates as the first branch, followed by right carotid artery, and right subclavian artery (labels 1–3). In non–mirror-image right aortic arch (see Fig. 23-16B), the sequence of branching is left carotid artery, right carotid artery, right subclavian artery, then left subclavian artery (the fourth branch of the aorta; labels 1–4). The left (aberrant) subclavian artery originates from the proximal descending aorta often with a prominent diverticulum (of Kommerell) at its origin. The artery courses behind the esophagus and can produce a vascular ring with esophageal compression, which can be diagnosed by posterior impression of a barium-filled esophagus. Another variety of right aortic arch branching is the right arch with a left descending aorta. In this form, the

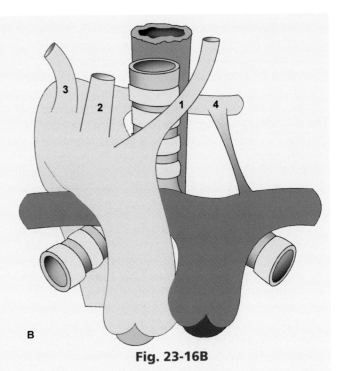

B

Fig. 23-16B

descending aortic arch crosses the midline toward the left side by a retroesophageal route.

13. ANSWER: A. There is limited data on the normal reference sizes of the ascending aorta in adults as measured by transthoracic echocardiography. From a recent large population study, the sizes of the ascending aorta closely correlate with age and body surface area. Over time, the ascending aorta shows a faster growth rate during early adulthood as compared to older age. In general, the diameter at the sinus of Valsalva is larger than the tubular portion of the ascending aorta (mean difference between the sinuses and tubular portion is 0.2 cm in men and 0.1 cm in women). Thus, the presence of a tubular ascending aorta of greater diameter than the reference sinus of Valsalva likely represents a pathologic process and abnormal aortic dilation.

14. ANSWER: B. Shone complex is a rare congenital heart disease comprised typically of four obstructive left heart lesions: supravalvular mitral ring, parachute-like mitral valve, subaortic stenosis, and aortic coarctation. Although coarctation of the aorta is common, obstruction of the left ventricular outflow can include subaortic stenosis, valvular aortic stenosis, and bicuspid aortic valve.

Turner syndrome (or gonadal dysgenesis) has commonly recognized cardiac malformations. The most common cardiac defects are coarctation of the aorta and bicuspid aortic valve. Other abnormalities associated with Turner syndrome can include aortic dissection, aortic sinus, and ascending aortic aneurysm. Noonan syndrome is a common genetic disease typified by facial anomalies, short stature, webbed neck, undescended

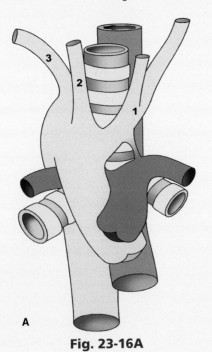

A

Fig. 23-16A

testes, and congenital heart defects. The classic cardiac malformations reported in Noonan syndrome are pulmonary stenosis and hypertrophic cardiomyopathy. Down syndrome (or trisomy 21) is frequently associated with congenital heart defects. The most common cardiac abnormalities are atrioventricular septal defects (or endocardial cushion defect), and ventricular septal defects. Other associated defects in Down syndrome include atrial septal defects and tetralogy of Fallot.

15. ANSWER: C. An aorta that is anterior to the pulmonary artery associated with atrioventricular concordance and ventricular-arterial discordance refers to the anatomic configuration of D-transposition of the great arteries. D-transposition (complete or uncorrected transposition) is a cyanotic congenital heart defect in which the aorta is anterior and to the right of the pulmonary artery. It is characterized by the aorta arising from the morphologic right ventricle and the pulmonary artery arising from the morphologic left ventricle, resulting in two separate circulatory systems. The condition is often diagnosed in utero by ultrasound, but if not, cyanosis upon birth will immediately lead to the diagnosis.

An aorta that is anterior to the pulmonary artery associated with atrioventricular discordance and ventricular-arterial discordance refers to L-transposition or congenitally corrected transposition. L-transposition is an acyanotic congenital heart defect in which the aorta is anterior and to the left of the pulmonary artery (Fig. 23-17). It is characterized by double discordance (a "double switch"), where the atrial and ventricular connections are discordant, and the ventricular connections to the great arteries are also discordant. Blood flow is from the right atrium into the right-sided morphologic left ventricle, through the pulmonary artery to the lungs and returning from the pulmonary veins into the left atrium, to the left-sided morphologic right ventricle, and to the aorta. Since circulation is physiologically corrected, patients survive into adulthood.

An aorta overriding the ventricular septum with a malaligned ventricular septal defect describes tetralogy of Fallot. This cyanotic heart defect is classically described by four malformations: a ventricular septal defect, pulmonary stenosis, an overriding aorta, and right ventricular hypertrophy. The degree of pulmonary stenosis varies and is the main determinant of disease severity and degree of cyanosis. This condition is often diagnosed at birth or during the first year of life, depending on cyanosis severity. A periductal aorta-pulmonary connection with normal pulmonary pressure refers to a patent ductus arteriosus. When a patent ductus remains untreated, depending on its size, pulmonary hypertension and heart failure can develop. In the absence of pulmonary hypertension, the condition is well tolerated and can persist into adulthood. Figure 23-17 demonstrates the orientation of the aortic and pulmonary valve as seen from the parasternal short axis view with normal

anatomy compared with D or L type transposition of the great arteries. AV = aortic valve; PV = pulmonic valve.

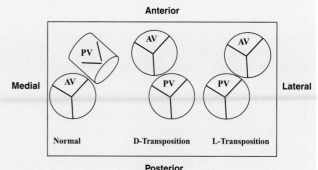

Fig. 23-17

16. ANSWER: B. The transesophageal echocardiographic image depicts a large mobile aortic thrombus in the distal aortic arch/proximal descending thoracic aorta in the absence of significant aortic atheroma. Although most sources of embolism from the aorta are related to atherosclerotic lesions, isolated free floating aortic thrombi can occur. A majority of these thrombi develop in areas of diffuse atheromatous disease, but in rare cases, they develop in an aorta free of overt atherosclerotic changes. When they develop, the common locations for aortic thrombi are the arch, near the ostium of the left subclavian artery, or on the posterior segment of the distal aortic arch near the isthmus. Frequently, the insertion site of the thrombus is at a small atherosclerotic plaque. In a fraction of cases, an underlying thrombophilic state exists, such as antiphospholipid antibody syndrome or malignancy. Although definitive therapy has not been well defined, an initial strategy of anticoagulant therapy appears reasonable. However, if recurrent embolic events occur, surgical removal of the aortic thrombi may be necessary.

Mobile aortic thrombi do not predispose to aortic dissection, although they may be seen in the presence of traumatic aortic disruption. Aortic aneurysms may be complicated by thrombus formation but in these cases, thrombi are usually of the mural, layered variety and rarely pedunculated. Systemic bacteremia may infect the aorta leading to an aortitis. However, this occurs in areas of significant aortic atheromatous burden.

17. ANSWER: A. The transesophageal echocardiographic image shown depicts severe aortic atheromatous plaque in the descending thoracic aorta. Plaque size can be graded on the basis of intimal thickness: 2–4 mm, mild, grade 1; >4 mm, moderate, grade 2; >4 mm with diffuse calcification, mobile plaques, or ulcerated lesions, grade 3. Plaque thickness as assessed by echocardiography has been identified as an independent risk factor for embolic events. Protruding aortic plaques of >4 mm are strongly associated with risk of ischemic stroke. Plaque composition and mobility have also been shown to predict embolic complications.

Noncalcified plaques and mobile plaque components present an even greater embolic risk.

18. ANSWER: B. The transesophageal image shows the descending thoracic aorta on a transverse plane. There is a large aortic atheromatous plaque on the posterior wall of the aorta (see white arrow in Fig. 23-3). The plaque protrudes ~0.7 cm and is only mildly calcified. As described in the prior question, plaque size can be graded on the basis of its thickness: 2–4 mm, mild, grade 1; >4 mm, moderate, grade 2; >4 mm with diffuse calcification, mobile component, or ulcerated lesion, grade 3. Embolic complications occur at a rate of nearly 20% per year in patients with large aortic atheromatous plaques. This echocardiographic characteristic (i.e., plaque thickness) can be a prognosticator of embolic events. Protruding aortic plaques >4 mm have been strongly associated with risk of ischemic stroke. Furthermore, plaques with little calcification and plaques with mobile components pose an even greater embolic risk.

The management of significant aortic atheromatous disease is controversial. The initial treatment of choice is geared at lipid lowering with statin drugs, and anticoagulation/antiplatelet therapy. Systemic anticoagulation with warfarin remains controversial, partly due to inadequate available prospective data. Whether complete systemic anticoagulation with warfarin is more effective than antiplatelet therapy in patients with aortic atheromatous disease for the prevention of vascular events is not clear. However, endovascular stent grafting is not considered a useful strategy in this setting.

Aortic atheromatous debris does not predispose to aortic instability, such as risk of aortic dissection or pseudoaneurysm formation. Its presentation is most often related to systemic embolic events. Fever, constitutional symptoms, and back pain are symptoms most attributable to an inflammatory aortic aneurysm. Rarely, bacterial aortitis can develop in aortic segments with advanced atheromatous disease; but echocardiographic findings would show highly mobile plaque components suggestive of infected atherothrombotic material (i.e., vegetations).

19. ANSWER: B. The continuous-wave Doppler signal is most consistent with a severe coarctation of the aorta. This aortic abnormality can be imaged best from the suprasternal view. Doppler assessment can yield information on the severity of the aortic narrowing, and the modified Bernoulli equation can be employed to estimate peak systolic pressure gradients. By imaging from the suprasternal notch, a continuous-wave Doppler signal will show elevated systolic velocities (in this case ~4.0 m/sec). When the coarctation is severe, persistent forward flow during diastole will occur and is detected by Doppler as pandiastolic flow velocity profiles (in this case ~1.5 m/sec). In cases of mild coarctation, there will be no significant residual blood flow moving antegrade during diastole.

In cases of severe aortic regurgitation and sinus of Valsalva aneurysm rupture with aortic fistula formation, there are significant Doppler flow reversals seen during diastole, which could be detected from sampling the arch or descending aorta from the suprasternal notch. However, elevated systolic velocity profile (>2.0 m/sec) sampling from this aortic site should not be detected.

20. ANSWER: B. The two-dimensional and Doppler images shown depict a pseudocoarctation of the aorta. Pseudocoarctation of the aorta is an anomaly characterized by a redundant and tortuous distal aortic arch with a kink that occurs just after the left subclavian artery. Unlike coarctation of the aorta, blood flow through the aorta is not obstructed; there should be no or minimal pressure gradient detected (as shown). Usually present in true coarctation of the aorta, collateral circulation is absent with pseudocoarctation. Anomalies associated with pseudocoarctation include Turner syndrome.

All of the other options shown are noted in true coarctation of the aorta: rib notching on plain chest radiograph due to well-developed collateral circulation; right arm hypertension from preductal coarctations; and ascending aortic aneurysms, which may be associated with coarctation and bicuspid aortic valve.

21. ANSWER: B. The short- and long-axis transesophageal images of the aortic root demonstrate a right coronary sinus of Valsalva aneurysm. Aortic sinus of Valsalva aneurysms are most commonly of congenital origin, although they can develop as a result of endocarditis, syphilis, or trauma. Males predominate with a male-to-female ratio of 3:1. The right sinus of Valsalva followed by the noncoronary sinus is the most common site of aortic sinus aneurysmal dilation. If they rupture, a fistula develops from the aortic sinus to the right ventricle (when the right sinus is involved) or to the right atrium (when the noncoronary sinus is involved).

22. ANSWER: C. As previously discussed, ascending aortic size correlates best with several anthropometric measures. The more precise determinants are age, body height, and body surface area. Normal reference sizes of the ascending aorta in adults as measured by transthoracic echocardiography have been recently published. The study findings underscore the importance of indexing aortic dimensions to age and body surface area.

Regarding indications for prophylactic aortic surgery, traditional cutoff values for aortic diameters are when the ascending aorta approaches >5.0–5.5 cm (Table 23-2). However, it is clear that at least 15% of patients have aortic dissection or rupture at a diameter of <5.0 cm. It is believed that indexing the aortic size to the patient's height or body surface area would take into account the likely greater risk of aortic instability for the same size in shorter compared with taller patients. Based on this logic, several ratios have been proposed to better discriminate the appropriate size

TABLE 23-2 Recommendations for Aortic Surgery in Asymptomatic Patients with Thoracic Aortic Aneurysm

Class I

- Degenerative thoracic ascending aortic aneurysm or aortic sinus diameter >5.5 cm.
- Marfan syndrome or genetic aorta (including bicuspid aortic valve) and ascending aortic diameter >4.0 to 5.0 cm (depending on the condition).
- Aortic growth rate of >0.5 cm/yr in an aorta <5.5 cm in diameter.
- Patients undergoing aortic valve surgery with an ascending aorta or aortic root >4.5 cm.
- Chronic dissection and a descending thoracic aortic diameter >5.5 cm
- Degenerative aneurysms and a descending thoracic aortic diameter >5.5 cm, endovascular stent grafting should be strongly considered when feasible.

Class IIa

- Marfan syndrome or genetic aorta (including bicuspid aortic valve) when the ratio of maximal ascending or aortic root area (πr^2) in cm^2 divided by the patient's height in meters exceeds 10.
- Loeys-Dietz syndrome or a confirmed TGFBR1 or TGFBR2 mutation when aortic diameter >4.2 cm by transesophageal echocardiogram or >4.4 to 4.6 cm by computed tomographic imaging and/or magnetic resonance imaging.
- Women with Marfan syndrome contemplating pregnancy and an ascending aortic diameter >4.0 cm.
- Low operative risk patients with isolated aneurysms of the aortic arch >5.5 cm.

(Adapted from the 2010 ACCF/AHA/AATS/ACR/ASA/SCA/SCAI/SIR/STS/SVM Guidelines for the Diagnosis and Management of Patients with Thoracic Aortic Disease)

for elective aortic surgery. The first ratio employs the aorta's maximal cross-sectional area divided by the patient's height in meters: Ratio = πr^2 (cm^2)/height (m). A ratio of >10 helps identify patients at greater risk of developing aortic dissection. The second ratio employs the aorta's maximal diameter divided by the patient's body surface area: Ratio = aortic diameter (cm)/body surface area (m^2). A ratio of >2.75 cm/m^2 confers moderate risk, and a ratio of >4.25 cm/m^2 confers the greatest risk of aortic dissection or rupture.

Thus regarding our patient in question, he is a 41-year-old man who is tall and with a large body surface area. An aortic diameter of 4.3 cm is within the normal range of limits based on his body size. The ascending aorta can be adequately imaged from transthoracic windows, namely the left parasternal position from various intercostal spaces. Because the aorta is subject to pulsatile blood flow, it should be ideally imaged during diastole.

23. ANSWER: D. The transthoracic long-axis image displays the ascending aorta. The aortic valve is seen at the left and the mid tubular portion of the ascending aorta on the right. The aortic segments of interest are the aortic annulus, sinuses of Valsalva, sino-tubular junction, proximal tubular aorta, and the mid tubular aorta. The mid tubular aorta is demarcated by the level of the right pulmonary artery (white arrow shown in Fig. 23-8). The right pulmonary artery courses behind the ascending aorta, perpendicular to its long axis, and thus is seen in cross-section in the transthoracic long-axis view.

24. ANSWER: D. In long-axis imaging of the ascending aorta, the aortic morphology is subdivided at the following levels: aortic annulus, sinuses of Valsalva, sino-tubular junction, proximal tubular aorta, and the mid tubular aorta. See Figure 23-18. With normal aortic structure, the diameter at the sinus of Valsalva is slightly larger than the tubular portion of the ascending aorta (mean difference between the sinuses and tubular portion is 0.2 cm in men and 0.1 cm in women). The image depicted shows a dilated aortic root at the sinuses of Valsalva (4.6 cm) with preserved sino-tubular junction architecture (no effacement) and a normal sized tubular ascending aorta (3.4 cm). Effacement of the aortic root is defined by the gradual increase in diameter from the sinuses of Valsalva into the ascending aorta, with the absence of a discernable sino-tubular junction (the landmark, which defines the transition between the root and the tubular ascending aorta). Effacement of the aortic root is suggestive of more advanced medial degeneration of aortic tissue and progressive aortic aneurysmal disease.

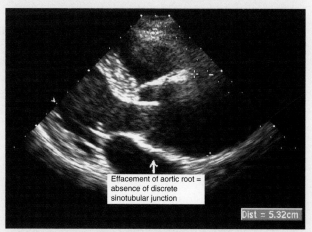

Fig. 23-18

25. ANSWER: C. Figure 23-10 shows the descending thoracic aorta in cross-section with a linear echodensity separating the lumen into two compartments, suggestive of an intimal flap. Given the location of the flap, the image is most consistent with a distal type B aortic dissection. Although there is no color Doppler confirmation, both compartments of the divided aorta seem echolucent, suggesting blood flow and patency.

The ascending aorta is not visualized at the 0-degree transverse plane in such proximity to the esophageal transducer. Therefore, a diagnosis of a proximal type A aortic dissection cannot be made on the basis of Figure 23-10. In an elephant trunk aortic surgery, the key element is that the distal anastomosis consists of a portion of the tube graft that is left suspended within the lumen of the proximal descending thoracic aorta. This elephant trunk portion is later used during the subsequent staged distal aortic surgery. The elephant trunk graft has a thicker and more echogenic appearance than an intimal flap and will appear circular or oval, an unusual shape for an intimal flap (Fig. 23-19).

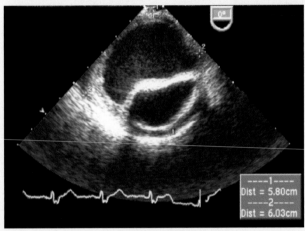

Fig. 23-19

26. ANSWER: A; 27. ANSWER: C. The transesophageal images show a case of proximal aortitis in association with reactive arthritis (Reiter syndrome). Aortic involvement is a well-recognized manifestation of systemic inflammatory conditions such as vasculitis (giant cell arteritis, Takayasu's) and the spondyloarthropathies (ankylosing spondylitis, reactive arthritis). When present, the inflammatory process involves the ascending aorta extending proximally to the sinuses of Valsalva, aortic leaflets, annulus, and aortic-mitral curtain. Complications of aortitis include significant aortic regurgitation and advanced heart block; progression to aortic dissection does not occur. In a series of patients with ankylosing spondylitis, more than half had aortic root thickening and one-fourth had thickening of the aortic-mitral curtain by transesophageal echocardiography.

In suspected acute aortic diseases, echocardiography plays a pivotal role in the initial evaluation of these patients. The finding of diffuse aortic wall thickening suggestive of aortitis can pose a diagnostic dilemma making it difficult to distinguish from other aortic conditions, such as periaortic abscess or intramural hematoma. Distinguishing features of intramural hematoma are displacement of intimal calcium, a crescent-shaped appearance of wall thickening, and when present, areas of echolucent spaces representing intramural blood. There are several echocardiographic features in this case, which favor the diagnosis of an inflammatory aortitis. The absence of aortic valve vegetations argues against an infectious etiology such as endocarditis. Primary bacterial aortitis most commonly occurs in aortic segments with advanced atheromatous disease (rarely the aortic root). The finding of diffuse aortic wall thickening extending to the annulus and anterior mitral leaflet (the aortic-mitral curtain), highlights a specific echocardiographic feature consistent with spondyloarthropathy-associated aortitis.

KEY POINTS:

- Proximal aortitis is a well-recognized manifestation of systemic inflammatory conditions, such as vasculitis and the spondyloarthropathies.
- Proximal aortitis can be diagnosed echocardiographically as diffuse aortic root thickening.
- Thickening extending to the aortic annulus and aortic-mitral curtain points out an echocardiographic feature suggestive of spondyloarthropathy-associated aortitis.

28. ANSWER: C; 29. ANSWER: C. The main abnormality on the transesophageal echocardiogram is a large periaortic echodense space with pockets of echolucencies. The aortic homograft appears well seated, but has mild aortic regurgitation which is valvular and centrally directed. The appearance of the large periaortic echodense space is most consistent with an organized fluid collection. Possibilities include blood/hematoma, purulent fluid, and serous edema. In the early postoperative period following aortic valve surgery, the clinical syndromes complicating this case may include periaortic abscess formation, massive peri-graft edema, and periaortic hematoma. With the presence of an aortic root homograft, the possibility of a proximal aortic dissection is very unlikely. Although placement of an aortic homograft is typically associated with some degree of edema and hematoma, the findings in this patient are extremely uncommon and cannot be considered expected postoperative changes. Similarly, if the changes represented an infection and abscess, it would be expected that the patient manifest systemic symptoms and therefore early endocarditis is unlikely.

The patient has mild aortic regurgitation which is valvular and centrally directed. The mechanism appears functional and not secondary to leaflet perforation, restriction, or aortic instability. Homograft aortic regurgitation may be acceptable and considered non-pathological at grades up to mild. A vena contracta of a central aortic regurgitant jet of 0.3 cm or, of an eccentric jet of 0.2 cm, is considered of mild severity. Most aortic homograft prostheses will generate mildly accelerated antegrade flows depending on their size, but in general range from 1.5–2.5 m/sec. A high velocity systolic flow in the left ventricular outflow tract is abnormal, and in the postoperative patient with an aortic homograft, highly suggestive of dynamic outflow obstruction due to systolic anterior motion of the mitral valve.

The fluid collection in this case was periaortic blood/hematoma, related to partial suture dehiscence and paravalvular leak at the annulus level. As a result, a fistulous communication developed between the outflow tract and the periaortic space where blood accumulated. With the use of a transcatheter closure device, the paravalvular deficiency was occluded and the hematoma resolved over time.

KEY POINTS:

■ Fluid collections in the periaortic space detected by echocardiography may represent blood/hematoma or purulent material such as abscess formation. Unless additional evidence for endocarditis exists (i.e., vegetations, leaflet perforation), distinguishing between these 2 entities is difficult and should be based on clinical grounds.

■ Up to a mild degree of aortic regurgitation from an aortic homograft is acceptable and common. However, high velocity systolic flow in the outflow tract after aortic valve surgery should raise suspicion for dynamic outflow obstruction due to mitral valve systolic anterior motion.

30. ANSWER: C; 31. ANSWER: A. The principal abnormality displayed by the transthoracic image is a calcified ascending aorta. In this case, the patient had a history of Hodgkin's lymphoma and underwent treatment with mantle radiation in his 20s. As a late consequence of radiotherapy, he developed radiation heart disease with coronary stenoses, aortic valve disease, and severe calcification of the aorta and great vessels.

It is well recognized that atherosclerosis and calcification of the aorta incrementally adds to the embolic complication risk of patients undergoing cardiac catheterization and heart surgery with aortic cross clamping. Both the severity and location of aortic atheroma have important implications for the neurological outcome of patients undergoing aortic manipulation. Aortic arch atheromatous disease has been linked to an increased risk of stroke after cardiac surgery, with a predilection for the left-hemisphere, further supporting the associated risk of arch atheroma.

How a calcified atheromatous aorta leads to an adverse neurological outcome after cardiopulmonary bypass is unclear but is believed to be in part related to cerebral embolization of aortic debris. Because of aortic manipulation, cannulation, and clamping, atheromatous debris becomes unstable, dislodges, and embolizes distally. As such, optimal detection of aortic atheroma, both severity and location, is paramount. Intraoperative transesophageal echocardiography is superior to manual palpation by the surgeon of the ascending aorta for the detection of atheromatous disease but epiaortic echocardiographic scanning appears to provide the most accurate results. The use of epiaortic imaging can help identify and, if possible, avoid zones of atheromatous debris in areas where aortic manipulations are planned. For those patients found to have significant atheromatous disease, aortic cannulation may carry a prohibitive embolic risk.

Consequently, alternative cannulation sites, such as the axillary or innominate artery, may be valid options.

KEY POINTS:

■ Atherosclerosis and calcification of the ascending aorta and aortic arch incrementally adds to the risk of stroke in patients after cardiac surgery.

■ Manual palpation of the aorta is inferior to transesophageal echocardiography in the detection of aortic atheromatous debris, whereas epiaortic echocardiographic imaging provides the most accurate results.

32. ANSWER: D; 33. ANSWER: C. The transesophageal image shows the descending thoracic aorta on a transverse plane. The findings are suggestive of a large intramural hematoma (>11 mm) involving the descending thoracic aorta. In this case, the aortic intramural hematoma is characterized by a crescent shaped thickening of the aortic wall with smooth margins, absence of an intimal flap, and evidence of displaced intimal calcium. In addition, an echolucent pocket in the aortic wall can be seen, which supports the finding of blood in the aortic media. Notable distinguishing features in this case favoring intramural hematoma are the smooth aortic wall contour (not often seen in severe atheromatous disease) and the echogenic intimal stripe from displaced intimal calcium.

Aortic intramural hematoma is a high mortality event, particularly when it involves the ascending aorta (type A), where its mortality is similar to that of classic aortic dissection. On the other hand, type B intramural hematoma carries an in-hospital mortality which approximates that of distal aortic dissection, around 8%–13%. Therefore, the management of type A intramural hematoma should involve surgical therapy without delay, whereas a more conservative medical approach can be taken with a type B hematoma. Several studies have evaluated the natural history of intramural hematoma and suggest that the most common long-term evolution is toward aortic aneurysm or pseudoaneurysm formation, although progression to classic aortic dissection is less common. Hematoma regression can occur and its best predictor is a normal aortic diameter upon initial presentation.

KEY POINTS:

■ In-hospital mortality of an acute type B aortic intramural hematoma is ~10%.

■ Most commonly, intramural hematoma will progresses on to aortic aneurysm or pseudoaneurysm formation.

34. ANSWER: A; 35. ANSWER: C. The transesophageal echocardiographic images reveal a patient with an acute type A aortic dissection presenting with a large pericardial effusion (hemopericardium). The long-axis images show an intimal flap at the level of the aortic root, confirming the diagnosis of a proximal dissection. Based on the clinical history, the patient is presenting with syncope, heart failure and evidence of cardiac tamponade. In this setting, the patient should be taken immediately to the operating room for aortic surgery. Small series have demonstrated concerns regarding pericardiocentesis in patients with cardiac tamponade and proximal dissection. In some cases after the removal of pericardial fluid, rapid decompensation and death have occurred, possibly related to augmented ventricular function and propagation of the dissection. Thus, when cardiac tamponade is present along with proximal aortic dissection, immediate surgery should be performed, unless a surgical team is not available and the patient is in extremis. Medications that decrease dP/dt, such as beta-blocker therapy are the initial agents of choice in aortic dissection; but given the patient's hypotension and tamponade, these agents should not be used.

In a modern day series of patients, the clinical and imaging characteristics and outcomes in acute aortic dis-

section have been reported. Overall in-hospital mortality for aortic dissection is ~27%. Most patients present with normal blood pressures or with hypertension, whereas only ~16% present with either hypotension or shock. Although not common, heart failure was the presenting sign in ~9% and pulse deficits noted in ~19% of acute proximal dissections. Important to keep in the differential diagnosis of syncope is aortic dissection, as ~12% of patients with proximal dissection present with a syncopal attack.

KEY POINTS:

■ When cardiac tamponade is present along with proximal aortic dissection, immediate surgery is indicated. Pericardiocentesis should not be performed in this setting unless rapid clinical deterioration is imminent.

■ In 1 in 10 patients, acute proximal dissection may present with congestive heart failure or syncope.

SUGGESTED READINGS

Biaggi P, Matthews F, Braun J, et al. Gender, age, and body surface area are the major determinants of ascending aorta dimensions in subjects with apparently normal echocardiograms. *J Am Soc Echocardiogr*. 2009;22:720–725.

Cohen A, Tzourio C, Bertrand B, et al. FAPS Investigators: French Study of Aortic Plaques in Stroke. Aortic plaque morphology and vascular events: a follow-up study in patients with ischemic stroke. *Circulation*. 1997;96:3838–3841.

Djaiani G, Fedorko L, Borger M, et al. Mild to moderate atheromatous disease of the thoracic aorta and new ischemic brain lesions after conventional coronary artery bypass graft surgery. *Stroke*. 2004;35:e356–e358.

Evangelista A, Mukherjee D, Mehta RH, et al. International Registry of Aortic Dissection (IRAD) Investigators. Acute intramural hematoma of the aorta: a mystery in evolution. *Circulation*. 2005; 111:1063–1070.

Fazel SS, Mallidi HR, Lee RS, et al. The aortopathy of bicuspid aortic valve disease has distinctive patterns and usually involves the transverse aortic arch. *J Thorac Cardiovasc Surg*. 2008;135: 901–907.

Ganaha F, Miller DC, Sugimoto K, et al. Prognosis of aortic intramural hematoma with and without penetrating atherosclerotic ulcer: a clinical and radiological analysis. *Circulation*. 2002;106: 342–348.

Hagan PG, Nienaber CA, Isselbacher EM, et al. The International Registry of Acute Aortic Dissection (IRAD): new insights into an old disease. *JAMA*. 2000;283:897–903.

Isselbacher EM, Cigarroa JE, Eagle KA. Cardiac tamponade complicating proximal aortic dissection. Is pericardiocentesis harmful? *Circulation*. 1994;90:2375–2378.

Kühl HP, Hanrath P. The impact of transesophageal echocardiography on daily clinical practice. *Eur J Echocardiogr*. 2004;5: 455–468.

Laperche T, Laurian C, Roudaut R, et al. Mobile thromboses of the aortic arch without aortic debris: a transesophageal echocardiographic finding associated with unexplained arterial embolism. The Filiale Echocardiographie de la Société Française de Cardiologie. *Circulation*. 1997;96:288–294.

Roldan CA, Chavez J, Wiest PW, et al. Aortic root disease and valve disease associated with ankylosing spondylitis. *J Am Coll Cardiol*. 1998;32:1397–1404.

Smith MD, Cassidy JM, Souther S, et al. Transesophageal echocardiography in the diagnosis of traumatic rupture of the aorta. *N Engl J Med*. 1995;332:356–362.

Song JM, Kim HS, Song JK, et al. Usefulness of the initial noninvasive imaging study to predict the adverse outcomes in the medical treatment of acute type A aortic intramural hematoma. *Circulation*. 2003;108:II-324–II-328.

Svensson LG, Kim KH, Lytle BW, et al. Relationship of aortic cross-sectional area to height ratio and the risk of aortic dissection in patients with bicuspid aortic valves. *J Thorac Cardiovasc Surg*. 2003;126:892–893.

Svensson LG, Labib SB, Elsenhauer AC, et al. Intimal tear without hematoma: an important variant of aortic dissection that can elude imaging techniques. *Circulation*. 1999;99:1331–1336.

The French Study of Aortic Plaques in Stroke Group. Atherosclerotic disease of the aortic arch as a risk factor for recurrent ischemic stroke. *N Engl J Med*. 1996;334:1216–1221.

2010 ACCF/AHA/AATS/ACR/ASA/SCA/SCAI/SIR/STS/SVM Guidelines for the diagnosis and management of patients with thoracic aortic disease. A Report of the American College of Cardiology Foundation/American Heart Association Task Force on Practice Guidelines, American Association for Thoracic Surgery, American College of Radiology, American Stroke Association, Society of Cardiovascular Anesthesiologists, Society for Cardiovascular Angiography and Interventions, Society of Interventional Radiology, Society of Thoracic Surgeons, and Society for Vascular Medicine. Hiratzka LF, Bakris GL, Beckman JA, Bersin RM, Carr VF, Casey DE Jr, Eagle KA, Hermann LK, Isselbacher EM, Kazerooni EA, Kouchoukos NT, Lytle BW, Milewicz DM, Reich DL, Sen S, Shinn JA, Svensson LG, Williams DM; American College of Cardiology Foundation/American Heart Association Task Force on Practice Guidelines; American Association for Thoracic Surgery; American College of Radiology; American Stroke Association; Society of Cardiovascular Anesthesiologists; Society for Cardiovascular Angiography and Interventions; Society of Interventional Radiology; Society of Thoracic Surgeons; Society for Vascular Medicine. *J Am Coll Cardiol* 2010;55:e27–e129.

Atrial Fibrillation

Susie N. Hong-Zohlman, David I. Silverman, and Warren J. Manning

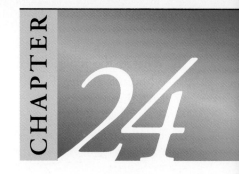

1. What is the estimated prevalence of left atrial (LA) thrombus in nonrheumatic atrial fibrillation (AF)?
   A. 0%–10%.
   B. 10%–20%.
   C. 20%–30%.
   D. 40%–50%.
   E. >50%.

2. A 75-year-old man with a history of hypertension is admitted after a transient ischemic attack and is found to be in AF. He is referred for a trans-esophageal echocardiogram (TEE). Which echo findings are associated with an increased likelihood of LA thrombus?
   A. Patent foramen ovale.
   B. LA appendage (LAA) velocities greater than 50 cm/sec.
   C. LA volume index of 25 ml/m².
   D. Spontaneous echo contrast (SEC).
   E. Anomalous pulmonary veins.

3. Which LA measurements best correlate with the maintenance of sinus rhythm after cardioversion?
   A. LA volume index of 30 ml/m² and LA appendage velocity 40 cm/sec.
   B. LA volume index of 30 ml/m² and LA appendage velocity 50 cm/sec.
   C. LA volume index of 40 ml/m² and LA appendage velocity 40 cm/sec.
   D. LA volume index of 40 ml/m² and LA appendage velocity 30 cm/sec.

4. *E/e'* best estimates pulmonary capillary wedge pressure (PCWP) in a patient with which cardiac pathology?
   A. Mitral annuloplasty ring.
   B. Severe mitral annular calcification (MAC).
   C. AF.
   D. Mechanical mitral valve.

5. What is the estimated prevalence of right atrial appendage (RAA) thrombus in patients with AF?
   A. <1%.
   B. 1%–6%
   C. 7%–10%
   D. 11%–15%
   E. 16%–20%

6. What is the prevalence of cardioversion-related thromboembolism in patients with nonvalvular AF of less than 48 hours without screening TEE?
   A. <1%.
   B. 1–5%.
   C. 6–10%.
   D. 11–15%.
   E. 16–20%.

7. Approximately what percent of patients with recent nonrheumatic AF and prior LA thrombus on TEE will have thrombus resolution after 4 weeks of therapeutic anticoagulation?
   A. 25%.
   B. 50%.
   C. 75%.
   D. 100%.

8. What is the reported sensitivity of transthoracic echocardiography (TTE) in identifying LA or LAA thrombi?
   A. 0–20%.
   B. 40–60%.
   C. 70–90%.
   D. >90%.

9. What is hypothesized to be the reason for a lower prevalence of RAA thrombus in patients with AF?
   A. RAA velocities are usually higher than those in the LAA.
   B. LAA neck is larger and "traps" thrombi.
   C. RAA width is larger and lacks anatomic remodeling during AF.
   D. RAA is resistant to clot formation.
   E. RAA does not fibrillate.

10. In which patient would the development of AF be most hemodynamically compromising?
   A. Hypertrophic cardiomyopathy (HCM) with a resting left ventricular outflow tract (LVOT) outflow velocity of 4 m/sec.
   B. Bicuspid aortic valve with a peak velocity of 3 m/sec.
   C. Ventricular septal defect with a peak velocity of 5 m/sec across the defect.
   D. Mitral annular calcification with a mean gradient of 5 mm Hg across the mitral valve.
   E. Mild to moderate mitral regurgitation with a peak velocity of 6 m/sec.

11. Which statement regarding AF postcardiac surgery is true?
   A. It is more frequent after coronary artery bypass surgery (CABG) than after mitral valve surgery.
   B. CABG combined with valvular surgery decreases the incidence of AF.
   C. It occurs in less than 5% of cardiac transplantation.
   D. Prophylaxis with beta blockade significantly decreases the risk of stroke postoperatively.
   E. Warfarin should be initiated if AF lasts more than 24 hours for a total of 4 weeks.

12. A 63-year-old woman with a history of chronic AF is referred for an echocardiogram prior to cardioversion. However, the patient refuses to undergo a TEE. What alternative may be offered to this patient to evaluate for LAA thrombi?
   A. Color M-mode through the left and right atrium.
   B. Pulse wave Doppler through the LAA.
   C. Cardiac magnetic resonance (CMR) imaging without gadolinium.
   D. TTE with harmonic imaging with intravenous (IV) contrast.
   E. Electron Beam Computed Tomography (EBCT).

13. A 55-year-old woman with a history of hypertension and new onset AF is hospitalized after 3 days of worsening palpitations. She is started on a heparin drip and beta blockade for rate control and referred for a TEE prior to cardioversion. TEE reveals a mildly dilated LA and is free of thrombi. Upon removal of the TEE probe, she spontaneously converts to sinus rhythm. What should be recommended to this patient upon discharge?
   A. Discontinue heparin and discharge with low-dose aspirin.
   B. Repeat TEE and discontinue anticoagulation if there are no thrombi.
   C. Anticoagulate with warfarin with a goal International Normalized Ratio (INR) of 2–3 for 4 weeks.
   D. Refer for LAA ligation.
   E. Pulmonary vein isolation.

14. A 67-year-old woman with chronic AF is admitted for acute shortness of breath and transient hypoxemia. Her INR is subtherapeutic at 1.3. A TEE is performed for possible electrical cardioversion. A thrombus is noted in the right atrium (RA) during TEE and the tricuspid regurgitation (TR) velocity is noted to be 4 m/sec. What would you recommend at this time?
   A. Immediate electrical cardioversion.
   B. Bolus amiodarone intravenously and follow with a continuous infusion.
   C. Surgical removal of the RA thrombus.
   D. Add aspirin and plavix and perform electric cardioversion.
   E. Start heparin drip, defer cardioversion, and evaluate for pulmonary embolus.

15. Which is a true statement with regard to spontaneous echo contrast (SEC)?
    A. It is only found in patients with AF.
    B. If not seen on initial TEE, there is a low likelihood it will be seen on a subsequent TEE.
    C. It is thought to be due to platelet aggregation similar to what occurs in ruptured plaques.
    D. Warfarin therapy does not affect the presence of SEC.
    E. It is only seen in the left atrium.

16. A 68-year-old woman with AF is referred for TEE due to a transient ischemic attack. Which of the following is true about her TEE finding in Figure 24-1?

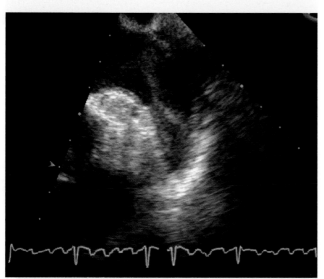

Fig. 24-1

    A. Its prevalence is the same for both AF and atrial flutter.
    B. Mitral regurgitation worsens this finding.
    C. There is an association with LA myxoma.
    D. It is an independent predictor of thromboembolic risk.
    E. Its prevalence declines with warfarin.

17. What can be inferred from these Doppler findings (Figure 24-2)?
    A. There is a high probability of maintaining sinus rhythm after cardioversion.
    B. This is associated with an increased risk of thromboembolism.
    C. There is severe pulmonary hypertension.

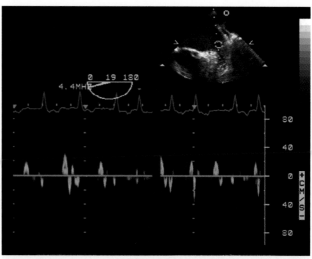

Fig. 24-2

    D. The patient should be referred for pulmonary vein isolation (PVI).
    E. It is associated with minimal to no spontaneous echo contrast.

18. A 22-year-old man presents with increasing dyspnea and decreased exercise tolerance that has limited his ability to participate in his basketball league. A TTE is performed (Figure 24-3). What would confirm the diagnosis?

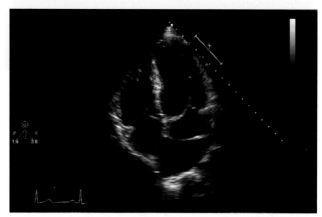

Fig. 24-3

    A. Increased gradient across the mitral valve.
    B. LAA contiguous with the basal (proximal) chamber.
    C. LAA contiguous with the apical (distal) chamber.
    D. Increased pulmonary vein velocity.
    E. Normal apical two-chamber view (e.g., this is an artifact).

25. A 55-year-old man is referred for electrical cardioversion for symptomatic AF/atrial flutter. Based on the Doppler findings in Figure 24-10, what would be expected immediately postcardioversion?

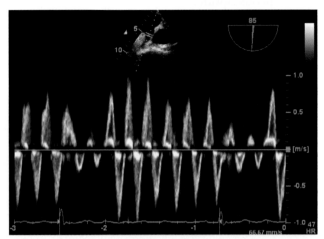

Fig. 24-10

A. Resolution of SEC.
B. Decreased risk of thromboembolism.
C. Recurrence of AF.
D. Improvement of LA function.
E. Decreased velocities in the LAA.

CASE 1:

A 65-year-old woman with a history of rheumatic fever as a child presents with dyspnea on exertion. A TEE is performed.

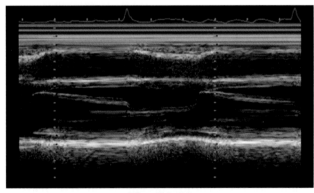

Fig. 24-11

26. Based on the M-mode in Figure 24-11, what is her estimated annual thromboembolic risk?
   A. 1%.
   B. 5%.
   C. 10%.
   D. 20%.
   E. 30%.

27. Increasing age and what other risk factors are independent predictors of AF in multivariate analysis of patients with this pathology?
   A. LA dimension.
   B. Ejection fraction.
   C. Mitral regurgitation.
   D. Tricuspid stenosis.
   E. Tricuspid regurgitation.

28. What is the preferred imaging modality to evaluate for LA thrombi?
   A. TTE.
   B. TTE with IV-administered contrast agent and harmonic imaging.
   C. Three-dimensional (3D) TTE.
   D. TEE.
   E. Pulsed wave Doppler through the LAA.

CASE 2:

A 50-year-old man is referred for PVI for treatment of paroxysmal AF. A TEE is ordered prior to his procedure.

29. What is the specificity of TEE for LA thrombus?
   A. <75%.
   B. 75%–80%.
   C. 80%–85%.
   D. 85%–90%.
   E. >90%.

30. The patient undergoes a successful PVI procedure. Three months postprocedure, he develops progressive shortness of breath with exertion. He is referred for TEE which demonstrates the findings in Figure 24-12.

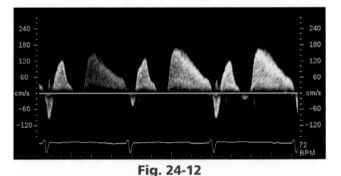

Fig. 24-12

Based on these Doppler findings, what is the likely etiology of his shortness of breath?
   A. Mitral stenosis.
   B. AF.
   C. Severe mitral regurgitation.
   D. Pulmonary vein stenosis.

CASE 3:

A 72-year-old man with paroxysmal AF presents with a transient ischemic attack and is referred for a TEE. The LA is normal in size on the images in Figure 24-13.

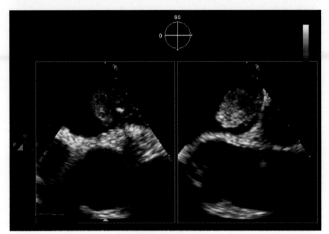

Fig. 24-13

31. Based on these findings, what would you recommend?
    A. Start warfarin with a goal INR of 3–4 and re-image in 3 weeks.
    B. Emergent PVI.
    C. Nothing, this is an artifact.
    D. Refer for cardiac surgery.
    E. Percutaneous transeptal removal.

32. What is a true statement regarding this finding on echocardiogram?
    A. There is no risk of recurrence after resection.
    B. It is usually malignant.
    C. Embolic phenomenon is rare.
    D. It is only found attached to the interatrial septum.
    E. It is commonly found in the left atrium.

33. Figure 24-13 combined with what other pathology is found in patients with Carney Complex?

A. Schwannomas.
B. Anomalous pulmonary veins.
C. Truncus arteriosis.
D. Right-sided aorta.
E. Bovine arch.

CASE 4:

A 38-year-old man presents with dizziness and shortness of breath during exercise. The M-mode in Figure 24-14 is taken during his TTE.

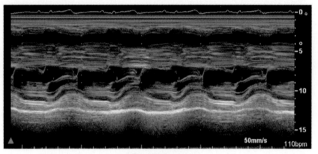

Fig. 24-14

34. What should be performed next?
    A. TEE to look for thrombus in the LA.
    B. Refer to cardiac surgery for mitral valve repair.
    C. Calculate gradient across the LVOT at rest and with exercise.
    D. Refer for PVI for symptomatic paroxysmal AF.
    E. Start empiric antibiotic therapy.

35. The patient is referred for stress echocardiogram and during exercise develops AF with rapid ventricular rate. He becomes extremely short of breath and hypotensive. How would you manage this patient?
    A. Perform TEE to rule out LA thrombus and refer for PVI.
    B. Bolus with IV furosemide.
    C. Emergent cardiac surgery for mitral valve repair.
    D. Immediate cardioversion.
    E. Coronary angiogram.

ANSWERS

1. ANSWER: B. Transesophageal echocardiographic (TEE) evidence of left atrial (LA) thrombi is seen in approximately 13% of patients presenting with nonrheumatic atrial fibrillation (AF) of more than 3 days duration.

2. ANSWER: D. Spontaneous echo contrast (SEC) is present in over 50% of all patients with AF and in over 80% of those with left atrial appendage (LAA) thrombi or a recent thromboembolic event.

3. ANSWER: B. LA size is important prognostically in AF. Progressive enlargement is associated with a decreased probability of maintaining sinus rhythm. LAA velocity is also thought to be a predictor of the likelihood of maintaining sinus rhythm after cardioversion.

Choice B has the smallest LA size and highest LAA velocity and is therefore the best option.

4. ANSWER: C. AF is the best choice among these options. *E/e'* should not be used to determine pulmonary capillary wedge pressure (PCWP) in patients with a mitral valve prosthesis or severe mitral annular calcification, as e' velocities may be inaccurate.

5. ANSWER: B. Although much less common than left atrial (LA) thrombi in patients with AF, right atrial (RA) or right atrial appendage (RAA) thrombi occur in 3%–6% of cases (versus 11%–15% for LA thrombi). The majority of patients with RA thrombi also have LA thrombi. Cardioversion should be deferred even if patients have isolated RA thrombi due to the theoretical risk of thromboembolism to the pulmonary artery.

6. ANSWER: A. In a consecutive series of more than 350 hospitalized patients with nonvalvular AF, the incidence of cardioversion-related thromboembolism was 0.8% in patients without screening TEE and AF of less than 48 hours. Of note, these patients were not on anticoagulation at the time of their thromboembolic event (anticoagulation was not initiated or was stopped shortly after admission). All thromboembolic events occurred in patients who had spontaneously converted to sinus rhythm.

7. ANSWER: C. In a study looking at patients with nonrheumatic AF, resolution of thrombi occurred in approximately 75% after 4 weeks of anticoagulation therapy.

8. ANSWER: B. The ability of TTE to identify or exclude LA or LAA thrombi is limited, with a reported sensitivity of 39%–63%. This is largely due to poor visualization of the LAA.

9. ANSWER: C. The larger RAA width and lack of anatomic remodeling may partially explain the substantially lower prevalence of RAA thrombus found among patients with AF. All the other choices are false statements.

10. ANSWER: A. The patient in choice A has a resting gradient of 64 mm Hg across the left ventricular outflow tract (LVOT), which is significantly elevated. Patients with hypertrophic cardiomyopathy (HCM) and LVOT obstruction often have compromised left ventricular (LV) filling due to abnormal relaxation secondary to myofibril disarray. Additionally, systolic anterior motion of the anterior leaflet of the mitral valve, which results in outflow tract obstruction and mitral regurgitation, can severely compromise cardiac output. The development of AF in such a patient would compromise LV filling significantly. Choices B–D are essentially mild forms of their respective pathologies.

11. ANSWER: E. The ACC/AHA recommends that warfarin should be initiated if AF lasts more than 24 hours for a total of 4 weeks postcardiac surgery. AF and atrial flutter occur frequently after cardiac surgery. The prevalence of AF is more frequent in valvular surgery than in CABG and greatest when combined (CABG plus valve surgery). AF is reported to be between 15% and 40% after CABG, 37%–50% after valve surgery, and up to 60% in CABG plus valve replacement. AF is reported to occur in 11%–24% after cardiac transplantation. Despite the reduction of AF with prophylactic medical therapy, the reduction in stroke has been found to be statistically nonsignificant.

12. ANSWER: D. The CLOTS Multicenter Pilot Trial found that the combination of harmonic imaging with IV contrast was useful in the detection of the thrombus by TTE. Although cardiac-computed tomography with iodinated contrast and delayed imaging could be used to evaluate LAA thrombi, EBCT would not, as it is not used with IV contrast and primarily used for calcium scoring. Cardiac magnetic resonance (CMR) without gadolinium has poor visualization of the LAA and would be suboptimal in the evaluation for LAA thrombi in patients with AF.

13. ANSWER: C. Although this patient spontaneously converted into sinus rhythm, she remains at risk for thromboembolism in the immediate postcardioversion period and should remain anticoagulated. The ACC/AHA/ESC guidelines recommend that warfarin therapy be continued for at least 4 weeks after cardioversion with a target INR of 2.5 (range 2.0–3.0) after being in AF for 48 hours.

14. ANSWER: E. This patient's history and TEE findings are suggestive of a pulmonary embolus (PE). Cardioversion should be deferred, especially with a known RA thrombus, and treatment with a workup for a PE should be instituted immediately.

15. ANSWER: D. Warfarin leads to thrombus resolution and a lower incidence of thromboembolism, but does not affect the presence of SEC. Serial TEE studies have shown that SEC subsequently develops in many patients with AF (44% in one report) who do not have SEC on initial TEE. SEC is thought to reflect increased erythrocyte aggregation caused by low shear rate due to altered atrial flow dynamics and uncoordinated atrial systole. Erythrocyte aggregation is mediated by plasma proteins, especially fibrinogen, which promotes red cell rouleaux formation by moderating the normal electrostatic forces (due to negatively charged membranes) which keep erythrocytes from aggregating. Thrombi can be seen in both the left and right atrium.

16. ANSWER: D. Figure 24-1 shows prominent spontaneous echo contrast (SEC) in the LAA. SEC is an independent predictor of thromboembolic risk and associated with an increase in embolic rate in patients with AF. Mitral regurgitation appears to lessen the frequency of SEC. Warfarin does not impact the prevalence of SEC. There is a strong association between LA

SEC and LA thrombi. The prevalence of SEC occurs more frequently in AF than in atrial flutter. There is no known association between SEC and LA myxoma.

17. ANSWER: B. The risk of stroke is increased with marked reductions in blood flow velocity, particularly in the LAA or posterior LA. A low-appendage ejection flow velocity is associated with the presence of appendage thrombus and with dense SEC. LA blood flow velocity (>40 cm/sec) is thought to be a predictor of the likelihood of maintaining sinus rhythm after cardioversion. There are no definitive findings that suggest that this patient has severe pulmonary hypertension or should be referred for PVI based on atrial appendage velocities.

18. ANSWER: C. Cor-triatriatum sinister is differentiated from a supravalvular mitral ring by the position of the LAA (Fig. 24-15, white arrow). In cor-triatriatum sinister, the left appendage is part of the distal (mitral valve) atrial chamber, while the LAA is part of the proximal (pulmonary vein) atrial chamber in patients with a supravavlular ring.

Cor-triatriatum may be associated with other congenital abnormalities (atrial septal defect, persistence of left superior vena cava), but is commonly seen in isolation when found in an adult. It may be associated with increased gradients across the membrane, leading to this patient's symptoms. However, this finding lacks specificity and does not confirm a diagnosis. Pulmonary vein stenosis is not commonly associated with cor-triatriatum and would not confirm a diagnosis.

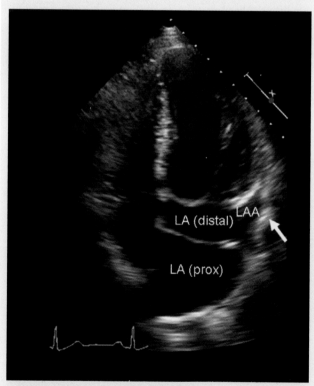

Fig. 24-15

Given Figure 24-15 and this patient's symptoms, an artifact cannot be assumed. Such a finding should be further investigated with multiple views, with and without Doppler. If TTE findings are ambiguous, a TEE may be warranted.

19. ANSWER: C. Figure 24-4 reveals a complex aortic plaque (pedunculated with mobile components). Patients who experience a cerebral event should be aggressively treated for secondary prevention with aspirin, statins, blood pressure control, smoking cessation, and glycemic control (if diabetic). Patent foramen ovale closure is not warranted given this patient's age and complex aortic atheroma. Although there is controversy with regards to warfarin therapy and aortic arch plaque, this patient is already therapeutic on antithrombotic agents for his AF. There is no data to demonstrate that a goal INR of 3-4 will improve the outcome of patients with aortic atheroma. Confirmation by chest CT is not warranted as Figure 24-4 represents atheroma and not aortic dissection.

20. ANSWER: D. Fluoroscopy reveals that the patient has mechanical valves (Bjork Shiley) in both the aortic and mitral positions. Due to the mitral position of his mechanical valve, anticoagulation with warfarin with a goal INR 2.5–3.5 is recommended. Additionally, low-dose aspirin (75–100 mg), concomitantly with warfarin, is recommended as per the 2008 ACC/AHA guidelines (Class I).

21. ANSWER: C. This M-mode reveals that this patient is in coarse AF. In a patient with new-onset AF, reversible causes of AF (e.g., hyperthyroidism) should be investigated and treated, if possible. There are no findings on this M-mode that would suggest that cardiac surgery, thrombolytics, cardiac CT, or alcohol septal ablation would be appropriate in this patient.

22. ANSWER: E. This four-chamber TTE demonstrates a prominent Eustachian valve and is a normal variant. The Eustachian valve is a remnant of the embryologic valve responsible for directing inferior vena caval blood across the atrial septum to the LA. It is a rigid and protuberant structure that arises along the posterior margin of the inferior vena cava to the border of the fossa ovalis. Although usually immobile, it may occasionally demonstrate independent motion within the RA and can be confused with tumors, vegetations, or thrombi. This should be differentiated from a Chiari network, which is a delicate-appearing, highly mobile, membranous structure arising near the orifice of the inferior vena cava. A Chiari network serves as the valve of the coronary sinus and is usually fenestrated. Like the Eustachian valve, the Chiari network has little clinical significance but may be confused with pathologic structures, such as vegetations or thrombi.

23. ANSWER: A. This is a pulsed wave Doppler of the LAA revealing AF/flutter. AF occurs transiently in 6%–10% of patients with an acute myocardial infarction, presumably due to atrial ischemia or atrial stretching secondary to heart failure. These patients have a worse prognosis than those who have acute myocardial infarctions without AF.

24. ANSWER: D. This finding on TEE represents lipomatous hypertrophy of the interatrial septum. In this condition, there is an unencapsulated accumulation of mature adipose tissue in the interatrial septum with sparing of the fossa ovale, which gives it the classic "dumb-bell" appearance on both TTE and TEE. It is thought to be a normal variant and is generally considered benign. This finding alone would not be a contraindication for cardioversion.

25. ANSWER: E. Immediately postcardioversion, there is an initial increase in SEC and thus an increased risk of thrombus formation/thromboembolism. This has been described with spontaneous conversion as well as following electrical and pharmacologic cardioversion. These findings are thought to be due to the reduction of LA function ("atrial stunning"), which can last for several weeks after successful cardioversion. Relatively high atrial appendage ejection velocity suggests shorter duration AF, and thus a higher likelihood of long-term maintenance of sinus rhythm. Additionally, there is a reduction in LAA function, demonstrated by decreased velocities through the LAA.

26. ANSWER: C. This M-mode demonstrates mitral stenosis and AF. Patients with mitral stenosis and AF have a stroke risk between 7% and 15% per year.

27. ANSWER: A. In a multivariate analysis of patients with mitral stenosis, only two independent risk factors for AF were found: LA dimension and increasing age.

28. ANSWER: D. The vast majority of atrial thrombi among patients with AF are located in the LAA. TTE has a reported sensitivity of 39%–63% in identifying or excluding LAA. Although there is improvement of visualization of the LA and the LAA with IV contrast and harmonic imaging with TTE, TEE still remains the gold standard to evaluate the LA and especially the LAA for thrombi.

KEY POINTS:

- Recognize mitral stenosis by M-mode and know there is an increase in stroke risk in patients with AF associated with rheumatic valvular disease.
- Only LA dimension and increasing age are independent predictors for AF in patients with mitral stenosis based on multivariate analysis.
- TEE remains the gold standard in the evaluation for LA thrombi.

29. ANSWER: E. The specificity of TEE for LA thrombi is reported to be between 90% and 100%.

30. ANSWER: D. Pulsed wave Doppler at the ostium of the pulmonary vein shows elevated velocities and spectral broadening both in systole and diastole, consistent with pulmonary vein stenosis. On TEE, normal right upper pulmonary vein S and D wave velocities are ~50–70 cm/s. The mean onset of pulmonary vein stenosis occurs between 2 and 5 months postprocedure.

Pulmonary vein stenosis is one of the potential complications of PVI. Early experience with PVI reported PV stenosis rates of up to 38%. More recent studies report the incidence to be only 1%–3%. The decline is likely related to a modification of the procedure with ablation now occurring in the body of the LA rather than within the pulmonary vein. A "retrograde" A wave is present confirming sinus rhythm.

KEY POINTS:

- TEE has both high sensitivity and specificity for LA thrombi.
- Pulmonary vein stenosis is a potential complication of PVI and should be suspected in those who present with shortness of breath after they have undergone this procedure. Interrogation by pulsed wave Doppler through the ostia of all four pulmonary veins should be performed to properly evaluate and rule out this condition.

31. ANSWER: D. This is a myxoma that is attached to the interatrial septum via a stalk, which is identified by calcification (the area of increased echogenicity (Fig. 24-16, white arrow)). Given this patient's history, this myxoma is likely responsible for an embolic phenomenon and should be removed surgically. That it is not an artifact can be seen in two different views (Fig. 24-16). While it is possible that this may also represent a thrombus, it is unlikely given the patient's normal sized LA and clearly demarcated stalk in the interatrial septum. Ao represents Aorta.

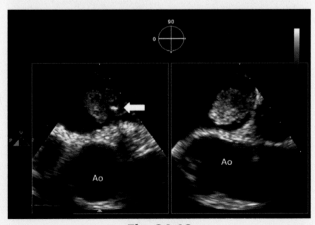

Fig. 24-16

32. ANSWER: E. Myxomas are benign tumors and the most common primary cardiac neoplasm. Almost 80% originate in the left atrium. While they commonly are found attached to the interatrial septum, they may be attached anywhere in the heart. Some patients are at risk for recurrence of the myxoma, which may occur in 2%–5% or the development of additional lesions. Systemic embolization has been reported up to 29%.

33. ANSWER: A. The Carney complex is an inherited, autosomal dominant disorder characterized by multiple tumors. These include atrial and extracardiac myxomas, schwannomas, and various endocrine tumors. Additionally, patients have a variety of pigmentation abnormalities, including pigmented lentigines and blue nevi.

KEY POINTS:

▨ This is not an artifact as it can be seen in two views (Fig. 24-13).

▨ Myxomas most commonly occur in the left atrium attached to the interatrial septum by a stalk (with calcification at the attachment).

▨ Myxomas should be removed in the setting of embolic phenomenon.

34. ANSWER: C. This is an M-Mode through the mitral valve, which shows a thickened septum with systolic anterior motion (SAM) of the anterior mitral valve leaflet (Fig. 24-17, white arrow), consistent with HCM. The patient is symptomatic during exercise, likely from LVOT obstruction and significant mitral regurgitation. Given this patient's age, history, M-mode findings, and likely diagnosis of HCM, embolic phenomenon and paroxysmal AF as the etiology of this patient's symptoms is less likely. While this patient has evidence of SAM and probable moderate to severe mitral regurgita-

tion, surgical repair of the mitral valve itself will not correct this patient's underlying pathology of HCM.

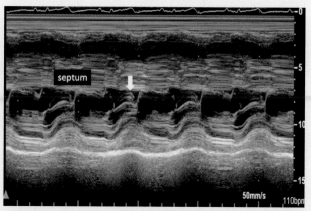
Fig. 24-17

35. ANSWER: D. This patient is hemodynamically unstable in the setting of AF and should be immediately cardioverted, without delay. Performing a TEE in this setting would be inappropriate. Patients with HCM are preload-dependent, especially those with LVOT obstruction, SAM, and severe mitral regurgitation. Patients who develop AF can become hemodynamically compromised upon losing their atrial kick. Giving diuretics would worsen this patient's condition given his poor stroke volume due to decreased filling. There is no indication for either emergent cardiac surgery or coronary angiogram.

KEY POINTS:

▨ Recognize HCM and SAM on M-mode.

▨ Emergent cardioversion in the setting of hemodynamically unstable AF is warranted and should not be delayed for TEE.

SUGGESTED READINGS

Antonielli E, Pizzuti A, Palinkas A, et al. Clinical value of left atrial appendage flow for prediction of long-term sinus rhythm maintenance in patients with nonvalvular atrial fibrillation. *J Am Coll Cardiol.* 2002;39:1443–1449.

Bonow RO, Carabello BA, Chatterjee K, et al. 2008 Focused Update incorporated into the ACC/AHA 2006 Guidelines for the Management of Patients With Valvular Heart Disease: a report of the American College of Cardiology/American Heart Association Task Force on Practice Guidelines (Writing Committee to revise the 1998 Guidelines for the Management of Patients With Valvular Heart Disease). Endorsed by the Society of Cardiovascular Anesthesiologists, Society for Cardiovascular Angiography and Interventions, and Society of Thoracic Surgeons. *J Am Coll Cardiol.* 2008;52:e1–e142.

Carabello BA. Modern management of mitral stenosis. *Circulation.* 2005;112:432–437.

Collins LJ, Silverman DI, Douglas PS, et al. Cardioversion of nonrheumatic atrial fibrillation. Reduced thromboembolic complications with 4 weeks of precardioversion anticoagulation are related to atrial thrombus resolution. *Circulation.* 1995;92:160–163.

Corti R, Fuster V, Fayad ZA, et al. Effects of aggressive versus conventional lipid-lowering therapy by simvastatin on human atherosclerotic lesions: a prospective, randomized, double-blind trial with high-resolution magnetic resonance imaging. *J Am Coll Cardiol.* 2005;46:106–112.

Crystal E, Garfinkle MS, Connolly SS, et al. Interventions for preventing post-operative atrial fibrillation in patients undergoing heart surgery. *Cochrane Database Syst Rev.* 2004;(4):CD003611.

de Divitiis M, Omran H, Rabahieh R, et al. Right atrial appendage thrombosis in atrial fibrillation: its frequency and its clinical predictors. *Am J Cardiol.* 1999;84:1023–1028.

Eagle KA, Guyton RA, Davidoff R, et al. ACC/AHA 2004 Guideline Update for Coronary Artery Bypass Graft Surgery: summary article. A report of the American College of Cardiology/American Heart

Association Task Force on Practice Guidelines (Committee to Update the 1999 Guidelines for Coronary Artery Bypass Graft Surgery). *J Am Coll Cardiol.* 2004;44:e213–e310.

Echocardiographic predictors of stroke in patients with atrial fibrillation: a prospective study of 1066 patients from 3 clinical trials. *Arch Intern Med.* 1998;158:1316–1320.

Fatkin D, Kelly RP, Feneley MP. Relations between left atrial appendage blood flow velocity, spontaneous echocardiographic contrast and thromboembolic risk in vivo. *J Am Coll Cardiol.* 1994;23:961–969.

Fatkin D, Loupas T, Low J, et al. Inhibition of red cell aggregation prevents spontaneous echocardiographic contrast formation in human blood. *Circulation.* 1997;96:889–896.

Fuster V, Ryden LE, Cannom DS, et al. ACC/AHA/ESC 2006 Guidelines for the Management of Patients With Atrial Fibrillation—executive summary: a report of the American College of Cardiology/American Heart Association Task Force on Practice Guidelines and the European Society of Cardiology Committee for Practice Guidelines (Writing Committee to Revise the 2001 Guidelines for the Management of Patients With Atrial Fibrillation). *Circulation.* 2006;114:e257–e354.

Ito T, Suwa M, Nakamura T, et al. Influence of warfarin therapy on left atrial spontaneous echo contrast in nonvalvular atrial fibrillation. *Am J Cardiol.* 1999;84:857–859, A858.

Klein AL, Grimm RA, Murray RD, et al. Use of transesophageal echocardiography to guide cardioversion in patients with atrial fibrillation. *N Engl J Med.* 2001;344:1411–1420.

Manning WJ, Silverman DI, Katz SE, et al. Impaired left atrial mechanical function after cardioversion: relation to the duration of atrial fibrillation. *J Am Coll Cardiol.* 1994;23:1535–1540.

Manning WJ, Silverman DI, Keighley CS, et al. Transesophageal echocardiographically facilitated early cardioversion from atrial fibrillation using short-term anticoagulation: final results of a prospective 4.5-year study. *J Am Coll Cardiol.* 1995;25:1354–1361.

Manning WJ, Silverman DI, Waksmonski CA, et al. Prevalence of residual left atrial thrombi among patients with acute thromboembolism and newly recognized atrial fibrillation. *Arch Intern Med.* 1995;155:2193–2198.

Manning WJ, Weintraub RM, Waksmonski CA, et al. Accuracy of transesophageal echocardiography for identifying left atrial thrombi. A prospective, intraoperative study. *Ann Intern Med.* 1995;123:817–822.

Packer DL, Keelan P, Munger TM, et al. Clinical presentation, investigation, and management of pulmonary vein stenosis complicating ablation for atrial fibrillation. *Circulation.* 2005;111:546–554.

Sallach JA, Puwanant S, Drinko JK, et al. Comprehensive left atrial appendage optimization of thrombus using surface echocardiography: the CLOTS multicenter pilot trial. *J Am Soc Echocardiogr.* 2009;22:1165–1172.

Sanders P, Morton JB, Morgan JG, et al. Reversal of atrial mechanical stunning after cardioversion of atrial arrhythmias: implications for the mechanisms of tachycardia-mediated atrial cardiomyopathy. *Circulation.* 2002;106:1806–1813.

Sohn DW, Kim YJ, Kim HC, et al. Evaluation of left ventricular diastolic function when mitral E and A waves are completely fused: role of assessing mitral annulus velocity. *J Am Soc Echocardiogr.* 1999;12:203–208.

Subramaniam B, Riley MF, Panzica PJ, et al. Transesophageal echocardiographic assessment of right atrial appendage anatomy and function: comparison with the left atrial appendage and implications for local thrombus formation. *J Am Soc Echocardiogr.* 2006;19:429–433.

Transesophageal echocardiographic correlates of thromboembolism in high-risk patients with nonvalvular atrial fibrillation. The Stroke Prevention in Atrial Fibrillation Investigators Committee on Echocardiography. *Ann Intern Med.* 1998;128:639–647.

Tunick PA, Kronzon I. Atherosclerosis of the aorta: a risk factor, risk marker, or an innocent bystander? *J Am Coll Cardiol.* 2005; 45:1907; author reply 1907.

Weigner MJ, Caulfield TA, Danias PG, et al. Risk for clinical thromboembolism associated with conversion to sinus rhythm in patients with atrial fibrillation lasting less than 48 hours. *Ann Intern Med.* 1997;126:615–620.

Wong CK, White HD, Wilcox RG, et al. New atrial fibrillation after acute myocardial infarction independently predicts death: the GUSTO-III experience. *Am Heart J.* 2000;140:878–885.

Appendix: Determining Stroke Risk and Antithrombotic Treatment for AF

TABLE 24-1 Stroke Risk in Patients With Nonvalvular AF Not Treated With Anticoagulation According to the CHADS$_2$ Index

CHADS$_2$ Risk Criteria	Score
Prior stroke or TIA	2
Age >75 y	1
Hypertension	1
Diabetes mellitus	1
Heart failure	1

Patients (N = 1,733)	Adjusted Stroke Rate (%/y)[a] (95% CI)	CHADS$_2$ Score
120	1.9 (1.2–3.0)	0
463	28 (2.0–3.8)	1
523	4.0 (3.1–5.1)	2
337	5.9 (4.6–7.3)	3
220	8.5 (6.3–11.1)	4
65	12.5 (8.2–17.5)	5
5	18.2 (10.5–27.4)	6

[a]The adjusted stroke rate was derived from multivariate analysis assuming no aspirin usage. (Data are from van Walraven WC, Hart RG, Wells GA, et al. A clinical prediction rule to identify patients with atrial fibrillation and a low risk for stroke while taking aspirin. *Arch Mem Med* 2003;163:936–943; and Gage BF. Waterman AD. Shannon W, et al. Validation of clinical classification schemes for predicting stroke: results from the National Registry of Atrial Fibrillation. *JAMA* 2001;285:2864–2870.)

AF indicates atrial fibrillation; CHADS$_2$, Cardiac Failure, hypertension, age, diabetes, and stroke (doubled); CI, confidence interval; and TIA, transient ischemic attack.

TABLE 24-2 Antithrombotic Therapy for Patients With AF

Risk Category	Recommended Therapy
No risk factors	Aspirin, 81–325 mg daily
One moderate-risk factor	Aspirin, 81–325 mg daily or warfarin (INR 2.0–3.0, target 2.5)
Any high-risk factor or more than one moderate-risk factor	Warfarin (INR 2.0–3.0, target 2.5)[a]

Less Validated or Weaker Risk Factors	Moderate-Risk Factors	High-Risk Factors
Female gender	Age greater than or equal to 75 y	Previous stroke, TIA, or embolism
Age 65–74 y	Hypertension	Mitral stenosis
Coronary artery disease	Heart failure	Prosthetic heart valve[a]
Thynotoxicosis	LV ejection fraction 35% or less, diabetes mellitus	

[a]If mechanical valve, target INR greater than 2.5.

INR indicates international normalized ratio; LV, left ventricular; and TIA, transient ischemic attack.

TABLE 24-3 Risk-Based Approach to Antithrombotic Therapy in Patients With AF

Patent Features	Antithrombotic Therapy	Class of Recommendation
Age less than 60 y, no heart disease (lone AF)	Aspirin (81–325 mg per day) or no therapy	I
Age less than 60 y, heart disease but no risk factors[a]	Aspirin (81–325 mg per day)	I
Age 60–74 y, no risk factors[a]	Aspirin (81–325 mg per day)	I
Age 65–74 y with diabetes mellitus or CAD	Oral anticoagulation (INR 2.0–3.0)	I
Age 75 y or older, women	Oral anticoagulation (INR 2.0–3.0)	I
Age 75 y or older, men, no other risk factors	Oral antlcoagulation (INR 2.0–3.0) or aspirin (81–325 mg per day)	I
Age 65 or older, heart failure	Oral anticoagulation (INR 2.0–3.0)	I
LV EF less than 35% or fractional shortening less than 25%, and hypertension	Oral anticoagulation (INR 2.0–3.0)	I
Rheumatic heart disease (mitral stenosis)	Oral anticoagulation (INR 2.0–3.0)	I
Prosthetic heart valves	Oral anticoagulation (INR 2.0–3.0 or higher)	I
Prior thromboembolism	Oral anticoagulation (INR 2.0–3.0 or higher)	I
Persistent atrial thrombus on TEE	Oral anticoagulation (INR 2.0–3.0 or higher)	IIa

[a]Risk factors for thromboembolism include heart failure (HF), left ventricular (LV) ejection fraction less than 35%, and history of hypertension.

AF indicates atrial fibrillation; CAD, coronary artery disease; INR, international normalized ratio; and TEE, transesophageal echocardiography.

Right Ventricular Disease and Pulmonary Hypertension

CHAPTER 25

Sherif F. Nagueh

1. Which of the following is an abnormal right ventricular (RV) dimension in an adult 30 years old?
   A. Basal RV diameter of 2.5 cm.
   B. Mid RV diameter of 3.8 cm.
   C. Right ventricular outflow tract (RVOT) diameter above the aortic valve of 2.6 cm.
   D. Base to apex RV length of 7.5 cm.

2. Which is an abnormal finding in an adult 30 years old?
   A. Tricuspid annular excursion of 2.0 cm.
   B. RV end-diastolic area of 26 cm^2.
   C. RV end-systolic area of 19 cm^2.
   D. RV fractional area change of 40%.

3. Which of the following is true concerning right atrial (RA) dimensions/area?
   A. RA volumes can be measured in low parasternal views.
   B. RA minor axis dimension of 4.8 cm is normal.
   C. RA volumes can be increased in patients with normal RV filling pressures.
   D. A dilated right atrium is an early marker of pulmonary hypertension.

4. Which of the following is an abnormal finding pertaining to the inferior vena cava (IVC) diameter?
   A. IVC diameter of 2.3 cm in a 23-years-old swimmer.
   B. IVC diameter of 1.1 cm in a 51-year-old woman with pulmonary hypertension.
   C. IVC diameter of 1.2 cm with 80% collapse during spontaneous breathing in a 61-year-old woman with systemic hypertension.
   D. IVC diameter of 2 cm and 40% collapse in a 35-year-old woman with exertional dyspnea.

5. A 46-year-old woman with 3-year duration of primary pulmonary hypertension is expected to have which of the following measurements?
   A. RA volume of 30 ml.
   B. D-shaped interventricular septum in diastole.
   C. RV free wall thickness of 1 cm.
   D. Long acceleration time of systolic flow through the RVOT.

6. Which of the following is characteristic of RV structure and function in patients with longstanding arrhythmogenic RV dysplasia (ARVD)?
   A. RV regional dysfunction in RVOT and apical segments.
   B. RV fractional area change of 50%.
   C. Tricuspid regurgitation (TR) jet by continuous-wave Doppler of 3.6 m/s.
   D. Left ventricular (LV) ejection fraction (EF) of 26%.

7. Which of the following tissue Doppler velocities is expected in a 36-year-old patient with primary pulmonary hypertension of 4-year duration?
   A. Septal mitral annulus systolic ejection velocity of 16 cm/sec.
   B. Lateral mitral annulus early diastolic velocity of 14 cm/sec.

C. Septal mitral annulus early diastolic velocity of 13 cm/sec.

D. Tricuspid systolic ejection velocity of 15 cm/sec.

E. Tricuspid early diastolic velocity of 13 cm/sec.

8. Which of these is an abnormal finding?
   A. Predominant forward hepatic vein diastolic flow in a 25-year-old man.
   B. A hepatic vein atrial reversal velocity of 20 ms duration.
   C. A tricuspid *E/A* ratio of 1.8 in a 34-year-old woman.
   D. A hepatic vein systolic velocity to diastolic velocity ratio of 0.3 in a 70-year-old man.
   E. Hepatic vein midsystolic reversal velocity of 15 cm/sec.

9. Which of the following is *not* a limitation for utilizing hepatic venous flow to predict RA pressure?
   A. A 55-year-old man with mid-diastolic rumble/holosystolic murmur at the lower left sternal border.
   B. A 61-year-old woman with postoperative dyspnea and paradoxical pulse.
   C. A 65-year-old man with a heart rate of 40/min after bypass surgery and cannon "a" waves in his jugular venous pulse.
   D. A 53-year-old man with low-voltage EKG, postural hypotension, and LV posterior wall thickness of 18 mm.
   E. A 45-year-old man who received a heart transplant 6 months ago.

10. Which of the following is compatible with advanced RV disease in patients with cardiac amyloidosis?
    A. RV free wall thickness of 7 mm.
    B. Deceleration time of tricuspid E velocity of 260 ms.
    C. Tricuspid *E/A* ratio of 1.
    D. A hepatic venous systolic velocity to diastolic velocity ratio of 0.6.
    E. Inspiratory venous and atrial flow reversals.

11. What is the pulmonary artery (PA) systolic pressure in a patient with a peak TR velocity of 3 m/sec and a jugular venous pressure of 15 cm?
    A. PA systolic pressure = 51 mm Hg.
    B. PA systolic pressure = 36 mm Hg.
    C. PA systolic pressure = 46 mm Hg.
    D. PA systolic pressure = 40 mm Hg.

12. Which of these patients has the highest pulmonary vascular resistance?
    A. TR jet of 3.6 m/sec and time velocity integral of RVOT systolic flow of 13 cm.
    B. TR jet of 3.3 m/sec and time velocity integral of RVOT systolic flow of 13 cm.
    C. TR jet of 3.6 m/sec and time velocity integral of RVOT systolic flow of 18 cm.
    D. TR jet of 3.5 m/sec and time velocity integral of RVOT systolic flow of 14 cm.

13. What is the mean PA pressure in this patient with TR peak velocity of 3 m/sec, pulmonary regurgitation (PR) end diastolic velocity of 2 m/sec, and RA pressure of 10 mm Hg?
    A. PA mean pressure = 26 mm Hg.
    B. PA mean pressure = 21 mm Hg.
    C. PA mean pressure = 33 mm Hg.
    D. PA mean pressure = 40 mm Hg.

14. What is the PA systolic pressure of this patient with pulmonary stenosis, where peak TR velocity is 4 m/sec, peak velocity across pulmonic valve = 3 m/sec, and RA pressure = 10 mm Hg?
    A. PA systolic pressure = 46 mm Hg.
    B. PA systolic pressure = 74 mm Hg.
    C. PA systolic pressure = 38 mm Hg.
    D. PA systolic pressure = 50 mm Hg.

15. Which of these supports the diagnosis of increased RV systolic pressure?
    A. Acceleration time of 120 ms in systolic flow recorded at RVOT.
    B. PR peak velocity of 1.5 m/sec, and RA pressure of 5 mm Hg.
    C. TR peak velocity of 3.5 m/sec.
    D. Flat interventricular septum during diastole only.

16. Which of the following is most compatible with the hepatic venous flow in Figure 25-1?

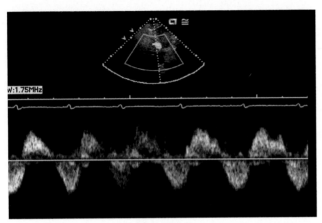

Fig. 25-1

A. 56-year-old man with systemic hypertension under control with medical therapy.
B. 39-year-old woman with hypotension in the setting of acute inferior wall MI.
C. 25-year-old man with recurrent septic pulmonary embolism.
D. 63-year-old man in atrial fibrillation.

17. Which of the following is compatible with the hepatic venous flow in Figure 25-2?

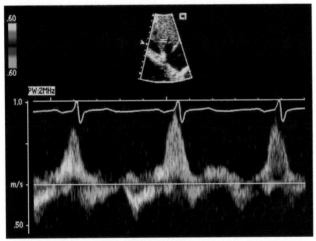

Fig. 25-2

A. 49-year old man with dilated cardiomyopathy and systemic and pulmonary congestion.
B. 29-year-old woman with pulmonary hypertension and systemic congestion.
C. 55-year-old man with cardiac amyloidosis and lower extremity swelling.
D. 65-year-old woman with hypertrophic cardiomyopathy and RV hypertrophy.

18. Which of the following is the most accurate conclusion about the continuous wave (CW) signal in Figure 25-3?

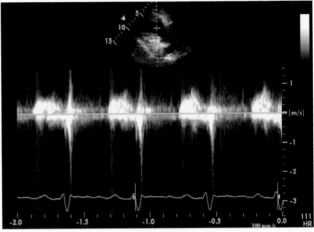

Fig. 25-3

A. PA systolic pressure can be reliably estimated.
B. PA systolic pressure is at least 25 mm Hg.
C. Intravenous saline is recommended for reliable assessment of PA systolic pressure.
D. With normal RV size and septal shape, PA systolic pressure is normal.

19. Which of the following is correct about Figure 25-4?

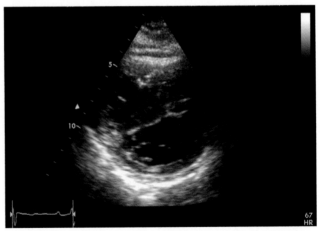

Fig. 25-4

A. It is seen in patients with systemic sclerosis, if noted only at end diastole.
B. It is seen in patients with fixed wide splitting of the second heart sound, if noted only at end diastole.
C. It is seen in patients with pulmonary embolism, if noted only at end diastole.
D. It is seen in patients with pulmonary stenosis, if noted only at end diastole.

20. What is the PA diastolic pressure in this patient with dyspnea on exertion (Fig. 25-5)? The IVC is dilated and does not collapse with sniffing.

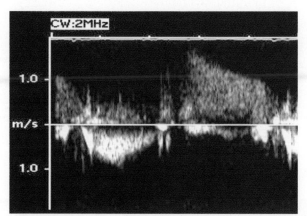

Fig. 25-5

A. PA diastolic pressure = 14 mm Hg.
B. PA diastolic pressure = 9 mm Hg.
C. PA diastolic pressure = 24 mm Hg.
D. PA diastolic pressure = 19 mm Hg.

21. Which is true about this patient with PR, (Fig. 25-6)?

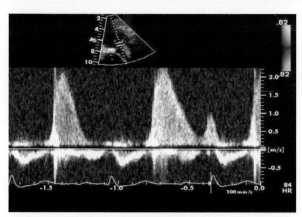

Fig. 25-6

A. Right ventricular end diastolic pressure (RVEDP) is normal.
B. RV stiffness is increased.
C. Systolic reversal in the hepatic veins is present.
D. Tricuspid E/A ratio is 0.6.

22. Choose the correct conclusion about LV diastolic function in this patient with pulmonary hypertension (Fig. 25-7).

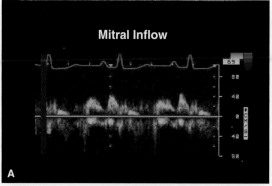

Fig. 25-7A

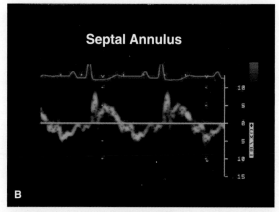

Fig. 25-7B

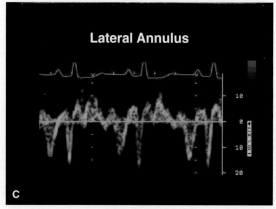

Fig. 25-7C

A. Mean left atrial pressure is increased.
B. LV relaxation is impaired.
C. Successful treatment with Bosentan will lead to an increase in mitral E/A ratio.
D. Left ventricular end diastolic pressure (LVEDP) is increased.

23. Choose the correct conclusion about LV diastolic function in this patient with pulmonary hypertension (Fig. 25-8).

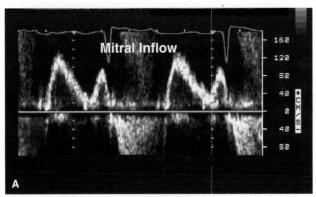

Fig. 25-8A

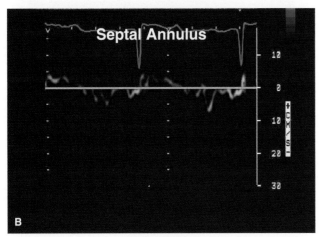

Fig. 25-8B

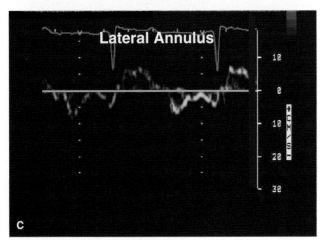

Fig. 25-8C

A. Mean left atrial (LA) pressure is normal.
B. LV relaxation is impaired and LA pressure is increased.
C. Treatment with diuretics will lead to an increase in mitral *E/A* ratio.
D. LVEDP is normal.

24. Choose the correct conclusion about LV and RV pressures in this patient with a holosystolic murmur at the left sternal border and a blood pressure of 150/80 mm Hg. The Doppler is obtained from VSD flow at the parasternal short-axis view at the level of the aortic valve (Fig. 25-9).

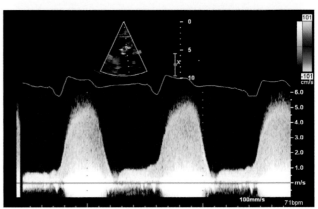

Fig. 25-9

A. RVEDP is higher than LVEDP.
B. RV systolic pressure is higher than LV systolic pressure.
C. If the peak velocity is approximately 5.5 m/sec, PA systolic pressure is 29 mm Hg in the absence of pulmonary stenosis.
D. The findings are compatible with a peak TR velocity of 3.5 m/sec in the absence of pulmonary stenosis.

25. What is the PA systolic pressure in this patient, where the TR peak velocity is 2.8 m/sec (Fig. 25-10)? Hepatic venous flow shows an *S/D* velocity ratio of 0.35.

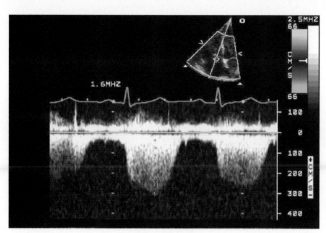

Fig. 25-10

A. PA systolic pressure = 31–36 mm Hg.
B. PA systolic pressure = 46–51 mm Hg.
C. PA systolic pressure = 41–46 mm Hg.
D. PA systolic pressure = 36–41 mm Hg.

CASE 1:

An echocardiogram is performed to evaluate hypotension in a patient with CAD after coronary artery bypass surgery. There are limited windows (see Video 25-1).

26. Concerning Video 25-1, which of the following is 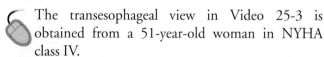 true?
   A. RV function is normal.
   B. LV size is normal.
   C. LV stroke volume is reduced.
   D. Patient can benefit from an intraaortic balloon pump.

27. Concerning Figure 25-11, which of the following is true?

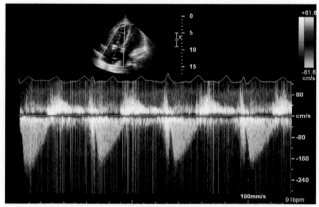

Fig. 25-11

A. PA systolic pressure can be reliably estimated based on the TR jet.
B. Midsystolic reversal is present in the hepatic veins.
C. RV systolic pressure is very close to RA "v" wave pressure.
D. Similar hemodynamic findings are noted in patients with longstanding ASD.

CASE 2:

The apical views in Videos 25-2A and B were obtained from a 36-year-old man with complaints of recurrent focal weakness of the right upper extremity, and reduced arterial O_2 saturation with exertion.

28. Which of the following is true?
   A. RV size is enlarged.
   B. LV EF appears reduced.
   C. A short-axis view would show a D-shaped septum in systole.
   D. RA "v" wave pressure is increased.

29. Which is true concerning the symptoms of the patient in question 28?
   A. Definity injection can help determine the underlying etiology.
   B. No further evaluation is needed at this time.
   C. An increase in LV filling pressures accounts for the exertional hypoxemia.
   D. He is likely to have an abnormal brain MRI examination.

CASE 3:

The transesophageal view in Video 25-3 is obtained from a 51-year-old woman in NYHA class IV.

30. Which of the following is true?
   A. The right atrium appears enlarged.
   B. There is predominant left-to-right shunting.
   C. LA pressure is higher than RA pressure.
   D. The lesion is not amenable to percutaneous closure.

31. Which is true concerning the TR jet and the pulmonary venous flow signals obtained from the same patient in question 30 (Fig. 25-12)?

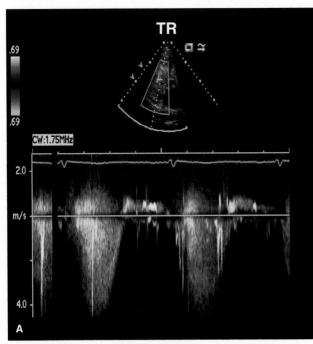

Fig. 25-12A

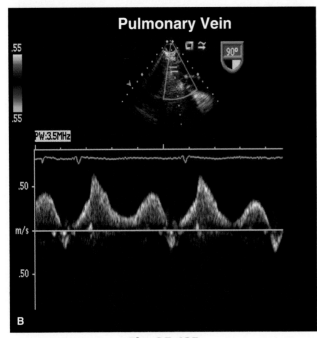

Fig. 25-12B

A. Pulmonary vascular resistance is normal.
B. Septal systolic velocity by tissue Doppler is probably reduced.
C. Diastolic dysfunction is the etiology of dyspnea.
D. Mitral regurgitation is the likely etiology of dyspnea.

CASE 4:

 The parasternal views (see Videos 25-4A and B) were obtained from a patient with a systolic murmur since birth.

32. Which is true?
   A. PA systolic pressure is normal.
   B. RV free wall thickness is likely 4 mm.
   C. LV EF is 50%–54%.
   D. Color Doppler shows severe PR.

33. Which of the following is true about the CW signal recorded at the RVOT obtained from the same patient (Fig. 25-13)?

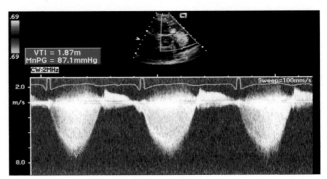

Fig. 25-13

A. Pulmonary vascular resistance is increased.
B. Peak TR velocity is likely 4.5 m/sec.
C. Hepatic veins will have a prominent atrial reversal signal after RA contraction.
D. The lesion is not amenable to percutaneous intervention.

CASE 5:

 The parasternal views in Videos 25-5A and B were obtained from a 36-year-old man with lower extremity swelling.

34. Which is true?
   A. RV volumes are normal.
   B. RV systolic pressure is increased.
   C. LV EF is mild to moderately depressed.
   D. Positive history of congenital heart disease.

35. Which of the following is true about the CW signal recorded at the RVOT obtained from the same patient (Fig. 25-14)?

A. Pulmonary vascular resistance is increased.

B. Percutaneous commissurotomy can be considered.

C. RV septum that is flat in diastole and systole is likely present.

D. Increased RV diastolic pressures.

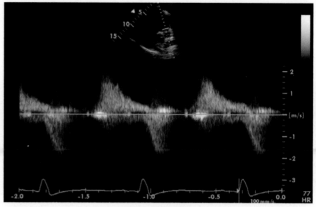

Fig. 25-14

ANSWERS

1. ANSWER: B. All of the measurements are within the range of normal values except for the mid-right ventricular (RV) diameter, which is consistent with moderate enlargement. The normal range for the latter diameter is 2.7–3.3 cm. For basal RV diameter, the normal range is 2–2.8 cm, and for the RV diameter above the aortic valve level, it is 2.5–2.9 cm. The long axis of the RV is normally between 7.1 and 7.9 cm (Table 25-1). Note that these measurements are obtained at end diastole and require parallel alignment of the septum and the ultrasound beam, and no foreshortening.

TABLE 25-1 Summary of Normal RV Dimensions

RV Dimensions	
Basal RV diameter, cm	2.0–2.8
Mid-RV diameter, cm	2.7–3.3
Basal-to-apical length, cm	7.1–7.9
Right ventricular outflow tract (RVOT) diameters	
Above aortic valve, cm	2.5–2.9
Above pulmonic valve, cm	1.7–2.3

2. ANSWER: C. The tricuspid annular descent is normally in the range of 1.5–2 cm. RV end-diastolic area in normal subjects ranges between 11 and 28 cm^2, whereas end-systolic area is between 7.5 and 16 cm^2. RV fractional area change is normally between 32% and 60%.

3. ANSWER: C. Right atrial (RA) dimensions and volumes can be measured to draw conclusions about RA size. RA volumes should be measured in an apical four-chamber view. The minor axis diameter is measured between RA lateral border and the interatrial septum in a perpendicular direction to RA long axis, and normally ranges between 2.9 and 4.5 cm. Changes in RV myocardial function as detected by myocardial imaging are the earliest abnormalities in patients with pulmonary hypertension; and in early stages, the RA volume is often normal. Similar to left atrial (LA) volumes, RA volumes are not sensitive markers to acute changes in filling pressures. Accordingly, a dilated right atrium can be seen in patients with normal RV filling pressures. In addition, increased flow as seen with athlete's heart or left-to-right shunts may increase RA size without increasing filling pressures. On the other hand, RA volumes are a better reflection of chronic changes of RV filling pressures.

4. ANSWER: D. Inferior vena cava (IVC) diameter is measured in the subcostal views at 1–2 cm from its drainage into the RA. The measurement is performed in a perpendicular direction to its long axis. A diameter <1.2 cm is indicative of normal to reduced RA pressure (RAP) (Table 25-2). Athletes can have a dilated IVC which exceeds 2 cm. In patients with normal RAP, the IVC has a normal diameter which decreases by >50% with inspiration. However, if spontaneous breathing is not accompanied by such a change, sniffing should be performed. The change in IVC diameter with sniffing, in addition to IVC diameter at baseline, should be used to predict RAP. When the RAP is mildly elevated in the range between 5 and 10 mm Hg, the IVC diameter is usually increased (>2.1 cm) with a collapse index, that is at least 50%.

TABLE 25-2 Summary of RAP Estimation Using IVC Collapse Index and Hepatic Venous Flow

Mean RAP	IVC% Collapse	Hepatic Veins
0–5 mm Hg	≥50%	$V_S > V_D$
5–10 mm Hg	≥50%	$V_S = V_D$
10–15 mm Hg	<50%	$V_S < V_D$
≥20 mm Hg	<50%	Flow only with V_D

IVC = inferior vena cava.
V_S = forward systolic velocity in hepatic venous flow.
V_D = forward diastolic velocity in hepatic venous flow.

5. ANSWER: C. In patients with pulmonary hypertension of 3-year duration, RA and RV enlargement are often present, along with increased RV free wall thickness. With RV enlargement, both long axis and minor dimensions are increased. RV free wall thickness is most reliably measured in the subcostal views and normally is up to 0.5 cm. In pulmonary hypertension, the interventricular septum is D-shaped both in systole and diastole. These patients also have a short acceleration time for systolic flow in the RVOT. Mean pulmonary artery (PA) pressure can be estimated using the regression equation: 80–0.5 (acceleration time).

6. ANSWER: A. In this cardiomyopathy, there are frequent abnormalities in RV regional and global function. The regional dysfunction is commonly noted in the RVOT, apex, and basal RV free wall in the region of the "triangle of dysplasia." RV dilatation and depressed global systolic function also occur, though not in all patients early on. In one study, dilatation of the RVOT was noted in all patients with arrhythmogenic RV dysplasia (ARVD) and may occur as an isolated finding. Other abnormalities include abnormally bright moderator band, RV sacculations (or diastolic outpouchings), aneurysm (systolic outpouchings), and trabecular derangements. left ventricular (LV) ejection fraction (EF) is characteristically normal in most patients with ARVD although infrequently a left-sided cardiomyopathy may occur. Given the presence of RV systolic dysfunction, PA pressures are usually normal and not elevated. Therefore, a peak tricuspid regurgitation (TR) velocity of 3.6 m/sec is not consistent with ARVD.

7. ANSWER: B. RV systolic and diastolic functions are depressed in patients with pulmonary hypertension. Because of the RV contribution to septal function, both septal systolic and diastolic mitral annulus tissue Doppler velocities are reduced. Likewise, tricuspid annulus velocities at the lateral side of the tricuspid annulus are reduced in these patients. On the other hand, LV function is preserved, and early diastolic velocities at the lateral side of the mitral annulus are usually normal.

8. ANSWER: D. The flow in the hepatic veins is largely determined by RAP during the cardiac cycle (Table 25-2). In normal subjects, antegrade flow from the hepatic veins to the RA occurs in systole (S) and diastole (D). With RA contraction, brief retrograde late diastolic flow (Ar), as well as late systole flow (Vr), occurs into the hepatic veins. It is feasible to record high-quality signals by transthoracic imaging from the subcostal window in most ambulatory patients. Hepatic vein flow velocities can be used to asses RAP. In general, a lower proportion of forward systolic flow is indicative of increased RAP, except in healthy young subjects where this finding is normal. Similar to mitral inflow, young subjects have an *E/A* ratio that is >1 with a short DT, and reduced RA contribution to RV filling.

9. ANSWER: D. There are limitations to using hepatic venous flow to predict RAP. These include the presence of tricuspid valve stenosis or regurgitation, pericardial compression syndromes, high-grade AV block, and heart transplants. The presence of a restrictive cardiomyopathy is not a limitation. Option A is consistent with tricuspid stenosis/regurgitation. Option B is consistent with a postoperative pericardial compression syndrome. The patient in option C has high-grade heart block, and option E is a heart transplant. The presentation in D is consistent with amyloid where the patient has cardiac disease and peripheral neuropathy.

10. ANSWER: E. With advance RV disease in patients with cardiac amyloidosis, RV free wall thickness is >7 mm, and tricuspid inflow shows a restrictive filling pattern. Hepatic venous flow at this stage is characterized by reduced forward systolic flow, increased forward diastolic flow, and inspiratory diastolic flow reversal.

11. ANSWER: C. PA systolic pressure is given by $4(V_{TR})^2$ + RAP. A jugular venous pressure of 15 cm water corresponds to 15 × 0.7 or 10–11 mm Hg, since 1 cm water corresponds to 0.7 mm Hg. Accordingly, PA systolic pressure is given by $4(3)^2$ + 10, or 46 mm Hg.

12. ANSWER: A. Pulmonary vascular resistance (PVR) is derived invasively as: (mean PA pressure − wedge pressure)/cardiac output. It can be estimated noninvasively by using the ratio between peak velocity of TR jet (as a surrogate of PA pressure), and time velocity integral of RVOT systolic flow (as a surrogate of cardiac output). Options A and C have the highest peak velocity, while option A has the least time velocity integral of RVOT systolic flow.

13. ANSWER: C. Mean PA pressure is given by PA diastolic pressure + 1/3 pulse pressure. This patient has a PA systolic pressure of $4(3)^2$ +10 or 46 mmHg. PA diastolic pressure = $4(2)^2$ +10 or 26 mmHg. Pulse pressure is given by 46 − 26 or 20 mm Hg. Accordingly, mean PA pressure = 26 + (20/3), or 33 mm Hg. Mean PA pressure can also be estimated using the regression equation: 80–0.5 (acceleration time).

14. ANSWER: C. RV systolic pressure is given by $4(V_{TR})^2$ + RAP, where V_{TR} is the peak velocity of the TR jet. Therefore, RV systolic pressure = 64 + 10, or 74 mm Hg. The gradient between RV systolic pressure and PA systolic pressure is given by RV systolic pressure − PA systolic pressure = $4(V_{PV})^2$, where V_{PV} is the peak velocity across the pulmonary valve. Therefore, PA systolic pressure = 74 − 36, or 38 mm Hg.

15. ANSWER: C. Mean PA pressure can be estimated using the regression equation: 80–0.5 (acceleration time). Therefore, the patient in A is predicted to have a mean PA pressure of 20 mm Hg, which is normal. Mean PA pressure can also be estimated using the peak velocity of pulmonary regurgitation (PR) to which an estimate of right ventricular end diastolic pressure (RVEDP), or RAP, is added. Therefore, the mean PA pressure in B can be predicted to be: $4(1.5)^2 + 5$ or 14 mm Hg, which is normal. In C, the peak systolic pressure is at least: $4(3.5)^2$, or 49 mm Hg, which is consistent with pulmonary hypertension. With increased RV systolic pressure, a D-shaped septum is present in both systole and diastole, and not only during diastole.

16. *ANSWER: C.* The hepatic venous flow shows holosystolic reversal compatible with severe TR, as in the setting of infective endocarditis of the tricuspid valve (option C). A patient with controlled blood pressure has normal RA pressure and predominant forward systolic flow, not systolic reversal. In the setting of RV infarction and acute inferior wall MI, RV filling pressures are increased and there is predominant forward diastolic flow in the hepatic veins. Systolic flow is reduced, but not reversed in atrial fibrillation.

17. *ANSWER: D.* The hepatic venous flow shows large Ar signal compatible with normal RA systolic function in the presence of increased RVEDP. In early stages of RV diastolic dysfunction, RVEDP is increased, whereas mean RAP is normal. This hemodynamic finding is compatible with option D. Systemic congestion occurs with increased RA mean pressure and predominant forward diastolic flow in all other choices.

18. *ANSWER: C.* This is an incomplete TR jet that should not be used to predict PA systolic pressure. Intravenous saline injection can be used however. Depending on the level of pulmonary hypertension and its duration, RV size and function and septal morphology can appear normal despite an increased PA systolic pressure.

19. *ANSWER: B.* When the interventricular septum is D-shaped in systole and diastole, RV systolic pressure is increased (options A, C, and D). If the D-shaped septum is noted only during diastole, RV volume overload is present as in patients with an atrial septal defect (option B).

20. *ANSWER: C.* The PA diastolic pressure is given by $4v^2$ + RA pressure, where v is the end-diastolic velocity of the PR jet. The patient with a dilated IVC that does not collapse with inspiration is consistent with an RA pressure of 20 mm Hg. Accordingly, the PA diastolic pressure is given by $4(1)^2 + 20$ or 24 mm Hg.

21. *ANSWER: B.* The PR signal is steep indicating rapid equilibration of pressure between the PA and the RV. When RV stiffness is increased, RV diastolic pressure rises rapidly leading to a PR signal that is similar to that seen in this case. These patients have increased RVEDP

and RAP. Tricuspid inflow is characterized by predominant early filling with an *E/A* ratio >1, and a steep deceleration time of tricuspid *E* velocity. Hepatic venous flow shows predominant forward flow in diastole (not systolic reversal).

22. *ANSWER: C.* The Doppler tracings show a mitral *E/A* ratio <1, a normal lateral e' velocity, and a reduced septal e' velocity. Collectively, these findings are seen in patients with pulmonary hypertension of a noncardiac etiology. The presence of a lateral *E/e'* ratio <10 is indicative of normal or reduced LV filling pressures. A mitral *E/A* ratio <1 is not due to impaired LV relaxation, but reduced LV filling due to pulmonary hypertension and dilated RV. With the reduction in pulmonary vascular resistance with Bosentan, LV filling increases as well as mitral *E/A* ratio.

23. *ANSWER: B.* This patient has a pseudonormal LV filling pattern, and a lateral *E/e'* ratio > 10. Collectively, the findings are consistent with pulmonary hypertension secondary to a cardiac etiology. LV relaxation is impaired given the reduction in lateral e' velocity. The increase in mitral *E/e'* ratio is consistent with increased LV filling pressures. Treatment with diuretics leads to a reduction in LV filling and the mitral *E/A* ratio.

24. *ANSWER: C.* The flow is obtained from a ventricular septal defect (VSD) signal showing flow between the LV and the RV during systole and diastole. This is compatible with a higher left ventricular end diastolic pressure (LVEDP) than RVEDP, as well as a higher LV systolic pressure than RV systolic pressure. RV systolic pressure is the same as PA systolic pressure in the absence of pulmonary stenosis. Accordingly, PA systolic pressure can be computed as PA systolic pressure = LV systolic pressure − $4(V_{VSD})^2$, where v is in m/sec and represents the peak velocity of the VSD jet by continuous-wave Doppler. In this case, PA systolic pressure = $150 − 4(5.5)^2 = 29$ mm Hg. This is not compatible with a TR jet of 3.5 m/sec, which indicates an RV/PA systolic pressure of at least 49 mm Hg.

25. *ANSWER: C.* The PA systolic pressure is given by $4v^2$ + RA pressure, where v is the peak velocity of the TR jet. The patient with predominant forward diastolic flow is compatible with an RA pressure of 10–15 mm Hg. Accordingly, the PA systolic pressure is given by $4(2.8)^2 + 10–15$ mm Hg, or 41–46 mm Hg.

26. *ANSWER: C.* The parasternal long-axis view shows a LV with reduced end-diastolic dimension, but increased wall thickness. While LV fractional shortening is normal, there is almost no change during the cardiac cycle in the RV area seen in Video 25-1. The latter observation is indicative of a severely depressed RV systolic function. Because of severe RV systolic dysfunction, LV filling and stroke volume are reduced, as can be inferred from the reduced aortic valve leaflet separation in this view. Since LV function is normal, and the patient an intraaortic balloon pump already (seen in Video 25-1, the descending aorta posterior to the left atrium), option D is wrong.

27. *ANSWER: C.* Figure 25-11 shows the TR jet by CW recorded from a low left parasternal position. The signal is dense, triangular in shape, and shows early peaking with a peak velocity of only 160 cm/sec. These findings are consistent with severe TR, and an RV pressure that is very similar to RA "v" wave pressure. The patient would be expected to have holosystolic, and not just midsystolic, reversal in the hepatic venous flow. In this patient, the correct estimation of PA systolic pressure is challenging and is highly dependent on the accurate assessment of RAP, and not the TR jet peak velocity. In patients with longstanding atrial septal defect (ASD), secondary pulmonary hypertension develops with a much higher peak velocity of TR by CW Doppler.

KEY POINTS:

■ RV systolic dysfunction can be diagnosed by the change in RV dimensions and area by 2-D echocardiography.

■ Severe TR by CW Doppler is characterized by a dense signal with early peaking.

■ In patients with severe TR and a small systolic transvalvular pressure gradient, the accurate assessment of PA systolic pressure is highly dependent on the correct estimation of RAP.

28. ANSWER: D. The apical four-chamber views were obtained from a patient with Ebstein's anomaly. The tricuspid valve leaflets are seen close to the RV apex, and color Doppler shows moderately severe TR. LV EF appears normal, though additional views are needed for confirmation. RA, but not RV, size is increased because of the apical displacement of tricuspid valve leaflets in this condition. Because of reduced pulmonary blood flow, PA pressures are reduced to low normal, unless coexisting disease is present that can lead to pulmonary hypertension. Therefore, the patient would not show a D-shaped septum during systole.

29. ANSWER: D. Patients with Ebstein's disease frequently have interatrial shunting. This can result in systemic embolic events which may manifest with recurrent transient ischemic attacks and silent strokes that can be identified by brain MRI studies. Likewise, shunting is usually the cause of exertional hypoxemia, and not LV diastolic dysfunction. Further evaluation with saline contrast is needed to identify the site of shunting, but Definity injection is best avoided in these patients and generally contraindicated with interatrial shunts.

KEY POINTS:

■ Ebstein's disease is characterized by apical displacement of tricuspid valve leaflets. As a result, RA volume is increased and anatomic RV size is reduced.

■ Tricuspid regurgitation of varying severity is frequently present in this condition.

■ Interatrial shunting via PFO or ASD can occur and lead to transient ischemic attacks and systemic embolic events.

30. ANSWER: A. TEE shows a large RA with predominantly right-to-left shunting across the interatrial septum. The PFO shown in the TEE can be closed percutaneously. The presence of an RA to LA shunt supports the conclusion that RAP is higher than LA pressure.

31. ANSWER: B. The TR jet has a peak velocity close to 4 m/sec. This corresponds to a PA systolic pressure that is at least 64 mm Hg. Pulmonary venous flow shows predominant systolic flow and small atrial reversal velocity with LA contraction. The pulmonary venous flow pattern is consistent with normal LV filling pressures, and the absence of significant MR (which would have led to systolic reversal). Patients with pulmonary hypertension have increased pulmonary vascular resistance. The increased RV afterload (and RV systolic dysfunction later on) leads to reduced RV systolic velocities that can be recorded at the interventricular septum as the septal systolic velocity, and the RV free wall.

KEY POINTS:

■ Color Doppler can be used to identify the presence of a shunt across interatrial septum.

■ In patients with a noncardiac etiology of pulmonary hypertension and reduced LV filling, pulmonary venous flow shows predominant forward systolic flow and a small atrial reversal (Ar) signal.

32. ANSWER: A. The short-axis view shows a D-shaped interventricular septum in systole and diastole, consistent with increased RV systolic pressure. Color Doppler shows flow acceleration across the pulmonic valve consistent with pulmonary stenosis. Therefore, PA systolic pressure is possibly normal. Color Doppler shows mild PR, whereas 2-D imaging shows a hyperdynamic LV EF that is >70%. There is RV hypertrophy, and free wall thickness cannot be normal in this patient.

33. ANSWER: C. The CW signal indicates the presence of severe pulmonary stenosis with a peak velocity >6 m/sec. TR peak velocity should therefore be closer to that value. The patient does not have pulmonary hypertension and pulmonary vascular resistance is not increased. With RV hypertrophy, RV stiffness and late diastolic pressures are increased which lead to a prominent Ar signal in hepatic venous flow with RA contraction. Percutaneous commissurotomy can be used to treat pulmonary valve stenosis with good results.

KEY POINTS:

■ Patients with significant pulmonary stenosis have increased RV systolic pressure and RV hypertrophy. Therefore, a D-shaped septum would be noticed in systole and diastole.

■ RV hypertrophy is associated with increased RV stiffness and late diastolic RV pressures. RV diastolic dysfunction can be identified by increased Ar velocity and duration in hepatic venous flow.

■ Pulmonary stenosis can be diagnosed by CW Doppler using the peak velocity and the contour of the spectral envelope.

34. ANSWER: D. The parasternal long-axis view shows an LV with normal size and function but a dilated RV. Color Doppler shows some acceleration across the pulmonic valve in systole indicating increased systolic flow across the valve. However, the most important finding by color Doppler is the presence of severe PR. This lesion

is common after surgery for the repair of Tetralogy of Fallot, and does not lead to increased RV systolic pressure.

35. ANSWER: D. The CW signal is indicative of severe PR and the small increase in velocity across the pulmonic valve is largely due to increased transvalvular flow, and not valve stenosis. Patients with severe PR have a steep rise in RV diastolic pressure that leads to the rapid equalization of the pressure gradient between the PA and the RV in early diastole, and therefore a PR signal with steep deceleration and short pressure halftime. Severe PR leads to increased RV diastolic, not systolic, pressures. Therefore, a flat septum would be noted only in diastole, and not systole.

KEY POINTS:

■ Patients with significant PR have a dilated RV with eccentric hypertrophy.

■ Interventricular septal motion is characterized by an RV volume overload pattern, with a flat septum only in diastole.

■ Color Doppler can be used to assess the severity of PR.

■ Severe PR by CW Doppler shows rapid deceleration with short pressure halftime.

SUGGESTED READINGS

Abbas AE, Fortuin FD, Schiller NB, et al. A simple method for non-invasive estimation of pulmonary vascular resistance. *J Am Coll Cardiol.* 2003:1021–1027.

Appleton CP, Hatle LK, Popp RL. Demonstration of restrictive ventricular physiology by Doppler echocardiography. *J Am Coll Cardiol.* 1988;11:757–768.

Appleton CP, Hatle LK, Popp RL. Superior vena cava and hepatic vein Doppler echocardiography in healthy adults. *J Am Coll Cardiol.* 1987;10:1032–1039.

Appleton CP, Jensen JL, Hatle LK, et al. Doppler evaluation of left and right ventricular diastolic function: a technical guide for obtaining optimal flow velocity recordings. *J Am Soc Echocardiogr.* 1997;10:271–292.

Baumgartner H, Hung J, Bermejo J, et al. Echocardiographic assessment of valve stenosis: EAE/ASE recommendations for clinical practice. *J Am Soc Echocardiogr.* 2009;22:1–23.

Kircher BJ, Himelman RB, Schiller NB. Non-invasive estimation of right atrial pressure from the inspiratory collapse of the inferior vena cava. *Am J Cardiol.* 1990;66:493–496.

Lang RM, Bierig M, Devereux RB, et al. American Society of Echocardiography's Nomenclature and Standards Committee; Task Force on Chamber Quantification; American College of Cardiology Echocardiography Committee; American Heart Association; European Association of Echocardiography, European Society of Cardiology Recommendations for Chamber Quantification. *Eur J Echocardiogr.* 2006;7:79–108.

Masuyama T, Kodama K, Kitabatake A, et al. Continuous-wave Doppler echocardiographic detection of pulmonary regurgitation and its application to noninvasive estimation of pulmonary artery pressure. *Circulation.* 1986;74:484–492.

Nagueh SF, Appleton CP, Gillebert TC, et al. Recommendations for the Evaluation of Left Ventricular Diastolic Function by Echocardiography. *J Am Soc Echocardiogr.* 2009;22:107–133.

Nagueh SF, Kopelen HA, Zoghbi WA. Relation of mean right atrial pressure to echocardiographic and Doppler parameters of right atrial and right ventricular function. *Circulation.* 1996;93:1160–1169.

Oh JK, Hatle LK, Seward JB, et al. Diagnostic role of Doppler echocardiography in constrictive pericarditis. *J Am Coll Cardiol.* 1994;23:154–162.

Quinones MA, Otto CM, Stoddard M, et al. Recommendations for Quantification of Doppler Echocardiography: A Report from the Doppler Quantification Task Force of the Nomenclature and Standards Committee of the American Society of Echocardiography. *J Am Soc Echocardiogr.* 2002;15:167–184.

Ruan Q, Nagueh SF. Clinical application of tissue Doppler imaging in patients with idiopathic pulmonary hypertension. *Chest.* 2007;131:395–401.

Rudski LG, Lai WW, Afilalo, J, et al. Guidelines for the echocardiographic assessment of the right heart in adults: A report from the American Society of Echocardiography. *J Am Soc Echocardiogr.* 2010;23:685–713.

Simonson JS, Schiller NB. Sonospirometry: a non-invasive method for estimation of mean right atrial pressure based on two dimensional echocardiographic measurements of the inferior vena cava during measured inspiration. *J Am Coll Cardiol.* 1988;11:557–564.

Zoghbi WA, Enriquez-Sarano M, Foster E, et al. American Society of Echocardiography. Recommendations for Evaluation of the Severity of Native Valvular Regurgitation with Two-Dimensional and Doppler Echocardiography. *J Am Soc Echocardiogr.* 2003;16:777–802.

Zoghbi WA, Habib JB, Quiñones MA. Doppler assessment of right ventricular filling in a normal population: comparison with left ventricular filling dynamics. *Circulation.* 1990;82:1316–1324.

CHAPTER 26

Cyanotic Congenital Heart Disease

Nishant Shah and Richard A. Humes

1. Which is the most common *cyanotic* congenital heart disease?
   A. Transposition of great arteries.
   B. Total anomalous pulmonary venous return.
   C. Truncus arteriosus.
   D. Tetralogy of Fallot (TOF).
   E. Tricuspid atresia.

2. A 22-year-old well-known patient with Ebstein's anomaly of the tricuspid valve is seen in the office for a routine visit and complains of exertional dyspnea. Pulse oximetry reveals that his resting oxygen saturation is 89%. Review of his previous visits reveals that the last time this was checked at age 14, the saturation was 95%. This relative drop in his oxygen saturation is most likely produced by what abnormality of intracardiac hemodynamics seen on his echocardiogram?
   A. Ventricular septal defect (VSD).
   B. Pulmonary valve stenosis.
   C. Atrial septal defect (ASD).
   D. Aortic valve regurgitation.
   E. Coarctation of the aorta.

3. A newborn infant is evaluated because of a heart murmur. The echocardiogram reveals a large VSD with an overriding great vessel and a single large great artery giving rise to the aorta and the pulmonary artery. What is a TRUE statement about this congenital heart defect?
   A. There is a higher incidence of chromosomal abnormalities.
   B. Survival is dependent upon a patent ductus arteriosus (PDA).
   C. Survival is dependent upon an ASD.
   D. The oxygen saturation is normal.
   E. Surgical repair may be deferred for up to 2 years.

4. An echocardiogram is done on a 4-year-old patient with unrepaired TOF. He has a loud heart murmur at the upper right sternal border. The parasternal long-axis view reveals a typical large VSD with an overriding great aorta. The pulmonary arteries appear to be confluent and normal in size. There is right-to-left shunting at the ventricular level with no turbulence seen. Doppler interrogation of the tricuspid regurgitant signal reveals a velocity of 4.5 m/sec. What can be said about this patient's heart disease?
   A. He has developed pulmonary hypertension.
   B. A tricuspid valve problem has developed.
   C. This is an expected finding of no concern.
   D. The VSD is becoming restrictive with time.
   E. The Doppler signal from the tricuspid valve is incorrect.

5. An echocardiogram is done on an infant with cyanosis and no heart murmur. The parasternal long-axis view reveals a large VSD with right-to-left shunt. The posterior great artery appears to bifurcate into two arteries. There is a patent foramen ovale with a small left-to-right shunt. A large PDA is seen with bidirectional shunt. What is the most likely cause of the cyanosis?
   A. Abnormalities of the great arteries.
   B. Pulmonary arterial hypertension.
   C. Coarctation of the aorta.
   D. Decreased pulmonary blood flow.
   E. Total anomalous pulmonary venous return.

6. Which of the following cyanotic congenital heart defects is MOST likely to escape detection in childhood?
A. TOF.
B. Supracardiac total anomalous pulmonary venous return.
C. Transposition of the great arteries.
D. Tricuspid valve atresia.
E. Ebstein's anomaly of the tricuspid valve.

7. Cyanotic congenital heart disease is MOST frequently produced by what abnormality of intracardiac hemodynamics?
A. Abnormal great artery position.
B. Pulmonary venous anomalies.
C. Arteriovenous connections.
D. Pulmonary hypertension.
E. Decreased pulmonary blood flow.

8. Common echocardiographic features of Ebstein's anomaly include all of the following EXCEPT:
A. Atrial level shunting.
B. Apical displacement of the septal tricuspid leaflet.
C. Tricuspid regurgitation.
D. VSD.
E. Abnormal septal motion.

9. Which of the following pulmonary venous connections is NOT a form of total anomalous pulmonary venous return?
A. Connection to the innominate vein.
B. Connection to the right atrium.
C. Connection to the hepatic veins.
D. Connection to the coronary sinus.
E. Connection to the left atrium.

10. An echocardiogram is done on an infant with a heart murmur. The parasternal long-axis view reveals a large VSD with an overriding great vessel. The next important step in identifying this heart disease should be:
A. Examine for the presence of an ASD.
B. Identify the pulmonary artery connection.
C. Find the side of the arch.
D. Measure the size of the VSD.
E. Perform Doppler on the tricuspid valve.

11. A 2-month-old infant is seen for a heart murmur. The child is doing clinically well. The oxygen saturation is found to be 90% by pulse oximetry. Echocardiography reveals tricuspid valve atresia. What is a TRUE statement about this congenital heart defect?
A. An ASD or patent foramen ovale (PFO) is present.
B. A PDA must be present for survival.
C. The great arteries are transposed.
D. The great arteries are normally related.
E. A right aortic arch is usually present.

12. Which of the following cyanotic congenital heart defects is NOT dependent upon a PDA for survival in infancy?
A. TOF with pulmonary valve atresia.
B. Infradiaphragmatic total anomalous pulmonary venous return.
C. Transposition of the great arteries.
D. Pulmonary valve atresia with intact ventricular septum (hypoplastic right heart syndrome).
E. Severe Ebstein's anomaly of the tricuspid valve.

13. What is the echocardiographic feature of Ebstein's anomaly which is of most value to the cardiovascular surgeon in determining the possible success of tricuspid valvuloplasty?
A. Atrial level shunting.
B. Apical displacement of the septal tricuspid leaflet.
C. Presence of tricuspid regurgitation.
D. Presence of a VSD.
E. Mobility of the anterior tricuspid leaflet.

14. An echocardiogram done on a newborn infant reveals a normal appearing left heart with a small right ventricle, diminutive tricuspid valve, and no identifiable pulmonary valve. There is moderately severe tricuspid regurgitation with a severely enlarged right atrium. The pulmonary arteries are seen to be confluent and of near-normal size, supplied by a large PDA. Prostaglandin E1 is begun intravenously. Which of the following is a reasonable next step in clinical management?
A. Stop prostaglandin therapy.
B. Begin dobutamine.
C. Closed or interventional pulmonary valvotomy.
D. Tricuspid valvuloplasty.
E. Waterston shunt.

15. An infant is born with transposition of the great arteries with intact ventricular septum. A PDA is present and the baby is placed on prostaglandin E1 to maintain this. The infant remains cyanotic with an arterial saturation of 60%–63%. Which area of the heart should be studied thoroughly with echocardiography that would most likely account for this problem?

A. The pulmonary venous return.
B. The ductus arteriosus.
C. The aortic arch.
D. The systemic venous return.
E. The atrial septum.

16. A 2-week-old newborn is being evaluated for cyanosis and murmur. Echocardiography was performed as shown in Figure 26-1A (apical four-chamber view) and Figure 26-1B (parasternal short-axis view). The diagnosis of congenital heart disease was made. Based on these echocardiographic findings, what is the best guess of right ventricular systolic pressure?

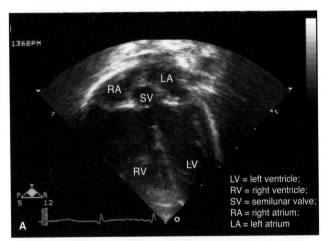

LV = left ventricle;
RV = right ventricle;
SV = semilunar valve;
RA = right atrium;
LA = left atrium

Fig. 26-1A

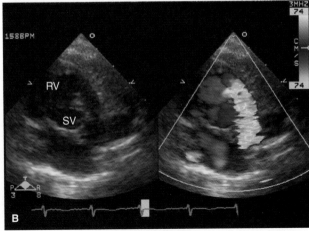

Fig. 26-1B

A. ½ systemic.
B. ¾ systemic.
C. Near systemic.
D. Systemic.
E. Suprasystemic.

17. A 2-day-old baby was found to have a decreased oxygen saturation of 84%. Echocardiography was performed to rule out any congenital heart disease. Figure 26-2 demonstrates color flow in the atrial septum from a subcostal view. This color flow pattern is seen throughout the cardiac cycle. Based on Figure 26-2, which one of the following defects would most likely produce this?

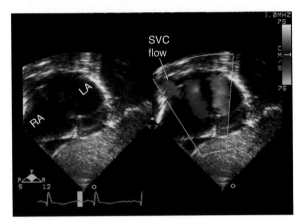

Fig. 26-2

A. Total anomalous pulmonary venous return (TAPVR).
B. Truncus arteriosus.
C. Critical aortic stenosis.
D. TOF.
E. D-Transposition.

18. A young adult was found to have an abnormal echocardiogram during evaluation of palpitations. The area marked with stars in Figure 26-3 demonstrates:

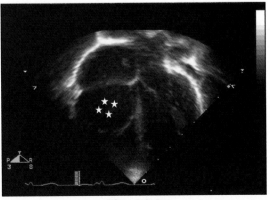

Fig. 26-3

A. Sail-like elongation of anterior tricuspid valve.
B. Atrialized portion of right ventricle.
C. Absence of tricuspid valve.
D. Hypoplastic right ventricle.
E. Left ventricular volume overload.

19. A 1-day-old newborn is transferred from the newborn nursery to the NICU because of cyanosis. His oxygen saturation is 75% and does not improve with 100% FiO$_2$. Echocardiography is as shown in Figure 26-4A (parasternal long-axis view) and Figure 26-4B (parasternal short-axis view). Both ventricles (left ventricle = LV; right ventricle = RV) and both semilunar valves (aortic valve = AV; pulmonary valve = PV) are labeled. Which one of the following combinations is correct in this condition?

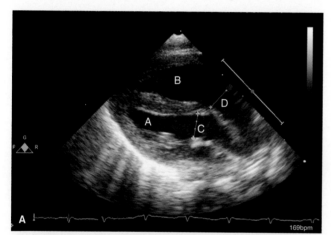

Fig. 26-4A

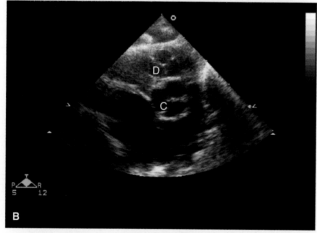

Fig. 26-4B

A. a = LV; b = RV; c = AV; d = PV.
B. b = RV; a = LV; c = AV; d = PV.
C. a = LV; b = RV; c = PV; d = AV.
D. a = RV; b = LV; c = PV; d = AV.

20. A 4-week-old girl presents to her primary care physician with parental complaints of bluish discoloration particularly with crying. On evaluation, her saturation is in the high 70's to low 80s. She was also found to have an ejection systolic murmur. Echocardiography was performed as shown in Figure 26-5A (parasternal long axis) and Figure 26-5B (parasternal short axis). Based on this information, which pathology will determine this girl's oxygen saturation?

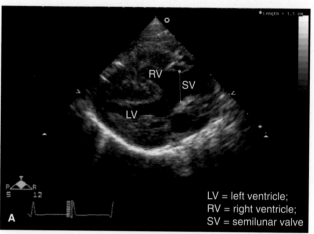

LV = left ventricle;
RV = right ventricle;
SV = semilunar valve

Fig. 26-5A

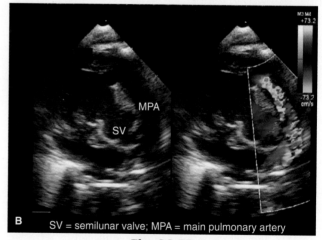

SV = semilunar valve; MPA = main pulmonary artery

Fig. 26-5B

A. Degree of right ventricular outflow tract obstruction.
B. Size of the VSD.
C. Degree of overriding of aorta.
D. Size of the ASD.

21. A 19-year-old young man was referred to cardiology clinic for evaluation of easy fatigability with sports and exercise activity. His vitals were within normal limits except oxygen saturation which was 86%. Echocardiography was performed as shown in Figure 26-6 (apical view). Which one of the following describes the patient's condition?

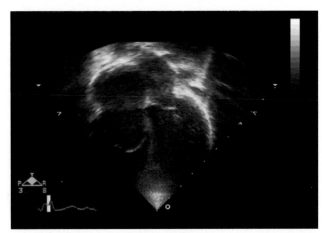

Fig. 26-6

A. Tricuspid atresia.
B. Pulmonary hypertension.
C. Uhl's anomaly.
D. Ebstein's anomaly.
E. Large ASD.

22. A 6-week-old male infant was referred to the pediatric cardiology clinic for an ejection systolic murmur which was found during a routine clinic visit in the primary pediatrician's office. He was born at full term and was discharged home on the second day of life. His parents mentioned that he had frequent episodes of bluish discoloration particularly associated with crying. Detailed examination showed a normal growth pattern for his age. He was breathing comfortably with an oxygen saturation of 86% at room air. The lungs were clear to auscultation. He had a normal S1 and S2 along with an ejection systolic murmur at the upper left sternal border. There was no organomegaly. His pulses were equal without any radiofemoral delay. His echocardiogram was performed which is shown in Figure 26-7.

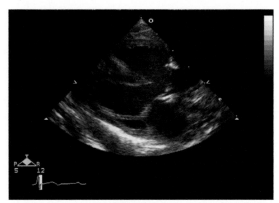

Fig. 26-7

Based on his clinical presentation and echocardiography, the most likely defect is:
A. Truncus arteriosus.
B. TOF.
C. D-Transposition of great arteries with a VSD.
D. Tricuspid atresia.
E. Perimembranous VSD.

23. A 6-week-old infant was admitted to the PICU with poor feeding, respiratory distress, and mild cyanosis. Chest x-ray showed pulmonary congestion. Echocardiography was performed and is shown in Figure 26-8A (parasternal long axis) and Figure 26-8B (apical view). Which of the following best describes this child's condition?

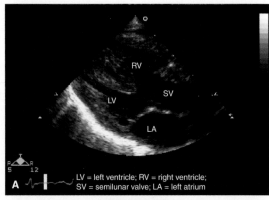

LV = left ventricle; RV = right ventricle;
SV = semilunar valve; LA = left atrium

Fig. 26-8A

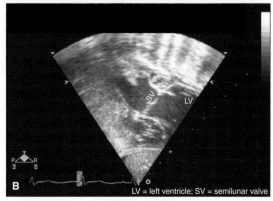

LV = left ventricle; SV = semilunar valve

Fig. 26-8B

A. The findings are consistent with a diagnosis of TOF.
B. The findings suggest a lesion in which both great arteries arise from the right ventricle.
C. The findings suggest a single artery giving rise to the systemic and pulmonary arteries.
D. This condition is frequently seen in trisomy 21.
E. The child has anomalies of pulmonary venous return.

24. You are called for an echocardiogram in the NICU on a newborn infant whose saturation is 80% at room air. Parasternal short-axis views were performed as shown in Figures 26-9A and B (systole and diastole, respectively). What is the next most important piece of information you would like to find out in this patient that will define proper diagnosis of this condition, natural history of this lesion, and future surgical management?

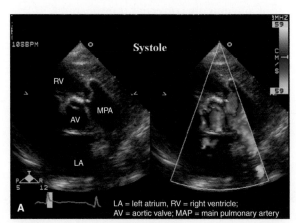

Fig. 26-9A

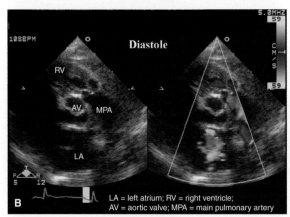

Fig. 26-9B

A. Evaluation of the atrial septum.
B. Evaluation of the ventricular septum.
C. Size of the left ventricle.
D. Evaluation of the aortic arch.
E. Evaluation of the pulmonary veins.

25. Echocardiography was performed on a 48-hour-old newborn because of persistent cyanosis. Figure 26-10 (apical view) is shown. Based on this, what is the diagnosis?

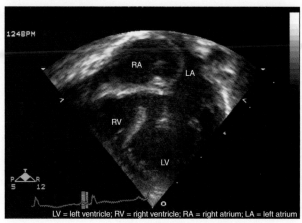

LV = left ventricle; RV = right ventricle; RA = right atrium; LA = left atrium

Fig. 26-10

A. TAPVR.
B. Complete atrioventricular canal defect.
C. Tricuspid atresia.
D. Ebstein's Anomaly.
E. Transposition of the great arteries.

26. A 3-week-old female infant presents to her physician with respiratory distress. Her oxygen saturation is in 80s. Echocardiography was performed. A subcostal picture is shown in Figure 26-11. The arrows in Figure 26-11 is suggestive of:

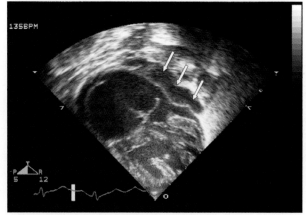

Fig. 26-11

A. Localized posterior pericardial effusion.
B. Truncus arteriosus.
C. Pulmonary venous confluence.
D. A mediastinal mass.
E. Descending aorta.

CASE 1:

A 4-week-old male infant was referred to a pediatric cardiology clinic for an ejection systolic murmur found during a routine clinic visit at the primary pediatrician's office. His echocardiography is shown in Video 26-1A (apical) and Video 26-1B (parasternal short axis).

27. Based on his clinical presentation and echocardiography, the most likely diagnosis is:
    A. Truncus arteriosus.
    B. TOF.
    C. D-Transposition of great arteries with a VSD.
    D. VSD.
    E. Pulmonary stenosis.

28. At 3 months of age, his parents noticed frequent episodes of bluish discoloration when the child was crying. According to the parents, there is no history suggestive of any lethargy, tiredness, or respiratory distress. He was brought to the pediatrician's office where his saturation is now 75% as compared to 86% at 4 weeks of life. Other than that, he was playful and active in the doctor's office. Echocardiography is shown in Video 26-1C. Which of the following will be the most likely finding in his echocardiography?
    A. Decreased blood flow across the pulmonary valve.
    B. Dynamic right ventricular outflow tract obstruction suggestive of tetralogy spells.
    C. Decreased right-to-left shunting across the VSD.
    D. Decreased left ventricular function.
    E. Increased blood flow across the pulmonary valve.

29. This infant is now 5 months of age and he has increasing cyanosis. He has moderate to severe right ventricular outflow tract obstruction along with a hypoplastic pulmonary valve. He is scheduled for surgery which includes relief of right ventricular outflow tract obstruction, trans-annular patch, and closure of a VSD. Which of the following associated conditions play a major role in determining the aforementioned surgery?
    A. Right aortic arch.
    B. ASD.
    C. Coronary anomalies.
    D. Additional muscular VSD.
    E. Size of the VSD.

30. The single anatomic hallmark responsible for each of the anatomic components in this condition is:
    A. Hypertrophy of RV muscle bundles.
    B. Anterior deviation of the outlet septum.
    C. Dysplasia of the pulmonary valve.
    D. Posterior deviation of the outlet septum.
    E. Distortion of the branch pulmonary arteries.

CASE 2:

A 2-day-old baby boy was transferred to a tertiary care center and was found to have a decreased oxygen saturation before discharge. His oxygen saturation was 80% and did not improve with 100% O$_2$. Echocardiography is as shown in Video 26-2A (parasternal view) and Video 26-2B (apical view).

31. What is the diagnosis?
    A. Double outlet right ventricle.
    B. Anomalous origin of coronary arteries.
    C. Congenitally corrected transposition.
    D. D-Transposition of great arteries.
    E. Truncus arteriosus.

32. What is the most common associated anomaly with this condition?
    A. Left ventricular outflow tract obstruction.
    B. Coarctation of the aorta.
    C. VSD.
    D. ASD.
    E. Coronary anomalies.

33. In this condition, what is a TRUE statement about the best source of intracardiac mixing?
    A. At the atrial level through a large ASD.
    B. At the ventricular level via a large VSD.
    C. At the great arterial level through a large PDA.
    D. The degree of mixing is more influenced by defect size than location.

CASE 3:

A 12-year-old boy was sent to the cardiology clinic for shortness of breath with exertion. In the clinic, his saturation was 79%. Echocardiography was done and is shown in Videos 26-3A and B.

34. What is the cause of desaturation?
   A. Pulmonary arteriovenous malformation.
   B. Right-to-left shunting at the atrial septal level.
   C. Pulmonary hypertension.
   D. Right ventricular dysfunction.

35. The most diagnostic echo feature of this condition is:
   A. Displacement index >8 mm/m^2.
   B. Sail-like anterior tricuspid leaflet.
   C. Posterior leaflet tethering to right ventricular free wall.
   D. Dilated tricuspid valve annulus.
   E. Right ventricular dilatation.

36. What is the most common condition associated with this abnormality of the tricuspid valve?
   A. Accessory conduction pathway.
   B. VSD.
   C. Pulmonary stenosis.
   D. Presence of left superior vena cava.
   E. ASD/Patent foramen ovale.

CASE 4:

Echocardiography was performed on a 48-hour-old newborn because of persistent cyanosis. Videos 26-4A (apical view), B, and C (parasternal short axis) are shown.

37. Based on these findings, which one of the following best describes this patient's problem?
   A. About 75% of the cases are associated with D-transposition of great arteries.
   B. Coarctation of aorta is usually not present in this condition.
   C. An obligatory left-to-right shunt is seen at the ASD level.
   D. The size of the VSD is extremely important in this lesion.
   E. Coronary artery anomalies are frequently seen.

38. Which is a correct statement about this problem?
   A. This is a ductal-dependent lesion.
   B. The great artery position is irrelevant clinically.
   C. Right ventricular pressure may be estimated by the tricuspid regurgitant Doppler method.
   D. An ASD is necessary for survival.
   E. The pulmonary artery branches are frequently enlarged.

CASE 5:

39. What is a true statement about the type of TAPVR shown in the suprasternal view in Video 26-5?
   A. Obstruction is never present in this type of TAPVR.
   B. It is almost always associated with pulmonary venous obstruction.
   C. It is associated with an intact atrial septum.
   D. This is the most common form of TAPVR.
   E. This form of TAPVR produces profound cyanosis of the newborn.

40. Which of the following echocardiographic features describes this condition?
   A. The left atrium is usually normal in size.
   B. The right ventricle is dilated in all types of TAPVR.
   C. The atrial and ventricular septum bow into the right side of heart.
   D. Doppler is usually not helpful to establish pulmonary venous connection.
   E. The pulmonary artery is often mildly hypoplastic.

41. An infant with mild cyanosis and cardiomegaly on chest x-ray is having an echocardiogram to examine the source of the cyanosis. There are four chambers and four valves with a normal great artery relationship. TAPVR is suspected when the right heart is noted to be large and a right to left atrial shunt is seen. In order to identify the location of the pulmonary veins, the echocardiographer needs to examine:
   A. The right ventricle.
   B. The left ventricle.
   C. The systemic veins.
   D. The aorta.
   E. The ductus arteriosus.

ANSWERS

1. ANSWER: D. Congenital heart disease is found in about 0.5%–0.8% of live births. Tetralogy of Fallot (TOF) is the fourth most common form of congenital heart disease, comprising about 10% of the total cases. Transposition of the great arteries would be the next most common in frequency, accounting for about 5%. Truncus arteriosus, tricuspid atresia, and total anomalous pulmonary venous return are relatively rare, accounting for only about 1%–2% of the total cases of congenital heart disease, respectively. A common mnemonic for remembering this has been that all forms of cyanotic disease begin with the "T." This is a reasonable way to remember the ones listed earlier, but this trick does not hold true completely. Additionally, the initial presentation for patients with "cyanotic" congenital heart disease, may not always be clinical cyanosis, even though these patients may eventually become cyanotic over time.

2. ANSWER: C. 50%–70% of patients with Ebstein's anomaly also have an atrial septal defect (ASD). Ventricular septal defects (VSD) and pulmonary atresia are also seen, but rarely. Left-sided heart lesions, such as aortic valve stenosis or coarctation of the aorta, are very uncommon in Ebstein's anomaly. The direction of shunting across this ASD can change during a patient's lifetime. During the newborn period, these patients will often be profoundly cyanotic due to right-to-left shunting. As pulmonary resistance drops and right ventricular compliance increases, the shunting will change to left-to-right and the cyanosis may disappear until young adulthood when the right ventricle stiffens and the right-to-left shunting resumes. From a clinical perspective, a patient with known Ebstein's anomaly who has any degree of cyanosis may be presumed to have an ASD.

3. ANSWER: A. The anatomic description is consistent with truncus arteriosus. There is also a malalignment VSD with override of the semilunar valve, in this case referred to as the "truncal" valve. Up to 33% of patients with truncus arteriosus will have DiGeorge syndrome, characterized by abnormal facies, thymic hypoplasia, and parathyroid hypoplasia or aplasia resulting in hypocalcemia. A large proportion (70%) of patients with DiGeorge syndrome have microdeletions of 22q11. This is so prevalent that DiGeorge syndrome and 22q11 deletion have become almost synonymous, although that is not completely accurate. Truncus arteriosus is not generally a ductal-dependent lesion, as the pulmonary artery blood supply is usually vigorous. Ductal-dependent lesions include defects which compromise great artery flow such as aortic or pulmonary valve atresia. Atrioventricular valve atresia will usually require an ASD for survival. The oxygen saturation is likely to slightly decrease in truncus arteriosus, due to mixing at the great artery level. However, patients with truncus arteriosus are not usually profoundly cyanotic and

may have near-normal saturations. Surgical repair is often carried out as a newborn, and should not be deferred for longer than a few months, if at all, due to a fairly high incidence of pulmonary vascular obstructive disease or Eisenmenger's syndrome, if it is not corrected early. Due to the absence of a main pulmonary artery, surgical repair involves closure of the VSD and placement of a right ventricle to pulmonary artery conduit—an important point for the future since the conduit may require multiple replacement operations during the lifetime of the patient.

4. ANSWER: C. The tricuspid regurgitant signal predicts a pressure in the right ventricle of about 90 mm Hg, using the modified Bernoulli equation. A patient with TOF will generally have a large VSD which has no real chance of closure or restriction. Therefore, the pressures in the right and left ventricles will equalize at systemic levels and the finding of a high tricuspid regurgitant velocity is expected in all cases. It is very unlikely (but not impossible) that pulmonary hypertension could develop in tetralogy patients. However, the usual presence of pulmonary valve and subvalvular stenosis generally protects the pulmonary arterial bed from hypertension. The presence of a loud murmur in the pulmonary area supports the presence of this finding.

5. ANSWER: A. This scenario describes a patient with transposition of the great arteries and VSD. The VSD is usually large in this scenario, so pulmonary pressures will be at systemic levels and pulmonary "hypertension" is technically present. This does not imply the presence of pulmonary vascular obstructive disease, which would be unlikely in an infant. Coarctation of the aorta, even if present, is an answer of no significance. Most patients with transposition actually have somewhat increased pulmonary blood flow with newborn transposition, despite the cyanosis. Total anomalous pulmonary venous return may produce cyanosis but would require a right-to-left atrial shunt and there is nothing in this scenario which points in that direction.

6. ANSWER: E. Detection of congenital heart disease can occur for many reasons. An increasing number of patients are detected prenatally by ultrasound examination. Even though these problems are "cyanotic" problems, cyanosis may be relatively mild as a clinical clue and go undetected. All of the diagnoses listed in the question might go undetected for a period of time. Transposition of the great arteries usually presents with profound cyanosis as a newborn. However, those patients with transposition and VSD may be less cyanotic and may present later with a heart murmur. This scenario is rare. TOF frequently presents as an asymptomatic heart murmur. However, the heart murmur is not subtle and usually brings the patient to attention in the first few weeks of life. A patient with

TOF with pulmonary atresia might be the silent exception. Tricuspid valve atresia may also present later in infancy with a heart murmur, but it is very rare for these patients to escape detection until adulthood. Supracardiac total anomalous pulmonary venous return will frequently have very mild, if any, clinical cyanosis. The heart murmur is soft and can be subtle. Some patients will escape detection in the first months of life and a very few patients have been known to escape detection until adulthood, but this is also fairly rare. Ebstein's anomaly can be very mild and patients may have little if any murmur. If there is no ASD, then they will not be cyanotic or have much exercise intolerance. Ebstein's can present with severe cyanosis as a newborn. However, mild forms of Ebstein's anomaly represent the most subtle of the choices and the most likely answer.

7. ANSWER: E. The spectrum of anomalies producing cyanosis is fairly broad and all of the reasons given may account for the clinical phenomenon of cyanosis. Realize that clinically cyanosis is due to a bluish discoloration of the skin. This is seen when the deoxyhemoglobin levels exceed about 4 gm%–5 gm%. Therefore, cyanosis may also be affected by the overall hemoglobin levels in the body since an oxygen saturation of 70% (30% of the hemoglobin will be desaturated as in the "deoxy" state) will reach the 5 gm% level much easier in a polycythemic patient than in an anemic patient. Patients who have decreased pulmonary flow and an intracardiac shunt, will be cyanotic because the amount of saturated pulmonary vein flow returning to the heart is diminished. Additionally, patients with simple shunts or even mixing lesions will not necessarily be cyanotic since they will have exuberant pulmonary flow and excessive pulmonary venous return. However, the answer is based more on the frequency of anomalies producing cyanosis. Tetralogy is common and has decreased pulmonary flow. Added to this are numerous other complex defects for which pulmonary stenosis is also a component. Patients with cyanosis due to great artery position or pulmonary vein anomalies are much rarer.

8. ANSWER: D. Ebstein's anomaly is characterized by apical displacement of the septal and inferior leaflets of the tricuspid valve. An established criterion for diagnosis of Ebstein's anomaly is apical displacement of the tricuspid valve septal leaflet from the crux of the heart by greater than 8 mm/m^2 body surface area. In addition, an elongated ("sail-like") anterior leaflet is present. Because of its anatomical derangement, the malformed tricuspid valve is typically regurgitant (and in rare cases stenotic). An atrial-level communication (ASD or patent foramen ovale) is present in up to 75% of cases. The volume overload of the right heart caused by the tricuspid regurgitation commonly leads to paradoxical septal motion. VSDs are seen in about 5% of patients with Ebstein's anomaly, but they are not common, thus the correct answer is "(D)."

9. ANSWER: E. Anomalous pulmonary venous connections are to the systemic venous system and may occur in a variety of ways. The most common is connection to the innominate vein (supracardiac). There may also be connections to the right atrium or coronary sinus. Connections below the diaphragm to the hepatic veins, through the liver, are frequently severely obstructed, creating a surgical emergency. A connection to the left atrium would be normal, and not anomalous, making this the answer.

10. ANSWER: B. There are a number of congenital defects which may present with a large malalignment VSD and overriding great vessel. The most common of these would be TOF. However, the great vessel is not always the aorta. Other "look-alikes" for this particular view might be truncus arteriosus, double-outlet right ventricle, D-transposition with VSD, or pulmonary atresia with VSD. In each case, the parasternal view may be similar but the key is identifying the position and status of the pulmonary artery. This is the key for both the proper diagnosis as well as aiding in predicting the clinical course. The presence of an ASD and the position of the arch may be important adjunctive items to add to the overall imaging picture but they do not have great clinical significance. The size of the VSD in this situation is virtually always one of a large and unrestricted flow. Tricuspid valve Doppler adds little in this situation.

11. ANSWER: A. All forms of tricuspid valve atresia must have some type of atrial communication to decompress the right atrium and allow for egress of blood from that chamber. Tricuspid atresia does not have to be ductal-dependent. This is more likely to be the case in instances of outflow obstruction rather than inflow obstruction. In cases of tricuspid atresia with transposition, there is frequently aortic coarctation present and this might become ductal-dependent if it is severe. However, ductal dependency is generally a phenomenon of early infancy, which comes to light after ductal closure in the first day or two of life–not a very common likelihood in a 2-month-old patient. Tricuspid atresia will present anatomically in two forms: 1) normally related great arteries (75%) and 2) transposition of the great arteries (25%). With either great artery position, there is complete mixing of pulmonary venous and systemic venous blood at atrial and ventricular levels and saturations overall will depend upon the amount of pulmonary blood flow. In this instance, the saturation is fairly high, suggesting vigorous pulmonary blood flow, but one cannot specifically distinguish between normal or transposed great arteries based on that finding alone. The arch position is irrelevant, but it is very rare to see a right aortic arch with tricuspid atresia.

12. ANSWER: B. The ductus arteriosus connects the main pulmonary artery and the aorta and can provide flow from one to the other when that flow is compromised by a serious congenital heart defect. Most of the time the defects which are "ductal-dependent" will be defects involving outflow obstruction or atresia such as: aortic atresia, pulmonary atresia, severe or critical aortic stenosis, or critical pulmonary stenosis. Transposition of the great arteries may or may not be ductal-dependent depending upon all of the features of anatomy, but it can be in some cases. Inflow atresia like mitral or tricuspid atresia may or may not be ductal-dependent if they have concomitant outflow problems or atresia. Ebstein's anomaly in the newborn is unusual because there is often no outflow atresia anatomically, but the poor antegrade flow through the pulmonary valve created by the abnormal tricuspid valve and right ventricle, often makes then ductal-dependent until the pulmonary resistance falls after a few days or weeks. Total anomalous pulmonary venous return below the diaphragm (infradiaphragmatic) is a severe lesion with often obstructed pulmonary venous return. However, the hemodynamics has nothing to do with the ductus arteriosus. Indeed, keeping the ductus open with prostaglandin E1 in this situation is often detrimental by increasing pulmonary artery flow into an obstruction.

13. ANSWER: E. Ebstein's anomaly is characterized by apical displacement of the septal and inferior leaflets of the tricuspid valve. The anterior leaflet is enlarged, elongated, and will have varying degrees of tethering to the right ventricular free wall which can limit the mobility of the valve. Echocardiographically, physicians often concentrate on the unusual apical displacement of the septal leaflet and the degree of tricuspid regurgitation. However, most surgical repairs (as opposed to replacement) of Ebstein's valves utilize the anterior leaflet as the primary portion of the apparatus which provides information about any valvular integrity. As such, this portion of the valve needs to be fairly mobile so that it can function as a "monocusp" valve after valvuloplasty. Therefore, the preoperative imaging must include multiple views of the anterior leaflet to be able to assess this mobility. Choices (A)–(D) are all features that may be present in Ebstein's anomaly but their presence does not necessarily determine success of a valvuloplasty.

14. ANSWER: D. The echocardiogram describes a patient with pulmonary valve atresia with an intact ventricular septum, often called the "hypoplastic right heart syndrome." This terminology is losing favor because there are other anatomic forms of congenital heart disease that may also have a small right ventricle which are markedly different and do not belong to the same category as noted earlier. There is a wide variety of anatomic situations within this group which include varying degrees of right ventricular hypoplasia. In the simplest form, with right ventricular hypoplasia that is not severe, patients may be treated with either surgical or even catheter-based pulmonary valvuloplasty. This approach addresses the primary problem of pulmonary valve atresia and potentially allows the patient to have a course of therapy which will lead to a four-chamber repair with two usable ventricles. Stopping prostaglandin therapy would be inadvisable in this setting. This is a ductal-dependent lesion and keeping the ductus arteriosus open with prostaglandin E1 is essential. Dobutamine is usually not needed unless there is decreased cardiac output. In this example, there is no clinical information to support that. In many instances, a Blalock-Taussig shunt (subclavian artery to pulmonary artery) is done either in isolation or in addition to the pulmonary valvuloplasty to augment the pulmonary blood flow. A Waterston shunt would do the same thing but these are almost never done any more because of difficulties controlling pulmonary blood flow. Patients with diminutive right ventricles may also have very high pressure (suprasystemic) in that chamber which can lead to the development of coronary fistulae and retrograde flow into the left coronary system. This "RV-dependent coronary circulation" can be an ominous sign and is associated with arrhythmia and sudden death. In these instances, a heart transplant may be the best viable option. Frequently, there may be significant tricuspid regurgitation and subsequent right atrial enlargement. Despite this, the tricuspid valve is usually left alone. Decreasing the tricuspid regurgitation may be a goal later in the course of management but it would never be the next step at this stage. Ultimately, the decisions would be to: 1) proceed with a four-chamber repair (if the right ventricle is big enough), 2) go the pathway of a single ventricle repair with an ultimate Fontan operation, and 3) heart transplant. All of these widely variant options make the decision tree for these patients very interesting and individualized.

15. ANSWER: E. Patients with transposition of the great arteries have two parallel circulations and survive with areas where the systemic and pulmonary circulations can mix. These include the atrial septum, the ventricular septum, and the ductus arteriosus. The atrial septum is by far the most effective place for infants with transposition to have mixing. If the atrial defect is small and constricted, this will likely result in more cyanosis, even if the ductus arteriosus is widely patent. Infants with a large VSD may also have problems mixing at the ventricular level. In this case, the ductus arteriosus should be examined, but prostaglandin is generally an effective drug and keeps the ductus widely patent. Checking the dosage, route of delivery, and status is always a good idea and would be a close second to the atrial septum as a place to check right away. The aortic arch should not have any bearing on cyanotic or hypoxemic issues. Anomalies of systemic and pulmonary venous return may be involved in cyanosis, but are less likely as answers here.

16. ANSWER: D. This patient has TOF. Figure 26-12A shows mal-aligned VSD and overriding of aorta. Figure 26-12B shows right ventricular outflow tract obstruction in the form of infundibular (subpulmonary) narrowing. TOF is a conotruncal anomaly that is classically defined as having the following four components: 1) right ventricular hypertrophy, 2) VSD, 3) overriding aorta, and 4) pulmonary stenosis. Tetralogy occurs in approximately 9% of children born with congenital heart defects. The VSD in TOF is usually large and nonrestrictive. Only in rare cases, will it be restrictive. In Figure 26-12, the VSD appears to be typically large and nonrestrictive. This will result in equalization of pressure between the ventricles. Since the left ventricle will always pump systemic pressure, this will also be the pressure in the right ventricle.

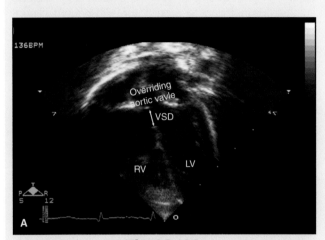

Fig. 26-12A

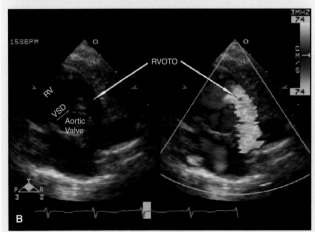

Fig. 26-12B

17. ANSWER: A. This example shows an intra-atrial shunt which is right to left and is present throughout the cardiac cycle. This suggests that the patient has an exclusive right-to-left shunt at the atrial level. In TAPVR, all of the venous return (systemic and pulmonary) comes to the right atrium. Some of the returning blood must be shunted through an ASD and enter into the left side of the heart and into the systemic circulation. Thus, in TAPVR, the only source of blood into the left atrium, is from the right atrium resulting from an obligatory right-to-left shunt at the atrial level. It would be quite unusual for the other cyanotic lesions listed to have right-to-left atrial shunting. However, in tricuspid atresia, the only egress from the right atrium is through the atrial septum to the left atrium, and in Ebstein's anomaly the right heart antegrade flow is impaired. So, in TAPVR, tricuspid atresia, and early in Ebstein's anomaly, the shunt at the atrial level is right to left as seen in this patient. In critical aortic stenosis, the shunt at the atrial level is predominantly left to right. There is a bidirectional shunt at the atrial septal level in truncus arteriosus.

18. ANSWER: B. This patient has Ebstein's anomaly of the tricuspid valve. This lesion was initially described in 1866 by the German physician Wilhelm Ebstein. Characteristic pathologic findings include apical displacement of the septal and posterior leaflets of the tricuspid valve into the right ventricle to varying degrees. The arrowheads in Figure 26-13 show the tricuspid valve annulus. The portion of the right ventricle between the true valve annulus and the apically displaced valve leaflets forms an "atrialized" portion of the right ventricle that is continuous with the true right atrium. Although the atrialized portion of the right ventricular anterior wall may be thin, the distal unaffected portion of the right ventricular wall is usually normal in thickness.

In Ebstein's anomaly, the effective right ventricular size is reduced depending upon the severity of the tricuspid valve displacement. However, it is not associated with hypoplasia of the right ventricle. The choice (C) is incorrect as the tricuspid valve is seen to be displaced apically. The anterior leaflet of the tricuspid valve cannot be seen in the apical four-chamber view. Instead, the posterior and septal leaflets are very well seen in Figure 26-13.

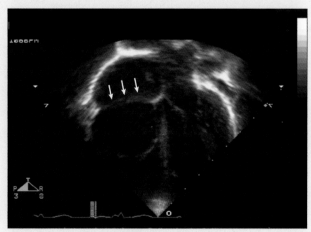

Fig. 26-13

19. ANSWER: C. This patient has D-transposition of great arteries. Transposition is defined as a connection of the aorta to the right ventricle and the pulmonary artery to the left ventricle. This abnormal ventricular arterial connection is also termed "ventriculo-arterial discordance" and probably results from abnormal conotruncal septation. Transposition occurs in approximately 4%–8% of children born with congenital heart defects. "D-transposition" is a term which refers to the way the conotruncal septum rotates in utero ("D" for dextro) and has been commonly applied to this entity. In transposition, the aorta arises from the right ventricle, usually in a position which is anterior and rightward of the pulmonary valve (Fig. 26-4B in the case). The two great arteries course parallel to one another; a distinctly different arrangement from the normal pulmonary artery crossing over the aortic root (Fig. 26-4A in the case).

Figure 26-14 demonstrates the position of the great arteries as commonly seen from the echocardiographic perspective of the parasternal short-axis view. Great artery position is a key to identifying the type of transposition. Normally, the pulmonary artery wraps around the aorta anteriorly as it courses posteriorly (Fig. 26-14B). With D-transposition, the great arteries assume a parallel course, and the aorta is located anterior and rightward of the centrally located pulmonary artery (Fig. 26-14A). In L-transposition, the great arteries are again parallel, but the aorta is anterior and leftward (Fig. 26-14C). It is important to note that in normally related great vessels, the pulmonary valve and aortic valve are not in the same plane while in any form of transposition, they are usually in the same plane as shown in Figure 26-4B as D and C, respectively, because of the generally more parallel course of the great arteries in transposition.

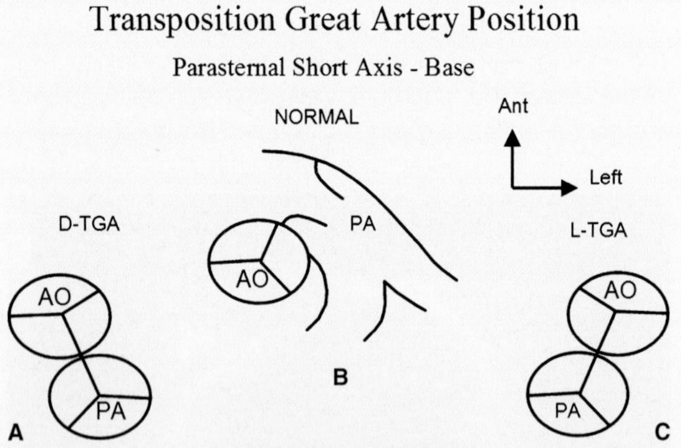

Transposition Great Artery Position

Parasternal Short Axis - Base

Fig. 26-14 (A-C)

20. ANSWER: A. Figure 26-5A illustrates a mal-alignment of the VSD with overriding of aorta. Figure 26-5B shows the narrowing of right ventricular outflow tract, hypoplastic pulmonary valve, and hypoplastic main pulmonary artery. This is consistent with the diagnosis of

TOF. The oxygen saturation is determined by how much blood goes across the right ventricular outflow tract (RVOT) into the pulmonary artery and thereby the degree of RVOT obstruction. It is important to note that RVOT obstruction can be at any level and can be at multiple levels—subvalvar, valvar, and or supravalvar. The degree of aortic override is usually about 50% but has been observed to range from 15% to 95% in one echocardiographic study. However, neither the VSD nor the degree of overriding of the aorta determines the level of saturation in TOF. An ASD/patent foramen ovale is present in most cases of TOF. The presence of an ASD is important to know for surgical purposes, but it does not have any role in the determination of oxygen saturation in TOF.

Based on the severity of right ventricular outflow tract obstruction, TOF can present in mainly three different forms. These clinical/anatomic variables (Fig. 26-15) include: a. "Pink" Tetralogy; b. Classic tetralogy; and c. Pulmonary atresia/VSD (tetralogy with pulmonary atresia). It is important to recognize that these descriptions refer to a starting point at the time of diagnosis and are helpful in trying to predict the subsequent clinical course. In the "pink" form of TOF, there is minimal narrowing/RVOT obstruction. This infant will have very little or no cyanosis at all and may even exhibit some symptoms of pulmonary overcirculation. The right ventricular outflow obstruction in tetralogy tends to change and worsen with time, causing more severe restriction of pulmonary blood flow. In the classic form of TOF, there is less blood flow to the lungs, the peripheral saturation will be lower than normal, and some infants are cyanotic. These patients may need a shunt surgery (Blalock-Taussig shunt) in the early period of their life to provide adequate pulmonary blood flow. Patients may start life "pink" and progress to a cyanotic stage with time. However, in practical terms, this happens infrequently in the modern age because infant surgery is generally available to address this trend. Early primary repair is often carried out within the first few months of life. Patients with pulmonary atresia are ductal-dependent and represent a very complex spectrum of tetralogy patients. There may be many anatomic variables in this group depending upon the anatomy of the pulmonary blood supply.

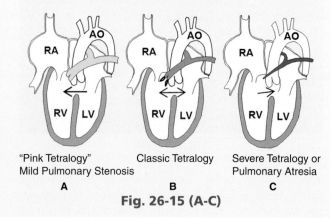

"Pink Tetralogy" Mild Pulmonary Stenosis   Classic Tetralogy   Severe Tetralogy or Pulmonary Atresia

A   **B**   **C**

Fig. 26-15 (A-C)

21 ANSWER: D. Ebstein's anomaly is a severe deformity of the tricuspid valve which results from failure of the normal development of the septal and posterior leaflets. These leaflets become displaced apically and are adherent to the septum and wall of the right ventricle, respectively. The anterior leaflet becomes enlarged and "sail-like" with variable attachments to the trabecular portion of the right ventricle and outflow area. The apical displacement of the valve reduces the effective volume of the right ventricle available for pumping function. In addition, the Ebstein's valve usually is quite insufficient. All of these factors contribute to tricuspid regurgitation, poor forward flow, and the potential for right-to-left shunt through an ASD or foramen ovale. Thus, patients with severe Ebstein's anomaly may be profoundly cyanotic, particularly as newborns. This cyanosis usually resolves after several weeks once pulmonary resistance starts to drop after the birth of the child. Patients with a less severe form of Ebstein's anomaly may be clinically quite well for many years till young adulthood such as given in the case.

This is not a case of tricuspid atresia as the tricuspid valve is seen displaced apically. Patients with pulmonary hypertension (primary or secondary to Eisenmenger's syndrome) can present with low saturation and limitation of exercise capacity, but they do not have the anatomical abnormality of the tricuspid valve as shown in the figure. A large ASD can lead to dilation of the right atrium and right ventricle secondary to a large left-to-right shunt. Less than 7%–10% of patients with large ASDs can develop Eisenmenger's syndrome in their late adulthood or in old age. Nonetheless, they also will not have such an anatomical abnormality of the tricuspid valve. Uhl's anomaly is an extremely rare congenital heart disease characterized by an almost total absence of the right ventricular myocardium. Less than 20 cases have been reported so far. It was first described in 1980. In Uhl's anomaly, the tricuspid valve is normal.

22. ANSWER: B. Echocardiography shows overriding of the aorta with a malaligned VSD. Although patients with tricuspid atresia present with cyanosis and heart murmur, they do not have such echocardiographic findings. Patients with truncus arteriosus, D-transposition of great arteries with VSD, and simple VSD might have similar appearing echocardiographic features; but they usually present with the symptoms of pulmonary overcirculation such as respiratory distress, hepatomegaly, and poor weight gain.

This is a typical presentation of a classic form of TOF. TOF is the most common cause of cyanotic congenital heart disease in children. The salient feature of this defect is an anterior deviation of the infundibular septum which narrows the right ventricular outflow tract leading to subpulmonary stenosis. The anterior deviation of the infundibular septum also is responsible for the mal-alignment of the VSD and the overriding (dextroposition) of the aorta. The VSD in tetralogy is virtually always large and nonrestrictive, leading to systemic pressures in the right ventricle. The pulmonary stenosis in tetralogy is highly variable but usually *increases in severity* with age. Progressive subvalvular (infundibular) pulmonary stenosis leads to increasing obstruction to pulmonary blood flow. With such an obstruction, two things happen: 1) right-to-left shunting occurs at the ventricular level, 2) relatively less blood gets to the lungs to become oxygenated. The combination of these two effects results in increasing cyanosis. The severity of pulmonary stenosis generally determines the magnitude of the right-to-left shunt. Unlike isolated large VSDs, patients with TOF will be relatively protected from the high-pressure damage to the lung vasculature because the pulmonary stenosis restricts lung flow and pressure and does not present with signs and symptoms of pulmonary overcirculation. Patients with TOF present most often with an asymptomatic heart murmur heard at the first office visit to the pediatrician or family practitioner. Some will also be picked up in the newborn period, but the murmur is often much softer at that time because 1) the subpulmonary stenosis has not developed significantly to produce turbulence and 2) pulmonary resistance is high and flow is decreased in the first day of life as the infant goes through normal transition. The children usually remain asymptomatic early in life, with normal growth and development. Symptoms develop with increasing desaturation and cyanosis.

23. ANSWER: C. This infant has truncus arteriosus. The parasternal long-axis view shows the malalignment VSD and overriding great vessel, similar to many other conotruncal abnormalities. The modified apical view in Figure 26-16A shows that the great artery divides into two segments, typical of truncus arteriosus.

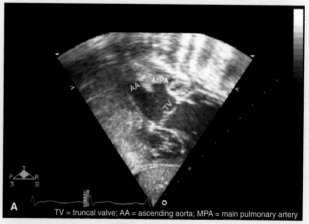

TV = truncal valve; AA = ascending aorta; MPA = main pulmonary artery

Fig. 26-16A

Color flow Doppler can help to illuminate the division of the great artery as shown in Figure 26-16B.

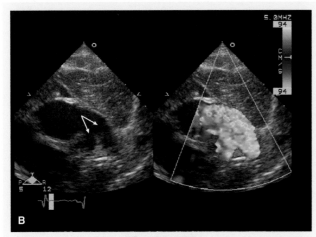

Fig. 26-16B

The arrows demonstrate the division of the common trunk into the anterior aorta and the more posterior pulmonary artery segment. This is more often better seen from a parasternal short-axis view as shown in Figure 26-16C.

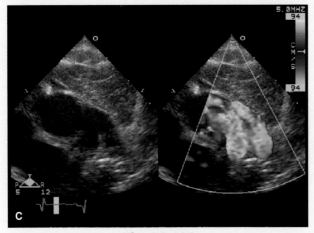

Fig. 26-16C

Truncus arteriosus is an uncommon congenital heart defect of the outflow tract of the heart. A single arterial vessel gives rise to the systemic, pulmonary, and coronary arteries. By definition, there is always a large malalignment VSD and the presence of a truncal valve instead of separate pulmonary and aortic valves. During normal embryology, the common arterial trunk undergoes septation to allow the aorta to arise from the left ventricle and the main pulmonary artery to arise from the right ventricle. An absent or abnormal conotruncal septation leads to persistence of truncus arteriosus.

Choices A and B are both incorrect, as in both conditions, the pulmonary artery arises from the right ventricle instead of a single truncal artery. Truncus arteriosus is associated with DiGeorge syndrome not with Trisomy 21 (VSD and complete atrioventricular canal defect are associated with Trisomy 21). There is

nothing in the images which suggests the presence of anomalous pulmonary venous return, although the scenario of pulmonary congestion and cyanosis would potentially suggest this entity.

24. ANSWER: B. This example demonstrates pulmonary valve atresia. There is no forward flow or regurgitation in the pulmonary valve region, establishing the atresia. Even though what appears to be a valve seen in the pulmonary position, it never opens.

Pulmonary valve atresia is divided into two broad categories based on the presence or absence of VSD. These two categories actually describe very different anatomic entities. These are: 1) pulmonary atresia with intact ventricular septum (PA/IVS) and 2) pulmonary atresia with VSD (PA/VSD). PA/IVS is also commonly referred to as the "hypoplastic right heart syndrome," although this is an older terminology, not used commonly. PA/IVS will have varying degrees of right ventricular hypoplasia and will frequently need to be repaired as a single ventricle. PA/VSD is a severe form of TOF. However, because of the wide variety of sources of pulmonary blood flow which may be encountered in PA/VSD, it is often described separately from tetralogy patients.

Usually, left ventricular size is adequate in all cases of pulmonary atresia. Choice D is incorrect because it is very unlikely to have pulmonary atresia and aortic arch abnormalities, such as coarctation of aorta or interrupted aortic arch. A right aortic arch may be seen more frequently in PA/VSD, but this is unlikely to help clinically in any great way. Evaluation of the atrial septum is useful but the presence or absence of an atrial septal defect will not change the diagnosis, natural history, or future surgical management. The pulmonary veins should always be examined but anomalies in this area are infrequent with any form of pulmonary atresia and are therefore of lesser importance.

25. ANSWER: C. The primary anatomic feature of tricuspid atresia, as shown in Figure 26-10, is the absence of the tricuspid valve, which prevents normal flow of right atrial blood directly into the right ventricle. The resulting membrane is usually muscular but may be fibrous. This membrane is very well seen in Figure 26-10, where the mitral valve is open with a membrane in place of the tricuspid valve. An ASD must be present to allow blood out of the right atrium. Tricuspid atresia provides a good example of the concept of downstream obstruction. When stenosis or atresia occurs at one level (in this case at the tricuspid valve level), obstruction or hypoplasia is often present downstream or in the path where blood would normally have flowed. For this question, it is common to have hypoplasia of the right ventricle, particularly the inlet portion. The development of a trabecular portion of the right ventricle and pulmonary arteries depends upon the presence of a VSD.

Total anomalous pulmonary venous return will produce an echo picture of right heart enlargement and perhaps relative left heart hypoplasia, with right-to-left shunting at the atrial level. Complete atrioventricular canal defect includes a common AV valve, large inlet VSD, and primum ASD which are not shown in Figure 26-10. Choices (D) and (E) are also incorrect as in these conditions, the tricuspid valve is present.

26. ANSWER: C. Figure 26-11 is highly suspicious of TAPVR. In TAPVR, the pulmonary veins usually converge in the midline posterior and superior to the left atrium (Fig. 26-11). There is no direct connection of the pulmonary veins to the left atrium. The convergence of pulmonary veins is called a pulmonary venous confluence. Right-sided pulmonary veins can be seen very well entering into the venous confluence.

In approximately 36% of cases, the confluence drains to the heart by way of an ascending vein to the innominate vein or SVC and then to the right atrium (supracardiac type, most common). In approximately 16%, the confluence drains directly to the coronary sinus (coronary sinus type) and in 15% the veins connect directly to the right atrium (cardiac type). In approximately 13%, the confluence drains by way of a descending vein, below the diaphragm, to the portal vein, hepatic vein, inferior vena cava, or ductus venosus (infracardiac type).

A mediastinal mass would usually appear as a bright echogenic area. This area is behind the left atrium, meaning it is a posterior structure and is hypoechoic. Truncus arteriosus is anterior structure arising from one or both ventricles. It is very unlikely to develop such a localized pericardial effusion and this would have a questionable association with any desaturation.

27. ANSWER: B. Video 26-1A shows an overriding of the aorta with malaligned VSD. Video 26-1B shows an infundibular narrowing along with a hypoplastic pulmonary valve and pulmonary artery. This combination of findings is diagnostic of TOF.

28. ANSWER: A. The description given in the case suggests a relatively normal, natural progression of the disease. In TOF, signs and symptoms generally progress secondary to hypertrophy of the infundibular septum. As the child grows, right ventricular outflow tract obstruction increases. Worsening of the right ventricular outflow tract obstruction leads to right ventricular hypertrophy, increased right-to-left shunting, and systemic hypoxemia and thereby worsening of cyanosis. Worsening of cyanosis can be a major determinant of the timing of surgical repair. Cyanosis is more pronounced when the child cries. In tetralogy spells, hypercyanosis persists even when the child is not crying and it is also associated with hyperpnea.

Hypercyanotic spells are also called hypoxemic episodes or tetralogy spells. These occur due to an acute increase in right-to-left shunting at the VSD. Various etiologies have been proposed, such as dynamic obstruction at infundibular level, increase in pulmonary vascular resistance, and decrease in systemic vascular resistance. Severe and often prolonged decrease in arterial saturation occurs which may lead to metabolic acidosis. Episodes are characterized by severe cyanosis and hyperpnea which is in response to the acute hypoxia and secondary metabolic acidosis. Prolonged episodes may be life threatening. Clinically, the murmur of pulmonary stenosis may become diminished or completely disappear suggesting diminished blood flow to pulmonary arteries. The child will have hyperpnea and cyanosis along with some irritability and or lethargy. Left ventricular function remains unchanged until a very late stage where it can become compromised secondary to severe metabolic acidosis.

29. ANSWER: C. There are a number of associated anomalies in TOF which may have clinical significance. In addition to the classic tetrad, the following anomalies may coexist:

- Valvular pulmonary stenosis (50%–60%).
- Right aortic arch (25%)—usually mirror image branching.
- ASD (15%).
- Coronary anomalies (esp. LAD from the right coronary) (5%).
- Additional muscular VSD (2%).
- Unilateral absent pulmonary artery (rare).

In current practice, surgical correction of TOF consists of relieving the right ventricular outflow tract obstruction and patching the VSD. The right ventricular outflow tract obstruction is relieved with or without a transannular patch. Patients with infundibular narrowing with an adequate pulmonary valve and pulmonary artery size can undergo infundibular muscle resection without a transannular patch. In such cases, pulmonary valve function may be preserved. In patients with RVOT obstruction along with a hypoplastic pulmonary valve (as in our case), transannular patch is inevitable. These patients will not have a functional pulmonary valve after surgery resulting in free pulmonary insufficiency. Pulmonary valve sparing operations in infancy may be possible when pulmonary valve annulus Z-scores are ≤4. This may be accomplished with acceptable postoperative right ventricular pressures and low reoperation rates.

Coronary abnormalities include:

1. A large conal branch or accessory left anterior descending artery (10%–15%).
2. Left anterior descending artery coming from right coronary artery (5%).
3. A single origin of the coronary arteries (4%).
4. Two coronary ostia arising from the same truncal sinus.
5. High ostial origin.

From a surgical perspective, the most important coronary anomaly is the origin of the left anterior descending artery from the right coronary artery. It subsequently runs anteriorly across the right ventricular outflow tract. In surgery with a transannular patch, the incision is placed in this area. To avoid transection of the vessel, surgeons may be required to vary their approach in relieving subpulmonic obstruction, or, possibly, to use a right ventricle to pulmonary artery conduit. From an echocardiography standpoint, it is important to identify these vessels preoperatively. Videos 26-1C and D show an example of an LAD from the right coronary artery.

In a small group of patients, particularly neonates with severe pulmonary artery hypoplasia, a palliative procedure such as modified Blalock-Taussig (BT) shunt may be needed initially to provide adequate pulmonary blood flow and allow the child to grow before performing a complete repair. This strategy was routinely performed in the past before the advent of infant surgical techniques. A modified BT shunt is performed by placing a Goretex® tube between the subclavian artery and the ipsilateral pulmonary artery. A right aortic arch is seen approximately in 25% of cases. Arch sidedness can affect the choice of the BT shunt side but it does not have great clinical importance. The presence of an ASD will not change the plan of surgery, though the surgeon has to close it during surgery. Additional muscular VSDs are usually small in size and are left alone in most cases. However, their presence must be known preoperatively. A large unrecognized muscular VSD found after operation may have significant negative clinical impact. The usual outlet, malalignment VSD in tetralogy is large and does not play a role in determining the surgical timing.

30. ANSWER: B. The infundibular obstruction found in TOF has been postulated to be a result of the anterior displacement of the bulbotruncal ridges with unequal separation of the developing outflow tracts and anterior deviation of the outlet septum. Anterior deviation of this septum results in misalignment of the outlet and trabecular portion of the ventricular septum causing a malaligned VSD and subsequent straddling of the aorta over the malaligned ventricular septum.

When stenosis or obstruction occurs at one level (in this case, at the right ventricular infundibular level), hypoplasia is often present downstream or in the path where blood would normally have flowed. In this case, it is common to have hypoplasia of the pulmonary valve and pulmonary arteries. Right ventricular hypertrophy is secondary to right ventricular outflow tract obstruction which has resulted from anterior displacement of the outlet septum. Posterior deviation of the outlet septum is seen in the Taussig-Bing variety of double-outlet right ventricle, not in TOF.

31. ANSWER: D. Definition: Transposition is defined as connection of the aorta to the right ventricle and the pulmonary artery to the left ventricle. There is atrioventricular concordance but ventriculoarterial discordance. Transposition occurs in approximately 4%–8% of children born with congenital heart defects. "D-transposition" is a term which refers to the way the conotruncal septum rotates in utero ("D" for dextro) and has been commonly applied to this entity. Transposition also occurs in children with other complex forms of congenital heart disease.

Anatomy: In transposition, the aorta arises from the right ventricle, usually in a position which is anterior and rightward of the pulmonary valve. The two great arteries course parallel to one another; a distinctly different arrangement from the normal pulmonary artery **crossing over** the aortic root. Echocardiographically, the posterior great artery, which is the pulmonary artery, will be seen taking an immediate posterior course, typical of the pulmonary arteries.

32. ANSWER: C. VSD is common and present in about 40% to 45% cases of D-TGA. There are basically two forms of transposition: Figure 26-17A with intact ventricular septum and Figure 26-17B with VSD (usually perimembranous).

D-Transposition of the Great Arteries

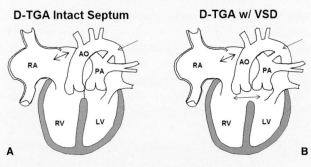

D-TGA Intact Septum   **D-TGA w/ VSD**

Fig. 26-17 (A-B)

Nearly half of the hearts with TGA have no other anomaly except a persistent patent foramen ovale or a patent ductus arteriosus (PDA). LVOT obstruction is present in 5% and 10% of cases of D-TGA with an intact ventricular septum and D-TGA with VSD, respectively. The coronary anatomy is normal in approximately 2/3 of the cases of D-TGA. Common coronary abnormalities are a circumflex from the right coronary artery, single coronary artery, or an inverted arrangement of coronary arteries (listed in decreasing frequency).

Other Associated Defects:

• ASD.
• Pulmonary stenosis—subvalvular, valvular.
• PDA.
• Coarctation of the aorta.

33. *ANSWER: A.* In D-transposition, desaturated blood returning to the right ventricle enters the aorta and returns to the systemic circulation ("parallel" circulation). This causes severe systemic desaturation (cyanosis). In a similar manner, fully saturated pulmonary venous blood returns to the left atrium, enters the left ventricle, and then the pulmonary artery. This oxygenated blood then returns to the lungs where further saturation with oxygen cannot occur. It is important to remember that desaturated blood needs to go from the systemic circulation into the pulmonary circulation in order to get oxygenated. At the same time, oxygenated blood needs to enter the systemic circulation in order to supply oxygen to the body. Without intracardiac mixing of systemic venous or pulmonary venous blood, this physiology results in fatal hypoxia. Survival in children with transposition depends on the presence of intracardiac (ASD, VSD) or extracardiac (PDA) shunts that allow mixing of systemic venous and pulmonary venous blood. The level of arterial oxygen saturation is influenced primarily by the pulmonary-to-systemic blood flow ratio. This ratio, in turn, depends on adequate size of anatomic shunting sites, local pressure gradient, and vascular resistance in each of the circulations. In the presence of a large shunting site, atrial level shunting is affected the least out of all three shunting sites by vascular resistance in systemic and pulmonary circulation. The pressure gradient between the two atria will be minimal, if any, whereas that is not true for VSD and PDA shunting sites. In summary, given the choices, an atrial level shunt is the best source for intracardiac shunting in D-TGA both theoretically as well as in clinical practice. It is very important to evaluate the adequate size of any atrial septal communication. In the case of a restrictive atrial septal communication, the child may need emergency balloon atrial septostomy to establish an area of adequate mixing and thereby adequate saturation. Video 26-2C shows a balloon septostomy done for a restricted atrial septal communication. After balloon steptostomy, adequate ASD is seen without any flow acceleration (Video 26-2D).

KEY POINTS:

■ Transposition of the great arteries produces profound early cyanosis.
■ The posterior great artery is the pulmonary artery and courses posteriorly from its origin.
■ VSD is a common associated anomaly.
■ Areas of potential mixing at atrial, ductal, and ventricular levels are important for survival preoperatively and need to be identified.

34. *ANSWER: B.* This patient has Ebstein's anomaly of the tricuspid valve. The desaturation results primarily from a right-to-left shunt at the atrial level. The video clips establish the diagnosis, although they do not specifically show this phenomenon (Fig. 26-18 and Video 26-3C).

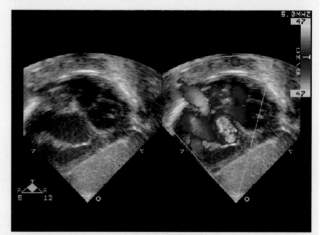

Fig. 26-18

Right-to-left shunting is often a little deceptive on echo imaging of the atrial septum—primarily because the user is not used to seeing a blue-colored flow pattern from this area. The right-to-left shunt is a result of many factors including a higher right atrial pressure than that of the left atrium and elevated total pulmonary resistance. This is caused by several factors including abnormal right ventricular filling by the redundant tricuspid valve leaflets and tricuspid valve insufficiency. Furthermore, right ventricular filling may be impeded by the abnormal contraction pattern of the atrialized portion of the right ventricle. During atrial systole, blood flows from the true right atrium into the atrialized portion of the right ventricle (the atrialized portion of right ventricle does not contract with the true atrium). However, during ventricular systole, much of the blood present in the atrialized right ventricle is propelled back into the true right atrium rather than passing forward into the true right ventricle. This results in decreased effective forward flow to the right side of the heart.

Pulmonary arteriovenous malformations and pulmonary hypertension are not seen usually in Ebstein's anomaly. Typically, right-to-left atrial shunting (and hypoxemia) will be present in the newborn. This resolves and left-to-right shunting may ensue as right ventricular compliance increases and pulmonary resistance decreases. In teen years, the right ventricular compliance may begin to decrease and tricuspid regurgitation may increase, resulting in a resumption of right-to-left atrial shunting.

35. ANSWER: A. All of the choices may be considered to be features seen in Ebstein's anomaly. From time to time, clinicians may encounter abnormalities of the tricuspid valve which have the appearance of Ebstein's anomaly. One proposed criterion for making the distinction between Ebstein and "Ebsteinoid" valves has been the measurement of the apical displacement of the septal leaflet >8 mm/m^2 BSA as measured along the septum from the insertion point of the mitral valve annulus to be diagnostic of Ebstein's anomaly.

Other echocardiographic findings are:

M-mode

• Paradoxical ventricular septal motion
• Delayed closure of tricuspid valve leaflets more than 65 milliseconds after mitral valve closure

Two-dimensional

• Tethering of posterior leaflet
• Abnormal morphology of tricuspid valve leaflet
• ASD
• Dilated right atrium
• Dilated tricuspid valve annulus
• Dilated right ventricle
• Left-sided cardiac abnormality in 25% of cases

Doppler studies

• Varying degrees of tricuspid regurgitation
• Varying degrees of tricuspid stenosis
• Right to left/bidirectional shunting at atrial level

Interestingly, it is the anterior leaflet of the tricuspid valve which may be the most important portion to image. This relative degree of involvement, tethering, and mobility of the anterior leaflet will determine suitability for repair versus replacement at surgery.

36. ANSWER: E. An interatrial communication (ASD/PFO) is almost always present in a patient with Ebstein's anomaly. An accessory conduction pathway is seen in approximately 25% of cases. Pulmonary stenosis and VSD are present occasionally but not as frequent as ASD/PFO. The presence of a left superior vena cava is not associated with Ebstein's anomaly.

KEY POINTS:

■ Ebstein's anomaly is a rare anomaly of the tricuspid valve produced by significant apical displacement of the tricuspid septal and posterior leaflets.

■ An ASD is associated with cyanosis in Ebstein's anomaly due to right-to-left atrial shunting.
■ The septal tricuspid leaflet displacement makes the diagnosis, but the anterior leaflet should be studied for surgical repair.

37. ANSWER: D. This newborn has tricuspid atresia. The presence of an imperforate linear echo density in the location of the normal tricuspid valve confirms the diagnosis of tricuspid atresia. Tricuspid atresia is divided into three categories: Type I—with normally related great arteries (75% of cases); Type II—D-transposition of great arteries (20%–25%); and Type III—is more complex disease with L-transposition or malposed great arteries (uncommon, 3%). Further subclassification of types I and II are described in Table 26-1.

TABLE 26-1	**Types of Tricuspid Atresia**
Type I	Normally related great arteries
	a. Intact ventricular septum with pulmonary atresia
	b. Small VSD and pulmonary stenosis
	c. Large VSD without pulmonary stenosis
Type II	Transposition of the great arteries
	a. Intact VSD with aortic atresia
	b. Small VSD with aortic stenosis and/or coarctation
	c. Large VSD without aortic stenosis or coarctation

Do not forget the simple rule in cardiac development! When stenosis or atresia occurs at one level (in this case, at the tricuspid valve level), obstruction or hypoplasia is often present downstream or in the path where blood would normally have flowed. In type I, the size of VSD will determine development of the outlet portion of the right ventricle, pulmonary valve, and pulmonary artery. Similarly in type II, the VSD size will determine development of the aortic valve and size of aorta as well as downstream problems such as coarctation.

In tricuspid atresia, there will be obligatory right to left shunt at the atrial level. Coarctation of the aorta is the most significant associated cardiac abnormality and occurs in approximately 8% of patients with tricuspid atresia. Coronary anomalies are rare in this lesion and generally are not clinically significant.

38. ANSWER: D. In tricuspid valve atresia, blood flows into the right atrium and must egress through an ASD. This lesion is frequently not dependent upon a ductus arteriosus for survival, although this may be true in some cases. Ductal dependence is more frequently seen in outlet stenosis or atresia, not inlet atresia. As noted in the previous question, the great artery position is of great importance clinically because downstream structures are affected which can greatly alter the clinical presentation from right heart obstruction to aortic obstruction. There is no tricuspid regurgitation in this lesion, so Doppler techniques will not apply here. The pulmonary branches are generally normal in size or hypoplastic. The latter is particularly true with tricuspid atresia and normally related great arteries with significant restriction at the level of the VSD.

KEY POINTS:

▨ Tricuspid atresia exists in two basic forms; normally related great arteries and transposition.

▨ Identifying the path of blood flow is crucial to establishing the clinical state.

▨ An ASD is needed for egress of blood out of the right atrium and flow will always be right to left.

39. ANSWER: D. Echocardiography shows TAPVR of the supracardiac type. In supracardiac TAPVR, the pulmonary venous confluence drains to the heart by way of an ascending vein to the innominate vein or SVC and then to the right atrium. This is the most common form seen in 35%–50% of cases. In approximately 20% of cases, the confluence drains directly to the coronary sinus or the veins connect directly to the right atrium (cardiac type). In approximately 20%, the confluence drains by way of a descending vein, below the diaphragm, to the portal vein, hepatic vein, inferior vena cava, or ductus venosus (infracardiac type). A mixed type of TAPVR may also be seen and is a combination of the other forms. The mixed type accounts for about 10% of TAPVR cases. Obstruction of venous return is virtually always present when the pulmonary venous return is below the diaphragm or infracardiac. In the supracardiac type, some form of obstruction is present in 50% of cases, but it is often mild. Obstruction is rarely seen in the cardiac type of TAPVR. In all forms of TAPVR, some form of atrial communication is almost always present. Profound cyanosis is unusual at any age. Some forms of TAPVR may go undetected until later in life, although this is unusual.

40. ANSWER: B. TAPVR is cyanotic congenital heart disease with right-sided volume overload. The right atrium will receive systemic as well as pulmonary venous return. This results in dilatation of right atrium and right ventricle as well as the pulmonary arteries. This is true for all types of TAPVR. In obstructed TAPVR, development of pulmonary hypertension can also lead to right ventricular hypertrophy. On the contrary, left-sided structures, left atrium, and/or left ventricle are often smaller in size. Also remember that a part of left atrium is formed by absorption of pulmonary veins which does not happen in TAPVR, resulting in a smaller left atrium. The atrial and ventricular septum bow into the left side because of volume and/or pressure overload on the right side. Doppler, particularly color flow Doppler, is very useful to establish the connection of pulmonary veins in normal hearts as well as in cases of TAPVR.

41. ANSWER: C. The scenario presented here is typical of a case of TAPVR. The first thing which needs to occur is an index of suspicion. In the case of small left heart or enlarged right heart or both, TAPVR should be suspected. When this is combined with right to left atrial shunting, a very strong suspicion for this entity should be present. The next phase of the echocardiographic evaluation involves a search of the systemic venous system for sources of abnormal flow. This includes the superior caval system and innominate vein, the coronary sinus, the liver and hepatic veins, and the right atrium. Color flow Doppler interrogation of the flows in these areas is essential to identifying the abnormal veins. Often, the abnormal flow will produce very turbulent flow in some of these areas as well as unusually large venous structures. An example of infradiaphragmatic TAPVR is shown in Videos 26-5B and C with an unusual, obstructed flow signal in the liver and hepatic veins which eventually drains into the IVC. Spectral Doppler interrogation is also important when obstruction is suspected from the color flow exam.

KEY POINTS:

▨ Total anomalous pulmonary venous return drains to the systemic veins, which should be the focal point of the echo examination.

▨ There are several different types of TAPVR.

▨ TAPVR may be obstructed before returning to the heart.

▨ Shunt flow at the atrial level will be right-to-left.

SUGGESTED READINGS

Allen HD, Driscoll JD, Shaddy RE, Feltes TF (eds). *Moss & Adam's Heart Disease in Infants, Children, and Adolescents: Including the Fetus and Young Adult.* 7th ed. Philadelphia: Lippincott Williams & Wilkins, 2008.

Anderson RH, Weinberg PM. The clinical anatomy of tetralogy of Fallot. *Cardiol Young.* 2005;15:38–47.

Attenhofer Jost CH, Connolly HM, Dearani JA, et al. Ebstein's anomaly. *Circulation.* 2007;115:277–285.

Castaneda-Zuniga W, Nath HP, Moller JH, et al. Left-sided anomalies in Ebstein's malformation of the tricuspid valve. *Pediatr Cardiol.* 1982;3:181–185.

Need LR, Powell AJ, del Nido P, et al. Coronary echocardiography in tetralogy of fallot: diagnostic accuracy, resource utilization and surgical implications over 13 years. *J Am Coll Cardiol.* 2000; 36:1371–1377.

Paranon S, Acar P. Ebstein's anomaly of the tricuspid valve: from fetus to adult: congenital heart disease. *Heart.* 2008;94:237–243.

Park MK. *Pediatric Cardiology for Practitioners.* 5th ed. Philadephia: Mosby, 2008.

Sommer RJ, Hijazi ZM, Rhodes JF. Pathophysiology of congenital heart disease in the adult: part III: complex congenital heart disease. *Circulation.* 2008;117:1340–1350.

Stewart RD, Backer CL, Young L, et al. Tetralogy of Fallot: results of a pulmonary valve-sparing strategy. *Ann Thorac Surg.* 2005;80: 1431–1438; discussion 1438–1439.

Warnes CA. Transposition of the great arteries. *Circulation.* 2006; 114:2699–2709.

Noncyanotic Congenital Heart Disease

CHAPTER 27

Benjamin W. Eidem

1. Which echocardiographic scan plane is most optimal to define a secundum atrial septal defect (ASD)?
   A. Suprasternal long-axis view.
   B. Parasternal long-axis view.
   C. Parasternal short-axis view.
   D. Subcostal four-chamber view.
   E. Apical four-chamber view.

2. Which of the following is the most common associated anatomic lesion found with a sinus venosus ASD?
   A. Anomalous right pulmonary venous connection.
   B. Inlet ventricular septal defect (VSD).
   C. Bicuspid aortic valve (AV).
   D. Persistent left superior vena cava.
   E. Coarctation of the aorta.

3. Which of the following associated congenital heart defects is most common in a patient with Down syndrome and an atrioventricular septal defect (AVSD)?
   A. Coarctation of the aorta.
   B. Total anomalous pulmonary venous connection.
   C. AV stenosis.
   D. Tetralogy of Fallot.
   E. Left ventricular (LV) hypoplasia.

4. Which of the following is the most common anatomic finding in a complete AVSD?
   A. Cleft in posterior leaflet of mitral component of AV.
   B. Medial rotation of LV papillary muscles.
   C. Ratio of LV inlet to outlet distance >1.0.
   D. Left ventricular outflow tract (LVOT) is "sprung" anteriorly.
   E. Left and right atrioventricular valve attachments are present at different levels.

5. The best echocardiographic view to delineate a subpulmonary (supracristal) VSD is:
   A. Parasternal long-axis view.
   B. Apical four-chamber view.
   C. Suprasternal long-axis view.
   D. Parasternal short-axis view.
   E. Apical five-chamber view.

6. Which of the following is the most characteristic acquired lesion resulting from a subpulmonary (supracristal) VSD?
   A. Aortic insufficiency.
   B. LVOT obstruction.
   C. Right ventricular (RV) outflow tract obstruction.
   D. Pulmonary valve stenosis.
   E. AV stenosis.

7. Which of the following is the most characteristic physiologic effect of a large VSD?
   A. RV volume overload.
   B. Low pulmonary arterial pressure.
   C. Equal RV and LV pressure.
   D. Increased systemic blood flow.
   E. Decreased pulmonary blood flow.

8. The most common anatomic type of subaortic stenosis is:
   A. Tunnel-type.
   B. Discrete membrane.
   C. Asymmetric septal hypertrophy.
   D. Systolic anterior motion of mitral valve.
   E. Anomalous mitral chordal insertion within the LVOT.

9. A neonate with valvar pulmonary stenosis has a peak Doppler velocity by continuous-wave Doppler of 4.1 m/sec. The estimated peak instantaneous Doppler gradient is:
   A. 67 mm Hg.
   B. 77 mm Hg.
   C. 72 mm Hg.
   D. 50 mm Hg.
   E. Cannot be calculated.

10. The most common associated cardiac abnormality in a patient with coarctation of the aorta is:
    A. Bicuspid AV.
    B. VSD.
    C. ASD.
    D. Pulmonary valve stenosis.
    E. Coronary artery anomaly.

11. In patients with coarctation of the aorta, systemic arterial pressure begins to be significantly affected when the overall aortic lumen is narrowed by:
    A. 20%.
    B. 30%.
    C. 50%.
    D. 75%.
    E. 90%.

12. The most common type of VSD that is associated with coarctation of the aorta is:
    A. Apical muscular.
    B. Anterior malalignment.
    C. Perimembranous.
    D. Inlet.
    E. Subpulmonary (supracristal).

13. The Doppler phenomenon often seen in patients with supravalvar aortic stenosis has been demonstrated to be a high-velocity poststenotic jet that hugs the aortic wall and preferentially transfers kinetic energy into the right innominate artery. Which of the following best describe this Doppler finding?
    A. Coanda effect.
    B. Ohm's law.
    C. Continuity equation.
    D. Poiseuille's law.
    E. Bernouilli's equation.

14. Interruption of the aortic arch is most common in which syndrome?
    A. DiGeorge.
    B. Down.
    C. Turner.
    D. Alagille's.
    E. Holt-Oram.

15. A Type A interruption of the aortic arch occurs:
    A. Between the right innominate and left common carotid arteries.
    B. Proximal to the right innominate artery.
    C. Between the left common carotid and left subclavian arteries.
    D. Distal to the left subclavian artery.
    E. Just distal to the sinotubular junction in the ascending aorta.

16. An echocardiogram is obtained on a 3-month-old with a loud cardiac murmur. The parasternal short-axis scan in Figure 27-1 is obtained. Which of the following best describes the cardiac defect?

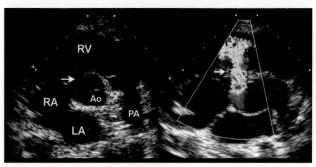

Fig. 27-1

    A. Large membranous VSD.
    B. Large muscular VSD.
    C. Ruptured sinus of Valsalva aneurysm.
    D. Severe valvar pulmonary stenosis.
    E. Severe AV insufficiency.

17. An echocardiogram is obtained after interventional device closure of a VSD (Fig. 27-2). What anatomic type of VSD has been closed with this procedure?

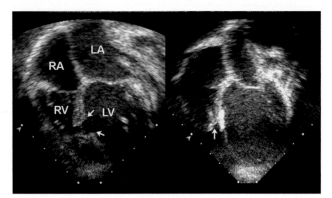

Fig. 27-2

A. Membranous VSD.
B. Inlet VSD.
C. Subpulmonary (supracristal) VSD.
D. Trabecular muscular VSD.
E. Anterior malalignment VSD.

18. What anatomic type of VSD is demonstrated in the parasternal short-axis image in Figure 27-3?

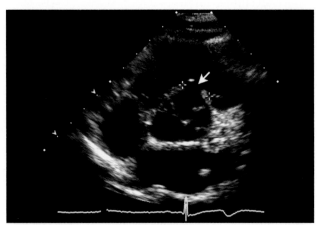

Fig. 27-3

A. Membranous VSD.
B. Inlet VSD.
C. Subpulmonary (supracristal) VSD.
D. Trabecular muscular VSD.
E. Anterior malalignment VSD.

19. A 1-month-old infant undergoes an echocardiogram secondary to a cardiac murmur. What aortic to pulmonary artery peak pressure gradient is predicted by the Doppler tracing in Figure 27-4?

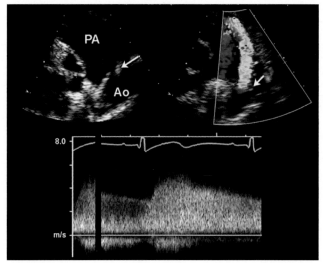

Fig. 27-4

A. 16 mm Hg.
B. 36 mm Hg.
C. 48 mm Hg.
D. 64 mm Hg.
E. The peak aorta to pulmonary artery gradient cannot be calculated.

20. A 2-day-old infant undergoes an echocardiogram because of respiratory distress. What anatomic lesion and hemodynamic physiology is demonstrated in Figure 27-5?

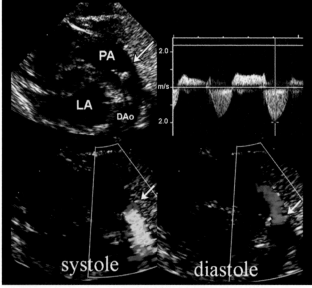

Fig. 27-5

A. Patent ductus arteriosus (PDA) with exclusive left-to-right shunting.

B. Aortopulmonary window with bidirectional shunting.

C. Severe coarctation of the aorta with exclusive right-to-left shunting through the ductus arteriosus.

D. PDA with bidirectional shunting.

E. Aortopulmonary collateral vessel with exclusive right-to-left shunting.

21. The parasternal long-axis image in Figure 27-6 is obtained in a 12-year-old with a new onset cardiac murmur. Which of the following cardiac diagnoses best describes this image?

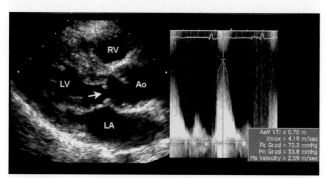

Fig. 27-6

A. Severe AV stenosis.

B. Subaortic membrane with moderate stenosis.

C. Systolic anterior motion of the mitral valve with mild stenosis.

D. Cardiac rhabdomyoma within the LVOT with moderate obstruction.

E. Anomalous mitral valve chordal insertion with severe LVOT obstruction.

22. A 2-year-old with Down syndrome presents for cardiac evaluation. The echocardiographic images in Figure 27-7 are obtained. What cardiac defect is best demonstrated by color Doppler (arrow)?

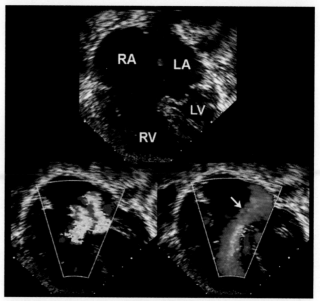

Fig. 27-7

A. Primum ASD.

B. Inlet VSD.

C. Sinus venosus ASD.

D. Persistent left superior vena cava to dilated coronary sinus.

E. Malalignment outlet VSD.

23. A previously healthy 6-year-old girl presents due to a recent episode of syncope with exercise. The suprasternal images in Figure 27-8 are obtained. Which of the following best describes her cardiac diagnosis?

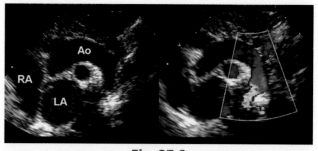

Fig. 27-8

A. Left pulmonary artery stenosis.

B. PDA.

C. Coarctation of the aorta.

D. Interruption of the aortic arch.

E. Transposition of the great arteries.

24. The Doppler pattern in Figure 27-9, in the abdominal aorta, is most consistent with:

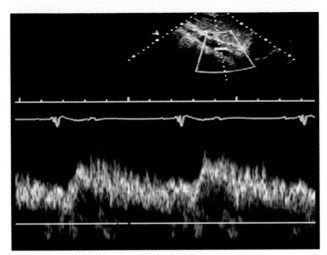

Fig. 27-9

A. Severe aortic insufficiency.
B. Large PDA.
C. Normal aortic flow pattern.
D. Coarctation of aorta.
E. Renal artery stenosis.

25. A 15-year-old presents for evaluation due to the presence of a cardiac murmur on auscultation. The echocardiographic images in Figure 27-10 are most compatible with which of the following diagnoses?

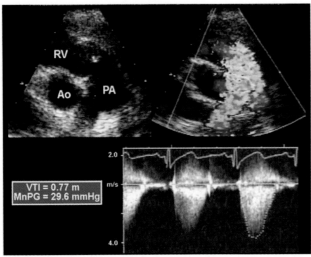

Fig. 27-10

A. Pulmonary valve stenosis.
B. Left pulmonary artery stenosis.
C. Dynamic right ventricle (RV) infundibular obstruction.
D. Tetralogy of Fallot with absent pulmonary valve.
E. Double-chambered RV.

CASE 1:

A neonate presents for evaluation secondary to a new cardiac murmur heard at his 2-week well-child outpatient visit. An echocardiogram was performed and the images in Figure 27-11 were obtained.

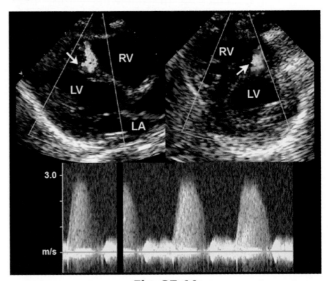

Fig. 27-11

26. Which of the following diagnoses are most consistent with these images?
    A. Small anterior muscular VSD with left-to-right shunting.
    B. Small posterior inlet VSD with left-to-right shunting.
    C. Large nonrestrictive muscular VSD with bidirectional shunting.
    D. Multiple "swiss cheese" VSDs with right-to-left shunting.
    E. Small outlet VSD with left-to-right shunting.

27. What is the peak LV to RV pressure gradient based upon the Doppler velocity displayed?
    A. 16 mm Hg.
    B. 36 mm Hg.
    C. 64 mm Hg.
    D. 100 mm Hg.
    E. The peak pressure gradient cannot be calculated.

28. What is the likelihood of spontaneous closure of this defect during childhood?
A. 5%–10%.
B. 20%–30%.
C. 40%–50%.
D. 60%–70%.
E. 80%–90%.

CASE 2:

A 7-year-old boy presents to your office with exercise intolerance. You note a 3/6 systolic ejection murmur at the left upper sternal border with a widely split S2 and a soft middiastolic rumble. The echocardiographic image in Figure 27-12 is obtained.

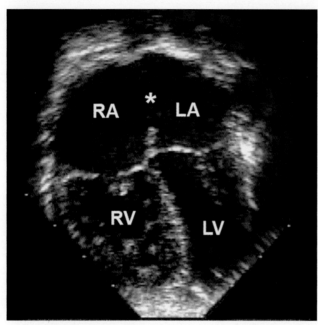

Fig. 27-12

29. Which of the following diagnoses is correct?
A. Primum ASD.
B. Secundum ASD.
C. Sinus venosus ASD.
D. Coronary sinus ASD.
E. Atrial septal aneurysm.

30. The direction in which blood flows across an ASD is primarily related to which of the following anatomic or hemodynamic factors?
A. Relative compliances of the ventricles.
B. Pulmonary vascular resistance.
C. Systemic vascular resistance.
D. Relative atrial pressures.
E. Size and morphology of the ASD.

31. The family is interested in repair of this defect but does not want him to undergo surgical repair. In your discussion with this family, which of the following defects would you tell them would be amenable to interventional device closure?
A. Primum ASD.
B. Secundum ASD.
C. Sinus venosus ASD.
D. Coronary sinus ASD.
E. AVSD.

CASE 3:

A 3-week-old infant presents to the Emergency Department with tachypnea and a cardiac murmur. These echocardiographic images in Figure 27-13A and Videos 27-1A–C are obtained.

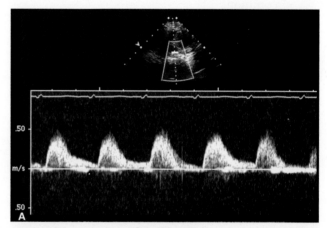

Fig. 27-13A

32. What is the most likely diagnosis?
A. Coarctation of the aorta.
B. Interruption of the aortic arch type A.
C. Supravalvar aortic stenosis.
D. Valvar aortic stenosis.
E. Subaortic stenosis.

33. After the echocardiogram is completed, the on-call resident performs four-extremity blood pressure measurements. The findings are as follows:

Right leg: 40/25 mm Hg.

Left leg: 42/22 mm Hg.

Right arm: 48/27 mm Hg.

Left arm: 72/35 mm Hg.

Which of the following is the most likely diagnosis?

A. Interruption of the aortic arch with restrictive PDA.

B. Coarctation of the aorta with VSD.

C. Coarctation of the aorta with aberrant right subclavian artery.

D. Truncus arteriosus with pulmonary artery ostial stenosis.

E. Normal aortic arch with stenosis of the left subclavian artery.

34. Which of the following statements regarding coarctation of the aorta is correct?

A. It is caused by formation of an anterior ledge of thickened aortic wall media tissue.

B. The most common site of coarctation is opposite the ductal insertion.

C. Involvement of the left subclavian artery is very common.

D. It commonly presents in the neonatal period with systemic hypertension and LV hypertrophy.

E. It is rarely associated with other congenital heart abnormalities.

35. The aforesaid patient undergoes a follow-up echocardiogram following initiation of PGE. The Doppler profile in Figure 27-13B is obtained. What is the most likely explanation?

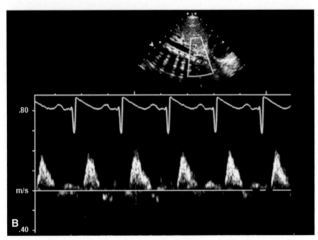

Fig. 27-13B

A. Significant aortic insufficiency is present.

B. PDA is now open.

C. Cardiac output is extremely low.

D. Pulmonary hypertension is present.

E. Thrombus is present in the descending aorta.

CASE 4:

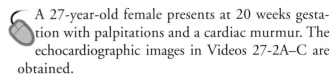

A 27-year-old female presents at 20 weeks gestation with palpitations and a cardiac murmur. The echocardiographic images in Videos 27-2A–C are obtained.

36. What is the underlying cardiac diagnosis:

A. Complete AVSD with large primum ASD and large inlet VSD.

B. Large secundum ASD.

C. Large primum ASD.

D. Large sinus venosus ASD.

E. Large malalignment outlet VSD.

37. The image of the left atrioventricular valve in Video 27-2D is obtained. What abnormality is demonstrated?

A. Double-orifice mitral valve.

B. Mitral arcade.

C. Cleft mitral valve.

D. Mitral valve prolapse.

E. Normal mitral valve anatomy.

38. The offspring of this female is born at term. The images in Video 27-2E and F are obtained shortly after delivery. What is the cardiac abnormality demonstrated in this newborn?

A. Complete AVSD.

B. Sinus venosus ASD.

C. Secundum ASD.

D. Tetralogy of Fallot.

E. Large outlet muscular VSD.

CASE 5:

A 6-year-old boy presents to you for evaluation of a cardiac murmur. His mom says that he has had the murmur "all his life" but it was felt to be functional. The patient does not complain of any symptoms but he is not very active. The only sport he seems interested in is basketball but he is too short. When you ask about the family history, they mention that there were a paternal uncle, grandfather, and great grandfather who had a very "thick heart muscle." On exam, you note short stature, a triangular face, an obvious chest deformity, a webbed neck, a RV lift, and a soft short systolic ejection murmur at the left upper sternal border without a click. He has normal distal pulses.

39. What is the finding demonstrated on echocardiography (Videos 27-3A–E)?
A. Bicuspid AV with coarctation of the aorta.
B. Discrete supravalvular aortic stenosis.
C. Thickened pulmonary valve with hypoplastic annulus.
D. Severe branch pulmonary artery stenosis.
E. Large PDA.

40. Which of the following would be the most expected cardiac abnormality in Noonan syndrome:
A. Pulmonary valve stenosis.
B. Dilated cardiomyopathy.
C. Supravalvar aortic stenosis.
D. Coarctation of the aorta.
E. AV stenosis.

41. Percutaneous pulmonary valvotomy was performed in this patient (Videos 27-3F–I). Cardiac hemodynamics obtained during the catheterization are shown in Table 27-1 (mm Hg):

TABLE 27-1

	Prevalvotomy	Postvalvotomy
RA (mean)	10	9
RV (systolic/EDP)	125/10	62/11
MPA	15/7	13/7
Systemic BP	86/60	80/60

After the procedure, you note a grade 4/6 late-peaking harsh systolic murmur at the left upper sternal border, which is increased in intensity from his admission exam, and a new, soft diastolic murmur. His systemic blood pressure is 80/60. On echocardiography, the predicted RV systolic pressure is 60 mm Hg. The postcath angiogram is shown in Videos 27-3H and I. Which of the following is the most likely underlying cause of these findings?
A. Significant residual pulmonary valve stenosis.
B. RV infundibular obstruction.
C. Hypovolemia with systemic hypotension.
D. Distal pulmonary artery branch stenosis.
E. Severe pulmonary regurgitation.

ANSWERS

1. ANSWER: D. The subcostal imaging window is optimal to demonstrate the atrial septum and any associated atrial septal defects (ASDs) that may be present. To visualize the atrial septum without potential drop-out, the imaging plane of sound should be perpendicular to the cardiac structure of interest. With respect to the atrial septum, the imaging plane that is optimally perpendicular is the subcostal four-chamber and sagittal views. ASDs can be demonstrated in other imaging windows including the parasternal short axis, apical four-chamber, and high right parasternal views but care must be taken not to diagnose an ASD when the plane of sound is more parallel to the atrial septum creating the potential for false drop-out in the two-dimensional image. The addition of color Doppler and spectral Doppler interrogation in these views may also facilitate the diagnosis of an ASD.

2. ANSWER: A. Sinus venosus ASDs are most commonly associated with anomalous connection of the right pulmonary veins. Either a single right upper pulmonary vein or the right upper and middle pulmonary veins insert anomalously to the superior vena cava (SVC) or the SVC-right atrial junction. Sinus venosus defects are found most commonly in the superior portion of the atrial septum creating a "biatrial" insertion of the SVC. These defects can also be located inferiorly near the entrance of the inferior vena cava into the right atrium.

3. ANSWER: D. Patients with Down syndrome (trisomy 21) have an almost 50% incidence of congenital heart disease, with atrioventricular septal defects (AVSDs) being the most common cardiac anomaly in this cohort. AVSD in association with tetralogy of Fallot is a common constellation of cardiac anomalies in patients with Down syndrome. Obstruction of the left ventricular outflow tract (LVOT) and coarctation of the aorta are also common cardiac abnormalities in patients with AVSD but are not as common in Down syndrome patients. Left ventricular (LV) hypoplasia can also occur in the setting of AVSD ("unbalanced AVSD with right ventricular [RV] dominance") but is less commonly seen in this cohort. Aortic valve stenosis and anomalous pulmonary venous connections are uncommon.

4. ANSWER: D. Anatomic hallmarks of AVSDs include a cleft in the anterior leaflet of the left atrioventricular valve, lateral rotation of the LV papillary muscles, and attachments of the left and right atrioventricular valves at the same level at the cardiac crux. In addition, due to the absence of the atrioventricular septum in these defects, the LV inflow is shortened and the LV outflow is elongated ("goose-neck deformity") creating a ratio of LV inlet to LV outlet ratio <1. Due to the presence of a common atrioventricular valve, the aortic valve is no longer "wedged" between the tricuspid and mitral valves and is pushed anteriorly ("sprung").

5. ANSWER: D. Subpulmonary ventricular septal defects (VSDs) are located adjacent to the pulmonary valve and aortic valve and have been termed subpulmonary, supracristal, or doubly committed defects. These defects can be optimally demonstrated in the parasternal short-axis scan plane but can also be demonstrated from the subcostal and apical windows with appropriate angulation into the right ventricular outflow tract (RVOT).

6. ANSWER: A. Aortic insufficiency is the most common associated abnormality because of prolapse of the aortic cusp into a subpulmonary VSD. While this associated prolapse of aortic tissue limits the size of the VSD and can lessen the left-to-right shunt, the progression of aortic insufficiency due to distortion of the aortic valve is well-recognized. If this regurgitation is significant and progresses, then surgical closure is indicated (and is not dependent upon the size of the left-to-right shunt).

7. ANSWER: C. Large VSDs result in equalization of right and left ventricular pressures as well as elevated pulmonary arterial pressure. Left-to-right shunting at the ventricular level results in a substantial increase in pulmonary blood flow with left atrial and ventricular volume overload. Systemic blood flow is not significantly increased in this setting.

8. ANSWER: B. The most common type of subaortic stenosis is related to a discrete membrane proximal to the aortic valve within the LVOT. This membrane is most often circumferential and can be adherent to both the aortic valve as well as the anterior leaflet of the mitral valve. LVOT obstruction in the setting of hypertrophic cardiomyopathy is often related to asymmetric septal hypertrophy in combination with systolic anterior motion of the mitral valve chordal and leaflet tissue. Anomalous mitral chordal insertions within the LVOT can be isolated or found in association with congenital heart disease and may result in obstruction but are not as common as discrete membranes.

9. ANSWER: A. Utilizing the modified Bernoulli equation to obtain the peak instantaneous gradient across the pulmonary valve, $4 \times [velocity]^2$, then $4 \times [4.1]^2 = 67$ mm Hg.

10. ANSWER: A. Bicuspid aortic valve is the most commonly associated cardiac finding in patients with simple coarctation with some studies showing as high

as an 80% occurrence in patients with coarctation. ASDs and VSDs are also common in patients with coarctation. Pulmonary valve stenosis and coronary arterial anomalies are much less frequent in this cohort.

11. ANSWER: C. The aortic lumen must be narrowed by at least 50% to significantly affect systemic arterial pressure.

12. ANSWER: C. The most common VSD associated with coarctation is a perimembranous defect. While less common, a posterior malalignment VSD often results in severe coarctation or interruption of the aortic arch. Muscular VSD as well as inlet VSD can also occur in the setting of coarctation, in particular with an unbalanced RV-dominant AVSD.

13. ANSWER: A. The systolic jet in patients with supravalvar aortic stenosis propagates further than the jet originating with aortic valvar stenosis and has a tendency to be entrained along the aortic wall thereby transferring its kinetic energy into the right innominate artery. This physical principle often is expressed clinically in these patients by marked discrepancy in upper arm blood pressures, with the right arm pressure higher than the left arm blood pressure.

14. ANSWER: A. Interruption of the aortic arch is most commonly found in DiGeorge syndrome and is a deletion in chromosome 22q11. This chromosome deletion results in conotruncal defects, with interruption of the aortic arch type B being the most frequent cardiac abnormality. Down syndrome (trisomy 21) is frequently associated with congenital heart disease, most commonly atrioventricular canal defects and VSDs. Turner syndrome (46 XO) has coarctation and bicuspid aortic valve as hallmark lesions while Holt-Oram is associated with secundum ASDs. Alagille's syndrome is most characteristically associated with pulmonary branch stenosis or RVOT obstruction.

15. ANSWER: D. Type A interruption of the aortic arch occurs distal to the origin of the left subclavian artery. Type B interruption occurs between the left common carotid and left subclavian arteries. Type C interruption occurs between the right innominate and left common carotid arteries.

16. ANSWER: A. The parasternal short-axis image in Figure 27-1 demonstrates a defect in the membranous portion of the ventricular septum adjacent to the tricuspid valve. The color Doppler image demonstrates a high-velocity mosaic jet from the left ventricle to the right ventricle.

17. ANSWER: D. The apical four-chamber image in Figure 27-2 demonstrates the muscular ventricular septum with a midmuscular defect occluded by a closure device. The apical four-chamber view demonstrates the inlet portion of the ventricular septum (near the atrioventricular valves) and the mid and apical muscular septum.

18. ANSWER: C. The parasternal short-axis image in Figure 27-3 demonstrates a defect in the subpulmonary region (supracristal) of the ventricular septum adjacent to the pulmonary valve. This defect has also been termed an infundibular or conal VSD due to the defect's position within the infundibular muscular septum.

19. ANSWER: D. The high left parasternal short-axis image in Figure 27-4 demonstrates a patent ductus arteriosus. Color Doppler is consistent with a left-to-right shunt from the aorta to the pulmonary artery (red color flow). Continuous-wave Doppler confirms an exclusive left-to-right shunt in both systole and diastole. The peak Doppler velocity is approximately 4.0 m/sec predicting a peak instantaneous pressure gradient of 64 mm Hg utilizing the simplified Bernoulli equation:

$$4 \times [velocity]^2, \text{ then } 4 \times [4.0]^2 = 64 \text{ mm Hg}.$$

20. ANSWER: D. The high left parasternal short-axis image in Figure 27-5 demonstrates a patent ductus arteriosus (PDA). Color Doppler is consistent with a bidirectional shunt from the aorta to the pulmonary artery (right-to-left shunting in systole and left-to-right shunting in diastole). Continuous-wave Doppler confirms bidirectional low-velocity shunting.

21. ANSWER: B. The parasternal long-axis image in Figure 27-6 demonstrates a circumferential subaortic membrane within the LVOT. Note the significant narrowing of the LVOT and the association of the membrane with the anterior leaflet of the mitral valve. The peak Doppler velocity obtained from a high right parasternal location predicts a mean gradient of ~34 mm Hg (moderate stenosis).

22. ANSWER: A. The apical four-chamber image in Figure 27-7 demonstrates a large primum ASD. The large left-to-right shunt is demonstrated across this defect by color flow imaging (arrow). Both atrioventricular valves are inserted at the same level at the cardiac crux consistent with an AVSD with a large primum component. No shunt is evident at ventricular level. Significant atrioventricular valve regurgitation is also demonstrated by color Doppler.

23. ANSWER: C. The suprasternal long-axis image of the aortic arch in Figure 27-8 demonstrates a juxtaductal coarctation of the aorta. Note the posterior shelf present in the descending aorta in the two-dimensional image and the area of coarctation demonstrated with color Doppler.

24. ANSWER: D. Pulsed-wave Doppler interrogation is demonstrated in the descending aorta. The Doppler pattern in Figure 27-9 demonstrates classic findings in coarctation of the aorta with delayed arterial upstroke and prominent diastolic runoff. Also note the absence of an early diastolic Doppler flow reversal, another hallmark of significant aortic obstruction.

25. ANSWER: A. The parasternal short-axis images in Figure 27-10 demonstrate a thickened pulmonary valve with prominent color flow acceleration originating at the pulmonary valve consistent with valvar stenosis. Continuous-wave Doppler predicts a mean gradient of ~30 mm Hg suggesting a moderate degree of stenosis.

26. ANSWER: A. The parasternal long-axis and short-axis scans in Figure 27-11 demonstrate a small anterior muscular VSD in the midmuscular septum. The continuous-wave Doppler velocity of ~3 m/sec suggests a restrictive defect. Remember, pulmonary vascular resistance in the neonate does not fall completely until 2–3 months of age so it would be expected with this small defect that the Doppler velocity will increase over the first few months of life consistent with a hemodynamically small defect. No additional VSDs are demonstrated by color Doppler imaging; however, the ventricular septum should be imaged by many different scan planes (parasternal long axis, parasternal short axis, apical four-chamber, and subcostal views) to assure no additional defects are present.

27. ANSWER: B. Utilizing the modified Bernoulli equation to obtain the peak instantaneous gradient across the VSD, $4 \times [velocity]^2$, then $4 \times [3.0]^2 = 36$ mm Hg.

28. ANSWER: E. Small trabecular muscular VSDs have a very high likelihood of spontaneous closure, typically 80%–90%. The majority will close within the first few years of life but spontaneous closure with these muscular defects can occur later in childhood and even in adulthood.

KEY POINTS:

▪ Muscular VSDs can be characterized as restrictive if the Doppler velocity through the defect is elevated consistent with a large pressure gradient and small-sized hole.

▪ Most (80%–90%) of muscular VSDs close spontaneously by late childhood.

29. ANSWER: B. The clinical examination in this patient suggests a large ASD. The apical four-chamber image in Figure 27-12 demonstrates an enlarged right atrium and right ventricle consistent with a significant left-to-right atrial shunt. While not the optimal echocardiographic view to evaluate the entire atrial septum (this scan plane is more parallel than perpendicular to the atrial septum), it does appear that there is a large dropout in the atrial septum consistent with a secundum

ASD (*). The primum septum is intact inferiorly and is confirmed by noting that the atrioventricular valves are inserted at different levels at the cardiac crux (atrioventricular septum is present). This apical view is not optimal to demonstrate a sinus venosus ASD. Lack of dilatation of the coronary sinus does not exclude a coronary sinus ASD but makes it much less likely. No atrial septal aneurysm is demonstrated in this image.

30. ANSWER: A. The direction of atrial level shunting is primarily related to the compliance of the ventricles. The right ventricle is typically more compliant than the left ventricle with characteristic left-to-right shunting being most common. These other factors also contribute to the degree and direction of atrial level shunting but ventricular compliance is most important.

31. ANSWER: B. Interventional device closure is performed in secundum ASDs of appropriate size and with adequate tissue rims. Sinus venosus, primum, and coronary sinus defects are not amenable to device closure due to their proximity to other cardiac structures (most notably the atrioventricular valves and the systemic and pulmonary veins).

KEY POINTS:

■ A secundum ASD will have an intact cardiac crux with insertion of the atrioventricular valves at different levels.

■ The direction of atrial shunting is largely dependent on the relative compliance of the ventricles.

  Only the secundum-type ASD is amenable to interventional device closure.

32. ANSWER: A. The images presented in Figure 27-13 are consistent with coarctation of the aorta. The suprasternal long-axis views demonstrate a juxtaductal coarctation of the aorta in the proximal descending aorta. Aliased color flow is demonstrated at the area of discrete narrowing. The parasternal long-axis images do not demonstrate any evidence of subaortic, valvar, or supravalvar aortic stenosis. A midmuscular VSD, however, is seen in this video. The pulsed-wave Doppler image from the descending aorta demonstrates diastolic runoff consistent with significant proximal obstruction (i.e., coarctation).

33. ANSWER: C. In patients with coarctation of the aorta, the brachiocephic vessels proximal to the coarctation typically have normal or increased systemic blood pressure while those vessels distal to the obstruction have decreased blood pressure. In a patient with a typical juxtaductal coarctation, the blood pressure in the arms is significantly higher than blood pressures recorded in the lower extremities. The blood pressures

in the patient listed in this question are decreased in the right and left legs (as one would expect in coarctation) but the right arm also has decreased pressure. This is most likely due to an aberrant right subclavian artery that originates distal to the coarctation from the descending aorta.

34. ANSWER: B. The most common site of coarctation of the aorta in infants and children is juxtaductal—the narrowing is opposite the insertion site of the ductus arteriosus. This is accompanied by a posterior infolding ("ledge") of thickened aortic wall media tissue. The left subclavian artery is most often not involved in the narrowing but can be in some cases. The typical neonatal presentation of severe coarctation is cardiovascular collapse when the patent ductus closes. Systemic hypertension and LV hypertrophy often present later in childhood with coarctation. Coarctation is often associated with other congenital heart lesions including bicuspid aortic valves, VSDs, and additional left heart obstructive lesions.

35. ANSWER: B. With the initiation of prostaglandin E, the ductus arteriosus has reopened allowing pulsatile flow to the descending aorta (from the pulmonary artery). In the presence of a large patent ductus arteriosus, the classic findings of "coarctation" in the abdominal aortic Doppler tracings will be absent because pulsatile flow can bypass the juxtaductal area of obstruction.

KEY POINTS:

■ The most common site of coarctation of the aorta is in the juxtaductal region.

■ Other associated congenital heart lesions with coarctation of the aorta include bicuspid aortic valves, VSDs, and additional left heart obstructive lesions.

■ The presence of a large PDA will eliminate the classic findings on the abdominal aortic Doppler tracing of coarctation of the aorta.

36. ANSWER: C. The apical four-chamber images in Videos 27-2A–C demonstrate a large primum ASD. Note that the atrioventricular valves are inserted at the same level at the cardiac crux consistent with the absence of the atrioventricular septum resulting in a large ASD. While there appears to be a small inlet VSD, there is no ventricular level shunt demonstrated by color Doppler. This potential area of shunting has been obliterated by atrioventricular valve leaflet and chordal tissue.

37. ANSWER: C. This parasternal short-axis image demonstrates a cleft in the anterior leaflet of the mitral valve. This defect is characteristic in patients with primum ASDs. Other mitral valve anomalies, such as a double-orifice mitral valve or mitral arcade, can occur in the setting of a primum ASD but are rare.

38. *ANSWER: A.* The apical four-chamber view demonstrates a large primum ASD and a large inlet VSD. The subcostal view nicely demonstrates the common atrioventricular valve in this complete AVSD.

KEY POINTS:

▨ A typical characteristic of a primum ASD is the insertion of the atrioventricular valves at the same level consistent with the absence of the atrioventricular septum.

▨ Primum ASD is associated with mitral valve anomalies, most notably a mitral valve cleft.

39. *ANSWER: C.* This patient has a physical examination and family history suggestive of Noonan syndrome. This autosomal dominant syndrome has phenotypic features including short stature, webbed neck, pectus excavatum, and triangular facies. Cardiovascular abnormalities are common in this syndrome and include pulmonary valve stenosis, hypertrophic cardiomyopathy, and ASDs. The patient's family history is suggestive of hypertrophic cardiomyopathy. The patient's physical exam is consistent with pulmonary valve stenosis.

Common echocardiographic features of pulmonary valve stenosis are included in Videos 27-3A–E. The subcostal (A & B) and parasternal short-axis scans (C & D) demonstrate thickening and restricted mobility of the pulmonary valve with color Doppler aliasing at the valve level consistent with stenosis. The apical four-chamber scan (E) demonstrates the marked hypertrophy in this child with severe valvar pulmonary stenosis.

40. *ANSWER: A.* The cardiovascular anomaly characteristic of Noonan syndrome is valvar pulmonary stenosis. Other cardiac abnormalites common in this syndrome include hypertrophic cardiomyopathy and ASDs. Supravalvar stenosis is commonly found in patients with Williams syndrome. Coarctation of the aorta and valvar aortic stenosis are common in Turner syndrome. Dilated cardiomyopathies are common in the muscular dystrophies, such as Duchenne muscular dystrophy, and in other metabolic disorders.

41. *ANSWER: B.* This patient's preprocedure (Videos 27-3F and G) and postprocedure angiograms (H & I) are included. The postangiography cines demonstrate significant dynamic RVOT obstruction after the relief of valvar pulmonary stenosis. The patient's physical examination is consistent with dynamic RVOT obstruction as well, demonstrating a loud late-peaking systolic murmur as well as the murmur of pulmonary regurgitation after the balloon dilatation of the pulmonary valve. Treatment with beta-blockade and eventual regression of RV hypertrophy often will significantly decrease the degree of dynamic obstruction in these patients with successful relief of pulmonary valve obstruction.

KEY POINTS:

▨ Clinical features of Noonan's syndrome include short stature, webbed neck, pectus excavatum, and triangular facies.

▨ Cardiovascular features of Noonan's syndrome include pulmonary valve stenosis, hypertrophic cardiomyopathy, and ASDs.

SUGGESTED READINGS

Atrial Septal Defects

Cetta F, Seward JB, O'Leary PW. Echocardiography in congenital heart disease: an overview. In: Oh J, Seward J, Tajik A, eds. *The Echo Manual*. 3rd ed. Philadelphia: Lippincott Williams & Wilkens, 2006:334–339.

Ettedgui J, Siewers R, Anderson R, et al. Diagnostic echocardiographic features of the sinus venosus defect. *Br Heart J*. 1990; 64:329–331.

McMahon C, Feltes T, Fraley J, et al. Natural history of growth of secundum atrial septal defects and implications for transcatheter closure. *Heart*. 2002;87:256–259.

Murphy J, Gersh B, McGoon M, et al. Long-term outcome after surgical repair of isolated atrial septal defect. Follow up at 27 to 32 years. *N Engl J Med*. 1990;13:1645–1660.

Van Praagh S, Carrera M, Sanders S. Sinus venosus defects: unroofing of the right pulmonary veins, anatomic and echocardiographic findings and surgical treatment. *Am Heart J*. 1994; 128:365–379.

Ventricular Septal Defects

Allan L. Abnormalities of the ventricular septum. In: Allan L, Hornberger LK, Sharland G, eds. *Textbook of Fetal Cardiology*. London: Greenwich Medical Media, 2000:195–209.

Corone P, Doyon F, Gaudeau S, et al. Natural history of ventricular septal defect. A study involving 790 cases. *Circulation*. 1977; 55:908–915.

Eroglu AG, Oztunc F, Saltik L, et al. Evolution of ventricular septal defect with septal reference to spontaneous closure rate, subaortic ridge and aortic valve prolapse. *Pediatr Cardiol*. 2003; 24:31–35.

Ge Z, Zhang Y, Kang W, et al. Noninvasive evaluation of interventricular pressure gradient across ventricular septal defect: a simultaneous study of Doppler echocardiography and cardiac catheterization. *Am Heart J*. 1992;124:176–182.

Hagler DJ, Edwards WD, Seward JB, et al. Standardized nomenclature of the ventricular septum and ventricular septal defects, with applications for two-dimensional echocardiography. *Mayo Clinic Proc*. 1985;60:741–752.

Hijazi Z. Device closure of ventricular septal defects. *Catheter Cardiovasc Interv.* 2003;60:107–114.

Marx GR, Allen HD, Goldberg SJ. Doppler echocardiographic estimation of systolic pulmonary artery pressure in pediatric patients with interventricular communications. *J Am Coll Cardiol.* 1985;6:1132–1137.

McDaniel NL, Gutgesell HP. Ventricular septal defects. In: Allen HD, Gutgesell HP, Clark EB, Driscoll DJ, eds. *Moss and Adams' Heart Disease in Infants, Children and Adolescents.* 6th ed. Philadelphia: Lippincott William & Wilkins, 2001:636–651.

Murphy DJ Jr, Ludomirsky A, Huhta JC. Continuous-wave Doppler in children with ventricular septal defect: noninvasive estimation of interventricular pressure gradient. *Am J Cardiol.* 1986;57: 428–432.

Mori K, Matsuoka S, Tartara K, et al. Echocardiography evaluation of the development of aortic valve prolapse in supracristal ventricular septal defect. *Eur J Pediatr.* 1995;154:176–181.

Ooshima A, Fukushige J, Ueda K. Incidence of structural cardiac disorders in neonates: an evaluation by color Doppler echocardiography and the results of a 1-year follow-up. *Cardiology.* 1995;86: 402–406

Soto B, Becker AE, Moulaert AJ, et al. Classification of ventricular septal defects. *Br Heart J.* 1980;43:332–343.

Snider AR, Serwer GA, Ritter SB. Defects in cardiac septation. In: *Echocardiography in Pediatric Heart Disease.* 2nd ed. St. Louis: Mosby, 1997:246–277.

van den Bosch AE, Ten Harkel DJ, McGhie JS, et al. Feasibility and accuracy of real-time 3-dimensional echocardiographic assessment of ventricular septal defects. *J Am Soc Echocardiogr.* 2006; 19:7–13.

Patent Ductus Arteriosus

Allen HD, Goldberg SJ, Valdes-Cruz LM, et al. Use of echocardiography in newborns with patent ductus arteriosus: a review. *Pediatr Cardiol.* 1982;3:65–70.

Huhta JC, Cohen M, Gutgesell HP. Patency of the ductus arteriosus in normal neonates: two-dimensional echocardiography versus Doppler assessment. *J Am Coll Cardiol.* 1984;4:561–564.

Hiraishi S, Horiguchi Y, Misawa H, et al. Noninvasive Doppler echocardiographic evaluation of shunt flow dynamics of the ductus arteriosus. *Circulation.* 1987;75:1146–1153.

Musewe NN, Poppe D, Smallhorn JF, et al. Doppler echocardiographic measurement of pulmonary artery pressure from ductal Doppler velocities in the newborn. *J Am Coll Cardiol.* 1990;15: 446–456.

Sahn DJ, Allen HD. Real-time cross-sectional echocardiographic imaging and measurement of the patent ductus arteriosus in infants and children. *Circulation.* 1978;58:343–354.

Silverman NH, Lewis AB, Heymann MA, et al. Echocardiographic assessment of the ductus arteriosus shunt in premature infants. *Circulation.* 1974;50:821–825.

Swensson RE, Valdes-Cruz LM, Sahn DJ, et al. Real-time Doppler color flow mapping for detection of patent ductus arteriosus. *J Am Coll Cardiol.* 1986;8:1105–1112.

Atrioventricular Septal Defect

Anderson RH, Webb S, Brown NA, et al. Development of the heart: (2) septation of the atriums and ventricles. *Heart.* 2003;89: 949–958.

Cetta F, Minich LL, Edwards WD, et al. Atrioventricular septal defects. In: Allen HD, Driscoll DJ, Shaddy RE, Feltes TF, eds. *Moss and Adams: Heart Disease in Infants, Children, and Adolescents (Including the Fetus and Young Adult).* Philadelphia: Lippincott Williams and Wilkins, 2008:646–667.

Cohen MS, Jacobs ML, Weinberg PM, et al. Morphometric analysis of unbalanced common atrioventricular canal using two-dimensional echocardiography. *J Am Coll Cardiol.* 1996;28: 1017–1023.

Fesslova V, Villa L, Nava S, et al. Spectrum and outcome of atrioventricular septal defect in fetal life. *Cardiol Young.* 2002;12: 18–26.

Geva T, Ayres NA, Pignatelli RH, et al. Echocardiographic evaluation of common atrioventricular canal defects: a study of 206 consecutive patients. *Echocardiography.* 1996;13:387–400.

Snider AR, Serwer GA, Ritter SB. Defects in cardiac septation. In: *Echocardiography in Pediatric Heart Disease.* St. Louis: Mosby-Year Book, 1997:235–296.

Smallhorn JF, de Leval M, Stark J, et al. Isolated anterior mitral cleft. Two dimensional echocardiographic assessment and differentiation from "clefts" associated with atrioventricular septal defect. *Br Heart J.* 1982;48:109–116.

van Son JA, Phoon CK, Silverman NH, et al. Predicting feasibility of biventricular repair of right-dominant unbalanced atrioventricular canal. *Ann Thorac Surg.* 1997;63:1657–1663.

Coarctation of Aorta

Huhta JC, Gutgesell HP, Latson LA, et al. Two-dimensional echocardiographic assessment of the aorta in infants and children with congential heart disease. *Circulation.* 1984;70: 417–424.

Marx, GR, Allen HD. Accuracy and pitfalls for Doppler evaluation of the pressure gradient in aortic coarctation. *J Am Coll Cardiol.* 1986;7:1379–1385.

Morriss MJ, McNamara DG. Coarctation of the aorta and interrupted aortic arch. In: Garson A Jr, Bricker JT, Fisher DJ, Neish SR, eds. *The Science and Practice of Pediatric Cardiology.* 2nd ed. Baltimore: Lippincott Williams & Wilkins, 1998;1317–1346.

Shaddy RE, Snider AR, Silverman NH, et al. Pulsed Doppler findings in patients with coarctation of the aorta. *Circulation.* 1986;73:82–88.

Smallhorn JT, Huhta JC, Adams PA, et al. Cross-sectional echocardiographic assessment of coarctation in the sick neonate and infant. *Br Heart J.* 1983;50:349–361.

Snider AR, Silverman NH. Suprasternal notch echocardiography: a two-dimensional technique for evaluating congenital heart disease. *Circulation.* 1981;63:165–173.

Tawes, RL Jr, Aberdeen E, Waterston DJ, et al. Coarctation of the aorta in infants and children. A review of 333 operative cases, including 179 infants. *Circulation.* 1969;39:1173–1184.

Pulmonary Valve Stenosis

Burch M, Sharland M, Shinebourne E, et al. Cardiologic abnormalities in Noonan syndrome: phenotypic diagnosis and echocardiographic assessment of 118 patients. *J Am Coll Cardiol.* 1993;22: 1189–1192.

Lima OC, Sahn DJ, Valdes-Cruz LM, et al. Noninvasive prediction of transvalvular pressure gradient in patients with pulmonary stenosis by quantitative two-dimensional echocardiographic Doppler studies. *Circulation.* 1983;67:866–871.

Trowitzsch E, Colan SD, Sanders SP. Two-dimensional echocardiographic evaluation of right ventricular size and function in newborns with severe right ventricular outflow tract obstruction. *J Am Coll Cardiol.* 1985;6:388–393.

Weyman AE, Hurwitz RA, Girod DA, et al. Cross-sectional echocardiographic visualization of the stenotic pulmonary valve. *Circulation.* 1977;56:769–774.

Aortic Valve Stenosis & LVOT Obstruction

Bezold LI, Smith EO, Kelly K, et al. Development and validation of an echocardiographic model for predicting progression of discrete subaortic stenosis in children. *Am J Cardiol.* 1998;81: 314–320.

Bonow RO, Carabello BA, Chatterjee K, et al. ACC/AHA 2006 Guidelines for the Management of Patients with Valvular Heart Disease: A Report of the American College of Cardiology/American Heart Association Task Force on Practice Guidelines (Writing Committee to Revise the 1998 Guidelines for the Management of Patients with Valvular Heart Disease). *J Am Coll Cardiol.* 2006; 48:e1–148.

Colan SD, McElhinney DB, Crawford EC, et al. Validation and re-evaluation of a discriminant model predicting anatomic suitability for biventricular repair in neonates with aortic stenosis. *J Am Coll Cardiol.* 2006;47:1858–1865.

Fernandes SM, Sanders SP, Khairy P, et al. Morphology of bicuspid aortic valve in children and adolescents. *J Am Coll Cardiol.* 2004;44:1648–1651.

Geva A, McMahon CJ, Gauvreau K, et al. Risk factors for reoperation after repair of discrete subaortic stenosis in children. *J Am Coll Cardiol.* 2007;50:1498–1504.

Lofland GK, McCrindle BW, Williams WG, et al. Critical aortic stenosis in the neonate: a multi-institutional study of management, outcomes, and risk factors. *J Thorac Cardiovasc Surg.* 2001; 121:10–27.

Mäkikallio K, McElhinney DB, Levine JC, et al. Fetal aortic valve stenosis and the evolution of hypoplastic left heart syndrome: patient selection for fetal intervention. *Circulation.* 2006; 113:1401–1405.

Rhodes LA, Colan SD, Perry SB, et al. Predictors of survival in neonates with critical aortic stenosis. *Circulation.* 1991;84: 2325–2335.

Vlahos AP, Marx GR, McElhinney DB, et al. Clinical utility of Doppler echocardiography in assessing aortic stenosis severity and predicting need for intervention in children. *Pediatr Cardiol.* 2008;29:507–514.

Zoghbi WA, Enriquez-Sarano M, Foster E, et al. Recommendations for evaluation of the severity of native valvular regurgitation with two-dimensional and Doppler echocardiography: a report from the American Society of Echocardiography's Nomenclature and Standards Committee and the Task Force on Valvular Regurgitation. *J Am Soc Echocardiogr.* 2003;16: 777–802.

CHAPTER 28

Tumors/Masses

Shepard D. Weiner and Shunichi Homma

1. A structure found in the left atrium that can be misinterpreted as a pathologic mass is:
   A. Eustachian valve.
   B. Crista terminalis.
   C. Moderator band.
   D. Chiari network.
   E. Suture line following transplant.

2. The following is a Class IIb indication for performing echocardiography in patients with cardiac masses or tumors:
   A. Evaluation of patients with clinical syndromes and events suggesting an underlying cardiac mass.
   B. Follow-up or surveillance studies after surgical removal of masses known to have a high likelihood of recurrence.
   C. Screening persons with disease states likely to result in mass formation but for whom no clinical evidence for the mass exists.
   D. Evaluation of patients with underlying cardiac disease known to predispose to mass formation for whom a therapeutic decision regarding surgery or anticoagulation will depend on the results of echocardiography.
   E. Patients with known primary malignancies when echocardiographic surveillance for cardiac involvement is part of the disease staging process.

3. This tumor is a benign cardiac tumor:
   A. Angiosarcoma.
   B. Rhabdomyoma.
   C. Lymphoma.
   D. Mesothelioma.
   E. Prominent ventricular trabeculations.

4. It is uncommon for this tumor to metastasize to the heart:
   A. Renal cell carcinoma.
   B. Breast.
   C. Thyroid.
   D. Lung.
   E. Melanoma.

5. The most common mechanism by which cardiac papillary fibroelastomas cause symptoms is:
   A. Direct invasion of the myocardium, resulting in impaired contractility or arrhythmias.
   B. Embolization.
   C. Obstruction of blood across heart valves.
   D. Pericardial effusion leading to cardiac tamponade.

6. Lipomatous hypertrophy of the atrial septum:
   A. Does not commonly cause symptoms.
   B. Is caused by fibrosis.
   C. Has the same histologic pattern as lipomas.
   D. Can be seen on transthoracic echocardiography and is an indication for the performance of transesophogeal echocardiography.

7. Which statement appropriately describes fibromas?
   A. Fibromas are typically small tumors.
   B. Fibromas are benign connective tissue tumors derived from fibroblasts that occur predominantly in children.
   C. Fibromas are typically found in one of the atria.

D. Fibromas are usually asymptomatic.

E. No treatment is recommended for asymtomatic patients with cardiac fibromas.

8. Which mass is the most common benign cardiac tumor in infants and children?
   A. Atrial myxoma.
   B. Angiosarcoma.
   C. Teratoma.
   D. Hemangioma.
   E. Rhabdomyoma.

9. The clinical manifestations of the Carney complex include:
   A. Papillary fibroelastoma.
   B. Hemangioma.
   C. Epilepsy.
   D. Cardiac myxoma.
   E. Nevoid basal cell carcinoma.

10. The following are symptoms associated with cardiac myxoma:
    A. Palpitations and diarrhea.
    B. Syncope and diarrhea.
    C. Dyspnea and fever.
    D. Dyspnea and dysphagia.

11. Which of the following statements about tuberous sclerosis is true?
    A. Tuberous sclerosis is a syndrome characterized by hamartomas in several organs, epilepsy, cognitive impairment, and adenoma sebaceum.
    B. The genetic defect for tuberous sclerosis has not been identified.
    C. Only a minority of patients with cardiac rhabdomyomas have tuberous sclerosis.
    D. Surgical resection of the cardiac tumors is recommended in asymptomatic patients with tuberous sclerosis.

12. Papillary fibroelastomas:
    A. Cannot occur on the pulmonic valve.
    B. Are usually single rather than multiple.
    C. Exclusively occur on cardiac valves.
    D. Commonly result in valvular regurgitation.

13. The most common malignant tumor of the heart is:
    A. Angiosarcoma.
    B. Lymphoma.

C. Metastastic disease.

D. Leiomyosarcoma.

E. Myxoma.

14. A characteristic feature of a cardiac myxoma on two-dimensional echocardiography is:
    A. An associated pericardial effusion.
    B. A narrow stalk connected to the fossa ovalis.
    C. An intramural hyperechoic mass.
    D. A mobile mass with a short pedicle attached to a cardiac valve.

15. In patients with human immunodeficiency virus (HIV) infection and acquired immunodeficiency syndrome (AIDS), this tumor has been described to affect the heart:
    A. Lipoma.
    B. Kaposi sarcoma.
    C. Rhabdomyosarcoma.
    D. Angiosarcoma.
    E. Hemangioma.

16. A 36-year-old woman was diagnosed with leiomyosarcoma (Fig. 28-1 of a zoomed view of the left atrium on parasternal long axis). Which of the following statements about leiomyosarcoma is correct?

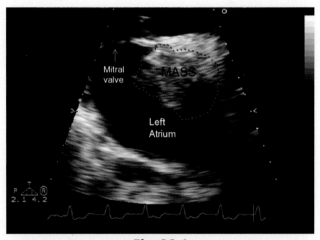

Fig. 28-1

A. Treatment of cardiac leiomyosarcomas consists solely of chemotherapy and radiation.
B. Leiomyosarcomas, like other malignant cardiac tumors, occur preferentially in the right heart.
C. Leiomyosarcomas typically present in their seventh decade.
D. Leiomyosarcomas are derived from smooth muscle cells.

17. A 40-year-old man with dyspnea is found to have a mass on transthoracic echocardiography (Fig. 28-2 of the right ventricular outflow tract in the pulmonic valve tilt view from parasternal long axis, and Video 28-1). Pathology at the time of surgery revealed an angiosarcoma. Which of the following accurately describes angiosarcomas?

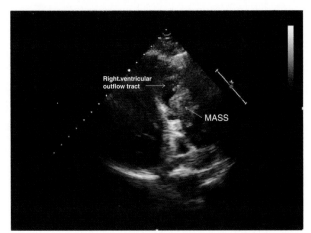

Fig. 28-2

A. Angiosarcomas usually are discovered late and typically have grown to be large or metastasized at the time of diagnosis.
B. Like other cardiac sarcomas, the gender distribution is equal (1:1).
C. Angiosarcomas most often occur in the left ventricle.
D. Patients usually present with tachyarrhythmias.

18. A 52-year-old woman presented with right flank pain and weight loss. Renal cell carcinoma was diagnosed. A transthoracic echocardiogram was performed (Fig. 28-3 of the parasternal long axis). Arrow points to a mass in the right ventricle. Which of the following statements about renal cell carcinoma is correct?

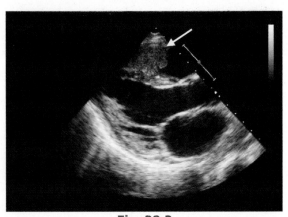

Fig. 28-3

A. Intravascular extension of the tumor is not a common manifestation of renal cell carcinoma.
B. Pulmonary embolization is not seen with metastatic renal cell carcinoma.
C. Metastatic renal cell carcinoma is rarely confused with thrombus on echocardiography.
D. The initial diagnosis of renal cell carcinoma can be made by detection of an intracardiac mass on echocardiography in some cases.

19. A 24-year-old man with synovial sarcoma had a transthoracic echocardiogram performed (Fig. 28-4 of the apical four-chamber view demonstrating a large pericardial effusion and mass abutting the lateral left atrial wall, and Video 28-2). Which of the following accurately characterizes synovial sarcomas?

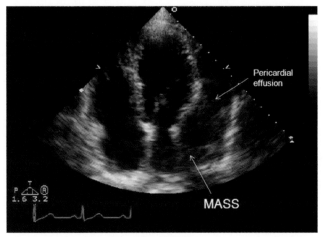

Fig. 28-4

A. Synovial sarcoma is caused by a translocation between chromosome 18 and the X chromosome.
B. Synovial sarcoma is not a malignant primary cardiac tumor.
C. Synovial sarcoma is a common type of cardiac tumor.
D. Synovial sarcoma has an excellent prognosis.

20. A 0.2 ml bolus of perflutren lipid microspheres was injected intravenously followed by a saline flush. A two-chamber view at 80 degrees on a transesophageal echocardiogram is show in Figure 28-5 and Video 28-3. Based on these images, which of the following conclusions is true about this patient's condition?

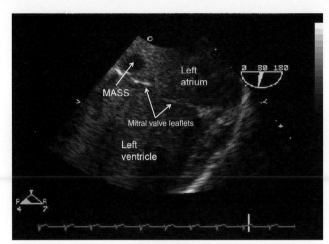

Fig. 28-5

A. The structure seen in the left atrium near the mitral annulus is likely to be an angiosarcoma.
B. The structure seen in the left atrium near the mitral annulus is likely to be a cystic structure.
C. The structure seen in the left atrium near the mitral annulus is likely to be a myxoma.
D. The structure seen in the left atrium near the mitral annulus is likely to be a papillary fibroelastoma.

21. An apical view from a transthoracic echocardiogram is shown in Figure 28-6 and Video 28-4. A prominent Chiari network is seen in the right atrium. Based on these images, which of the following statements is correct?

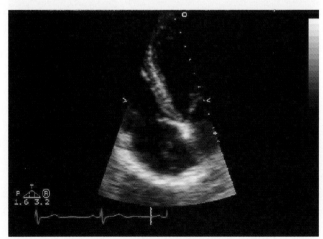

Fig. 28-6

A. A Chiari network is present in 20%–30% of normal hearts.
B. A Chiari network is associated with an increased risk of sudden cardiac death.
C. A Chiari network is a congenital remnant of the right valve of the sinus venosus.
D. A Chiari network is another name for crista terminalis.

22. A 62-year-old woman presented with worsening dyspnea on exertion and chest pain that began 4 months earlier. A transthoracic echocardiogram revealed a very large partially echodense fluid collection compressing the right atrium and right ventricle (Fig. 28-7 and Video 28-5). This structure was surgically removed and histology revealed a fibrovascular cyst with chronic inflammation consistent with a pericardial cyst. Which of the following statements about pericardial cysts is correct?

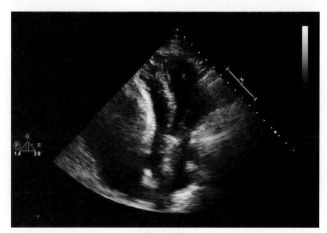

Fig. 28-7

A. The diagnosis of pericardial cyst can sometimes be suggested on chest radiograph by the identification of a rounded mass along the right heart border.
B. Pericardial cysts are the most common anterior mediastinal mass lesion.
C. Cysts are considered to be true neoplasms.
D. It is common for pericardial cysts to become large enough to cause compressive symptoms.

23. A 56-year-old man with persistent atrial fibrillation underwent a minimally invasive modified surgical Maze procedure with suture closure of the left atrial appendage. A transthoracic echocardiogram was performed 1 month later. Figure 28-8 and Video 28-6 show the left atrium at 30 degrees with a small mobile echodensity that appears to be attached to the left atrial wall. Color Doppler showed contiguous flow between the left atrium and left atrial appendage and the pulsed Doppler tracing was consistent with a left atrial appendage flow pattern (not shown). Which of the following statements is correct?

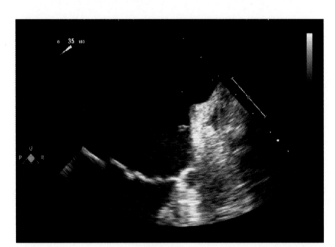

Fig. 28-8

A. The interpretation of masses found on echocardiography is not dependent on the clinical context in which it occurs.

B. There is a high occurrence of unsuccessful surgical left atrial appendage closure reported in the literature.

C. Transesophogeal echocardiography is not helpful in assessing the results of a surgical left atrial appendage closure procedure.

D. Residual communication between an incompletely closed left atrial appendage and the body of the left atrium is not a potential mechanism for thrombus formation and embolic events.

24. An 82-year-old man with a past history of an anterior wall ST segment elevation myocardial infarction had a transthoracic echocardiogram performed. A large left ventricular apical mass was seen (Fig. 28-9 of the apical four-chamber view) and the anterior wall and apex were akinetic. This mass most likely represents a:

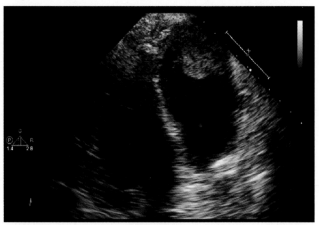

Fig. 28-9

A. Myxoma.
B. Rhabdomyosarcoma.
C. Thrombus.
D. Vegetation.

25. A 16-year-old boy was diagnosed with a single rhabdomyoma during his first year of life. He is asymptomatic. Figure 28-10, parasternal short axis, is from his most recent transthoracic echocardiogram. (See also Video 28-7.) Which of the following conclusions is true about this patient's condition?

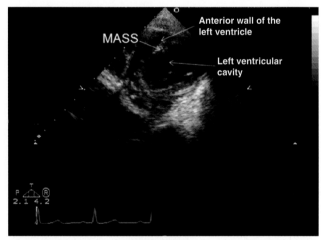

Fig. 28-10

A. The presence of a rhabdomyoma cannot be diagnosed before birth with fetal echocardiography.

B. The ventricular wall is a typical location for rhabdomyomas.

C. This patient should be referred to a cardiothoracic surgeon for removal of the rhabdomyoma.

D. This patient meets diagnostic criteria for tuberous sclerosis.

CASE 1:

A 55-year-old man with diabetes mellitus and hypertension is undergoing an evaluation for exertional dyspnea. An exercise echocardiogram is ordered. The baseline transthoracic echocardiogram is reported to reveal an intracardiac mass. The exercise portion of the exam is not completed and the patient is referred for a transesophogeal echocardiogram. Video 28-8 shows a zoomed-in view of the left atrium at zero degree. Figure 28-11 demonstrates the mass using real-time three-dimensional imaging.

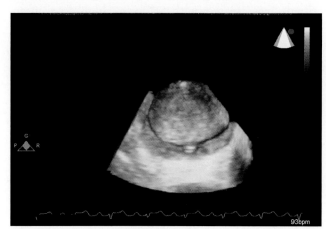

Fig. 28-11

26. Which of the following statements about Video 28-8 is correct?
   A. The size of the mass makes it most likely to be a metastatic tumor to the heart rather than a primary cardiac tumor.
   B. The left atrial location of this tumor and its attachment to the midportion of the atrial septum make it most likely a myxoma.
   C. This tumor may be found as part of a multisystem disease called tuberous sclerosis complex.
   D. This tumor type accounts for approximately 10% of all primary cardiac tumors.
   E. This tumor is characterized by infiltration of the atrial septum by lipomatous material.

27. Which statement accurately describes the tumor shown in the echocardiogram?
   A. It is typically recommended to surgically excise this tumor even if the patient is asymptomatic.
   B. This mass always prolapses through the mitral orifice in diastole.

C. This tumor most commonly presents in the elderly (greater than 65 years of age).
   D. A pericardial effusion is often associated with this tumor.
   E. This patient would be expected to have severely reduced left ventricular systolic function.

CASE 2:

A 66-year-old man presented with a transient ischemic attack. A transthoracic echocardiogram was performed. Video 28-9A shows the parasternal long-axis view. Video 28-9B shows the long-axis view at 129 degrees on the transesophageal echocardiogram. A diagnosis of papillary fibroelastoma is made.

28. Which of the following statements about papillary fibroelastomas is correct?
   A. Papillary fibroelastomas are usually easily distinguishable from vegetations.
   B. Papillary fibroelastomas are typically associated with significant valvular regurgitation.
   C. Papillary fibroelastomas usually attach to the upstream side of the valve.
   D. Papillary fibroelastomas account for the majority of valve-associated tumors.
   E. The major risk associated with papillary fibroelastomas is cardiac tamponade.

29. Which of the following statements about the treatment of papillary fibroelastomas is correct?
   A. After surgical resection, patients should be monitored closely with surveillance echocardiography performed every year since recurrence of papillary fibroelastomas is a common phenomenon.
   B. Tumor mobility does not impact the treatment decision for papillary fibroelastomas.
   C. Asymptomatic patients with immobile, small (<0.5 cm) papillary fibroelastomas should have surgical resection performed immediately.
   D. There is no role for anticoagulation in patients with symptomatic papillary fibroelastoma who are not surgical candidates.
   E. Symptomatic patients should be treated surgically because a successful and complete resection of papillary fibroelastomas is curative and the long-term postoperative prognosis is excellent.

30. Which statement accurately describes papillary fibroelastomas?
   A. Papillary fibroelastomas are the most common primary cardiac tumor in adults.
   B. The most commonly involved valve is the aortic valve, followed by the mitral valve.
   C. Papillary fibroelastomas are generally not visible by transthoracic echocardiography if they are less than 1 cm.
   D. The right ventricle is the predominant nonvalvular site involved.
   E. Multiple papillary fibroelastomas have been reported to be present in 50% of patients.

CASE 3:

A 71-year-old woman presented with fatigue and dyspnea in the setting of diarrhea and flushing for 5 months. Video 28-10A shows the tricuspid valve in the right ventricular inflow view. Video 28-10B is the same view with the addition of color flow imaging.

31. Which of the following statements about carcinoid heart disease is correct?
   A. Carcinoid affecting the tricuspid valve frequently results in tricuspid stenosis as the dominant lesion.
   B. Involvement of the left-sided valves usually occurs without a patent foramen ovale or high tumor activity.
   C. The valve pathology of carcinoid involves fibrosis, smooth muscle proliferation, and endocardial thickening which give the echocardiographic appearance of a thickened, retracted, and immobile valve.
   D. Treatment of carcinoid heart disease usually achieves cure with modern antitumor therapy and surgical intervention.
   E. Carcinoid heart disease typically causes severe symptoms shortly after the onset of the disease.

32. Which statement accurately describes carcinoid heart disease?
   A. Patients with carcinoid syndrome can have right-sided cardiac metastases without involvement of the liver.
   B. If valve replacement surgery is indicated and feasible, a mechanical prosthetic valve is always the preferred choice.
   C. On echocardiographic evaluation, right ventricular size in patients with carcinoid heart disease is usually normal.

D. Octreotride can be safely discontinued during the perioperative period.
   E. If there is pulmonic valve involvement, a continuous-wave Doppler signal through the pulmonary valve is an important part of the echocardiographic evaluation.

CASE 4:

A 30-year-old woman was diagnosed with malignant melanoma and underwent complete surgical excision with adequate margins. Given the depth of the melanoma, it was considered high risk and the patient was treated with adjuvant high-dose interferon. Two months later, the patient developed shortness of breath. Video 28-11A shows a right ventricular inflow view and Video 28-11B shows the apical view of the mass seen on transthoracic echocardiogram.

33. Which of the following is true about metastatic melanoma?
   A. It is uncommon for melanoma to metastasize to the heart.
   B. There is no role for surgery in patients with metastatic melanoma to palliate symptoms or prevent death from cardiac complications.
   C. The history of primary melanoma can be remote, occurring years prior to the discovery of the cardiac mass in some cases.
   D. Melanoma has a high propensity for metastasizing to the myocardium but not the pericardium.

34. Which statement accurately describes metastatic melanoma?
   A. "Charcoal" heart is the most common cardiac extension of melanoma.
   B. Melanoma accounts for the majority of metastatic cardiac tumors.
   C. The development of dyspnea in a patient with a history of melanoma is not a concerning symptom.
   D. The incidence of metastatic tumors to the heart has decreased during the last two decades.

CASE 5:

A 78-year-old woman was found to have a large intracardiac mass and pericardial effusion. Video 28-12A shows the apical four-chamber view. Pericardial fluid analysis and flow cytometry revealed diffuse large B-cell lymphoma. Chemotherapy was initiated promptly and a transthoracic echocardiogram was repeated two weeks later (Video 28-12B shows the apical four-chamber view).

35. Which of the following statements accurately characterizes primary cardiac lymphoma?
  A. It is rare to see a large pericardial effusion with primary cardiac lymphoma.
  B. Primay cardiac lymphoma is a common form of non-Hodgkin's lymphoma.
  C. Patients with primary cardiac lymphoma only present with cardiac tamponade.
  D. The histology of primary cardiac lymphoma in immunocompetent patients is diffuse large B-cell lymphoma in the majority of cases.

36. Which of the following statements about primary cardiac lymphoma is correct?
  A. Precordial chest pain is a symptom that can be seen with primary cardiac lymphoma.
  B. Establishing the diagnosis of primary cardiac lymphoma can be done definitively with non-invasive imaging.
  C. Without treatment, the median survival of patients with primary cardiac lymphoma is typically about 1 year.
  D. The median age of presentation is less than 40 years of age.

ANSWERS

1. ANSWER: E. There are many normal variants and benign conditions that can be misinterpreted on two-dimensional echocardiography as pathologic entities. A suture line following transplant is an example of a structure found in the left atrium that can be misinterpreted as a mass. The Eustachian valve, crista terminalis, and Chiari network are all normal structures found in the right atrium. The moderator band is a normal structure present in the right ventricle.

2. ANSWER: C. Screening persons with disease states likely to result in mass formation but for whom no clinical evidence for the mass exists is a Class IIb indication for performing echocardiography. Class I indications for echocardiography include evaluating patients with clinical syndromes suggesting an underlying cardiac mass, follow-up studies after surgical removal of masses known to recur, evaluating patients where treatment plans depend on the results of echocardiography, and assessing patients with known primary malignancies where surveillance for cardiac involvement is part of the disease staging process.

3. ANSWER: B. Rhabdomyoma is a benign cardiac tumor. Rhabdomyomas are usually small and lobulated, with diameters in the range of 2 mm to 2 cm. Rhabdomyomas are most often multiple and are strongly associated with tuberous sclerosis. Angiosarcoma, lymphoma, and mesothelioma are all malignant cardiac tumors. Prominent ventricular trabeculations can also be seen on echocardiography and represent either a normal variant, or, if severe enough, may indicate noncompaction.

4. ANSWER: C. It is uncommon for thyroid cancer to metastasize to the heart. Renal cell carcinoma, breast cancer, lung cancer, and melanoma all are known to metastasize to the heart. Table 28-1 lists the primary cancers that metastasize to the heart. Renal cell carcinoma spreads hematogenously to the inferior vena cava and right side of the heart. Breast cancer spreads to the heart by either hematogenous or lymphatic means. Lung cancer usually metastasizes to the heart via direct extension. Lymphoma spreads through the lymphatic system. Metastatic melanoma can result in intracavitary or myocardial involvement. Carcinoid typically results in tricuspid and pulmonic valve thickening.

TABLE 28-1 Tumors that Metastasize to the Heart

Primary Cancer	Route of Spread and/or Cardiac Manifestation
Renal cell carcinoma	Inferior vena cava to right side of the heart
Breast	Hematogenous or lymphatic spread; pericardial effusion common
Lung	Direct extension; pericardial effusion common
Melanoma	Intracavitary or myocardial involvement
Lymphoma	Lymphatic spread
Carcinoid	Tricuspid and pulmonic valve thickening

(Adapted from Armstrong WF, Ryan T, eds. *Feigenbaum's Echocardiography.* 7th ed. Philadelphia: Lippincott Williams & Wilkins, 2010.)

5. ANSWER: B. The most common mechanism by which papillary fibroelastomas cause symptoms is embolization. Other cardiac tumors may cause symptoms through several mechanisms, including direct invasion of the myocardium leading to impaired contractility or arrhythmias, obstruction, and pericardial effusions resulting in cardiac tamponade.

6. ANSWER: A. Lipomatous hypertrophy of the atrial septum does not commonly cause symptoms. This condition is thought to be benign although there is a reported association with atrial arrhythmias and superior vena cava obstruction if there is massive lipomatous hypertrophy. The atrial septum is infiltrated by lipomatous material that results in thickening of the inferior and superior portions. The fossa ovalis is spared and results in a "dumbbell-shaped" appearance on two-dimensional echocardiography. Lipomatous hypertrophy of the atrial septum is usually distinguishable by the highly refractile echogenic quality of fat. Although no absolute diagnostic criteria have been established, a septal thickness of 20 mm is often quoted. Lipomatous hypertrophy of the atrial septum represents a hamartoma. Pathologically, in contrast to true lipomas, lipomatous hypertrophy consists of a nonencapsulated accumulation of mature and fetal adipose tissue and atypical cardiac myocytes within the interatrial septum. The term hypertrophy is a misnomer since the condition is due to an increased number rather than an increased size of adipocytes. This condition can be seen on transthoracic echocardiography and its presence alone is not an indication for transesophogeal echocardiography.

7. ANSWER: B. Fibromas are benign connective tissue tumors derived from fibroblasts that occur predominantly in children. Fibromas are the second most common type of primary cardiac tumors occurring in the pediatric population. Most are detected in children younger than 10 years, and about one-third are diagnosed in infants younger than 1 year. Cardiac fibromas are typically large tumors, ranging from 3 to 10 cm in diameter. Cardiac fibromas usually occur within the ventricular myocardium, most commonly in the anterior wall of the left ventricle or interventricular septum. About 70% of patients with fibromas are symptomatic. Symptoms result from either obstruction, systolic dysfunction, or conduction abnormalities. The most common clinical manifestations are congestive heart failure and ventricular tachyarrhythmias. Given the risk of fatal arrhythmias, resection is usually recommended in asymptomatic patients. Sudden death has been reported to occur in approximately 15% of patients, typically in infants.

8. ANSWER: E. Rhabdomyomas are the most common benign cardiac tumor in infants and children, accounting for approximately half of the cardiac tumors in these age groups.

9. ANSWER: D. The diagnostic criteria for the Carney complex include having two of 12 recognized clinical manifestations or one clinical manifestation plus one of the two genetic criteria (see Table 28-2). Cardiac myxoma is a diagnostic clinical criterion for the Carney complex. The other clinical manifestations relate to either pigmented skin lesions or endocrine neoplasia. Familial myxomas, such as those seen in the Carney complex, account for a small percentage of all myxomas. Patients with familial myxomas tend to present earlier, are more likely to have myxomas in atypical locations, may have multiple myxomas, and are more likely to develop recurrent tumors. Epilepsy is associated with tuberous

sclerosis. Nevoid basal cell carcinoma is associated with cardiac fibroma in the Gorlin syndrome.

TABLE 28-2 Carney Complex Diagnostic Criteria

Clinical Criteria

1. Spotty skin pigmentation involving lips, conjunctiva, and genital mucosa
2. Myxoma (cutaneous and mucosal)
3. Cardiac myxoma
4. Breast myxomatosis
5. Primary pigmented nodular adrenocortical disease
6. Acromegaly
7. Sertoli cell tumor (or characteristic calcification on testicular ultrasound)
8. Thyroid carcinoma
9. Psammomatous melanotic schwannoma
10. Multiple epithelioid blue nevi
11. Multiple breast ductal adenoma
12. Osteochondromyxoma

Genetic Criteria

1. Affected first-degree relative
2. Inactivating mutation of PRKAR1 alpha gene

(Adapted from Stratakis CA, Kirschner LS, Carney JA. Clinical and molecular features of the Carney complex: diagnostic criteria and recommendations for patient evaluation. *J Clin Endocrinol Metab.* 2001;86:4041–4046.)

---

10. ANSWER: C. Myxomas present with symptoms resulting from intracardiac obstruction, systemic embolization, or constitutional symptoms. Dyspnea is the most common symptom. Syncope and palpitations are also seen. Constitutional symptoms, such as fever and weight loss, are also seen in approximately 15%–20% of patients. The association of constitutional symptoms with cardiac myxoma is likely due to the tumor's synthesis and secretion of interleukin (IL)-6. IL-6 is a proinflammatory cytokine that induces the acute phase response. Increased levels of IL-6 have been found in myxoma tissue and the constitutional symptoms resolve after removal of the myxoma. Diarrhea is seen in the carcinoid syndrome.

11. ANSWER: A. Histologic evidence suggests that cardiac rhabdomyomas are actually myocardial hamartomas or malformations that are composed of myocytes rather than true neoplasms. The microscopic hallmark is a large (<80 micrometer diameter) cell containing a central cytoplasmic mass that is suspended by myofibrillar processes, termed the Spider cell. Tuberous sclerosis is an autosomal-dominant hamartoma syndrome whose causative genes (TSC-1 and TSC-2) are tumor suppressor genes that encode a protein complex that regulates cell size. At least 80% of patients with cardiac rhabdomyomas have tuberous sclerosis. Fifty percent or more of cardiac rhabdomyomas regress spontaneously after infancy. Therefore, in the absence of symptoms, surgery is not indicated.

12. ANSWER: B. More than 90% of the time papillary fibroelastomas are single. Papillary fibroelastomas can occur on any valve. The aortic and mitral valve are most commonly involved in adults. Despite their valvular attachment, valve dysfunction is rare. Much less commonly, papillary fibroelastomas can occur on papillary muscle, chordae tendineae, or in the atria. The median diameter of papillary fibroelastomas is 8 mm and the largest reported is 40 mm. A short pedicle is seen approximately 50% of the time, and is more typical in tumors arising from the endocardium of a cardiac chamber.

13. ANSWER: C. Primary malignant tumors of the heart are much less common than metastatic tumors to the heart. In autopsy series, the incidence of primary tumors of the heart was only 0.02 percent. The relative incidence of primary tumors of the heart (both benign and malignant) is shown in Table 28-3.

TABLE 28-3 Relative Incidence of Primary Cardiac Tumors

Type of Tumor	Number	Percent
BENIGN	319	59.8%
Myxoma	130	24.4%
Lipoma	45	8.4%
Papillary fibroelastoma	42	7.9%
Rhabdomyoma	36	6.8%
Fibroma	17	3.2%
Hemangioma	15	2.8%
Teratoma	14	2.6%
Mesothelioma of AV node	12	2.3%
Other	5	1.0%
MALIGNANT	125	23.5%
Angiosarcoma	39	7.3%
Rhabdomyosarcoma	26	4.9%
Mesothelioma	19	3.6%
Fibrosarcoma	7	1.3%
Leiomyosarcoma	1	–
Synovial Sarcoma	1	–
Other	18	3.4%
CYSTS		
Pericardial cyst	82	15.4%
Bronchogenic cyst	7	1.3%

(Adapted from McAllister HA Jr, Fenoglio JJ Jr. *Tumors of the Cardiovascular System*. Washington: Armed Forces Institute of Pathology, 1978.)

14. ANSWER: B. Cardiac myxomas typically have a narrow stalk connected to the fossa ovalis. Approximately 75% of cardiac myxomas occur in the left atrium, where the site of attachment is almost always in the region of the fossa ovalis of the interatrial septum. Cardiac myxomas may occasionally be found on the posterior wall of the left atrium. However, this location within the left atrium should raise the suspicion for a malignant cardiac tumor. Approximately 15%–20% of cardiac myxomas occur in the right atrium, and less often they can be seen in the right or left ventricle. There are case reports of myxomas originating from the atrioventricular valves. Pericardial effusions are usually found in the setting of malignant cardiac tumors. Lipomas appear as an intramural hyperechoic mass. A mobile mass with a short pedicle attached to a cardiac valve is a papillary fibroelastoma.

15. ANSWER: B. Kaposi sarcoma, as well as malignant lymphoma, is recognized to occur in the setting of acquired immunodeficiency syndrome (AIDS). Cardiac involvement with Kaposi sarcoma usually occurs as part of a disseminated Kaposi sarcoma. The incidence of Kaposi sarcoma involving the heart has been estimated to be 12%–28% by autopsy studies.

16. ANSWER: D. Leiomyosarcomas are derived from smooth muscle cells and may originate from the smooth muscle cells lining the pulmonary veins. Although chemotherapy and radiation are part of the treatment plan, they are adjuncts to radical surgical resection. However, cardiac leiomyosarcomas have a poor prognosis, with a mean survival after surgery of less than 7 months. The majority of malignant tumors occur preferentially in the right side of the heart, with the exception of leiomyosarcoma, which often occurs in the left atrium. The preferential left atrial location and the frequently myxoid appearance of leiomyosarcomas makes them difficult to differentiate preoperatively from atrial myxomas. Unlike myxomas, leiomyosarcomas may originate from the posterior wall of the left atrium and involve the pulmonary veins. Patients with leiomyosarcoma typically present in their 30s, a decade younger than with other types of sarcomas.

17. ANSWER: A. Angiosarcomas usually are large or have metastasized at the time of diagnosis. Angiosarcomas often are not amenable to complete resection and have a very poor prognosis, even compared to the other cardiac sarcomas. Unlike other sarcomas, which have a 1:1, gender ratio, there appears to be a 3:1 male-to-female ratio among patients with angiosarcoma. Angiosarcomas have a strong predilection for the right heart, particularly the right atrium. They can be either intracavitary or diffuse and infiltrative. The common presentation is right-sided heart failure or cardiac tamponade as well as constitutional symptoms.

18. *ANSWER: D.* Some patients with renal cell carcinoma may present with symptoms related to cardiac metastases. The diagnosis of renal cell carcinoma may be first introduced by the echocardiogram. Intravascular extension of tumor is a common manifestation of renal cell carcinoma. Since vena caval and right heart involvement is known to occur with metastatic renal cell carcinoma, pulmonary embolism, either from tumor or thrombus, can be seen. The appearance of metastatic renal cell carcinoma itself can be confused with thrombus on echocardiography and sometimes cardiac magnetic resonance imaging is helpful to distinguish these entities.

19. *ANSWER: A.* Synovial sarcoma is caused by a translocation between chromosome 18 and the X chromosome. Synovial sarcoma is one of the malignant primary cardiac sarcomas. Synovial sarcoma is an extremely rare cardiac tumor. Like most cardiac sarcomas, the prognosis of synovial sarcoma is poor.

20. *ANSWER: B.* The use of myocardial contrast echocardiography to identify intracardiac tumors based on masses with vascularization has been described for both transthoracic echocardiography and transesophogeal echocardiography. The mass shown in Figure 28-5 does not opacify with the administration of perflutren lipid microspheres. This lack of uptake indicates a lack of vascularity. Given its echocardiographic appearance, this structure was considered to be consistent with a cyst rather than a thrombus or vegetation.

21. *ANSWER: C.* The Chiari network is a congenital remnant of the right valve of the sinus venosus. It consists of a network of fibers in the right atrium that originate from a region of the Eustachian valve at the orifice of the inferior vena cava with attachments to the upper wall of the right atrium or atrial septum. Chiari networks are present in 2%–3% of normal hearts. Chiari networks are usually not clinically significant although their role in cryptogenic stroke, in association with a patent foramen ovale or atrial septum aneurysm, is controversial.

22. *ANSWER: A.* The diagnosis of pericardial cyst can sometimes be suggested on chest radiograph by the identification of a rounded mass along the right heart border. Echocardiography or chest computed tomography is recommended to follow-up this finding to better establish the diagnosis. Primary cysts of the mediastinum account for approximately 20% of all mediastinal lesions. This group includes pericardial cysts, bronchogenic cysts, enteric cysts, thymic cysts, and thoracic duct cysts. Cysts are not considered to be true neoplasms. Cysts lack malignant potential, although the examination of tissue either by open, thoracoscopic, or percutaneous means is necessary to definitively exclude a neoplasm. However, conservative management of asymptomatic patients in whom noninvasive imaging is strongly suggestive of a pericardial cyst is also a reported approach. It is rare for pericardial cysts to become large enough to cause compressive symptoms and hemodynamic alterations.

23. *ANSWER: B.* In a series from the Cleveland Clinic, only 55 of 137 (40%) surgical left atrial appendage closures were successful. Successful left atrial appendage closure occurred more often with excision than suture exclusion and stapler exclusion. This clinical vignette highlights the importance of clinical correlation when interpreting echocardiographic images. In this case, the echodensity most likely represents suture material given the patient's history. Transesophogeal echocardiography is an excellent method for assessing the success of left atrial appendage closure procedures. Evidence suggests that the residual communication between an incompletely closed left atrial appendage and the body of the left atrium is a potential mechanism for thrombus formation and embolic events.

24. *ANSWER: C.* The development of a left ventricular thrombus is one of the more common complications of myocardial infarction. Thrombi are important clinically because they can lead to embolic complications. The likelihood of developing a left ventricular thrombus after an acute myocardial infarction varies with infarct location and size. Left ventricular thrombus is most often seen in patients with large anterior ST elevation infarctions with aneurysm formation and akinesis or dyskinesis. Transthoracic echocardiography has been the standard procedure for the diagnosis of left ventricular thrombus after acute myocardial infarction. Echocardiography can help identify those patients at high risk of thromboembolism. The two major echocardiographic risk factors for clinical thromboembolism are mobile thrombi and protruding thrombi. Echocardiography can also be used to monitor resolution of thrombus with anticoagulation. In patients with suboptimal acoustic windows or prominent trabeculations, the use of an intravenous contrast agent to opacify the left ventricular apex can sometimes be used to improve the sensitivity and specificity of thrombus detection. Alternatively, cardiac magnetic resonance imaging could be performed.

25. *ANSWER: B.* Rhabdomyomas are usually found in the ventricular walls or on the atrioventricular valves. The presence of a rhabdomyoma can be diagnosed before birth with fetal echocardiography. There is no evidence that these tumors undergo malignant transformation and no treatment is required for asymptomatic tumors. Although 80%–90% of rhabdomyomas are associated with tuberous sclerosis, cardiac rhabdomyomas can occur as an isolated finding as it has in this case.

26. ANSWER: B. The most common location for cardiac myxomas is the left atrium, with the attachment site at the atrial septum. Size is not a reliable way to distinguish between primary cardiac tumors and metastases. Cardiac myxoma may be found as part of a multisystem disease called the Carney complex. Cardiac myxoma is the most common primary cardiac tumor, accounting for 20%–30% of intracardiac tumors. Lipomatous hypertrophy is characterized by fatty infiltration of the atrial septum.

27. ANSWER: A. Once the likely diagnosis of cardiac myxoma is made based on echocardiography, resection is recommended because of the risk of embolization or cardiovascular complications. The operative mortality is reported to be fewer than 5 percent and the postoperative recovery is generally uneventful. Left atrial cardiac myxomas that are large enough may prolapse through the mitral orifice during diastole resulting in obstruction. This can result in the classically described auscultatory finding of the tumor "plop." The mean age at presentation for cardiac myxomas is 50 years of age. Pericardial effusion is not commonly seen in the setting of cardiac myxoma. Cardiac myxomas are not specifically associated with an impairment in left ventricular dysfunction.

KEY POINTS:

■ Cardiac myxomas are the most common primary cardiac tumor.

■ Cardiac myxomas usually occur in the left atrium, with the attachment site at the atrial septum.

28. ANSWER: D. Papillary fibroelastomas account for approximately 85% of valve-associated tumors. Papillary fibroelastomas are not easily distinguishable from vegetations. Papillary fibroelastomas are small, generally 0.5–2.0 cm in diameter, and are often confused with vegetations. The distinction between papillary fibroelastomas and vegetations can be difficult by echocardiography. Therefore, the correct diagnosis often depends on the clinical context. Although papillary fibroelastomas occur on valves, they usually do not result in significant valvular regurgitation. Papillary fibroelastomas most often attach to the arterial side of semilunar valves and the atrial surface of the atrioventricular valves. Symptoms of papillary fibroelastoma are usually caused by embolization, either of the tumor itself or an associated thrombus. The most common clinical presentation is cerebrovascular accident or transient ischemic attack.

29. ANSWER: E. Surgical resection is indicated for papillary fibroelastomas in patients who have had embolic events, complications that are directly related to tumor mobility (i.e., coronary ostial occlusion), and those with highly mobile or large (>1 cm) tumors. The recurrence of papillary fibroelastomas after surgical resection has not been reported. Asymptomatic patients with immobile, small (<0.5 cm) papillary fibroelastomas could be followed-up closely with periodic clinical evaluation and echocardiography. Surgical intervention should be considered when symptoms develop or the tumor becomes mobile, as tumor mobility is the independent predictor of death or nonfatal embolization. Symptomatic patients who are not surgical candidates could be offered long-term oral anticoagulation, although no randomized controlled data are available on its efficacy.

30. ANSWER: B. Papillary fibroelastomas most commonly involve the aortic valve, followed by the mitral valve. Papillary fibroelastomas are the second most common primary cardiac tumor in adults, following cardiac myxomas. Papillary fibroelastomas are generally not visible by transthoracic echocardiography if they are less than 0.2 cm. The left ventricle is the predominant nonvalvular site of involvement. Multiple papillary fibroelastomas have been reported to be present in 9%–10% of patients.

KEY POINTS:

■ Papillary fibroelastomas account for approximately 85% of valve-associated tumors.

■ Papillary fibroelastomas most often attach to the arterial side of semilunar valves and the atrial surface of the atrioventricular valves.

■ The most common clinical manifestation of a papillary fibroelastoma is a cerebrovascular accident or transient ischemic attack.

31. ANSWER: C. The valve pathology of carcinoid involves fibrosis, smooth muscle proliferation, and endocardial thickening which give the echocardiographic appearance of a thickened, retracted, and immobile valve. Appearances of the affected valve are pathognomic for carcinoid in the absence of exposure to the appetite suppressants fenfluramine and phentermine, ergot-derived dopamine agonists, and ergot alkaloid agents such as methysergide and ergotamine. In carcinoid heart disease, the tricuspid valve becomes nearly fixed in a partially open position resulting in severe tricuspid regurgitation. A "dagger-shaped" continuous-wave Doppler profile, resulting from severe tricuspid regurgitation that causes early peak pressure and rapid decline, representing equalization of right atrial and ventricular pressures, can be seen in severe disease. Involvement of the left-sided valves occurs in less than 10%–15% of cases and raises the likelihood of a concomitant patent foramen ovale, bronchial carcinoid, or high levels of circulating vasoactive substances.

Left-sided valve disease is usually less severe than right-sided valvular lesions. Serotonin is thought to be inactivated as it passes through lung parenchyma. Although there has been significant progress in the treatment of carcinoid heart disease and many patients survive for years, cure is rarely achieved. Carcinoid heart disease is remarkably well-tolerated initially despite severe right-sided valve lesions. Eventually, dyspnea on exertion, lower extremity edema, and fatigue (signs and symptoms of right heart failure) develop.

32. ANSWER: E. If there is pulmonic valve involvement, a continuous-wave Doppler signal through the pulmonic valve typically shows increased systolic peak velocity consistent with stenosis and evidence of pulmonary insufficiency. There usually is rapid dampening of the regurgitant signal with late diastolic reversal of flow consistent with pulmonary stenosis and elevated right ventricular pressure. Only carcinoid patients with liver metastases develop the distinctive lesions of the right-sided heart valves. When the primary carcinoid tumor is of a pulmonary bronchus, the carcinoid valvular lesions may be limited to the left-sided valves. Initial reports favored the use of mechanical prosthesis given the concern for bioprosthetic valve degeneration in the setting of damage by vasoactive substances. However, improvements in medical therapy with somastatin analogs may be more protective for bioprosthetic valves. Additionally, these patients usually have multiple liver metastases and associated coagulopathies making bio-prostheses more appealing. Mechanical prostheses may also be less than ideal since subsequent tumor resections are often required and may be complicated by the need for full anticoagulation. The choice of prosthesis should be tailored to the individual patient risk of bleeding, life expectancy, and future interventions. It is important to note that several series report high perioperative mortality, although the operative risk has declined from >20% in the 1980s to <10% in more recent studies. Since the tricuspid valve, with or without pulmonary valve involvement, is affected in most cases of carcinoid heart disease, the right ventricle typically enlarges. As the right ventricle becomes volume overloaded, paradoxical motion of the interventricular septum occurs. Right ventricular function seems to remain intact until later in the disease course. Carcinoid crisis characterized by hypotension, bronchospasm, and flushing can be precipitated by surgery. During the perioperative period, it may be difficult to make the distinction between carcinoid crisis and hypotension secondary to myocardial dysfunction. Perioperative octreotide, aimed at reducing serotonin release, is the most effective treatment for preventing carcinoid crisis during surgery. Intravenous octreotide (50–100 micrograms/hour) should be started at least 2 hours before surgery and the infusion should continue for 48 hours after surgery. Patients may require subcutaneous octreotide after this 48-hour period.

KEY POINTS:
- Only carcinoid patients with liver metastases develop right-sided carcinoid heart disease.
- In carcinoid heart disease, the tricuspid valve becomes nearly fixed in a partially open position resulting in severe tricuspid regurgitation.
- Involvement of the left-sided valves occurs in less than 10%–15% of cases and raises the likelihood of a concomitant patent foramen ovale, bronchial carcinoid, or high levels of circulating vasoactive substances.

33. ANSWER: C. Malignant melanoma can be diagnosed and initially treated years prior to the development and discovery of cardiac metastases. Metastatic melanoma involves the heart in more than 50% of cases. In select patients, there may be a role for surgery in patients with metastatic melanoma to palliate symptoms or prevent death from cardiac complications. Malignant melanoma may metastasize to the myocardium and/or pericardium.

34. ANSWER: A. "Charcoal" heart is the most common cardiac extension of melanoma. Although solid intracardiac metastasis from melanoma is well-described and evident in this clinical vignette, most commonly cardiac extension of melanoma is subclinical and manifests as "charcoal" heart, with tumor studding the pericardial surface. More common malignancies, such as breast and lung cancer, account for the greatest percentages of metastatic cardiac tumors. Even with a remote history of melanoma, there is concern for the subsequent development of cardiac metastasis and echocardiography should be performed for further evaluation. The incidence of metastatic tumors to the heart has increased over the last several decades due to advances in oncologic treatment and improvement in cancer patient outcomes.

KEY POINT:
- Malignant melanoma may metastasize to the myocardium and/or pericardium.

35. ANSWER: D. The histology of primary cardiac lymphoma in immunocompetent patients is diffuse large B-cell lymphoma in more than 80% of cases, whereas in patients with HIV, the histology is the more aggressive small noncleaved or immunoblastic lymphoma. Primary cardiac lymphoma evolves rapidly and has been considered an oncologic emergency requiring rapid tissue diagnosis to institute prompt chemotherapy. Primary cardiac lymphoma with diffuse large B-cell histology is sensitive to treatment with chemotherapy, as was illustrated in this case which revealed significant resolution of the intracardiac mass after chemotherapy. Approximately half of patients with primary cardiac lymphoma will have large pericardial effusions. Primary cardiac lymphoma is a rare form of non-Hodgkin's lymphoma often restricted to right-sided heart chambers and/or pericardium and accounts for 5% of primary malignant cardiac tumors. Patients with primary cardiac lymphoma may present with varying clinical presentations due to cardiac tamponade, pulmonary embolism, heart failure, neurologic symptoms, and arrhythmia, depending on the tumor location.

36. ANSWER: A. Although the most common presenting complaint by patients with primary cardiac lymphoma is right-sided heart failure (about 50% of patients), precordial chest pain is present in 15%–20% of these patients. The diagnosis of primary cardiac lymphoma can be challenging. Transthoracic echocardiography, followed by transesophogeal echocardiography, is usually the initial approach. However, magnetic resonance imaging appears to be the most sensitive imaging modality. Tissue diagnosis is essential for confirmation. Cytological analysis of pericardial fluid has been reported to have variable sensitivity, ranging from 14% to 67%. Transvenous endomyocardial biopsy has a sensitivity of only about 50%. Therefore, open biopsy is considered the gold standard. The median survival of patients with cardiac lymphoma who are not treated is less than 1 month. The median age of presentation is 64 years and the male-to-female ration is 3:1. Primary cardiac lymphoma is rare but the incidence has increased due to the number of patients with immunosuppresion due to AIDS or solid organ transplant.

KEY POINTS:

▓ Approximately half of patients with primary cardiac lymphoma will have large pericardial effusions.

▓ Primary cardiac lymphoma with diffuse large B-cell histology is sensitive to treatment with chemotherapy.

SUGGESTED READINGS

Armstrong WF, Ryan T, eds. *Feigenbaum's Echocardiography*. 7th ed. Philadelphia: Lippincott Williams & Wilkins, 2010.

Bhattacharyya S, Davar J, Dreyfus G, et al. Carcinoid heart disease. *Circulation*. 2007;116:2860–2865.

Castillo JG, Filsoufi F, Rahmanian PB, et al. Early and late results of valvular surgery for carcinoid heart disease. *J Am Coll Cardiol*. 2008;51:1507–1511.

Cheitlin MD, Alpert JS, Armstrong WF, et al. ACC/AHA Guidelines for the Clinical Application of Echocardiography: a Report of the American College of Cardiology/American Heart Association Task Force on Practice Guidelines (Committee on Clinical Application of Echocardiography) developed in collaboration with the American Society of Echocardiography. *Circulation*. 1997;95:1686–1744.

Gibbs P, Cebon JS, Calafiore P, et al. Cardiac metastases from malignant melanoma. *Cancer*. 1999;85:78–84.

Kanderian AS, Gillinov AM, Pettersson GB, et al. Success of surgical left atrial appendage closure: assessment by transesophogeal echocardiography. *J Am Coll Cardiol*. 2008;52:924–929.

Kwiatkowski DJ. Tuberous sclerosis: from tubers to mTOR. *Ann Hum Genet*. 2003;67:87–96.

McAllister HA Jr, Fenoglio JJ Jr. *Tumors of the Cardiovascular System*. Washington: Armed Forces Institute of Pathology, 1978.

Oh JK, Seward JB, Tajik AJ. *The Echo Manual*. 3rd ed. Philadelphia: Lippincott Williams & Wilkins, 2007.

Perez-Diez D, Estevez-Cid F, Barge-Caballero E, et al. Chewing gum inside the heart. *Circulation*. 2009;119:e525–e526.

Peters PJ, Reinhardt S. The echocardiographic evaluation of intracardiac masses: a review. *J Am Soc Echocardiogr*. 2006;19:230–240.

Pinede L, Duhaut P, Loire R. Clinical presentation of left atrial cardiac myxoma. A series of 112 consecutive cases. *Medicine* (Baltimore). 2001;80:159–172.

Pinto DS, Blair BM, Schwartzstein RM, et al. Clinical problem-solving. A sailor's heartbreak. *N Engl J Med*. 2005;353:934–939.

Premkumar V, Paimany B, Gopal AS. Primary large B-cell lymphoma. *J Am Soc Echocardiogr*. 2006;19:107.e1–107.e2.

Reynen K. Frequency of primary tumors of the heart. *Am J Cardiol*. 1996;77:107.

Schneider B, Hofmann T, Justen MH, et al. Chiari's network: a normal anatomic variant or risk factor for arterial embolic events? *J Am Coll Cardiol*. 1995;26:203–210.

Stratakis CA, Kirschner LS, Carney JA. Clinical and molecular features of the Carney complex: diagnostic criteria and recommendations for patient evaluation. *J Clin Endocrinol Metab*. 2001;86:4041–4046.

Sun JP, Asher CR, Yang XS, et al. Clinical and echocardiographic characteristics of papillary fibroelastomas: a retrospective and prospective study in 162 patients. *Circulation*. 2001;103:2687–2693.

Zanettini R, Antonini A, Gatto G, et al. Valvular heart disease and the use of dopamine agonists for Parkinson's disease. *N Engl J Med*. 2007;356:39–46.

Zipes DP, Libby P, Bonow RO, et al. *Braunwald's Heart Disease: A Textbook of Cardiovascular Medicine*. 7th ed. Philadelphia: Elsevier Saunders, 2005.

INDEX

Note: Page locators followed by f and t indicates figure and table respectively.